Introduction to Critical Care Nursing

Second Edition

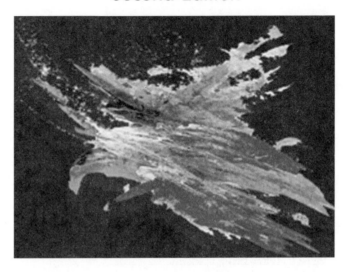

Jeanette C. Hartshorn, PhD, RN, FAAN
Professor and Associate Dean for Academic Administration
School of Nursing
University of Texas
Galveston, Texas

Mary Lou Sole, PhD, RN, CCRN
Associate Professor and Graduate Program Coordinator
University of Central Florida
School of Nursing
Orlando, Florida

Marilyn L. Lamborn, PhD, RN
Associate Professor and Chair
Department of Nursing
University of West Florida
Pensacola, Florida

W.B. SAUNDERS COMPANY
A Division of Harcourt Brace & Company
Philadelphia London Toronto Montreal Sydney Tokyo

W.B. SAUNDERS COMPANY
A Division of Harcourt Brace & Company

The Curtis Center
Independence Square West
Philadelphia, Pennsylvania 19106

Library of Congress Cataloging-in-Publication Data

Hartshorn, Jeanette.
Introduction to critical care nursing / Jeanette Hartshorn, Mary Lou Sole, Marilyn
Lamborn.—2nd ed.

    p.   cm.

Includes bibliographical references and index.

ISBN 0–7216–6218–8

1. Intensive care nursing.   I. Sole, Mary Lou.   II. Lamborn, Marilyn.
III. Title.
    [DNLM: 1. Critical Care.   2. Nursing Care.   WY 154 H335i 1997]

RT120.I5H37   1997   610.73′61—dc20

DNLM/DLC   96–16723

INTRODUCTION TO CRITICAL CARE NURSING, SECOND EDITION   ISBN 0–7216–6218–8

Printed in the United States of America.

Last digit is the print number: 9   8   7   6   5   4   3   2   1

ABOUT THE AUTHORS

Jeanette C. Hartshorn

Jeanette C. Hartshorn, Ph.D., R.N., FAAN, is Professor and Associate Dean for Academic Administration and Graduate Program Director at the University of Texas School of Nursing at Galveston. Previously, she was Associate Dean for Undergraduate Nursing at the University of Texas Health Science Center at San Antonio School of Nursing. She was also Associate Professor at the Medical University of South Carolina College of Nursing, where she headed a graduate program in critical care nursing. She received a diploma in nursing from Evanston Hospital, Evanston, Illinois; a B.S.N. from the Medical University of South Carolina; an M.S.N. from the University of South Carolina; and a Ph.D. in nursing from the University of Texas at Austin. She is active in several nursing organizations and is a past president of the American Association of Critical-Care Nurses. She has published more than 50 articles and book chapters. With 22 years of nursing experience, she has worked as a staff nurse, a clinical nurse specialist, and an administrator. In addition to her administrative responsibilities, she currently operates a nurse-managed clinic for individuals with epilepsy within the Department of Neurology at the University of Texas Medical Branch at Galveston.

Mary Lou Sole

Mary Lou Sole, Ph.D., R.N., CCRN, is Associate Professor and Graduate Coordinator at the University of Central Florida School of Nursing in Orlando. She also works per diem as a staff nurse. She has more than 20 years' experience in critical care education, practice, and research. She has taught critical care at both undergraduate and graduate levels and has worked as a critical care clinical nurse specialist. She received a diploma from the Ohio Valley General Hospital School of Nursing in Wheeling, West Virginia; a B.S.N. from Ohio University; a master's degree in nursing from The Ohio State University; and a doctorate in nursing from the University of Texas at Austin. She is active locally and nationally in the American Association of Critical-Care Nurses and Sigma Theta Tau. She is a member of the American Nurses Association, National League for Nursing, Phi Kappa Phi, Sigma Xi, and the Society for Critical Care Medicine. She has received local, state, and national awards for excellence in teaching as well as research. She has published extensively in critical care literature. She is Editor-In-Chief of *AACN Clinical Issues: Advanced Practice in Acute and Critical Care*.

Marilyn L. Lamborn

Marilyn Lamborn, PhD., R.N., is currently Chair and Associate Professor, Department of Nursing, at the University of West Florida in Pensacola. She has been involved in critical care education and clinical activities for more than 22 years. Past positions include staff nurse; head nurse; co-director of patient referral, education, and home health services; diabetic and cardiac educator; clinical specialist; and academic educator and administrator. She received a diploma in nursing from Georgia Baptist Hospital School of Nursing in Atlanta, a bachelor and master of science in nursing from the Medical College of Georgia, and a doctorate in nursing from the University of Texas at Austin. She is active in Sigma Theta Tau and was president of Delta Alpha chapter. She is a site visitor for the National League for Nursing and a member of the American Nurses Association, Phi Kappa Phi, and Sigma Xi.

CONTRIBUTORS

Jacqueline Fowler Byers, PhD, RN
Director, Quality Management and Performance, Orlando Regional Healthcare System. Visiting Assistant Professor, College of Nursing, University of Florida–Orlando Campus, Orlando, Florida.
Ventilatory Assistance; Code Management

Vicki L. Byers, PhD, RN
Clinical Nurse Specialist, Neuroscience Nursing, Center for Health Care Education Studies, Fort Sam Houston, Texas.
Nervous System Alterations

Nancy J. Crigger, PhD, RN
Assistant Professor, University of Central Florida School of Nursing, Orlando, Florida
Ethical and Legal Issues in Critical Care Nursing

Phyllis A. Enfanto, MS, RN, CCRN
Nurse Coordinator, Pediatric/Adolescent Services, Beth Israel and Childrens Hospital Medical Care Center, Lexington, Massachusetts.
Acute Respiratory Failure

Janet Goshorn, MSN, RN, CCRN
Clinical Nurse Specialist, Outcomes Management Project Facilitator, Orlando Regional Healthcare System, Orlando, Florida.
Acute Renal Failure

Elisabeth Greenfield, MS, RN, CCRN
Chief Nurse, U.S. Army Institute of Surgical Research, Fort Sam Houston, Texas.
Burns

Beth Hammer, BSN
Staff Nurse, Medical Intensive Care Unit, Clement J. Zablocki Veterans Affairs Medical Center, Milwaukee, Wisconsin.
Gastrointestinal Alterations

Jeanette C. Hartshorn, PhD, RN, FAAN
Professor and Associate Dean for Academic Administration, School of Nursing, University of Texas, Galveston, Texas.
Overview of Critical Care Nursing; Nervous System Alterations

Anne-Marie Jones, MSN, RN
Critical Care Consultant; Wright-Patterson Air Force Base, Ohio.
Hematological and Immune Disorders

Joanne M. Krumberger, MSN, RN, CCRN
Critical Care Clinical Nurse Specialist, Clement J. Zablocki Veterans Affairs Medical Center. Course Instructor, Marquette University, Milwaukee, Wisconsin.
Gastrointestinal Alterations; Endocrine Alterations

Marilyn L. Lamborn, PhD, RN
Associate Professor and Chair, Department of Nursing, University of West Florida, Pensacola, Florida.
Cardiac Alterations

Darlene "Cheyenne" Martin, PhD, RN
Director, Center for Ethics, Law and Policy, School of Nursing, University of Texas, Galveston, Texas.
Ethical and Legal Issues in Critical Care Nursing

Marsha Martin, MN, RN, CCRN
Cardiology Education Specialist, Orlando Regional Healthcare System, Orlando, Florida.
Code Management

Mary G. McKinley, MSN, RN, CCRN
Clinical Nurse Specialist, Critical Care, Ohio Valley Medical Center, Wheeling, West Virginia.
Shock

Nancy C. Molter, MN, RN, CCRN
Cardiovascular Clinical Nurse Specialist, St. Luke's Baptist Hospital, San Antonio, Texas.
Burns

Marthe J. Moseley, MSN, RNC, CCRN, CS
Clinical Nurse Specialist, Critical Care South Texas Veterans Healthcare System, Audie L. Murphy Memorial Division. Adjunct Faculty, Clinical Instructor, University of Texas Health Science Center of San Antonio, School of Nursing, San Antonio, Texas.
Cardiac Alterations

Cynthia Kline O'Sullivan, MSN, RN
Nurse Manager, Surgical Intensive Care Unit and
  Post-Anesthesia Care Unit, Boston University
  Medical Center Hospital, Boston, Massachusetts.
  Hemodynamic Monitoring

Suzanne S. Prevost, PhD, RN, CCRN, CNAA
Director, Outcomes Evaluation and Nursing
  Education, University of Texas Medical Branch,
  and Associate Professor, School of Nursing,
  Galveston, Texas.
  *Individual and Family Response to the Critical Care
    Experience*

Catherine F. Robinson, MS, RN, CCRN, CEN
Clinical Nurse Specialist, Emergency/Trauma, Ohio
  Valley Medical Center, Wheeling, West Virginia.
  Shock

Mary Lou Sole, PhD, RN, CCRN
Associate Professor and Graduate Program
  Coordinator, University of Central Florida School
  of Nursing, Orlando, Florida.
  *Overview of Critical Care Nursing; Ventilatory
    Assistance; Shock*

**Joan M. Vitello-Cicciu, MSN, RN, CCRN, CS,
FAAN**
Critical Care Clinical Nurse Specialist, Boston
  University Medical Center Hospital, Boston,
  Massachusetts.
  Hemodynamic Monitoring

Linda G. Waite, MN, RN
Instructor, University of San Francisco, San
  Francisco, California
  Endocrine Alterations

Stephanie Woods, PhD, RN, CCRN
Assistant Professor, University of the Incarnate
  Word, San Antonio, Texas.
  Dysrhythmia Interpretation

Susan Zorb, MSN, RN, CCRN, ANP
Lung Transplant Coordinator, Massachusetts
  General Hospital, Boston, Massachusetts.
  Acute Respiratory Failure

REVIEWERS

Kathleen E. Andrews, MN, RN, CCRN
Missouri Western State College
St. Joseph, Missouri

Betty Nash Blevins, MSN, RN, CCRN, CS
Bluefield State College
Bluefield, West Virginia

Mary Sharon Boni, DNSc, RN, CCRN
Alderson Broaddus College
Philippi, West Virginia
St. Joseph's Hospital
Buckhannon, West Virginia

Claire B. Corbin, MS, RN
School of Nursing
Charlotte–Mecklenburg Hospital Authority
Charlotte, North Carolina

Patricia A. Dalleske, MSN, RN
Instructor, Department of Nursing
Youngstown State University
Youngstown, Ohio

Luann M. Daggett, MSN, RN
Program Coordinator
University of Southern Mississippi
Meridian, Mississippi

Diane Ford, MS, RN
Andrews University
Berrien Springs, Michigan

Diane E. Fritsch, MSN, RN, CCRN, CS
Clinical Nurse Specialist
Trauma/Critical Care Nursing
MetroHealth Medical Center
Cleveland, Ohio

Janet Goshorn, MSN, RN, CCRN
Clinical Nurse Specialist, Outcomes Management
  Project Facilitator, Orlando Regional Healthcare
  System
Orlando, Florida

Susan F. Klaus, MSN, RN, CCRN
Assistant Professor
Division of Nursing
Graceland College
Independence, Missouri

Deborah G. Klein, MSN, RN, CCRN, CS
Clinical Nurse Specialist
Trauma/Critical Care Nursing
MetroHealth Medical Center
Cleveland, Ohio

Marsha M. Martin, BSN, RN, CCRN
Cardiology Educational Specialist
Orlando Regional Healthcare System
Orlando, Florida

Diane R. McDougal, MNed, RN
Assistant Professor
Youngstown State University
Youngstown, Ohio

Patricia Gonce Morton, PhD, RN
Associate Professor
University of Maryland
School of Nursing
Baltimore, Maryland

Deborah Panozzo Nelson, MS, RN, CCRN
EMS Nursing Education
Tinley Park, Illinois

Deborah Raney Phillips, MSN, RN, CCRN
School of Nursing
Kent State University
Kent, Ohio

Teresita F. Proctor, MS, RN, CS
Instructor
Elizabeth General Medical Center School of
  Nursing
Elizabeth, New Jersey
Assistant Clinical Professor
Union County College
Cranford, New Jersey

Dolores A. Robertson, MSN, RN, CEN
Assistant Professor of Nursing
Graceland College
Independence, Missouri

Mary Russo, MSN, RNC
Maui Community College
Kahului, Hawaii

Maureen M. Tess, MS, RN, CCRN
Rush-Presbyterian–St. Luke's Medical Center
Chicago, Illinois

Pamela Becker Weilitz, MSN(R), RN, CS
Barnes and Jewish Hospitals
St. Louis, Missouri

Ann H. White, MSN, MBA, RN, CNA
Department of Nursing
University of Southern Indiana
Evansville, Indiana

Kathleen M. Zupan, MSN, RN
Frances Payne Bolton School of Nursing
Case Western Reserve University
Cleveland, Ohio

PREFACE

Patient acuity has changed dramatically during the past several years. Patients in critical care units, step-down units, and medical-surgical units are more acutely ill than ever. Long-term acute care hospitals provide services for patients previously cared for only in critical care settings. Patients are sent home earlier with technology that in the recent past was used only in hospital settings. Because of these changes in health care delivery, nurses must be prepared to care for critically ill individuals in a variety of settings.

The amount of information needed by the nurse to care for today's patients can be overwhelming. New knowledge is generated and disseminated at a rapid pace. Technology is continuously developed and improved to assist in monitoring and treating the patient. Pharmacological advances are introduced frequently.

A challenge for the nurse educator is to provide essential information related to critical care to nurses entering practice as well as to those changing specialties. This second edition of *Introduction to Critical Care Nursing* provides content essential for entry level practice in critical care, regardless of the setting. The book is not intended as a complete reference for critical care nursing practice. Content is focused toward the baccalaureate nursing student but is appropriate for other nursing education programs as well as staff development programs that educate nurses for critical care practice.

The first edition of *Introduction to Critical Care Nursing* was noted by both faculty and students for its usefulness in providing key points in an easy-to-read format. This edition builds on that strength and provides updated information and some new features. Each chapter includes a research applications box that summarizes and analyzes a research study related to chapter content to encourage the student to read research and value its importance in patient care. Critical thinking questions have been added to each chapter to stimulate class discussion.

The book is organized into three sections. Part 1, Fundamental Concepts, includes three chapters covering information basic to all types of critical care practice. These chapters include an overview of critical care nursing, individual and family responses to critical illness, and a new chapter on ethical-legal issues.

Part 2, tools for the Critical Care Nurse, provides information needed for routine patient care management. Chapter topics include dysrhythmia interpretation, ventilatory management, hemodynamic monitoring, and management of cardiopulmonary arrest. This information is essential, regardless of the practice setting.

The final nine chapters of the book complete Part 3, Nursing Care During Critical Illness. The nursing process is used as a framework for organizing content for these chapters. Diagrams of pathophysiological processes have been added to assist in understanding mechanisms leading to illness and consequences of illness. Tables summarizing pharmacological management of illness and disease processes have been added. Updated nursing care plans are included to assist the reader in understanding how the information fits together.

Caring for critically ill patients is challenging. Our goal for this second edition of *Introduction to Critical Care Nursing* is to provide a basic textbook that will be read and used by the student to gain essential information for practice.

Our hope is that this textbook will be used as the basis for development of a comprehensive knowledge of critical care nursing.

JEANETTE C. HARTSHORN
MARY LOU SOLE
MARILYN L. LAMBORN

BRIEF CONTENTS

DETAILED CONTENTS

NOTICE

Critical care nursing is an ever-changing field. Standard safety precautions must be followed, but as new research and clinical experience broaden our knowledge, changes in treatment and drug therapy become necessary or appropriate. The editors of this work have carefully checked the generic and trade drug names and verified drug dosages to ensure that the dosage information in this work is accurate and in accord with the standards accepted at the time of publication. Readers are advised, however, to check the product information currently provided by the manufacturer of each drug to be administered to be certain that changes have not been made in the recommended dose or in the contraindications for administration. This is of particular importance in regard to new or infrequently used drugs. It is the responsibility of the treating physician, relying on experience and knowledge of the patient, to determine dosages and the best treatment for the patient. The editors cannot be responsible for misuse or misapplication of the material in this work.

THE PUBLISHER

PART

1

Fundamental Concepts

1

Overview of Critical Care Nursing

Mary Lou Sole, Ph.D., R.N., CCRN
Jeanette C. Hartshorn, Ph.D., R.N., FAAN

OBJECTIVES

- Define critical care nursing.
- Discuss the purposes and functions of the American Association of Critical-Care Nurses.
- Describe the scope of practice of critical care nursing.
- Differentiate between structure, process, and outcome standards for critical care nursing.
- Identify current trends in critical care nursing.

Evolution of Critical Care

The first intensive care units were started in the 1950s to provide specialized care for critically ill patients, such as polio victims. In the 1960s, recovery rooms were established for the care of patients who had undergone surgery, and coronary care units were instituted for the care of individuals with cardiac problems. Critical care nursing evolved as a specialty in the 1970s with the development of general intensive care units. Since that time, critical care nursing has become increasingly specialized. Examples of specialized critical care units are cardiovascular surgery, neurological, trauma, transplantation, pediatric, and neonatal units.

Critical care nursing has expanded beyond the walls of the traditional critical care units. Acutely ill individuals with high technology requirements and/or complex problems, such as those who are ventilator dependent, are now cared for in stepdown units, in medical-surgical units, in long-term acute care hospi-

tals, and at home (AACN, 1996). Critical care nurses coordinate care for these acutely ill patients, regardless of the setting.

American Association of Critical-Care Nurses

Overview. The American Association of Critical-Care Nurses (AACN) is a professional organization that was established in 1969 and has grown to include more than 75,000 members. The mission of the organization is to advance the art and science of critical care nursing and to promote environments that facilitate comprehensive practice for critically ill individuals (AACN, 1990a). Values of the organization include education, research, and collaborative practice and are evident in membership benefits, such as continuing education offerings, educational advancement scholarships, research grants, and official publications: *Critical Care Nurse, American Journal of Critical Care,* and *AACN News*. (Individuals interested in learning more about AACN and/or joining the organization should contact AACN, 101 Columbia, Aliso Viejo, CA 92656.)

Certification. Critical care nurses are eligible for certification in the specialty; this certification is known as *CCRN*. CCRN certification is available for care of adult, pediatric, or neonatal populations. The purpose of certification is to protect the consumer—the patient and the family. The AACN Certification Corporation oversees the critical care certification process. Nurses who have cared for critically ill individuals for a designated period of time are eligible to take the CCRN examination. Once they pass the written examination, nurses may use the CCRN credential. Continuing education and ongoing care for critically ill patients are required for recertification.

Vision. The American Association of Critical-Care Nurses has adopted a vision to guide critical care nursing practice. The vision is for a "Healthcare system driven by needs of critically ill patients where critical care nurses make their optimal contributions" (AACN, 1993).

Professional Guidelines. The American Association of Critical Care Nurses has generated publications to guide the practice of critical care nursing. These include a definition of the practice, position statements, and standards for practice.

Definition of Critical Care Nursing

Critical care nursing is specifically concerned with human responses to life-threatening problems, such as trauma or major surgery, as well as the prevention of these problems. Prevention of health problems is also an important part of critical care practice. For example, a critical care nurse can teach a patient methods for lowering blood cholesterol levels, thereby potentially preventing a life-threatening problem.

The basis of this approach rests with the words *human responses*. Critical care nurses deal with the total human being and his or her response to actual and potential health problems. This suggests that the critical care nurse is involved with prevention as well as cure. The focus of the critical care nurse includes the family and its response in addition to the patient's response. Additionally, human response can be a physiological or psychological phenomenon.

Scope of Practice

A scope of practice statement provides a framework within which an individual can provide a particular service. The AACN's *Scope of Practice for Nursing Care of the Critically Ill Patient and Family* statement (AACN, 1996) provides a description of the practice of critical care nursing. Central to this statement is a belief in a patient-driven system in which nurses and other health care providers coordinate and provide care. The major components of practice include the dynamic interaction of the critically ill patient and family, the critical care nurse, and the practice environment (AACN, 1996).

The Critically Ill Patient and Family. The critically ill patient and family experience compromised health status in which they are less able to compensate, are more physiologically unstable, and are more dependent on caregivers. The patient is at a higher risk for complications and death. The critical care nurse provides leadership for the care of the patient, while incorporating the values and preferences of patients and families (AACN, 1996).

The Critical Care Nurse. The critical care nurse is responsible for ensuring that all critically ill patients and families receive optimal care. Unique aspects of critical care practice include the following: focusing on the patient and family, receiving a multitude of data and prioritizing information, providing research-based interventions, monitoring patients continuously to detect changes, collaborating frequently with members of the health care team, intervening proactively to prevent complications and exacerbations of illness, and promoting wellness (AACN, 1996).

In critical care nursing practice, the nurse must demonstrate caring behaviors, make skilled clinical judgments, act on behalf of others, and use teamwork and innovation. Collaboration and coordination with other health care providers are key elements of practice (AACN, 1996).

The Critical Care Environment. The critical care environment is viewed as any setting in which patient care involves complex assessment and therapy, high-intensity interventions, and vigilant nursing care. It is not limited to a critical care unit.

Standards

Standards serve as guides for clinical practice. They establish goals for patient care and provide mechanisms for nurses to assess the achievement of patient goals.

Three categories of standards exist: structure, process, and outcome. *Structure standards* present an organizational framework within which care is provided; these standards reflect the setting in which the process of care takes place. Examples of structure standards are administrative procedures and staffing levels.

Process standards are concerned with nurse performance, including implementation of the nursing process, patient education, and continuity of care (Foglesong, 1987). An example of process standards includes implementation of the nursing care plan.

The third type of standards, *outcome standards,* articulate expected patient goals and outcomes. Examples include patient health status and satisfaction with care. The current trend in health care focuses on evaluation of patient outcomes.

Standards for Critical Care Practice

The AACN *Standards for Nursing Care of the Critically Ill* (1989) contains both structure and process standards. Examples of these standards are shown in Table 1–1.

Another publication, *Outcome Standards for Nursing Care of the Critically Ill,* delineates those specific outcomes desired as a result of nursing care delivered (AACN, 1990b). The outcome standards suggested by the AACN contain several components, including nursing diagnosis, definition, defining characteristics, etiologies, outcome standards and criteria, interventions, monitoring, additional potential nursing diagnoses, and related medical conditions. Examples of AACN outcome standards are shown in Table 1–2.

This discussion of standards is designed to provide a brief overview of the available resources. The

---

Table 1–1. EXAMPLES OF AACN COMPREHENSIVE STRUCTURE AND PROCESS STANDARDS

Structure Standards
1. The critical care unit shall be designed to ensure a safe and supportive environment for critically ill patients and for the personnel who care for them.
2. The critical care unit shall be constructed, equipped, and operated in a manner that protects patients, visitors, and personnel from electrical hazards.

Process Standards
1. Data shall be collected continuously on all critically ill patients wherever they may be located.
2. The identification of patient problems/needs and their priority shall be based upon collected data.

American Association of Critical-Care Nurses. (1989). *Standards for nursing care of the critically ill* (2nd ed.). Norwalk, CT: Appleton & Lange.

Table 1–2. EXAMPLES OF OUTCOME STANDARDS

Powerlessness

Definition

The state in which an individual perceives a loss of control over certain events or situations.

Outcome Standard

Sense of control is perceived.

Outcome Criteria

Expresses control over events/situations
Participates in activities of daily living
Participates in decision making

Impaired Skin Integrity

Definition

The state in which an individual's skin is adversely altered or at risk of being adversely altered.

Outcome Standard

Skin is intact, or integrity is improved.

Outcome Criteria

Skin color, texture, turgor, moisture, and temperature are normal for patient.
Ulcers, lesions, or erythema is absent.
Tissue epithelialization/granulation at site of impaired skin integrity is evident.
Mucous membrane is intact.

Adapted from American Association of Critical-Care Nurses. (1990). *Outcome standards for nursing care of the critically ill.* Newport Beach, CA: Author.

---

reader is encouraged to review the two above-mentioned publications in some detail to gain a thorough understanding of the topic.

Trends and Issues

As changes in health care delivery evolve, critical care nursing continues to expand and develop to meet patients' needs. Several current trends are affecting practice. Critical care nurses must be aware of these and other emerging trends when caring for critically ill patients.

Critical illnesses are more complex and critically ill patients are more ill than ever before. The critical care nurse is challenged to provide care for individuals who have multisystem organ dysfunction and complex needs. Contributing to this trend is the increasing aging population. The elderly tend to have more multisystem organ failure, which requires longer hospital stays, higher cost, and more intense nursing care.

As care has become more complex, ethical issues have skyrocketed. Termination of life support, transplantation, and quality of life are just a few issues that nurses must address in everyday practice.

Costs for critical care services account for a large portion of an institution's budget. Critical care nurses are challenged to provide comprehensive services while reducing costs and length of stay. Changing nurse to patient ratios and using unlicensed assistive personnel are strategies being used to reduce costs. Additionally, care of the critically ill is becoming more standardized. Many institutions are hiring outcomes managers to monitor the quality and the cost of patient care.

Critical care nursing has always involved collaborative practice with other health care professionals. However, today's environment emphasizes collaborative practice teams for the care of patients. The goal of these teams is to provide comprehensive patient care in a cost-effective manner, while recognizing and using each others' talents and expertise.

Technology that assists in patient care is growing at a rapid pace. Technology must be balanced with caring and compassion. In addition, the use of expensive technology must be justified. Is it making a difference in patient outcomes?

Patients are being transferred from critical care units much earlier than before and are discharged from the hospital, often while still acutely ill. Critical care nurses are challenged to provide high-quality, cost-effective care for these individuals, regardless of the setting.

These and other trends will continue to shape the future of critical care practice. It is not known how ongoing health care reform will affect critical care practice. Each nurse must continue to monitor trends and stay informed. Participation in organized nursing is one of the best ways to influence practice in an ever-changing environment.

Summary

Because the boundaries of critical care have expanded, all nurses will be providing care for critically ill individuals. Knowledge of professional organizations and the scope and standards of practice is important for the nurse entering critical care practice. The purpose of this textbook is to provide fundamental information essential to the care of critically ill patients. The reader is challenged to apply the concepts discussed throughout this book to daily practice.

CRITICAL THINKING QUESTIONS

1. Discuss perceptions of critical care nursing practice.
2. Compare perceptions of critical care from the viewpoints of student, nurse, patient, and family.
3. Give examples of various environments of critical care nursing practice.

REFERENCES

American Association of Critical-Care Nurses. (1989). *Standards for nursing care of the critically ill* (2nd ed.). Norwalk, CT: Appleton & Lange.

American Association of Critical-Care Nurses. (1990a). *Mission statement* [Position statement]. Aliso Viejo, CA: Author.

American Association of Critical-Care Nurses. (1990b). *Outcome standards for nursing care of the critically ill.* Newport Beach, CA: Author.

American Association of Critical-Care Nurses. (1993). *Vision statement.* Aliso Viejo, CA: Author.

American Association of Critical-Care Nurses. (1996). *Scope of practice for nursing care of the critically ill patient and family* (working draft). Aliso Viejo, CA: Author.

Foglesong, D. (1987). Standards promote effective production. *Nursing Management, 18*(1), 24–27.

RECOMMENDED READINGS

Gordon, S. (1994). Inside the patient-driven system. *Critical Care Nurse, 14*(3)(Suppl.), 3–26.

Society of Critical Care Medicine, and the American Association of Critical-Care Nurses. (1994). *Joint position statement: Essential provision for critical care in health system reform.* Anaheim and Aliso Viejo, CA: Authors.

Smith, R. N., & Panting K. (1995). The changing and challenging ICU. *Nursing Dynamics, 4*(1), 10–15.

2

Individual and Family Response to the Critical Care Experience

Suzanne S. Prevost, Ph.D., R.N., CCRN, CNAA

OBJECTIVES

- List stressors that are common to the patient, family, and nurse in the intensive care unit setting.
- Relate the symptoms of powerlessness and anger in the critically ill population to selected nursing interventions.
- Define the causes and treatment of intensive care unit syndrome.

- Discuss the influence of individual personal characteristics on patients' responses to critical care.
- Describe the main needs of the family of the critically ill.
- Discuss techniques that the nurse can use to avoid burnout resulting from critical care nursing.

Introduction

Critical illness is a dramatic event for both the individual and the family. In a few situations, some psychological preparation may be possible. For example, patients undergoing open heart surgery frequently schedule the procedure and have an opportunity to learn about the critical care experience before it happens. Many other patients have no warning that a critical illness or injury will strike. Patients who experience trauma and are consequently admitted to the critical care unit have no opportunity to consider the critical care experience. Thus, a major psychological insult is superimposed on a major physiological insult. This psychological insult affects the family as well as the patient. The critical care nurse is in the most important position to understand this phenomenon and

to help both patients and families cope with the situation.

One of the most fundamental concepts that critical care nurses must understand is the interrelationship between psychological and physiological stressors and responses in the midst of critical illness. Life-threatening physical symptoms of critical illness, such as excruciating pain or hemorrhage, are coupled with dramatic and overwhelming psychological responses, such as fear, anxiety, and spiritual distress. Psychological responses can exacerbate, or worsen, physical symptoms. Similarly, effective nursing management of psychological responses can contribute to physiological healing.

Although other chapters in this text address the various physiological stressors and responses of critical illness, this chapter addresses the psychological realm of critical illness and its influence on patients, families, and nurses. Psychosocial interventions are as crucial for positive outcomes of the critical care experience as any physiological intervention.

The Patient

Patients admitted to the intensive care unit (ICU) face many stressors. Some obvious stressors related to the ICU environment include loss of privacy; artificial lighting 24 hours per day; constant noise from monitoring and life support machines; lack of meaningful stimuli, such as the personal touch of family members; and physical pain or discomfort resulting from serious illness.

Several nurse researchers have measured patients' perceptions of stressors in the ICU. Both Soehren (1995) and Pennock et al. (1994) found the presence of oral and nasal tubes to be the most significant stressor. Additional major stressors that have been identified include experiencing loss of control, missing one's spouse, not being able to talk, being tied down or not being able to move freely, being in pain, being

thirsty, being on a ventilator, and having sleep interruptions. Patients believe that life support and monitoring equipment attached to them restrict their movement. Being in pain and being thirsty are consequences of the injury or even the treatment of the critical care event. Reigel (1989) estimated that 30 to 70% of patients experience severe psychological stress, with resulting feelings of powerlessness, anger, and development of the ICU syndrome. Each of these patient responses is explored in greater detail later in this chapter. A summary of stressors, responses, and interventions for ICU patients is presented in Table 2–1.

The critical care nurse continuously monitors the patient's physical signs and symptoms; therefore, the nurse must remember that changes in physical status can be related to the psychological or environmental stressors of being in ICU as well as to the physical stressors of critical illness. For example, illness or medications may cause a patient to be disoriented. The nurse may respond by restraining the patient to prevent injury. The combined frustration of being disoriented and immobilized by restraints can increase the patient's frustration, agitation, and restlessness. It may also increase the blood pressure, pulse, and respirations.

Table 2–1. STRESSORS, RESPONSES, AND INTERVENTIONS FOR THE PATIENT IN THE INTENSIVE CARE UNIT

Stressors	Responses	Interventions
Physical	*Physical*	*Physical*
Oral/nasal tubes	Vital sign changes, (e.g., hypertension, tachypnea, tachycardia)	Monitor for physical symptoms
Pain/discomfort		Control pain
Thirst/hunger	Dysrhythmias	Promote physical comfort (e.g., back massage, oral hygiene, clean sheets)
Ventilator use	Dyspnea	
Sleep disruptions	Diaphoresis	
Needle sticks	Anorexia	Use sensory aids (e.g., glasses)
Dyspnea/shortness of breath	Nausea	Use comforting touch
	Changes in elimination patterns	Promote sleep
	Increased pain	Support circadian synchrony (see Table 2–3)
	Restlessness	
	Circadian desynchronization	
Psychological	*Psychological*	*Psychological*
Immobility/restraints	Anger	Explain procedures
Frequent examinations/ touching	Anxiety	Encourage family visits
	Fear	Instill hope
Lack of control	Hopelessness	Affirm healing progress
Missing spouse/family	Powerlessness	Provide familiar objects (e.g., photos, rosary)
Confusion	Spiritual distress	
Boredom	Intensive care unit syndrome	Provide chaplaincy or spiritual support
Environmental	*Environmental*	*Environmental*
Uncomfortable beds	Sensory overload	Promote privacy/dignity
Room too hot or cold	Sensory deprivation	Adjust temperature to suit patient
Constant light and noise	Intensive care unit syndrome	Control auditory/stimuli (e.g., alarms, beeping)
Lack of privacy		Use ``white noise'' (e.g., electric fans or tapes of ocean sounds)
Unpleasant sights, smells, sounds		Place clocks and calendars within visual range

Table 2–2. EXAMPLES OF BIOLOGICAL RHYTHMS

Circadian rhythms
  Sleep-wakefulness
  Body temperature
  Blood pressure
  Urine flow
Ultradian rhythms
  REM/NREM sleep
  Sinoatrial node firing
  Nerve action potential
Infradian rhythms
  Menstrual cycle
  Hibernation
  Aging

REM = rapid eye movement; NREM = non–rapid eye movement.

Therefore, nurses must critically analyze the relationships between physical and psychological stressors and must cautiously evaluate the risks and benefits of various interventions.

ALTERATION IN CIRCADIAN RHYTHMS

Circadian rhythms affect everything we do and are easily disrupted in the critically ill. The term *circadian rhythm* was first used to describe those biological rhythms whose cycles lasted about (Latin *circa*) 24 hours, or one day (Latin *dies*). Research has demonstrated the existence of rhythms less than 24 hours, termed *ultradian,* and rhythms greater than 24 hours, termed *infradian* (Lanuza and Dunbar, 1993). Table 2–2 lists examples of circadian, ultradian, and infradian rhythms (Moore-Ede et al., 1982).

The exact nature of circadian rhythms is a subject of continuing controversy. The primary synchronizer is thought to be the day-night cycle. Environmental temperature, humidity, noise, odors, food availability, and other factors are also thought to function as synchronizers. The term *desynchronization* refers to the disruption of the previous 24-hour pattern in a circadian rhythm. It is not surprising that this phenomenon is common in critically ill patients because little differentiation between day and night exists in the intensive care unit. Lights and noise tend to be constant, 24 hours per day.

A goal of the critical care nurse is to help the patient maintain circadian synchrony. Table 2–3 outlines some of the ways current knowledge of circadian rhythms can be used to enhance nursing practice by providing nursing interventions that support circadian synchrony.

POWERLESSNESS

Powerlessness is defined as a perceived lack of control over a current health-related situation or problem and the client's perception that any action he or she takes will not affect the outcome (Anderson, et al., 1994). Another definition, by Steinhart (1987), states that powerlessness is the inability to make decisions and control the environment. Patients often feel powerless when they are in the ICU.

The ICU environment contributes to the patient's feeling of powerlessness. First, the patient with a critical illness may feel a lack of control over the disease process. The illness is often of such a magnitude that the patient was unable to control it at home and needed medical intervention. The illness has led to an ICU admission that has further decreased the patient's control over his or her environment and activities of daily living. Because of the illness, the patient may have lost control over normal bodily functions. A ventilator

Table 2–3. NURSING INTERVENTIONS TO SUPPORT CIRCADIAN SYNCHRONY

1. Align interventions with individual's usual patterns of activity-rest and sleep-wakefulness to prevent desynchronization.
2. Evaluate temperature based on circadian peaks (4 PM–6 PM) and troughs (4 AM–6 AM).
3. Plan patient activities to coincide with peak cardiovascular responsiveness (late afternoon).
4. Closely monitor patients at risk for cardiovascular and pulmonary events during documented peak periods of morbidity (6 AM–noon) and mortality (4 PM–8 PM).
5. Evaluate serum and urine electrolyte levels and urine volume levels based on known circadian fluctuations. Urine volume and excretion peak from late morning to early afternoon.
6. Coordinate medication administration to coincide with the circadian fluctuations of systems they affect. Corticosteroid administration should be coordinated with endogenous corticosteroid peaks to prevent suppression of normal adrenal activity. Theophylline is most effective when given in a form that has maximum drug availability at night, when airway patency is at its trough.
7. Administer new medications in the morning, when histamine activity is at its lowest and corticosteroid levels are optimum, to reduce the likelihood of an allergic reaction.
8. Maintain consistent day-night patterns by control of lighting and temperature.

may be the means of breathing, and a Foley catheter, the means of emptying the bladder.

The patient also loses control of other activities of daily living. The nursing and medical staff control such fundamental activities as bathing and eating. If the patient is allowed to eat, the nurses determine when and whether assistance is needed. Restricted diets are often required, and the patient may not be allowed to choose foods he or she enjoys. Frequently, the patient is unable to eat and receives nutrition via an intravenous line or a nasogastric or gastric tube. Besides nutritional assistance, the patient must rely on the nursing staff for baths, turning, and other activities each of us take for granted.

Other areas in which the patient loses control are the frequency of family visits and the timing of treatments. The visiting hours are restricted, and the patient is unable to see significant others when or as often as desired. The patient frequently has no control of when treatments, such as breathing treatments, physical therapy, and occupational therapy, are performed.

Finally, the patient has a lack of knowledge. Knowledge is frequently a source of power because those who possess knowledge can often control a situation. The patient with inadequate knowledge about the disease and treatment may imagine the worst. Without adequate knowledge, the patient may think that he or she is dying, or that the equipment attached to his or her body is permanent.

When patients feel powerless, they may manifest certain behaviors. Common behaviors of the patient experiencing powerlessness include (Roberts, 1986) apathy, withdrawal, resignation, fatalism, lack of decision making, aggression, and anger.

Each patient may manifest different combinations of these behaviors. The powerless patient is often frightened, anxious, and frustrated. Activities and decisions that he or she was once capable of are now being performed by others. This frustration can lead to anger, hostility, withdrawal, or depression. These consequences can often delay the recovery period.

Several nursing interventions may be helpful. First, recognition of the potential for feelings of powerlessness is essential. Although not all patients experience the phenomenon to the same extent, they all experience it. Patients who are particularly at risk are those who are usually in positions of power or control in their daily lives. The nurse can help the patient decrease the feelings of powerlessness by restoring some control to the patient. If it is not harmful to the patient, the nurse can allow the patient to determine when treatments are given. For example, the patient can decide to have physical therapy in the morning or in the afternoon or can decide when to get out of bed

to sit in the chair or to bathe. Additionally, the nurse can allow the patient to decide where to place personal belongings, such as pictures and get-well cards. One of the most important responsibilities of the critical care nurse is to keep the patient informed about treatment options and prognoses and to encourage the patient's involvement in related decision making. As the patient's condition improves, increasing control can be given to the patient. The nurse must be vigilant in identifying situations in which the patient can exercise control.

ANGER

Anger is an emotional defense that protects the individual's integrity to a perceived threat and to an agent of harm (Roberts, 1986). Frustration frequently produces anger when a person is blocked from achieving a goal. Anger can have both negative and positive effects. Anger that is turned inward, or *internalized,* can lead to depression, whereas anger that is turned outward, or *externalized,* can motivate the individual.

The critical care environment has many factors that can lead to anger. The two most prominent factors are powerlessness and loss. Powerlessness, with its resulting frustration and anger, has already been discussed. The loss in this situation can be a loss of bodily function or a limb or the perceived loss of one's former life, owing to illness, disability, or disfigurement. Both powerlessness and loss can lead to anxiety and frustration. The patient responds to the anxiety and frustration with anger. The loss or powerlessness is viewed as a threat to the individual, and the individual responds with anger. The behaviors that may be displayed in anger include the following (Roberts, 1986):

- Clenching the muscles or the fist
- Turning away of the head or body
- Avoidance of eye contact
- Silence
- Sarcasm
- Insulting remarks
- Verbal abuse
- Argumentativeness
- Demanding behavior

Frequently, the health care team or family members become the scapegoats as the patient expresses anger. The patient may verbally or physically lash out at team members or family to cope with the situation. In other cases, the patient may be afraid to show anger for fear of reprisals. Some patients find it frightening to be angry at the people who are delivering the care because they are totally dependent on these people. If the patient is afraid of being angry at the staff, his or her anger may be directed at the family or it may be internalized. Internalized anger can contribute to physiological consequences, such as increased blood pressure and increased gastric acid secretion.

If the patient is unable to externalize the anger, he or she may become depressed. In this instance, the nurse must look for behaviors indicative of depression. Some of the obvious symptoms of depression are loss of interest in people, dissatisfaction, difficulty making decisions, and crying. Or the depressed patient may express that he or she feels like a failure, is being punished, or has suicidal ideations.

The patient who externalizes the anger may be able to use it as the motivation for getting well. The anger can motivate the patient to change the situation that is causing the frustration. For example, if the patient has experienced a myocardial infarction that was partially prompted by a high-cholesterol diet, high blood pressure, and lack of exercise, the anger may motivate the patient to change his or her existing unhealthy behaviors. The nursing staff can use this anger to assist the patient in getting well. However, the nurse must first assist the patient in identifying the source of the anger. Additionally, the nurse must give the patient "permission" to be angry and assist him or her in identifying appropriate ways to express the anger. Above all, the nurses and family must realize that anger is a normal response and can be a healthy indication of coping.

INTENSIVE CARE UNIT SYNDROME

Intensive care unit syndrome was first studied by Blachly and Starr (1964) and Egerton and Kay (1964). Their purpose was to study the psychosis experienced by patients who had undergone cardiotomy. Since then, many studies have examined the ICU syndrome. Some of the terms used to describe the ICU syndrome are *ICU psychosis, postcardiotomy delirium, postoperative psychosis, intensive care delirium, acute confusion, and impaired psychological response.*

The ICU syndrome is defined as a syndrome that usually occurs after 48 hours in the ICU. Symptoms can range from perceptual distortion to vivid hallucinations and paranoia. Common features of the syndrome are clouding of the consciousness, decreased attention span, disorientation, memory loss, and labile emotions. Although this syndrome can occur in any critically ill patient, it is particularly prevalent in patients who have had complicated cardiotomy surgeries. Incidence rates of 40 to 78% have been noted in patients who have cardiac valve surgery (Tess, 1991). It tends to clear within 48 hours after the patient is transferred out of the ICU. The syndrome was historically thought to be limited to adults, but it has recently been documented in critically ill children as well (Hughes, 1994).

The environmental factors identified as contributing to ICU syndrome include sleep deprivation, sensory deprivation, and sensory overload. Physiological factors include age, severity of illness, history of psychological problems, cardiopulmonary bypass, prolonged surgery and anesthesia time, electrolyte imbalances, hypothermia, endocrine disorders, and medications.

Sleep deprivation occurs in the ICU as a result of noise, pain, and frequent interruptions of the sleep cycle. Furthermore, the lights are on continuously for 24 hours, and many units do not have windows, which would help orient the patient to night and day. Studies on experimental sleep deprivation have shown symptoms similar to those of patients with ICU syndrome after 2 to 5 days of sleep deprivation. The symptoms dissipated after the subjects had one night of recovery sleep. Likewise, patients with ICU syndrome have a resolution of the symptoms within 1 to 2 days after being transferred out of the ICU.

Besides sleep deprivation, patients in the ICU are also faced with sensory deprivation. Sensory deprivation is a decrease in the amount of meaningful sensory input. In many units, few windows, clocks, or calendars are present that would help maintain time orientation. The constant noise, lights, technical language, and lack of familiar faces all contribute to sensory deprivation. The patient is deprived of the familiar touches, sounds, smells, and tastes of their usual environment. Everything around the patient is unfamiliar and strange; the familiar environment of home and the family is missing.

Although the constant noise and lights contribute to sensory deprivation, they also contribute to sensory overload. Not only is there a lack of meaningful input, there is also an overabundance of unfamiliar input. Sensory overload implies that two or more stimuli are confronting the patient at a level that is greater than normal. The term sensory overload also implies that too many stimuli are confronting the patient at one time and are thus causing confusion. The constant chatter of unfamiliar voices adds to this confusion as well.

All of these factors lead to the ICU syndrome. The behavioral changes one might notice in these patients are similar to the symptoms of sleep deprivation, sensory deprivation, and sensory overload. Symptoms commonly begin with perceptual distortions, such as interpreting a speckled pattern on the ceiling as insects or a piece of ICU equipment as an animal in the room. These symptoms may progress to full-blown, terrifying hallucinations. Patients can progress from restlessness and disorientation to paranoia and combativeness (Urban, 1993).

A main nursing goal for patients with ICU psychosis is to reduce the sleep deprivation, sensory deprivation, and sensory overload faced by the patient. The patient should be reoriented every 2 to 4 hours and should be addressed directly. Instead of repeatedly questioning the patient (e.g., "Do you know what day it is? Do you know where you are?"), a less demeaning and less frustrating way to reorient the patient is to incorporate this content into normal conversation (e.g., "It's 10:00 o'clock in the morning on the fifth of January. You are still in the intensive care unit. Your family will be here to see you in about 30 minutes.") (Matthiesen et al., 1994). Conversations about other patients and personal issues should be conducted outside the patients' hearing range because such information can increase the confusion. Activities should be planned to allow the patient to have 70- to 90-minute periods of uninterrupted sleep. Additionally, the nurses can decrease the noise level by decreasing the volume on alarms and limiting or decreasing the volume of idle conversations. Lighting should be adjusted to simulate night and day, an effect that helps orient the patient and introduce normal stimuli. A clock and calendar should be within the patient's visual field. The family should be encouraged to visit and bring personal items to place at the bedside. These interventions help decrease the sleep deprivation, sensory deprivation, and sensory overload that lead to the ICU syndrome.

INDIVIDUALIZED PATIENT RESPONSES

The previous discussion has reviewed some of the more common patient responses to the critical care experience. However, each individual's response is influenced by various factors, including age and developmental stage, prior experiences with illness and hospitalization, family relationships and social support, prior stressful experiences and coping mechanisms, and personal philosophies about life, death, and spirituality.

Some elderly patients have a diminished ability to adapt and cope with the major physical and psychological stressors of critical illness. This is often the result of multiple losses over the years, including loss of physical function, loss of family members, and loss of resources, such as homes and income. Yet some elderly patients with chronic illnesses, who have endured multiple ICU experiences, demonstrate amazing resilience. Patients who have survived a prior ICU stay generally have less anxiety during subsequent admissions. For other patients, their only prior experience with ICU may have ended with the death of a family member. This scenario can add considerably to the patient's fears and anxiety.

Families and Significant Others

Although the experience of being critically ill most directly affects the individual, family members and significant others also experience many changes. In caring for the critically ill, the nurse must recognize the influence of the family on the individual's recovery. When one family member is ill, all family roles and functions are affected. Serious illness precipitates a crisis within the family that can throw even a highly organized family into disequilibrium. The illness or injury of one family member influences all members of the family. The American Association of Critical-Care Nurses' (1989) standards emphasize the importance of assessment of the family and the continual involvement of the family in the patient's nursing care.

To begin to care successfully for the family, the nurse must identify the framework from which it operates (Greeneich and Long, 1993). Thus, the nurse can approach the situation through recognition of the need to provide care for the family as a unit. The nurse must be empathetic to what the family is experiencing in order to understand the family members and to provide guidance throughout the experience.

FAMILY ASSESSMENT

Once the patient has been admitted to the critical care unit, an assessment of the family will provide valuable information for the preparation of the nursing care plan. Assessment of the family structure is the first step and is essential before specific interventions can be designed. An evaluation of communication patterns within the family leads to an understanding of the role relationships within the family. For example, this assessment can help to reveal the individuals who are involved in making decisions and how conflicts are resolved within the family. Communication patterns may also illuminate role relationships within the family. As illness changes roles, the nurse begins to evaluate how these changes are implemented and whether or not they are acceptable to the individuals. For example, a wife who has been dependent on her husband for most decisions may be very uncomfortable accepting a more dominant role in the face of her husband's illness. During this time, it is also important to seek an evaluation of the family's values, goals, and aspirations.

Family functioning is another important area for the critical care nurse to assess. Observation of the family helps the nurse understand the interactions between family members. Answers to such questions as whether family members get along or whether the atmosphere surrounding the family is one of support and nurturance or one of competition provide important information about the family's ability to work together during a crisis. Other, more external factors, such as the availability of resources to support the family, is another important consideration. For example, the availability of child care or friends and neighbors to help with other aspects of daily life can help the family cope during the crisis of a critical illness.

FAMILY STRESSORS AND NEEDS

The critical care experience, including the observation of a loved one in a life-threatening situation, the overwhelming technology of the ICU, and separation from the family member in an ICU waiting area, produces numerous stressors for the family. Family members often ignore their own basic physical needs, such as the need to eat, sleep, or bathe, out of fear that the patient's status may change while they are away from the bedside or the waiting room. This lack of attention to their own needs decreases their ability to cope with the crisis at hand and to support the ill family member.

Many studies have been completed that identify the needs of families of the critically ill (Greeneich and Long, 1993; Hickey and Leske, 1992; Kleinpell, 1991; Leske, 1986; Molter, 1979; O'Neill-Norris and Grove, 1986). The results of these studies suggest that information is the highest-priority need for families. Throughout the patient's stay in the critical care unit, the family needs a constant flow of information concerning their loved one's status and progress. Several studies have also determined that families seek consistent methods for the delivery of information about the hospital stay. Families also report the need for updated information as the patient's status changes. A recent study (Davis-Martin, 1994) found that even after patients have been in the ICU for a long time (>2 weeks), the desire for information was still the top need of family members.

Another major area of need for the family is reassurance. Several studies identified that families wanted to experience "hope." That is, the family members wanted to know that there was a possibility for recovery for their loved one. They reported that they wanted to know that the staff cared about their relative and that the care delivered was the best possible. Some studies suggest that family members wanted to feel accepted by the staff so that their needs and questions would be heeded. Reassurance includes having the information needed to understand what is happening in the ICU in order to alleviate anxiety.

Families also reported that personal needs, including convenient availability of bathroom facilities, cafeteria, and telephone, were important during this time. Families also reported the need for areas where they could be alone or could privately consult with physicians, counselors, or religious leaders. Common stressors, responses, and interventions for families are listed in Table 2–4.

FAMILY RESPONSES

As with the patient, the family's response to the crisis of critical illness is dependent on many of the same personal characteristics, including age, prior experiences with illness and hospitalization, family relationships and social support, prior stressful experiences and coping mechanisms, and personal philosophies about life, death, and spirituality.

Fear and anxiety are among the most common responses of families. The foremost fear is the fear of death of their loved one. Additional sources of fear and anxiety include potential pain or discomfort; lack of understanding of the equipment, procedures and prognosis; financial concerns; and fears related to temporary or permanent changes in the roles of the patient and other family members. For some family members, fear and anxiety are so intense that they cannot physically or emotionally cope with the situation. They may exhibit physical symptoms, such as nausea or fainting, or they may avoid visiting entirely.

Families already experiencing signs of dysfunction may exhibit more pronounced symptoms during an episode of critical illness. For such families, responses may include argumentativeness, aggression, intoxication, guilt, blame, and in some cases, physical and verbal violence toward health care workers. These families tend to have great difficulty and conflict associated with treatment decisions for the patient.

INTERVENTIONS

The critical care nurse can use specific interventions while working with the family. Several options are available to help meet the informational needs of the family. Some facilities have used a daily telephone call to a family member or they have made a toll-free long-distance line available so that family members can be kept informed of the patient's status. Hodovanic et al. (1984) reported on a "telefamily" program in which a daily telephone call to one family member was made by a designated nurse. The purpose of this call was to provide continuous communication with the family. The consistent provision of nurses to work with the patient and family increases the family's sense of trust and security, as well as their ability to communicate effectively. Another method recommended both to provide information and to lessen anxiety is the support group (Harvey et al., 1995).

Adequate education about the experience of being

Table 2–4. STRESSORS, RESPONSES, AND INTERVENTIONS FOR FAMILIES IN THE INTENSIVE CARE UNIT

Stressors	Responses	Interventions
Physical	*Physical*	*Physical*
Exhaustion	Anorexia	Encourage health maintenance (e.g.,
Thirst/hunger	Restlessness	proper eating/sleeping)
	Sleeplessness	Provide comforting touch
Psychological	*Psychological*	*Psychological*
Lack of control	Anger	Provide orientation to unit
Lack of information	Anxiety	Provide consistent caregivers
Role reversal/changes	Avoidance	Explain patient appearance, devices,
Missing patient	Fear	and procedures
Separation from family	Guilt	Keep family informed of status changes
Financial concerns	Helplessness	Prepare patient to look ``normal'' (e.g.,
Boredom	Hopelessness	remove excess equipment before
	Ineffective coping: individual	visits, bathe and cover patient)
	and family	Encourage family visits
	Powerlessness	Encourage family to get close, touch,
	Spiritual distress	and talk to the patient
		Allow family participation in patient's
		care (e.g., bathing, massage)
		Instill hope
		Affirm healing progress
		Provide support groups
		Provide pastoral care services
Environmental		*Environmental*
Overwhelming technology		Provide orientation to unit, hospital
Uncomfortable furniture		area
Lack of seating in patient rooms/waiting		Promote privacy/dignity
areas		Provide seating near patient
Lack of sleeping accommodations		Control auditory stimuli (e.g., alarms,
Lack of hygiene facilities		beeping)
Constant light and noise		
Lack of privacy		
Unpleasant sights, smells, sounds		
Unfamiliar buildings or neighborhoods		

in a critical care unit may also help to meet the family's informational needs. A brochure describing the unit, the personnel caring for the patients, the usual activities, and other specifics is very helpful to the family. As specific questions arise, the family can refer back to the brochure and glean the necessary information. Because a high level of anxiety tends to limit the family members' recall, they should be encouraged to make notes regarding what the nurses and physicians have told them and regarding questions they would like to ask during their next interaction with the nurse or physician.

Several additional strategies may also be beneficial in working with the family. The nurse should begin by personalizing communication, that is, call family members by their names. This measure demonstrates the nurse's sincere interest in them and identifies the nurse as being responsible for the patient's care. The nurse must learn to recognize and respect the family members' usual role behaviors. For exam-

ple, the wife who is used to close physical contact with her husband appreciates opportunities to hold her husband's hand and participate in his care. This simple step is likely to greatly decrease her anxiety. Family members can participate in routine nursing interventions, such as feeding, bathing, and positioning the patient. Such activities help the family members feel useful and connected to the patient. The critical care nurse may also find it helpful to use role modeling for the family so that they will know how to interact with their loved one.

When the patient's behavior is surprising to the family (e.g., confusion), it is helpful to explain the reasons for the behavior to the family. Forewarning them before they enter the patient's room helps them keep the patient's behavior in perspective. The critical care nurse can also help the family recognize the temporary nature of the behavior.

One of the simplest, yet most important, interventions the nurse can provide for the family is allowing and encouraging their access to the patient, through open or individualized visiting hours. Increased visitation frequency tends to have positive physical and psychological effects on the patient (Dunbar and McLain, 1993) and a positive impact on the family's satisfaction with care (Laramee, 1995).

Ward et al. (1990) increased family satisfaction and decreased family anxiety through a structured visitation program. The program included educational classes for the nursing staff to help them understand family needs, written handouts and psychological support for family members, and individualized visiting intervention checklists to remind nurses of common family needs and related interventions.

A nursing faculty member (West, 1989) wrote of her 14-day vigil with her father in an ICU. She offers the following recommendations for critical care nurses based on her experience:

1. Always introduce yourself to the family.
2. Make sure that the patient appears as normal as possible.
3. Give the family a short status report with each visit.
4. Allow family members to visit as often and long as possible, without interrupting care.
5. If visiting is interrupted by a procedure or another crisis in the unit, be sure to explain the situation to the family as soon as possible.
6. Incorporate family interventions, as well as patient interventions, in the care plan.
7. Put yourself in the family's place and consider how you and your family would want to be treated.
8. Touch the family members to demonstrate your concern.

The Nurse

STRESSORS

The critical care unit can be a rewarding and satisfying area in which to work; however, it is not without its stressors. Although all areas of nursing are stressful, critical care is particularly known for the stress it places on nurses. Critical care units are highly technological areas in which nurses are required to make rapid life-sustaining and life-saving decisions. A survey of 577 ICU nurses identified the top work-related stressors as lack of reward, the crisis atmosphere, lack of experience of medical residents, shift rotation, and poor relationships with nursing administration (Robinson and Lewis, 1990).

Even very experienced critical care nurses experience the stressors found in the critical care unit. Stressors reported by nurses are outlined in Table 2–5. Shift work is stressful, but rotating of shifts is reported to be even more stressful. Rotation of shifts causes a disruption in the nurse's circadian rhythm. Working weekends while other family members and friends are involved in activities can also be a stressor. For example, even with every other weekend off, nurses often receive last-minute invitations from a friend on their scheduled work weekend. Many days are so busy that the nurse is unable to take a break or eat a meal. Constant interruptions disrupt the organization of the nurse, thereby adding to the stress.

Another stressor identified by nurses is the death of patients. Although death occurs routinely in the intensive care unit, witnessing patients who die without dignity is particularly stressful. An example of an undignified death is a confused 80-year-old woman from a nursing home who had diabetes and multisystem organ failure. She had a below-the-knee amputation that was bubbling with an infection. Her other leg was pulseless, and several infected areas existed on her toes, heel, and lower leg. The physicians continued aggressive therapy with talk of further amputation up to her hip. To add to the complexity of the situation, the family supported all aggressive treatment, despite the seemingly hopeless picture. Caring for this patient was extremely stressful for the nurses. The family and the physicians made sporadic visits, but the nurses were with the patient around the clock. The physicians and the family did not see the constant pain and suffering of the patient, but the nurses did. Sometimes, critical care nurses have a difficult time putting this type of situation into perspective and out of their thoughts after they leave the unit.

Emergency situations require rapid decision-making skills that place additional stress on many nurses. However, some nurses report that caring for long-term patients in the acute care setting places more stress on them than do emergency situations. Stress is very much an individualized phenomenon.

Other stressors in the work environment are exposure to infectious diseases, radiation, high noise levels, and cramped work areas. Other staff members displaying signs of burnout add stress to the critical care nurse. Nurses report that performing nonnursing duties, "floating" to other areas, low salary, and conflict with other departments are sources of stress. Administrators can cause stress when they are not supportive and do not seek nursing input into decisions that affect nursing practice. Although these factors are stressful to critical care nurses, they are also stressful to nurses working in other areas of the hospital. Obviously, stress is an expected part of the nurse's work. However, if the stress becomes overwhelming, the nurse may experience burnout.

Table 2–5. STRESSORS, RESPONSES, AND INTERVENTIONS FOR THE CRITICAL CARE NURSE

Stressors	Responses	Interventions
Physical	*Physical*	*Physical*
Shift rotation	Anorexia	Promote health maintenance (e.g., proper eating/sleeping)
Physical labor (e.g., lifting large patients and equipment)	Weight loss/gain	Exercise
Long hours (e.g., usually 12-hour shifts)	Sleep disturbances	
Missed breaks and meals		
Exhaustion		
Psychological	*Psychological*	*Psychological*
Need to think and act quickly	Anxiety	Use stress-reduction techniques
Crisis atmosphere	Apathy	Take breaks away from nursing unit
Long-term/chronic patients	Depression	Take time off/vacations
Death and dying	Ineffective coping: individual	Emphasize the positive aspects of the job
Ethical dilemmas	Isolation	Seek out positive feedback
Constant learning of new technology	Powerlessness	Develop interests beyond work
Lack of rewards	Chemical abuse/dependency	Participate in continuing education
Lack of control over work environment	Absenteeism	Attend assertiveness training
"Floating" to other departments	Burnout	Attend time management courses
Combination of work and home stressors		Develop problem-solving skills
Working weekends and holidays		Set realistic goals
Conflict with doctors or administrators		
Lack of experience of medical residents		
Environmental		*Environmental*
Constant light and noise		Maintain an organized work area
Crowded work areas		Control/reduce noise
Occupational hazards (e.g., chemicals, infectious diseases, radiation)		Use safeguards/precautions (e.g., universal precautions, radiation shields)
Unpleasant sights, smells, sounds		

Burnout

DEFINITION

Maslach (1982) defined burnout as "a syndrome of emotional exhaustion, depersonalization, and reduced personal accomplishment that can occur among individuals who do 'people work.' It is a response to the chronic emotional strain of dealing extensively with other human beings, particularly when they are troubled or having problems." The cause of burnout is failure to cope with job stressors. In addition, unrealistic goals, low self-esteem, self-criticism, and overcommitment are associated with burnout. Stechmiller and Yarandi (1993) surveyed 300 critical care nurses and found that health difficulties, family demands, lack of career commitment, and difficulty dealing with coworkers were also important factors. Burnout is widespread within the nursing profession, and every nurse is at risk for it.

SYMPTOMS

Burnout occurs gradually. Maslach (1982) described four stages of burnout: (1) emotional and physical exhaustion, (2) negativism and cynicism, (3) self-isolation, and (4) terminal burnout. In the first stage, the nurse shows signs of emotional and physical exhaustion. Emotionally, the nurse has difficulty going to work. Physically, the nurse feels tired and is prone to headaches and colds. In the second stage, the nurse feels cynical and negatively toward coworkers and patients. As burnout progresses into the third stage, the nurse isolates himself or herself and performs as little work as necessary. The nurse wants only to perform the job and go home. The final stage is terminal burnout, which is manifested by total disgust for humanity in general. According to Maslach (1982), burnout may have physiological, behavioral, and emotional symptoms (Table 2–6).

PREVENTION

Burnout can be prevented by recognition of stress overload. Because stressful conditions exist in critical care units, the nurse needs to learn stress-reduction methods. These methods can be as simple as taking a break and listening to a stress-reduction tape or practicing visual imagery (see Table 2–5). One nurse goes to his car and reads the newspaper on his break. He says that when he comes back into the hospital, he feels fresh, like he is coming in at the beginning of the shift. Nurses are encouraged to take breaks off of the unit, to take regular days off and vacations, and to take extra time off if signs of early burnout are observed.

Just as burnout is contagious, so is optimism. Nurses can work to surround themselves with optimistic coworkers. Praise by coworkers is one of the best defenses against burnout. Focusing on the positive rather than on the negative aspects of one's job and life may be helpful. Critical care nurses can improve their odds against burnout by making time for themselves (e.g., reading a favorite book, engaging in hobbies), attending assertiveness training and time-management courses, and developing problem-solving skills. Ceslowitz (1989) performed a study on burnout and coping in hospital staff nurses. The results showed lower burnout scores in nurses who used problem solving, used positive reappraisal, sought social support, and used self-controlled coping.

For the person with low self-esteem, Husted et al. (1989) recommended self-esteem enhancement to reduce the chances of burnout. Burnout can be prevented by recognition of its signs and symptoms. Awareness of the signs and symptoms of burnout is the first step in halting the process. Often, nursing colleagues recognize the symptoms before the individual recognizes them. Like an alcoholic who must first admit that he or she is an alcoholic for therapy to be successful, so must a nurse experiencing burnout admit to having feelings of burnout.

STRATEGIES FOR JOB SATISFACTION AND A SUCCESSFUL CAREER

Career Development

A career is defined as one's progress through life and a profession. Some nurses have many jobs but never have a career. Development of a professional career requires a more positive and futuristic mindset about one's work. It requires increasing the levels of responsibility and accountability at work as well as increasing attention to one's future professional development. Any nurse can have a job, but for nursing to be a profession, nurses need to develop careers. Development of nursing careers results in higher levels of satisfaction and more options for professional advancement.

Approaching critical care nursing from the perspective of a career rather than merely a job can begin within the first few weeks of employment. A nurse who was employed in a critical care unit for 1 year after graduation listed five tips for the new graduate in the critical care unit:

1. Ensure that a critical care course and a preceptor program will be provided.
2. Ensure that you feel comfortable with the pre-

Table 2–6. SYMPTOMS OF BURNOUT

Physiological	Behavioral	Emotional
Fatigue	Increased absenteeism	Withdrawal from work and family
Headaches	Impatience	Depression
Cold, clammy hands	Alcohol and drug addiction	Irritability
Nausea/vomiting	Rigidity	Anger
Diarrhea	Accident proneness	Indifference
Muscle tension	Low productivity	Detachment
Elevated blood pressure	Overactivity	Hostility
Excessive urination	Compulsive eating	Avoidance
Profuse sweating	Inability to eat	Pessimism
Increased respirations	Forgetfulness	Crying
Increased pulse rate	Restlessness	Anxiety
	Sleeplessness	Frustration
	Loss of interest	

Adapted from Maslach, C. (1982). *Burnout—the cost of caring.* Englewood Cliffs, NJ: Prentice-Hall.

ceptor. If not, do not worry about hurting someone's feelings. You need a good learning environment!

3. Attend seminars on self-image, communication, and assertiveness. These exercises will help you to present a more professional image, and you will feel more professional.

4. Always ask questions, no matter how stupid you think they may sound. It is more stressful to pretend you know something than to admit that you do not know and to learn it.

5. Do not work overtime for the first few months. This can be very stressful. Take time to rest and absorb what you have learned.

Continuing Education

Increased job satisfaction occurs when the nurse knows that he or she has made the best possible choices in the patient's care. Acquisition of knowledge through continuing education enables nurses to make these sound decisions. Many high-quality, low-cost seminars and courses are available to this end. Professional, career-oriented nurses often assume the responsibility for continuing education, including the costs, rather than relying on their employer for educational expenses and paid time off. Another alternative is to take advantage of seminars sponsored by their own institutions.

Summary

The experience of critical illness has a profound effect on the individual, the family, and the nurse. This chapter provides information concerning the responses of these groups to the critical care experience. By understanding the stressors, the responses, and the interventions, critical care nurses are able to achieve optimal patient and family outcomes and increased personal satisfaction.

CRITICAL THINKING QUESTIONS

1. When family members visit in the ICU, they often feel intimidated, nervous, and helpless. They want to provide some help or comfort to the patient, but they do not know how. How can family members be encouraged to participate in the care of the critically ill patients? What kind of things can they do to get involved and comfort the patient?

2. Nursing research has demonstrated that information is the highest-priority need for ICU family members. What kind of information should the nurse share with family members? What factors should the nurse consider before sharing information?

3. What are some of the most common stressors for ICU nurses, and how can nurses reduce the negative effects associated with each of these stressors?

RESEARCH APPLICATION

Article Reference

Tomlinson, P., Kirschbaum, M., Harbaugh, B., & Anderson, K. (1996). The influence of illness severity and family resources on maternal uncertainty during critical pediatric hospitalization. *American Journal of Critical Care, 5*(2), 140–146.

Study Methods and Findings

In this study, 40 mothers of critically ill children used standardized scales to rate their perceptions of uncertainty, family cohesion, and social support. Illness severity for the children was assessed by use of the Pediatric Risk of Mortality Scale. The study was conducted in a midwestern hospital with a 15-bed pediatric intensive care unit. The age of the children ranged from 1 to 14 years. The mean age of the mothers was 30 years. The authors were surprised to find that these subjects reported more than twice the amount of social support reported in previous studies, and family cohesion (not illness severity) had the greatest impact on maternal uncertainty.

Strengths/Weaknesses

Four well-established and validated instruments were used (Pediatric Risk of Mortality Scale, Mishel's Uncertainty of Illness Scale, the Family Adaptability and Cohesion Evaluation, and the Norbeck Social Support Questionnaire). The sample ($n=40$ pairs) was very small, and the study was limited to one setting. Perceptions of other family members (e.g., fathers) were not investigated.

Implications for Practice

In the midst of critical illness, if family function is deficient, mothers need considerable support from health care providers. The parents of the sickest child are not necessarily the ones who need the most support from staff. Intensive care unit nurses can help to reduce uncertainty by keeping mothers and other family members well informed.

REFERENCES

Anderson, K., Anderson, L., & Glanze, W. (Eds.). (1994). *Mosby's medical, nursing, and allied health dictionary* (4th ed). St. Louis, MO: C. V. Mosby Co.

American Association of Critical-Care Nurses. (1989). *Standards for nursing care of the critically ill* (2nd ed). Norwalk, CT: Appleton & Lange.

Blachly, P., & Starr, A. (1964). Postcardiotomy delirium. *American Journal of Psychiatry, 121,* 371–375.

Ceslowitz, S. B. (1989). Burnout and coping strategies among hospital staff nurses. *Journal of Advanced Nursing, 14*(7), 553–557.

Davis-Martin, S. (1994). Perceived needs of families of long-term critical care patients: A brief report. *Heart and Lung, 23*(6), 515–518.

Dunbar, S., & McClain, R. (1993). Family care. In M. Kinney, D. Packa, & S. Dunbar (Eds.), *AACN's clinical reference for critical care nursing* (3rd ed.) (pp. 411–425). St. Louis, MO: C. V. Mosby Co.

Egerton, N., & Kay, J. H. (1964). Psychological disturbances associated with open-heart surgery. *British Journal of Psychiatry, 110,* 1365–1370.

Greeneich, D., & Long, C. (1993). Using a model to assess family satisfaction. *Dimensions of Critical Care Nursing, 12*(5), 272–278.

Harvey, C., Dixon, M., & Padberg, N. (1995). Support group for families of trauma patients: A unique approach. *Critical Care Nurse, 15*(4), 59–63.

Hickey, M., & Leske, J. (1992). Needs of families of critically ill patients. *Critical Care Nursing Clinics of North America, 4*(4), 645–649.

Hodovanic, B. H., Reardon, D., Reese, W., & Hedges, B. (1984). Family crisis intervention program in the medical intensive care unit. *Heart and Lung, 13*(3), 243–249.

Husted, G. L., Miller, M. C., & Wilczynski, E. M. (1989). Retention is the goal: Extinguish burnout with self-esteem enhancement. *Journal of Continuing Education in Nursing, 20*(6), 244–248.

Hughes, J. (1994). Hallucinations following cardiac surgery in a pediatric intensive care unit. *Intensive and Critical Care Nursing, 10*(3), 209–211.

Kleinpell, R. (1991). Needs of families of critically ill patients: A literature review. *Critical Care Nurse, 11*(8), 34–40.

Lanuza, D., & Dunbar, S. (1993). Circadian rhythms: Implications for cardiovascular nursing and drug therapy. *Journal of Cardiovascular Nursing, 8*(1), 63–79.

Laramee, A. (1995). The satisfaction of family needs of critically ill patients: A comparison of visiting policies (Abstr). *American Journal of Critical Care, 4*(3), 252.

Leske, J. S. (1986). Needs of relatives of critically ill patients: A follow-up. *Heart and Lung, 15,* 189–193.

Maslach, C. (1982). *Burnout—The cost of caring.* Englewood Cliffs, NJ: Prentice-Hall.

Matthiesen, V., Sivertsen, L., Foreman, M., & Cronin-Stubbs, D. (1994). Acute confusion: Nursing intervention in older patients. *Orthopaedic Nursing, 13*(2), 21–29.

Molter, N. C. (1979). Needs of relatives of critically ill patients: A descriptive study. *Heart and Lung, 8,* 332–339.

Moore-Ede, M. C., Sulzman, F. M., & Fuller, C. A. (1982). *The clocks that time us: Physiology of the circadian timing system.* Cambridge, MA: Harvard University Press.

O'Neill-Norris, L., & Grove, S. K. (1986). Investigation of selected psychosocial needs of family members of critically ill patients. *Heart and Lung, 15,* 194–199.

Pennock, B., Crawshaw, L., Maher, T., Price, T., & Kaplan, P. (1994). Distressful events in the ICU as perceived by patients recovering from coronary artery bypass surgery. *Heart and Lung, 23*(4), 323–327.

Reigel, B. (1989). Stressors of critically ill patients. In B. Reigel, & D. Ehrenreich (Eds.). *Psychological aspects of critical care nursing* (pp. 17–29). Rockville, MD: Aspen Publishers.

Roberts, S. L. (1986). *Behavioral concepts and the critically ill patient* (2nd ed). East Norwalk, CT: Appleton & Lange.

Robinson, J., & Lewis, D. (1990). Coping with ICU work-related stressors: A study. *Critical Care Nurse, 10*(5), 80–88.

Soehren, P. (1995). Stressors perceived by cardiac surgical patients in the intensive care unit. *American Journal of Critical Care, 4*(1), 71–76.

Stechmiller, J., & Yarandi, H. (1993). Predictors of burnout in critical care nurses. *Heart and Lung, 22*(6), 534–541.

Steinhart, M. J. (1987). Psychosocial concerns of critically ill patients and their families. In I.A. Fein, & M.A. Strosberg (Eds.). *Managing the critical care unit* (pp. 325–337). Rockville, MD: Aspen Publishers.

Tess, M. (1991). Acute confusional states in critically ill patients: A review. *Journal of Neuroscience Nursing, 23*(6), 398–401.

Urban, N. (1993). Patient responses to the environment. In M.R. Kinney, D.R. Packa, & S.B. Dunbar (Eds.). *AACN's clinical reference for critical-care nursing* (pp. 117–128). St. Louis, MO: C. V. Mosby Co.

Ward, C., Constancia, P., & Kern, L. (1990). Nursing interventions for families of cardiac surgery patients. *Journal of Cardiovascular Nursing, 5*(1), 34–42.

West, A. (1989). Letter to the editor. *Heart and Lung, 18*(1), 103–104.

RECOMMENDED READINGS

Clark, C., & Heidenreich, T. (1995). Spiritual care for the critically ill. *American Journal of Critical Care, 4*(1), 77–81.

Corley, M. (1995). Moral distress of critical care nurses. *American Journal of Critical Care, 4*(4), 280–285.

Dossey, B. M., Guzzetta, C. E., & Kenner, C. V. (1992). Body-mind-spirit. In B.M. Dossey, C.E. Guzzetta, & C.V. Kenner (Eds.). *Critical care nursing: Body-mind-spirit* (pp. 1–16). Philadelphia, PA: J. B. Lippincott Co.

Evans, J., & French, D. (1995). Sleep and healing in intensive care settings. *Dimensions of Critical Care Nursing, 14*(4), 189–199.

Halm, M., & Alpen, M. (1993). The impact of technology on patients and families. *Nursing Clinics of North America, 28*(2), 443–457.

Krachman, S., D'Alonzo, G., & Criner, G. (1995). Sleep in the intensive care unit. *Chest, 107*(6), 1713–1720.

Lopez-Fagin, L. (1995). Critical care family needs inventory: A cognitive research utilization approach. *Critical Care Nurse, 15*(4), 21–26.

Morath, M. J., & Lynch, M. (1989). Intensive care psychosis. In M. S. Sommers (Ed.). *Difficult diagnosis in critical care nursing* (pp. 193–209). Rockville, MD: Aspen Publishers.

Wallace-Barnhill, G. (1989). Psychological problems for patients, families and health professionals. In W. Shoemaker, S. Ayers, A. Grenvik, P. R. Holbrook, & W. L. Thompson (Eds.). *Textbook of Critical Care* (2nd ed.) (pp. 1414–1420). Philadelphia: W. B. Saunders Co.

3

Ethical and Legal Issues in Critical Care Nursing

Darlene "Cheyenne" Martin, Ph.D., R.N.,
Nancy J. Crigger, Ph.D., R.N.

OBJECTIVES

- Discuss nurses' ethical obligations to patients in the critical care setting.
- Compare the components of a systematic ethical decision-making model.
- Describe the ethical and legal value of established ethical codes and standards of care.
- Define negligence and its relationship to legal malpractice claims.

- Identify three conditions that must be present for patients to give informed consent.
- Explain how advance directives ensure patients' rights to self-determination.
- Discuss the legal and ethical issues that surround organ and tissue transplantation.

Introduction

Critical care nurses are often confronted with ethical and legal dilemmas related to informed consent, withholding or withdrawal of life-sustaining treatment, transplantation, privacy, and, increasingly, justice in the distribution of health care resources. Many dilemmas are by-products of advanced medical technologies developed over the past several decades. Although technology provides substantial benefits to acutely and chronically ill patients, extensive public and professional debate occurs over the appropriate use of these technologies, especially those that are life sustaining. One of the primary concerns in critical care is whether or not patients' values and beliefs about treatment can be overridden by the "technological imperative," or the strong tendency to use technology because it is available.

Although many ethical dilemmas are not unique to critical care, they occur with greater frequency in critical care settings. Because nurses often establish close and extended relationships with critical care patients, they must be aware of situations that threaten the welfare of their patients. It is crucial that nurses examine the nature and scope of their ethical and legal obligations to patients.

The ethical and legal issues that frequently arise in the nursing care of critical care patients are examined in this chapter. The discussion includes problems that surround informed consent, the care of patients with the human immunodeficiency virus (HIV), the withholding and withdrawal of treatment, patient rights and nurse obligations, and malpractice. The elements of ethical decision making and the pivotal involvement of the nurse are discussed.

Ethical Obligations and Nurse Advocacy

Critical care nurses' ethical and legal responsibilities for patient care have increased dramatically during the past decade. As nurses assume expanded roles in clinical practice and develop greater professional autonomy, they have greater direct accountability for their practice. Evolving case law and current concepts of nurse advocacy and contractual relationships clearly indicate that nurses have substantial ethical and legal obligations to promote and protect the welfare of their patients.

The duty to practice ethically and to serve as an ethical agent on behalf of patients is an integral part of nurses' professional practice. The nurse's duty is clearly stated in the *Code for Nurses with Interpretive Statements,* which was adopted by the American Nurses Association (ANA) in 1976 and revised in 1985 (Table 3–1). The code for nurses delineates the moral principles that guide professional nursing practice. Nurses in all practice arenas, including critical care, must be knowledgeable about the provisions of the code and must incorporate its basic tenets into their clinical practice. The code is a powerful tool that shapes and evaluates individual practice as well as the nursing profession.

Nurses' ethical obligation to serve as advocates for their patients is derived from the unique nature of the nurse-patient relationship. Critical care nurses assume a significant care-giving role that is characterized by intimate, extended contact with persons who are often most vulnerable. Nurses in critical care settings become an important part of the patient's world and constantly monitor, assess, respond, comfort, and at times, accompany their patients to death (Martin, 1987).

The nurses' role as healer is powerful and creates prima facie duty of nurse advocacy. Bandman and Bandman (1995) referred to the duty to act as advocate for patients as having "standing." Standing is a legal concept applied to persons who have legitimate interest and authority to represent someone in a decision-making capacity. Critical care nurses have a moral responsibility to act as advocates on their patients' behalf because of their unique relationship to their patients and their specialized nursing knowledge.

Ethical Decision Making

As reflected in the ANA code of ethics (1985), one of the primary ethical obligations of professional

Table 3–1. THE AMERICAN NURSES ASSOCIATION CODE OF ETHICS

1. The nurse provides services with respect for human dignity and the uniqueness of the client unrestricted by considerations of social or economic status, personal attributes, or the nature of health problems.
2. The nurse safeguards the client's right to privacy by judiciously protecting information of a confidential nature.
3. The nurse acts to safeguard the client and the public when health care and safety are affected by the incompetent, unethical, or illegal practices of any person.
4. The nurse assumes responsibility and accountability for individual nursing judgments and actions.
5. The nurse maintains competence in nursing.
6. The nurse exercises informed judgment and uses individual competence and qualifications as criteria in seeking consultation, accepting responsibilities, and delegating nursing activities to others.
7. The nurse participates in activities that contribute to the ongoing development of the profession's body of knowledge.
8. The nurse participates in the profession's efforts to implement and improve standards of nursing.
9. The nurse participates in the profession's efforts to establish and maintain conditions of employment conducive to high quality nursing care.
10. The nurse participates in the profession's effort to protect the public from misinformation and misrepresentation and to maintain the integrity of nursing.
11. The nurse collaborates with members of the health professions and other citizens in promoting community and national efforts to meet the health needs of the public.

From American Nurses Association. (1985). *Code for nurses with interpretive statements.* Kansas City, MO: Author.

nurses is protection of their patients' basic rights. This obligation requires nurses to recognize ethical dilemmas that actually or potentially threaten patients' rights and to participate in the resolution of those dilemmas.

An ethical dilemma is a difficult problem or situation in which conflicts exist about the making of morally justifiable decisions (Davis and Aroskar, 1991). Whether or not all nurses on a unit should be informed that a newly admitted patient has a diagnosis of HIV infection is an example of an ethical dilemma. The conflicting principles in this example are the patient's right to privacy and the caregivers' right to information that might affect their ability to provide care.

Arriving at a morally justifiable decision in this situation can be difficult for patients, families, and health professionals. One helpful way to approach ethical decision making is to use a systematic, structured process, such as the one depicted in Figure 3–1. This

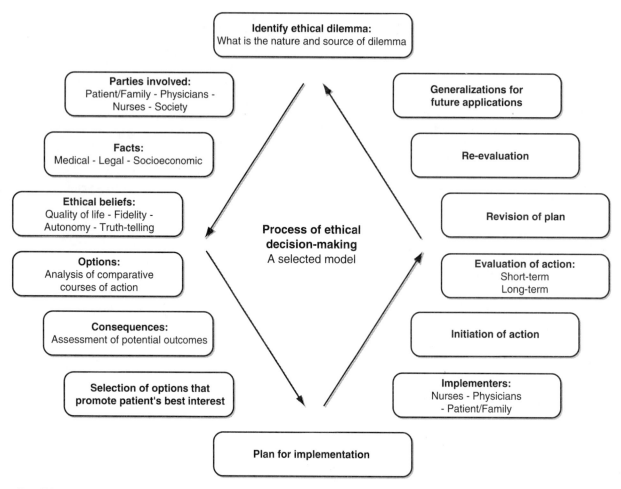

Note: This model is intended to provide a framework for discussion of ethical issues but is not intended as a "formula."

Figure 3-1. Process of ethical decision making.

model provides a framework for evaluation of the related ethical principles and the potential outcomes, as well as relevant facts concerning the patient's medical status, ethical beliefs, and treatment preferences. Using this approach, the patient, family, and health care team members evaluate choices and choose the option that promotes the patient's best interests.

Ethical decision making includes implementing the decision and evaluating the short-term and long-term outcomes. Evaluation provides meaningful feedback about decisions and actions in specific instances, as well as the effectiveness of the decision-making process. The final stage in the decision-making process is an assessment of whether or not the decision in a specific case can be applied to other dilemmas with similar circumstances. In other words, is this decision useful in similar cases? It is important to note that a systematic approach to decision making does not guarantee that morally justifiable decisions are reached or that the outcome is beneficial to the patient.

Ethical Principles

As reflected in the decision-making model noted above, relevant ethical principles should be considered. Principles facilitate moral decisions by guiding the decision-making process, but may conflict with each other and force a choice between the competing principles. Several ethical principles are significant in the critical care setting.

The principle of respect for persons states that each person should be treated as a unique individual and as a member of the human community. This principle emphasizes the substantial interdependence and interconnectedness of individuals in our society (Davis and Aroskar, 1991).

The principle of autonomy states that any person should be free to govern his or her life to the greatest degree possible. This principle implies a strong sense of self-determination and an acceptance of responsibility for one's own choices and actions. Autonomy is the opposite of paternalism, which is the interference with one's liberty. The threat of paternalism from health care providers has been reduced somewhat in recent years as the trend moves from unilateral to shared decision making (Kapp, 1989).

The principle of beneficence is the duty to provide benefits to others when in a position to do so and to help balance harms and benefits.

The principle of nonmaleficence is the explicit duty to not intentionally inflict harm on others. Nonmaleficence is derived from the Latin admonition to physicians: "primum non nocere"—above all, do no harm.

The principle of justice requires that health care resources be distributed fairly and equitably among groups of people.

The principle of veracity is upheld if persons tell the truth in their communication with others.

The principle of fidelity claims that one has a moral duty to be faithful to the commitments that one makes to others.

Increasing Nurses' Involvement in Ethical Decision Making

Although nurses play a significant role in the care of patients, they often report limited involvement in the formal processes of ethical decision making (Baggs, 1993; Martin, 1987; Winslow and Winslow 1991). Nurses' perception of limited involvement in the resolution of ethical dilemmas may be related to many factors, such as lack of formal educational preparation in ethics, lack of institutional mechanisms for review of dilemmas, perceived lack of administrative and/or peer support for involvement in decision making, concern about reprisals, and lack of perceived decision-making authority.

If nurses are to fulfill their advocacy obligations to patients, they must become active in the process of decision making at all levels. Ways for nurses to increase their participation in ethical decision making include involvement in institutional ethics committees, nursing ethics committees, multidisciplinary ethics forums and ethics rounds, peer review and quality assurance committees, and institutional review boards that review research protocols within their institutions. In addition, some hospitals have established ethics consultation services with nursing and medical ethicists to assist staff, patients, and families in responding to difficult ethical issues.

Nurses improve and update their knowledge through formal and continuing education courses in nursing ethics, as well as through telephone and computerized electronic consultation and reference services. Educational programs and ethics consultation services are available through several ethics and law centers in the United States, including the American Nursing Association Center for Ethics and Human Rights; the Center for Nursing Ethics, Law, and Policy at the University of Texas Medical Branch School of Nursing; the Joseph and Rose Kennedy Institute for the Study of Human Reproduction and Bioethics; and the Hastings Center (Table 3–2).

Legal Accountability in Nursing

In addition to ethical obligations, nurses in the critical care setting have legal responsibilities to patients. Legal responsibilities have expanded dramatically during the past two decades as nurses have assumed more comprehensive roles in clinical practice. The number of nurses named as defendants in legal suits alleging negligence has increased as the standard of care in state courts across the United States has steadily increased.

Preventing situations that compromise health is far preferred to defending one's actions in courts, but

---

Table 3–2. ETHICAL CONSULTATION SERVICES

1. American Nurses Association Center for Ethics and Human Rights
   600 Maryland Avenue, SW
   Suite 100W
   Washington, DC 20024-2571
   Telephone: (202) 651-7000
2. Hastings Center for Biomedical Ethics
   255 Elm Road
   Briarcliff Manor
   New York, NY 10510
   Telephone: (914) 762-8500
3. Center for Nursing Ethics, Law and Policy
   University of Texas Medical Branch School of Nursing at Galveston
   301 University Boulevard
   Galveston, TX 77555
   Telephone: (409) 772-1011
4. Joseph and Rose Kennedy Institute for the Study of Human Reproduction & Bioethics
   Kennedy Institute of Ethics
   Georgetown University
   Washington, DC 20057
   Telephone: (202) 687-8089

prevention is possible only if nurses have a clear, current knowledge of their legal obligations to patients. An awareness of evolving case law and judicial trends also helps nurses prevent allegations of negligence and malpractice. This section of the chapter briefly explores theories of negligence and malpractice as well as other legal doctrines relevant to clinical practice in critical care.

NEGLIGENCE

Negligence is a specific category of tort law. A tort is a legal wrong committed by an individual or individuals against the person or property of another. In order to recover monetary damages or other forms of compensation, the law provides that the injured person may bring a civil suit against the person who caused harm.

Negligence is the failure of a person to act in a reasonable and prudent manner. Two types of negligence exist: acts of commission (e.g., giving a wrong medication to a patient) or acts of omission (e.g., failing to raise the side rails on the bed of a sedated patient). The professional nurse's conduct is measured against a standard of care, or what other reasonably prudent nurses would do or not do in the same or similar circumstances. When negligent actions are committed by a professional nurse during the course of his or her professional duties, the nurse may be liable for malpractice.

ELEMENTS OF A MALPRACTICE CLAIM

In medical malpractice cases, the plaintiff (the person bringing the suit) has the burden of proving that the defendant (the person being sued) is liable, or responsible for an injury. For a malpractice claim against a nurse to be successful, the plaintiff must establish proof of the following elements: (1) the nurse had a specific professional duty to the patient, (2) the nurse did not carry out his or her duty, (3) the nurse caused injury to his or her patient, and (4) the patient's injury resulted from the nurse's negligent action. For example, a patient develops a corneal ulcer while unconscious. The nurse was negligent because he or she had a duty to assess and protect the patient's eye from injury. The nurse's failure to perform his or her duty resulted in injury, manifested as the corneal ulcer.

Professional Standards of Care

One of the most crucial aspects of malpractice cases involving nurses is the determination of standards of care by which the conduct of professional

nurses can be evaluated. From a legal perspective, a standard is defined as the general recognition of, and conformity to, established practice. Plaintiffs may win judgments against nurses if they are able to establish the nurse's failure to perform to an accepted standard of care.

Standards of professional nursing practice are derived from external sources, including expert nurse testimony, state nurse practice acts, the American Nurses Association standards of practice, accreditation standards and regulations, authoritative publications, and internal institutional policies and protocols. In addition, courts may review nursing job descriptions and nursing documentation. An important standard for critical care nurses is the *Outcome Standards for Nursing Care of the Critically Ill* (AACN, 1990) (see Chapter 1). Standards generally reflect a growing trend to evaluate nursing practice from national, rather than local, prevailing standards. The underlying assumption in today's technological society is that most nurses have access to similar educational materials and scientific information and can be held to a universal normative standard. Because baseline standards of care are continuously evolving, the critical care nurse has a responsibility to maintain current knowledge in his or her field.

ABANDONMENT

Nurses working in critical care settings are responsible for their patients' safe and continuous care. Abandonment by the nurse or by other health providers is defined as the severance of a professional relationship while a patient is still in need of health care. Although malpractice cases involving abandonment primarily involve physicians, existing case law indicates that nurses may be increasingly vulnerable to allegations of abandonment.

The potential for abandonment may increase as nurses assume more advanced clinical roles with direct contractual relationships with patients (Smith, 1991). Imagine that a nurse practitioner is the only health care provider in a small North Dakota town that is many miles from health care facilities. The practitioner's patient, who has lung cancer with metastatic disease, refuses to quit smoking. The nurse in turn refuses to treat the patient because he will not agree to follow her treatment plan. This case raises the possibility of abandonment on the part of the nurse practitioner in view of the limited availability of care and the patient's need for continued care.

Selected Ethical and Legal Issues
INFORMED CONSENT

Many complex dilemmas in critical care nursing concern informed consent. Consent problems arise because patients are experiencing acute, life-threatening illnesses that interfere with their ability to make decisions about treatment. The doctrine of informed consent is based on the principle that competent adults have the right to self-determination or to make decisions regarding their acceptance or rejection of medical or nursing treatment.

ELEMENTS OF INFORMED CONSENT

Three primary elements must be present for a person's consent or decline of medical treatment to be considered legally valid: capacity, voluntariness, and information (Rozovsky, 1995). *Capacity* refers to an individual's ability to understand information regarding a proposed medical or nursing treatment. A patient's ability to understand relevant information is an essential prerequisite to his or her participation in the decision-making process and should be carefully evaluated by physicians and nurses seeking consent. Some conditions that reduce a patient's capacity to understand include the diagnosis (e.g., shock; extreme anxiety; medications, such as sedatives; and drugs or prior existing disorders that result in mental status alterations, such as Alzheimer's disease, Down's syndrome).

Consent must be given voluntarily in order for the consent to be legally binding. *Voluntariness* requires that a person's consent be given without coercion, fraud, or extreme duress.

Persons who consent base their decision on sufficient knowledge. Basic *information* considered necessary for patients' decision making include the following (Rozovsky, 1995):

- A diagnosis of the patient's specific health problem and condition
- The nature, duration, and purpose of the proposed treatment or procedures
- The probable outcome of any medical or nursing intervention
- The benefits of medical or nursing interventions
- The potential risks that are generally considered hazardous or common
- Alternative treatments and their feasibility
- Short-term and long-term prognoses if the proposed treatment or treatments are not provided

INFORMED CONSENT OF ADOLESCENTS

In most states, persons younger than 18 years are considered to be minors and are unable to give consent for medical or nursing treatments. Consent must be obtained from a parent or legal guardian. Exceptions may be made if older children or adolescents have the ability to comprehend some aspects of the proposed treatments. Some ethicists believe that children or adolescents should be given the opportunity to participate in decisions that affect them (Holder, 1988). In addition, three exceptions to the requirement of parental consent are emergency care, care of emancipated minors, and minor treatment statutes.

Emergency Treatment

Virtually all states have statutes that provide for the emergency treatment of minors if a life-threatening condition occurs and if parents are unavailable to give consent. Once the emergency has passed, however, the parents' consent to continue the treatment must be obtained as quickly as possible.

Emancipated Minors

A second exception to parental consent involves emancipated minors. Although the exact definition of emancipation varies from state to state, it generally refers to adolescents who no longer live with their parents, who are able to economically support themselves, who are married, or who are in the military service. Because minors in these situations are no longer presumed to be subject to the control or regulation of their parents, they are able to make decisions independently regarding medical or nursing treatment.

Minor Treatment Statutes

A third exception to the parental consent requirement is the statutory provision that allows unemancipated minors to consent to specific types of medical care without parental notification. Minor treatment statutes were enacted to encourage adolescents to seek treatment for sexually transmitted disease and birth control. The statutes have been expanded to include treatment of substance abuse, rape, and emotional disorders.

Decisions Regarding Life-Sustaining Treatment

Care of persons who are terminally ill or in a persistent vegetative state raises profound questions about the constitutional rights of persons or surrogates (one who speaks for the patient) to make decisions related to death or life-sustaining care, as well as the rights of the state to intervene in treatment decisions (Table 3–3). These issues represent the ultimate test of civil liberties and freedom to make one's own decisions in the face of death.

Table 3–3. LIFE AND DEATH DEFINITIONS IN CRITICAL CARE ETHICS

Advance Directive—A statement in which competent individuals give direction for their care in the event that they lose the capacity to do so. Advance directives may be formal (e.g., living will) or informal.

Death—The process of degenerative and destructive changes occurring in tissues of a living organism that generally follow irreversible cessation of spontaneous ventilation and circulation.

Do Not Resuscitate (DNR) Order—A medical order that prohibits the use of cardiopulmonary resuscitation and emergency cardiac care to reverse signs of clinical death. The decision to order DNR status for a given individual may be made by the physician if resuscitation is deemed futile or in a joint decision of the physician, patient, and/or surrogate or family. The DNR order may or may not be specified in patients' advance directives.

Durable Power of Attorney—A family member or surrogate designated as the legal agent for another should that individual become incompetent or incapacitated.

Futility—A medical situation in which important goals of care are not achievable.

Irreversible Coma*—A condition in which the brain has no function with no chance for recovery.

Living Will—A specific request made by a competent individual that directs medical care in the event that the individual loses the capacity to do so. The living will is a formalized advanced directive that is held to be legally binding in some states.

Persistent Vegetative State—A condition in which an individual does not meet any of the criteria for brain death but displays profound neurological impairment with little to no choice of recovering a quality life.

Resuscitation—Intervention with the intent of preserving life, restoring health, or reversing clinical death.

Surrogate—An individual designated by the individual (when judged competent) or appointed to make medical decisions for the individual in the event that the individual loses the capacity to do so.

*As defined by the Ad Hoc Committee of the Harvard Medical School (1968). A definition of irreversible coma. *Journal of the American Medical Association*, 205(6), 337–340.

The issue of treatment for persons whose quality of life is severely compromised, as in irreversible coma or brain death, is often a byproduct of advanced biomedical technology. Technology frequently offers a means for sustaining life in persons who would have previously succumbed to their illnesses. The widespread use of advanced life-support systems and cardiopulmonary resuscitation has changed the nature and context of dying. A "natural death" in the traditional sense is rare, as evidenced by the fact that 80% of the 2 million people who die each year in the United States in acute or extended care facilities are considered to be candidates for cardiopulmonary resuscitation (Solomon et al., 1993).

The benefits derived from aggressive technological management often outweigh the negative effects, but the use of life-sustaining technologies for persons with severely impaired quality of life or for those who are terminally ill has stimulated intensive debate and litigation. Two key issues in this debate are the appropriate use of technology and the ability of the seriously ill person to retain decision-making rights.

At the heart of the technology controversy are conflicting beliefs about the morality and legality of allowing persons who are terminally ill or severely debilitated to request withdrawal or withholding of medical treatment. Two types of treatment are considered: extraordinary and maintenance of life support. Extraordinary or heroic treatment includes resuscitation efforts by cardiopulmonary resuscitation or emergency cardiac care and maintenance of life support. Examples of life support include ventilatory assistance and maintenance of nutrition.

EXTRAORDINARY TREATMENT

Resuscitation efforts are used to reverse the clinical signs of death: loss of spontaneous respiration and/or loss of cardiac function. No reliable clinical method exists for determining the extent of brain damage that has already occurred at the time that resuscitation efforts are initiated. Ethical questions arise about the use of cardiopulmonary resuscitation and emergency cardiac care. In what situations should resuscitation efforts be used? How long should efforts continue? A generally accepted position is that resuscitation should cease if the physician determines the efforts to be futile or hopeless. Futility constitutes sufficient reason for either withholding or ceasing extraordinary treatments. According to the American Heart Association (1994), physicians may withhold or stop resuscitation in the following medically futile circumstances:

- If cardiopulmonary resuscitation and emergency cardiac care were attempted without restoration of breathing and heartbeat
- If a patient's vital functions deteriorate despite maximal therapy
- If previous research indicates that no one could have survived under the same circumstances

Withholding or stopping extraordinary resuscitation efforts is ethically and legally appropriate if the patient or surrogate has previously made his or her preferences known through advance directives (see Advance Directives).

One type of resuscitation effort that is not ethical is referred to as "slow codes" or "show codes." This type of resuscitation is often used to deceive the family into thinking that the effort was legitimate. However, limited resuscitation, like administration of certain drugs or withholding of intubation, if requested by the patient or surrogate, is legal if the patient or surrogate is properly informed and requests the limitation in advance. Limited resuscitation orders must be documented in the physician's orders.

WITHHOLDING OR WITHDRAWAL OF LIFE SUPPORT

The Karen Ann Quinlan case (*In re Quinlan,* 1976) dramatically drew attention in the courts and the public arena to the issue of withdrawing life-sustaining treatment. The case raised substantial questions about the criteria used for withdrawal of treatment as well as the actual process of decision making. The New Jersey Supreme Court recognized the right of incompetent patients to be withdrawn from life-sustaining treatment, if such an act can be determined to be in their best interests. The court interpreted the constitutional right of privacy contained within the ninth amendment to be the basis for their decision and held that a person did not lose the right to decide whether or not life-sustaining treatment should be terminated merely because of incompetence.

After the Quinlan decision, several dozen court cases have grappled with the ethical issue of withdrawing treatment from persons who are either permanently brain damaged or dying. Judicial opinions in these cases tend to support the decisions of competent adult patients and families or surrogates to forego life-sustaining treatment if little chance exists for recovery (Meisel, 1995). The American Heart Association further delineates justification for withholding and withdrawal of life support in the adult or child who remains permanently unconscious, when the burden of treatment exceeds any benefit or when scientific evidence indicates that the chances for recovery are remote.

The courts endorsed the concept that persons have a limited right to refuse treatment, even if that decision may lead to death. The right to refuse life-sustaining treatment is not an absolute. In consideration of such a request, the decision has typically been weighed against four countervailing state interests: preservation of life, prevention of suicide, protection of innocent third parties, and maintenance of the integrity of the medical profession (Meisel, 1995).

Consensus does, however, exist on the rights of competent adult patients to make treatment decisions for themselves. However, concern exists when decisions are made by surrogates or family if the patient is incompetent. The courts have established stringent procedural safeguards that must be present before treatment can be terminated. The primary concern of the courts has been to protect the interests of patients

who are unable to articulate their views about life-sustaining treatment (New York State Task Force on Life and Law, 1992).

Although many cases deal with the removal or withholding of life-support technology, a new group of cases have focused attention on the cessation of artificial feeding and hydration. These cases have raised two questions: whether prolonged artificial feeding is an ordinary or an extraordinary form of medical treatment and whether nondying patients or their surrogates can decline such nourishment.

Several judicial responses to these issues have been made. The New Jersey Supreme Court upheld the judgment of a guardian to remove a nasogastric tube from an elderly, seriously ill patient so that she would not have to endure the pain of an intrusive tube. Ms. Conroy, aged 83 years, had been admitted to the hospital from a nursing home with severe decubitus ulcers on her foot as a result of diabetes. Her physicians had recommended that her left leg be amputated above the knee. Because Ms. Conroy had chronic brain syndrome, she was not able to communicate her wishes about treatment. Ms. Conroy's nephew, acting as her legal guardian, refused permission for the surgery and also later requested that her nasogastric tube be removed (Guarino and Antoine, 1990).

Barber v. Superior Court was a highly publicized case that raised the question of whether the withdrawal of nutritional support constituted murder on the part of physicians (Meisel, 1995). In this case, Mr. Clarence Herbert suffered a cardiac arrest in the recovery room after abdominal surgery. He was resuscitated and placed on a mechanical ventilator. After 3 days, his attending physicians, Drs. Barber and Nejdi, made a determination that Mr. Herbert was in an irreversible coma and suggested to his family that he be removed from ventilator support. Mr. Herbert's wife agreed with the physician, and Mr. Herbert was removed from the ventilator but subsequently began to breathe on his own. Two days later, the physicians ordered removal of Mr. Herbert's intravenous feeding lines, and, several days later, he died.

After Mr. Herbert's death, a nurse who provided care to him voiced her concern to the Los Angeles County District Attorney that Mr. Herbert's life support systems were removed precipitously. After a preliminary investigation, the district attorney issued a criminal complaint for first-degree homicide against Drs. Nejdi and Barber for removal of ventilator support and intravenous feedings because withdrawal constituted an act of murder. The California appeals court eventually dismissed all of the charges against the physicians, holding that cessation of life support was not illegal, because it fell within the scope of acceptable practice for patients in irreversible comas. Further, the court ruled that no difference existed between withholding respiratory treatment and intravenous feedings because both are a type of mechanical assistance.

The Nancy Cruzan case (Frader et al., 1990) is the most influential one to date regarding the removal of nutrition and hydration. Nancy Cruzan was injured in a motor vehicle accident in 1983 and within several weeks was determined to be in a chronic vegetative stage. She was confined to a Missouri state hospital for several years with no hope of recovery. In 1988, her parents petitioned the state courts for permission to terminate her enteral nutrition and hydration after hospital employees refused to do so without court approval. The family petitioned on the basis of the standard of "substitute judgment" and "best interest."

Permission to remove enteral nutrition and hydration was granted by the Missouri trial court based on Nancy's preaccident statement to a friend that she wished to die if no reasonable quality of life existed. However, on appeal, the Missouri Supreme Court reversed the lower court decision, rejected Nancy's statement as unreliable, and rejected her parent's request for termination of treatment. The court concluded that no one else can make that choice for an incompetent person in the absence of either a formal document such as a living will or "clear and convincing evidence" of the patient's wishes.

The case was appealed to the United States Supreme Court, which upheld the decision of the Missouri Supreme Court. The United States Supreme Court (*Cruzan v. Director,* 1990) concluded that the states have the right to adopt their own standards of proof to determine a patient's wishes regarding treatment. It also ruled that states are not required to recognize the right of a family to make decisions for the incompetent patient.

On November 1, 1990, the case was again heard by the original lower court in Missouri. Three witnesses provided testimony stating that they recalled specific conversations with Nancy in which she stated that she would not wish to live "like a vegetable." The trial court judge reaffirmed his decision to allow the feeding tube to be pulled, based on this new evidence concerning Ms. Cruzan's wishes. The family directed hospital authorities to remove the tube on December 14th, and Nancy died 2 weeks later (C. Cruzan, personal communication, 1995; Guarino and Antoine, 1990).

Several subsequent court decisions have upheld the privacy right of both competent and incompetent patients to have nutrition and hydration withheld based on a stringent test of the best interest standard. The contradictory court decisions regarding withdrawal of nutrition and hydration reflect society's ambivalence and the discomfort of many health professionals with this practice (Campbell and Thill-Baharozian, 1994). The traditional medical ethic has regarded the provision of sustenance as a fundamental act of caring; some may view this shift as a violation of medical and nursing codes.

PATIENT SELF-DETERMINATION ACT

In response to public concern about end-of-life decisions and the overall lack of consistent hospital policies, the United States Congress enacted the Patient Self-Determination Act in 1990. The act requires that all health care facilities that receive Medicare and Medicaid funding inform their patients about the patients' right to initiate an advance directive as well as the patients' right to consent to or refuse medical treatment.

ADVANCE DIRECTIVES

An advance directive is a communication that specifies a person's preference about medical treatment should he or she become incapacitated. Several types of advance directives exist, but the most common are living wills and durable powers of attorney for health care (Fig. 3–2).

The living will provides a mechanism by which an individual can authorize that specific treatments can be withheld in the event that he or she becomes incapacitated. Although living wills provide some direction to caregivers, problems exist with their use. In some states, living wills are not legally binding and are seen as advisory. In addition, some states require that death be "imminent" before a living will can go into effect. This requirement may exclude patients who are terminally ill but whose dying process is prolonged, or patients who are in a persistent vegetative state but are not dying.

The durable power of attorney for health care is more protective of patients' interests regarding medical treatment than is the living will. With this mechanism, patients legally designate an agent that they trust, such as a family member or friend, to make decisions on their behalf should they become incapacitated. Some legal commentators recommend the joint use of a living will and a durable power of attorney to give added protection to a person's preferences about medical treatment.

In the final analysis, if self-determination and informed consent are to have real value, patients or their surrogates must be given an opportunity to consider relevant options and to shape decisions that affect their life or death.

LIVING WILL AND DURABLE POWER OF ATTORNEY

(For Health Care)

Florida Registry &
Living Will Registry Of America, Inc.
Founded in 1988

A National Non-Profit
Information and
Registration Center

STATE OF FLORIDA
DECLARATION

Declaration made this _____ day of _____ , 19 _____

I, (name) _____

of (mailing address) _____ ,

(city, state) _____ (zip) _____

(Social Security Number) _____ (Phone) (_____) _____
willfully and voluntarily make known my desire that my dying not be artificially prolonged under the circumstances set forth below, and I do hereby declare;

If at any time I should have a terminal condition ((a) A condition caused by injury, disease, or illness from which there is no reasonable probability of recovery and which, without treatment, can be expected to cause death; or (b) A persistent vegetative state characterized by a permanent and irreversible condition of unconsciousness) and if two (2) physicians who have personally examined me, one of whom shall be my attending physician, have determined that there can be no recovery from such condition and that my death is imminent, I direct that life-prolonging procedures be withheld or withdrawn when the application of such procedures would serve only to prolong artificially the process of dying, and that I be permitted to die naturally with only the administration of medication or the performance of any medical procedure deemed necessary to provide me with comfort, care or to alleviate pain.

( ) I do desire that nutrition and hydration (food and water) be withheld or withdrawn when the application of such procedures would serve only to prolong artificially the process of dying. (No mark or check indicates my desire to be artificially tube fed.)

In the absence of my ability to give directions regarding the use of such life-prolonging procedures, it is my intention that this declaration be honored by my family and physician as the final expression of my legal right to refuse medical or surgical treatment and to accept the consequences for such refusal.

In the event I am unable to speak for myself, I hereby designate (name) _____ ,

my _____ at _____ (_____) _____
　　　　(relationship)　　　　　　　(city, state)　　　　　　　　(phone)
to serve as my durable power of attorney for health care, for the purpose of making medical treatment decisions for me. In the event that my first choice is unable to serve, I appoint as alternate:

(name) _____ , my _____
　　　　　　　　　　　　　　　　　　　　　　　　　　　　　　(relationship)

at _____ (_____) _____
　　　　(city, state)　　　　　　　　　　　　　　　　(phone)
This power of attorney shall remain effective in the event that I become incompetent or otherwise unable to make such decisions for myself. The appointment of this power of attorney as my agent for the purpose of making medical treatment decisions involves in no way any power to change the declaration of this living will.

Special request or instruction:

Other Alternates:

Figure 3–2. Example of a living will. (Used by permission of Florida Registry and Living Will Registry of America, Inc.)

29

Organ and Tissue Transplantation

Improved surgical methods and increasingly effective immunosuppressive drug therapy have improved the number and the type of successfully transplanted organs and tissues (Table 3–4). Despite the successes in transplantation, not enough organs exist to meet the growing demand. Congress enacted the Nation Organ Procurement and Transplantation Network to facilitate fair allocation of organs and tissues for transplantation. This network is administered by the United Network for Organ Sharing (UNOS), a group that maintains a list of individuals who are awaiting transplantation and helps coordinate the procurement of organs (UNOS Education Department, 1995).

Potential donors may agree to donate organs or tissues at any time by signing a donor card, but final consent for donation by the family or surrogate is needed before the donor is declared brain dead. In some situations, removal of the organ to be transplanted is not life threatening and can be accomplished without causing significant harm to the donor (e.g., kidneys and bone marrow). Other types of organ and tissue removal (e.g., heart) are harmful to the donor and are performed only in donors who meet the legal definition for brain death.

The concept of brain death is distinct from the concept of persistent vegetative state or irreversible coma. In brain death, complete and irreversible cessation of brain function occurs, whereas in irreversible coma or persistent vegetative state, some brain function remains intact. Tests to determine brain death are outlined in Table 3–5. If the patient is brain dead and is a designated donor, perfusion and oxygenation of organs is maintained until the organs can be removed. Even with optimal artificial perfusion and oxygenation, organs intended for transplantation must be removed and transplanted quickly.

The nurse is often the first person to have contact with family members or loved ones of the patient who is brain dead. Everyone in the United States has the legal right to donate organs. In order to uphold that right, the family or significant others must be given the opportunity to donate organs or tissues on behalf of their loved one.

Table 3–5. TESTS USED TO DETERMINE BRAIN DEATH*

1. Cessation of spontaneous respiration
2. Cessation of spontaneous heartbeat
3. Cessation of brain function, including absence of all function of the brainstem and cerebral hemispheres, and verified by

- No response on neurological examination
- Isoelectric electroencephalogram
- Absence of cerebral blood flow

in the absence of hypothermia or drug-induced states

*These tests are formalized into criteria for brain death by different institutions or groups, such as the Harvard Medical School Ad Hoc Committee or the National Institute of Health Collaborative Study of Cerebral Survival. No absolute standardization exists for "brain death criteria."

Table 3–4. ORGAN AND TISSUE TRANSPLANTATION

Material Transplanted	Necessitating Condition
Bone	Conditions requiring facial/bone reconstruction
Bone marrow	Leukemias
Brain tissue	Parkinson's disease
Cartilage	Conditions requiring facial/bone reconstruction
Corneas	Corneal damage, agenesis
Fascia	Conditions requiring repair of tendons, ligaments
Heart	End-stage cardiac myopathy
Heart valves	Diseased valves
Kidneys	End-stage renal disease
Liver	End-stage liver disease
Lungs	End-stage lung disease
Pancreas	Diabetes mellitus
Skin	Burns (temporary cover)
Veins	Diseased veins/arteries

ETHICAL CONCERNS SURROUNDING TRANSPLANTATION

Organ and tissue transplantation involves numerous and complex ethical issues. First consideration is given to the rights and privileges of all moral agents involved: the donor, the recipient, the family or surrogate, and all other recipients and donors. Important ethical principles that are useful in ethical decision making regarding transplantation include respect for persons and their autonomous choices, beneficence and nonmaleficence, utility, justice, and fidelity.

Three of the most controversial issues in transplantation are the moral value that should be placed on the human body part, the just distribution of a human body part, and the complex problems inherent in applying the concept of brain death to clinical situations.

Care of Persons with Human Immunodeficiency Virus or Acquired Immunodeficiency Syndrome

Profound ethical and legal issues often arise in providing nursing care to persons with HIV or AIDS in critical care settings. Many of these issues are related to fundamental civil rights, including the right to privacy and confidentiality, informed consent in treatment and research, professional duties to provide care, mandatory testing, the right to refuse treatment, and allocation of scarce resources.

This disease, perhaps more than any other, challenges health professionals to examine their own ethical beliefs about treatment as well as their professional obligations to persons who are often marginalized in society. Critical care nurses, in particular, provide care to patients with HIV or AIDS when they are often in the most acute stages of their illness and when they may be the most vulnerable.

DUTY TO TREAT

One of the most fundamental and emotionally charged issues that nurses must confront is the nature and extent of their professional duty to treat persons with HIV or AIDS. Several recent studies suggest that many nurses are reluctant to care for HIV patients out of concern for their own safety.

Very strong ethical and legal justifications support a nurse's duty to treat. From a legal perspective, a nurse's duty to provide care is derived from a contract with the employing agency as well as the historical tradition that the practice of professional nursing may involve certain acknowledged risks.

The American Nurses Association issued a strong position paper in 1988 stating that nurses have a moral obligation to care for HIV-infected patients when there is minimal risk of harm to themselves. That position has been echoed by the American Medical Association's Council on Ethical and Judicial Affairs, which stated, "A physician may not ethically refuse to treat a patient whose condition is within the physician's realm of competence, solely because the patient is seropositive."

Hospitals and other health care agencies have specific legal obligations to provide safe work environments for employees who care for persons with HIV or acquired immunodeficiency syndrome (AIDS) and other communicable diseases. The Occupational Safety and Health Administration requires that health care agencies use universal precautions and develop specific protocols and procedures for infection control, employee training related to universal precautions, and follow-up of employees who have been exposed to HIV or AIDS. Occupational Safety and Health Administration regulations also specify that employees be provided with personal equipment that can help prevent the transmission of HIV or AIDS from patients to health care workers (U.S. Office of Technology Assessment, 1992).

The Centers for Disease Control and Prevention does not support mandatory HIV testing of patients in acute care settings but does recommend that patients be offered the opportunity for voluntary, confidential testing.

Summary

The ethical and legal responsibilities of nurses who work in acute care settings have increased dramatically during the past decade. As nurses develop greater autonomy and assume more expanded roles in clinical practice, they also assume more responsibility and accountability for their practice.

It is clear from evolving case law, as well as from state nurse practice acts, that nurses are held to a high standard of care and are also held directly accountable for their individual nursing actions. An increase in professional standards is also reflected in the revised code of ethics that was recently adopted by the American Nurses Association. In response to these standards, nurses must maintain and continually update their knowledge base and clinical competencies. Failure to do so could not only cause harm to patients but also put nurses and their employers at risk for allegations of negligence.

CRITICAL THINKING QUESTIONS

1. You are taking care of Mrs. H., a 90-year-old patient with gastrointestinal bleeding. She has developed numerous complications and requires mechanical ventilation. She is unresponsive to nurses and family members. She has been in the hospital 2 weeks and requires a transfusion nearly every day to sustain adequate hemoglobin and hematocrit levels. Her prognosis is poor. Before this hospitalization, she lived independently at her own home. During visitation, her family tells you they are tired of seeing their mother suffer. How do you respond to the family, and what follow-up do you perform?

2. You are taking care of Mr. J., a 23-year-old man with a closed head injury. During your shift, you note a change in the level of consciousness at 3:00 AM. You call the physician, who tells you to watch Mr. J. until the physician attends rounds the next

---

RESEARCH APPLICATION

Article Reference

Sherman, D. A., & Branum, K. (1995). Critical care nurses' perception of appropriate care of the patients with orders not to resuscitate. *Heart and Lung, 24*, 321–329.

Study Overview

Do not resuscitate (DNR) orders may influence critical care nurses' perception of the appropriateness of other nonresuscitative elements of care. This study compared the differences in perceptions of appropriate levels of care of patients with and without DNR orders. The researchers developed the Appropriateness of Care Questionnaire (ACQ), in which nurses were asked to rate the appropriateness of 16 interventions for a woman with sepsis. Half of the distributed questionnaires indicated that the woman had a DNR order, and half noted that she did not have a DNR order. The ACQ interventions were divided into two subscales: physical interventions and psychological interventions.

Eighty-seven of the 317 ACQ forms distributed to critical care nurses were returned; the average length of critical care nursing experience of the nurses sampled was 8.5 years. The sample participants practiced all adult critical care settings: cardiac, medical, surgical, and neurological intensive care units. Of the returned questionnaires, 45 were of DNR type, and 42 were of the non-DNR type, so the questionnaires were weighted equally for statistical analyses.

Analysis of variance tested the hypothesis that a difference existed in the appropriateness scores for DNR and non-DNR scores. A significant difference in scores ($P=.0031$) was found between the DNR and non-DNR cases. Six of the 16 interventions were considered less appropriate for the DNR status patient. All six of the interventions were classified as physical rather than psychological.

The findings imply that DNR orders may be inconsistently interpreted by critical care nurses and that nurses perceive that aspects of care other than the resuscitation measures are influenced by DNR status.

Critique

The ACQ was well developed. The research question is relevant to nursing practice, and the research is well justified. Even though the sample was nonrandom, the low rate of return of the ACQ (27%) is of concern. A questionnaire that evaluates attitudes in a hypothetical case is an indirect measurement of what might occur in actual situations and limits the usefulness of study findings.

Nursing Implications for Practice

The inconsistency of what is meant by DNR suggests the need for a two-part approach of clarification and education. Health care institutions should clarify DNR policies and better educate nurses who are to adhere to these policies. Other health care team members, particularly physicians, could give better direction for patient care. Advanced directives of patients or family may also help delineate care for patients who have DNR orders.

The study also points to a need for further study of the factors that influence critical care nurses' perceptions of appropriate interventions. One variable suggested in the article was religious orientation of the nurse respondents. In addition, quantification of the interventions would be an important variable to evaluate because the appropriateness of some interventions depends on how often they are performed. For example, it might be appropriate to conduct a neurological assessment of the patient with a DNR order at eight-hour intervals, but not at 1-hour intervals.

---

morning. He tells you not to call him back. Mr. J.'s neurological status continues to deteriorate. What actions do you take?

REFERENCES

American Nurses Association. (1985). *Code for nurses with interpretive statements.* Kansas City, MO: Author.

American Heart Association. (1994). *Textbook of advanced cardiac life support* (R. O. Cummins, Ed.). Dallas, TX: Author.

Baggs, J. G. (1993). Collaborative interdisciplinary bioethical decision-making in intensive care units. *Nursing Outlook, 41*(3), 108–112.

Bandman, E. L., & Bandman, B. (1995). *Nursing ethics through the lifespan* (3rd ed). Norwalk, CT: Appleton & Lange.

Campbell, M. L., & Thill-Baharozian, M. (1994). Impact of the DNR therapeutic plan on patient care requirements. *American Journal of Critical Care, 3*(3), 202–207.

Cruzan v. Director, Missouri Dept. of Health, 58 USLW 49116 (US 1990).

Davis, A. J., & Aroskar, M. A. (1991). *Ethical dilemmas and nursing practice.* Norwalk, CT: Appleton & Lange.

Frader, J., Francis, L., Grodin, M., Hackler, C., & Jennings, B. (1990). Bioethicists' statement on the U.S. Supreme Court's Cruzan decision. *New England Journal of Medicine, 323*(10), 688.

Guarino, K. S., & Antoine, M. P. (1990). The case of Nancy Cruzan: The Supreme Court decision. *Critical Care Nurse, 2*(1).

Holder, A. (1988). Minor's rights to consent to medical care. *Journal of the American Medical Association, 257,* 400–403.

In re Quinlan, 70 NJ 10, 355 A 2d 647 (1976).

Kapp, M. B. (1989). Medical empowerment of the elderly. *Hastings Center Report, 19,* 5–7.

Martin, D. A. (1987). The legacy of Baby Doe: Nurses' ethical-legal responsibilities to handicapped newborns. In J. N. Humber & R. R. Almeder (Eds.), *Biomedical ethics reviews 1987* (pp. 15–30). Clifton, NJ: Humana Press.

Meisel, A. (1995). *The right to die* (2nd ed.). New York: John Wiley & Sons.

New York State Task Force on Life and Law: Recommendation, 1992.

Rozovsky, F. A. (1995). *Consent to treatment.* Boston: Little, Brown.

Smith, S. (1991). Three models of the nurse-patient relationship. In T. A. Mappes & J. S. Zembatzy (Eds.), *Biomedical ethics* (3rd ed.) (pp. 143–149). New York: McGraw Hill.

Soloman, M. Z., O'Donnell, L., Jennings, B., Gilfoy, V., Wolf, S. M., Nolan, K., et al. (1993). Decisions near the end of life: Professional views on life-sustaining treatments. *American Journal of Public Health, 83*(1), 14–23.

UNOS Education Department. (1995). *Between life and death.* Richmond, VA: United Network for Organ Sharing.

U.S. Office of Technology Assessment. (1992). HIV in the healthcare workplace: A background paper. *AIDS Patient Care, 6*(4), 169–185.

Winslow, B. J., & Winslow, G. R. (1991). Integrity and compromise in nursing ethics. *Journal of Medicine and Philosophy, 16,* 307–323.

RECOMMENDED READINGS

Asch, D. A. (1996). The role of critical care nurses in euthanasia and assisted suicide. *New England Journal of Medicine, 334,* 1374–1379.

Clarke, D. E., Goldstein, M. K., & Raffin, T. A. (1994). Ethical dilemmas in the critically ill elderly. *Clinics in Geriatric Medicine, 10*(1), 91–101.

Dooley, J., & Marsden, C. (1994). Healthcare Ethics Forum '94: Advance directives: The critical challenges. *AACN Clinical Issues in Critical Care Nursing, 5*(3), 340–345.

Jones, L. C. (1994). A right to die? *Intensive and Critical Care Nursing, 10*(4), 278–288.

Kee, C. (1995). Nurses' perceptions of informed consent. *AARN Newsletter, 51*(2), 23–27.

Marsee, V. (1994). Ethical dilemmas in the delivery of intensive care to critically ill oncology patients. *Seminars in Oncology Nursing, 10*(3), 156–164.

Noll, M. L., Merrell, R., & Byers, J. F. (1993). Mandatory HIV testing: A timely controversy. *Dimensions of Critical Care Nursing, 12*(2), 92–99.

Rozovsky, L. E. (1994). Canada: The high cost of waiting. *Hospital Health Network, 68*(13), 4.

Rushton, C. H. (1994). The critical care nurse as patient advocate. *Critical Care Nurse, 14*(3), 102–106.

Scanlon, C. (1996). Euthanasia and nursing practice—Right questions, wrong answer. *New England Journal of Medicine, 334,* 1401–1402.

Shekleton, M. E., Burns, S. M., Closhesy, J. M., Hanneman, S. K. G., & Ingersoll, G. L. (1994). Terminal weaning from mechanical ventilation: A review. *AACN Clinical Issues in Critical Care Nursing, 5*(4), 523–533.

Storch, J. L., & Dossetor, J. (1994). Public attitudes towards end-of-life treatment decisions. *Canadian Journal of Nursing Administration, 7*(3), 65–89.

Watne, K., & Donner, T. A. (1995). Distinguishing between life-saving and life-sustaining treatments: When the physician and spouse disagree. *Dimensions of Critical Care Nursing, 14*(1), 42–47.

PART

2

Tools for the Critical Care Nurse

CHAPTER

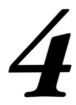

Dysrhythmia Interpretation

Stephanie Woods, Ph.D., R.N., CCRN

OBJECTIVES

- Explain the relationships between mechanical and electrical events in the heart.
- Interpret the basic dysrhythmias generated from the sinoatrial node, atrioventricular node, atria, and ventricles.

- Describe appropriate interventions for common dysrhythmias.
- Explain the basic concepts of cardiac pacing.

Introduction

The ability to analyze and interpret dysrhythmias is a fundamental skill that is required of the critical care nurse. The goal of this chapter is to provide a basic understanding of electrocardiography for the purpose of analyzing and interpreting cardiac dysrhythmias. Electrocardiography is the process of creating a visual tracing of the electrical activity of the cells in the heart. This tracing is called the electrocardiogram (ECG).

The critical care nurse often cares for patients whose cardiac rhythm is monitored. The nurse must have a clear understanding of electrocardiography and must be able to quickly assess and treat the patient's cardiac rhythm.

Basic Electrophysiology

AUTOMATICITY

The electrocardiographic tracing provides evidence that the cardiac muscle is generating electrical

activity. The basis for this electrical activity is automaticity. Automaticity is what makes the heart muscle different from other forms of muscle in the human body. Automaticity simply means that the cardiac muscle can generate its own electrical activity, even during brief times when blood supply or nervous stimulation is absent.

Students demonstrate the concept of automaticity in basic biology courses. When the heart of a small animal is dissected out of the body, it continues to beat, although blood and nervous supply have been removed. In the human body, special groups of cells generate automatic impulses for the purpose of exciting the remainder of the heart's muscle cells. Although this process is facilitated by blood flow from the coronary arteries and stimulation from the sympathetic and parasympathetic nervous systems, the heart can continue to generate electrical activity for a brief time after blood and nervous supply have ceased.

The Cardiac Cycle

The cardiac cycle is composed of both the electrical activity caused by automaticity and the mechanical, or muscular, response known as contraction. The electrical activity can be divided into two phases called depolarization and repolarization. The mechanical, or muscular, response is divided into diastole and systole. Depolarization is the active phase of electrical activity and is associated with systole. Repolarization is the resting phase and is associated with diastole.

Cardiac Action Potential

Depolarization and repolarization of the myocardium occur as a result of the movement of the electrolytes sodium and potassium across the cardiac cell membrane (Fig. 4–1). The interior of the cardiac cell is normally in a negatively charged state. This negative state is referred to as the cardiac cell's *resting membrane potential.* The normal resting membrane potential is −90 mV when the cell is in a repolarized state. Although the cardiac cell is normally in a negative state, it is the very presence of this negative state that stimulates the formation of an electrical impulse, or the beginning of depolarization.

Just before depolarization begins, sodium is found outside the cardiac cell, and potassium is found inside the cardiac cell. The movement of the positively charged sodium ions into the cardiac cell begins the active electrical process known as depolarization. Depolarization is considered an active process because cellular energy in the form of adenosine triphosphate (ATP) is required. In response to the influx of sodium, the positively charged potassium ions begin to move

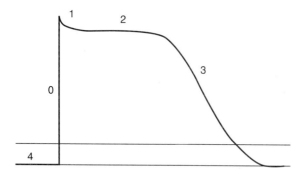

Figure 4–1. Cardiac action potential. The cardiac action potential represents the electrical phases of depolarization and repolarization. At phase 0, the cardiac cell is in a negative electrical state. Phase 1 occurs with the rapid movement of sodium into the cardiac cell. During phase 2, sodium continues to move inside the cell, and potassium begins to move outside the cell. During phase 3, potassium continues to move outside the cell. During phase 4, the sodium-potassium pump moves sodium back to extracellular space and potassium back to the intracellular space. One action potential occurs for each systole/diastole cycle.

to the outside of the cardiac cell. Potassium's movement out leads to a slightly less positive, or more negative, state preferred by the cardiac cell.

Toward the end of depolarization, sodium ceases its movement into the cardiac cell, and potassium continues its movement to the outside of the cardiac cell. The net result is a restoration of the normal resting membrane potential of −90 mV, and the resting phase, or repolarization, begins. Sodium and potassium are then returned to their proper places inside or outside the cell via the sodium-potassium pump. Again, it is this return to a resting, or repolarized, state that stimulates the next depolarization.

Repolarization of the cardiac cell leads to a resting state for the muscle. During repolarization, the ventricles are filled with blood from the atria. A sufficient time of rest is necessary for the ventricles to be adequately filled before the next depolarization and subsequent systole occurs.

RELATIONSHIP BETWEEN ELECTRICAL ACTIVITY AND MUSCULAR CONTRACTION

Under normal circumstances, depolarization is followed by contraction of a cardiac muscle fiber. The term *systole* refers to the contraction of the cardiac muscle.

The electrocardiographic tracing, or the ECG, is evidence of electrical activity only. The presence of an ECG pattern does not necessarily ensure that the patient's heart is also contracting. For confirmation that cardiac systole is occurring, clinical signs, such as a palpable pulse and the presence of an adequate blood pressure, are sought.

Nurses may encounter situations in which a patient is pronounced dead despite the fact that an ECG tracing can be obtained. These patients are most often suffering from terminal disease processes for which no cure is possible, or they may be the victims of unsuccessful resuscitation efforts. A patient is pronounced dead when no pulse or blood pressure can be established. Despite the fact that the heart is no longer contracting and pumping blood to the coronary arteries and the nervous tissues, the patient's heart may continue to generate electrical impulses, thereby creating an ECG tracing.

In this scenario, automaticity continues, despite the lack of blood and nervous supply. The length of time that the heart can continue to create electrical impulses varies, but the electrical activity usually ceases within minutes. In this case, electrical activity occurs without subsequent muscle contraction. This phenomenon is referred to as pulseless electrical activity (American Heart Association, 1994).

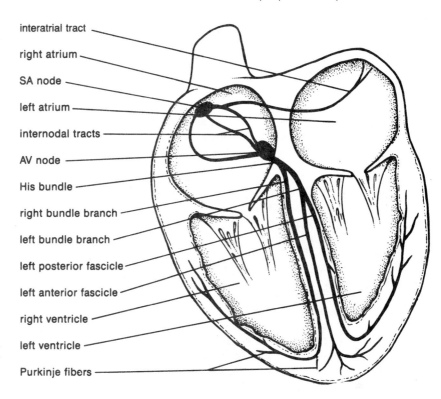

interatrial tract

right atrium

SA node

left atrium

internodal tracts

AV node

His bundle

right bundle branch

left bundle branch

left posterior fascicle

left anterior fascicle

right ventricle

left ventricle

Purkinje fibers

Figure 4–2. Normal cardiac conduction pathway. SA = sinoatrial; AV = atrioventricular (Adapted from Patel, J., McGowan, S., & Moody, L. (1989) *Arrhythmias: Detection, treatment, and cardiac drugs.* (p. 2.). Philadelphia: W. B. Saunders Co.)

NORMAL CARDIAC CONDUCTION PATHWAY

Theoretically, any cardiac cell can generate an electrical impulse. However, under normal conditions, special groups of cardiac cells are responsible for impulse generation and conduction. These special cells make up the normal cardiac conduction pathway (Fig. 4–2). The cardiac cells are networked so that depolarization can spread easily from cell to cell. Depolarization normally begins in the sinoatrial (SA), or sinus, node, a special group of cardiac cells located high in the right atrium. The SA node is often referred to as the master, or dominant, pacemaker of the heart. This dominance results from the SA node's anatomical position as well as its intrinsic ability to generate 60 to 100 beats per minute under normal circumstances. Once the impulse is formulated in the SA node, it is conducted through the atria via the internodal pathways. These pathways connect the SA and the atrioventricular (AV) nodes and are responsible for conducting the impulse throughout the right and left atria.

The atria serve as reservoirs that collect blood returning from the head, body, and lungs. The right atrium receives deoxygenated blood from the head via the superior vena cava and from the body via the inferior vena cava. The left atrium receives oxygenated blood that is returning from the lungs via the pulmonary veins.

Atrial depolarization precedes atrial contraction. The time during which atrial depolarization occurs correlates with the time the atria drain their blood into the ventricles. Most of this process occurs as a result of gravity flow. However, as depolarization ends, the atria contract, sending any remaining blood down to the ventricles. Contraction of the atria results in roughly a 30% increase in the volume of blood sent to the ventricles, thereby dramatically affecting stroke volume and cardiac output for the next ventricular systole (Guzzetta and Dossey, 1992). Many sources refer to atrial systole as "atrial kick."

From the atria, depolarization proceeds to the AV node, which is located between the atria and the ventricles. The AV node has two important functions. First, the AV node delays entry of the electrical impulse into the ventricles. If the impulse immediately proceeds into the ventricle, contraction occurs before the ventricles have had adequate time to fill with blood from the atria. The result is a decreased stroke volume for the next systole, and therefore a decrease in cardiac output. This delay in impulse conduction is very short, only 0.02 seconds; however, it allows for adequate ventricular filling.

A second important function of the AV node is to act as a back-up pacemaker for the heart should the SA node fail. When acting as the back-up pacemaker, the AV node generates 40 to 60 beats per minute under normal conditions. The AV node can emerge as the dominant pacemaker when the SA node's rate falls to less than 40 beats per minute or when automaticity is increased in the AV node.

Increased automaticity in the AV node can result in an increased heart rate. If the AV node is able to depolarize faster than the SA node, it can temporarily take over as the dominant pacemaker. Stress, caffeine, and nicotine are common causes of increased automaticity (Huszar, 1994).

Once ventricular filling has been accomplished, the impulse leaves the AV node and moves down into the ventricles via the common bundle of His. The bundle of His is a thick cord of nerve fibers that runs down the first third of the ventricular septum. The common bundle then divides into the right and left bundle branches. The right bundle branch runs down the right side of the ventricular septum, and the left bundle branch runs down the left. The bundle branches have divisions known as fascicles. The right bundle branch has one fascicle. The left bundle branch divides into two fascicles, the anterior-superior and the posterior-inferior. The large muscle mass of the left ventricle requires two fascicles for adequate depolarization, whereas the smaller, right ventricle requires only one (see Fig. 4–2).

The impulse first enters the left ventricle via the left bundle branch, then moves across the septum for conduction down the right bundle branch. The impulse enters the left ventricle first to allow more time for its depolarization. However, despite this slight lead time, the overall effect is virtually simultaneous depolarization of both ventricles. From the bundle branches, the electrical impulse is carried deep within the ventricular muscle by fine conductive fibers known as Purkinje fibers. The Purkinje fibers also act as a final back-up pacemaker for the heart. Should both the SA and the AV nodes fail, the Purkinje fibers can generate an intrinsic rhythm of 15 to 40 beats per minute.

In summary, any change in the normal generation or conduction of impulses leads to the development of dysrhythmias. Therefore, a thorough understanding of the normal conduction pathway and its intrinsic capabilities is prerequisite to an understanding of the genesis of dysrhythmias.

The Twelve-Lead ECG System

The 12-lead ECG system includes three standard limb leads, three augmented limb leads, and six precordial leads.

STANDARD LIMB LEADS

The three limb leads are designated as leads I, II, and III. Limb leads are placed anywhere on the arms

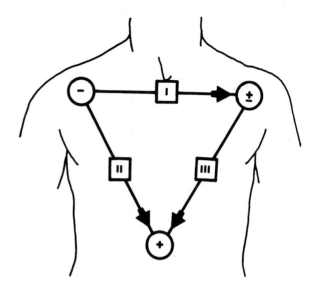

Figure 4–3. The bipolar limb leads. (From Abedin, Z., & Conner, R. (1989). *Twelve-lead ECG interpretation* (p. 15). Philadelphia: W. B. Saunders Co.)

and legs. These leads are bipolar, meaning that a positive lead is placed on one limb and a negative lead on another.

Electricity flows from negative to positive. Lead I records the flow of electricity from a negative lead on the right arm to a positive lead on the left arm. Lead II records activity between a negative lead on the right arm and a positive lead on the left leg. Lead III records activity between a negative lead on the left arm and a positive lead on the left leg (Fig. 4–3). The normal ECG waveforms are upright in the limb leads, with lead II producing the most upright waveforms.

AUGMENTED LIMB LEADS

The augmented limb leads are designated aVR, aVL, and aVF. These leads are unipolar, meaning that they record electrical flow in only one direction. A reference point is established in the center of the heart, and electrical flow is recorded from that reference point toward the right arm (aVR), the left arm (aVL), and the feet (aVF) (Fig. 4–4). The "a" in the names of these leads means augmented, and because these leads produce small ECG complexes, they must be augmented or enlarged for analysis. The ECG machine increases the size of these complexes 1.5-fold. Normally, the ECG complexes are upright, or positive, in lead aVF and downward, or negative, in aVR. Lead aVL usually produces an equiphasic QRS complex, meaning that half of the complex rises above the baseline and half falls below the baseline (Fig. 4–5).

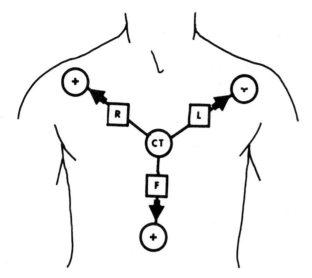

Figure 4-4. The unipolar limb leads. (From Abedin, Z., & Conner, R. (1989). *Twelve-lead ECG interpretation* (p. 15). Philadelphia: W. B. Saunders Co.)

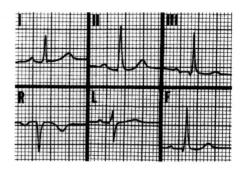

Figure 4-5. Note positive QRS complex in aVF and negative QRS complex in aVR. The QRS in aVL is equiphasic. Note that half of the QRS complex falls below the baseline and half rises above the baseline. (From Abedin, Z., & Conner, R. (1989). *Twelve-lead ECG interpretation* (p. 32). Philadelphia: W. B. Saunders Co.)

The augmented leads are monitored by use of the limb leads already in place.

PRECORDIAL LEADS

The six precordial leads are positioned on the chest wall directly over the heart. The landmarks for placement of these leads are the intercostal spaces, the sternum, and the clavicular and axillary lines. Positions for these six leads are as follows (Fig. 4–6):

V_1—fourth intercostal space, right sternal border
V_2—fourth intercostal space, left sternal border
V_3—halfway between V_2 and V_4
V_4—fifth intercostal space, midclavicular line
V_5—fifth intercostal space, anterior axillary line
V_6—fifth intercostal space, midaxillary lines

The precordial leads are particularly useful in the localization of anterior and lateral myocardial ischemia, injury, and infarction. Because these leads lie directly over the surface of the heart, changes in the normal ECG can indicate which areas of the heart have sustained damage. V_1 lies over the right ventricle; V_2 and V_3 lie over the ventricular septum; V_3 and V_4 lie over the anterior, or frontal, surface of the left ventricle; and V_5 and V_6 lie over the lateral, or side, surface of the left ventricle. None of the 12 leads records activity directly over the posterior, or back side, of the heart.

In most monitored settings, protocol dictates that a 6-second strip of the patient's rhythm be obtained and documented in the patient's chart every 4 hours.

In addition to scheduled times, a rhythm strip should be obtained when the practitioner assumes care of a patient and when a patient experiences any change in cardiac rhythm or has chest pain.

Whatever type of monitoring system is used, proper lead placement is necessary for the production of high-quality ECG tracings. In the early 1990s, Drew surveyed critical care nurses across the United States and found that the leads most frequently used were not always the best choice. Additionally, lead placement was often found to be incorrect (Drew, 1991). Limb leads should be placed on the body close to where the limbs join the torso. The right and left arm leads should be placed at the shoulder where the arms

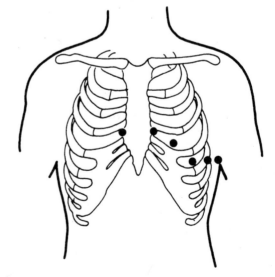

Figure 4-6. The precordial leads. (From Conover, M. B. (1988). *Understanding electrocardiography: Arrhythmias and 12-lead ECG*. St. Louis: C. V. Mosby Co.)

join the body. Inaccurate tracings result when electrodes are moved away from shoulders or placed on the lower torso toward the heart. The right and left leg leads can be placed on the lower abdomen closer to where the legs join the torso (Drew, 1993).

In the clinical setting, the standard limb leads are most often used for monitoring. Lead II, in particular, is preferred by most practitioners, since it produces upright, or positive, waveforms (Drew, 1991). Most leads are suitable for monitoring in patients with a normal width QRS complex. V_1 is recommended for use in patients with wide QRS complexes. Ideally, leads II and V_1 should be monitored simultaneously (Drew, 1993). If a monitor does not have the capability of producing V lead tracings, another useful cardiac lead is the modified chest lead, or MCL1. This lead simulates the precordial lead V_1. A negative electrode is placed on the left arm, below the clavicle. The positive electrode is placed at the right sternal border and between the fourth and fifth intercostal spaces. This is the same position as for V_1 (Fig. 4–7).

V_1 and MCL1 allow for earlier detection of changes associated with myocardial ischemia and for diagnosis of bundle branch blocks. V_1 is preferred over MCL1, if available (Drew, 1993). MCL1 and V_1 can also be helpful for differentiating whether abnormal beats are arising from the right versus the left ventricle. V_1 and MCL1 typically produce negative P, Q, R, S, and T waveforms (Alspach, 1991; Drew 1993).

Many bedside monitors in critical care units have the capability of performing 12-lead electrocardiography. With the ability to monitor any of 12 leads, the practitioner can choose the lead that produces the clearest waveforms and monitors areas of suspected heart damage. A complete 12-lead ECG is usually obtained daily in patients with cardiac disease and when the patient experiences a change in cardiac status, particularly chest pain.

Analyzing the Basic Electrocardiographic Tracing

MEASUREMENTS

Electrocardiographic paper has standard measures, whether a single-lead or a 12-lead rhythm strip is obtained (Fig. 4–8). ECG paper is used to measure time of conduction and height of waveforms. When ECG paper is used to measure time, the least unit of measure is the small box, which is equal to 0.04 second, or 40.0 milliseconds. The next greater unit of measure is the large box, which contains five small boxes. One large box represents 0.20 second, or 200 milliseconds. Five large boxes represents 1 second, or 1000 milliseconds.

The largest unit of measure is in seconds and is marked off at the top of the ECG paper by vertical hatch marks (see Fig. 4–8). There may be 1, 2, or 3 seconds between two hatch marks. Five large boxes between hatch marks equal 1 second. Ten large boxes between hatch marks equal 2 seconds. Fifteen large boxes between hatch marks equal 3 seconds. In the clinical setting, it is standard for 6-second rhythm strips to be obtained for analysis and mounting in the patient's chart. To obtain a 6-second strip, the clinician counts off the appropriate number of hatch marks.

The value of measuring time on the ECG tracing is that speed of depolarization and repolarization in the atria and ventricles can be determined. The normal conduction intervals are discussed in the next section.

Standardized ECG paper allows the practitioner to measure the height, or amplitude, of waveforms. Amplitude is measured by the number of small boxes (see Fig. 4–8). Amplitude is measured on the vertical axis of the ECG paper. Each small box is equal to 1 mm in amplitude. Waveform amplitude indicates the amount of electrical voltage being generated in the various areas of the heart. When waveforms are small, voltage is low. When waveforms are large, voltage is high. Low voltage and small waveforms are expected from the small muscle mass of the atria. High voltage and large waveforms are expected from the larger muscle mass of the ventricles.

WAVEFORMS AND INTERVALS

The normal ECG tracing is composed of P, Q, R, S, and T waves (Fig. 4–9). These waveforms emerge from a flat baseline called the isoelectric line. Isoelectric means neither positive nor negative, that is, a flat line. Any waveform that projects above the isoelectric line is considered positive, and any that projects below the line is considered negative.

P Wave. The P wave is an indication of atrial depolarization. It is usually upright in leads I and II and has a rounded configuration. The amplitude of the P wave is measured at the center of the waveform and should not exceed three boxes, or 3 mm, in height.

Normally, a P wave indicates that the SA node initiated the impulse that depolarized the atrium. However, a change in the form of the P wave can indicate that the impulse did not come from the SA node, but rather from an abnormal pacemaking site, such as the atria or AV node.

PR Interval. The P wave is connected to the next set of waveforms, the QRS complex, by the PR interval. The interval is measured from the beginning of the P wave, where the positive deflection of the P wave leaves the isoelectric line, to where the QRS complex begins. The PR interval measures the time it

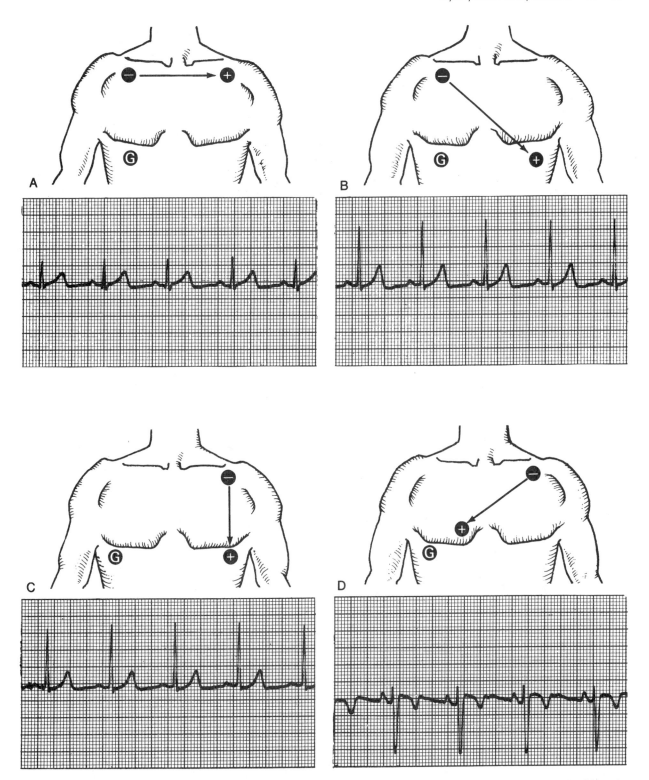

Figure 4–7. Limb leads and MCL1 electrode placement and their respective waveforms: *(A)* lead I, *(B)* lead II, *(C)* lead III, and *(D)* MCL1. (Reproduced with permission. ©*Textbook of advanced cardiac life support,* 1994 Copyright American Heart Association.)

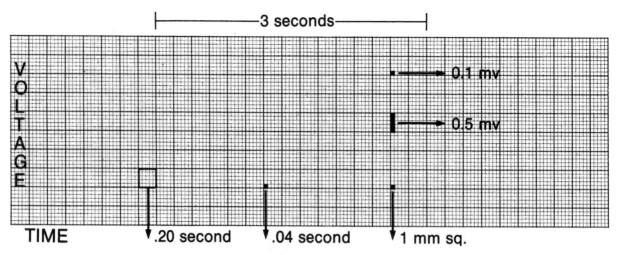

Figure 4–8. Standard ECG paper. (From Patel, J., McGowan, S., & Moody, L. (1989). *Arrhythmias: Detection, treatment, and cardiac drugs* (p. 10). Philadelphia: W. B. Saunders Co.)

takes for the impulse to depolarize the atria, travel to the AV node, and then dwell there briefly before entering the bundle of His. These activities normally take less than 0.20 seconds. The normal PR interval is 0.12 to 0.20 seconds, which is three to five small boxes

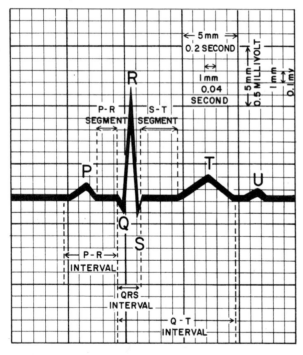

Figure 4–9. Normal ECG tracing: waveforms and intervals. (From Sanderson, R., & Kurth, C. (1983). *The cardiac patient: A comprehensive approach* (2nd ed.) (p. 149). Philadelphia: W. B. Saunders Co.)

wide (see Fig. 4–9). When the PR interval is longer than normal, the speed of conduction is abnormally slow. When the PR interval is shorter than normal, the speed of conduction is abnormally fast.

The word *dromotropy* is used to describe the speed of conduction. Many cardiac drugs increase the speed of conduction in the heart and are therefore called positive dromotropic agents. Drugs that decrease the speed of conduction are called negative dromotropic agents. Both types of drugs are discussed further in the section on treatment of dysrhythmias.

QRS Complex. The QRS complex is a set of three distinct waveforms that are indicative of ventricular depolarization (see Fig. 4–9). The term *QRS complex* is imprecise. The QRS complex is a generic term for the waveforms that indicate ventricular depolarization. However, many people do not have all three distinct waveforms, Q, R, and S, in their QRS complex (Fig. 4–10).

The textbook normal QRS complex begins with a negative, or downward, deflection immediately after the P wave. This negative deflection is known as a Q wave (see Fig. 4–9). If the initial waveform that follows the P wave is positive, the patient does not have a Q wave. The absence of a Q wave is not abnormal. Q waves are normally small waveforms and are usually present in the I, III, and aVL leads.

For a determination of whether the Q wave is of normal size, it is compared with the next positive waveform, which is called an R wave. A Q wave should be no larger than one fourth the size of the R wave. When Q waves exceed this normal size, they are referred to as *pathological*. Pathological Q waves are found on ECGs of patients who have had myocar-

DIFFERENT KINDS OF QRS COMPLEXES

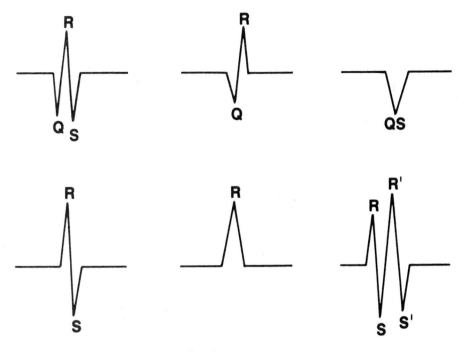

An R wave is a positive deflection.
A Q wave is a negative deflection before an R wave.
An S wave is a negative deflection after an R wave.

Figure 4–10. Different types of QRS complexes. (From Davis, D. (1985). *How to quickly and accurately master ECG interpretation* (p. 29). Philadelphia: J. B. Lippincott Co.)

dial infarctions. The deep Q wave in these patients indicates that an area of myocardial tissue has died. The ECG machine reads no electrical activity in the area, and this phenomenon creates a deep, negative waveform (Fig. 4–11).

The first positive, or upright, waveform that follows the P wave is designated the R wave. Again, a Q wave may or may not be present before the R wave. The R wave is normally tall and positive in lead II (see Fig. 4–9). The amplitude of the R wave varies across leads. Leads V₄ to V₆ usually have the tallest R waves because they measure electricity in the large muscle mass of the left ventricle. Some patients may have a second positive waveform in their QRS complex. If so, then that second positive waveform is called R prime (R′) (see Fig. 4–10).

The S wave is a negative waveform that follows the R wave. In an S wave, the waveform must go below the isoelectric line (see Fig. 4–9). The amplitude of the S wave is measured from the point it leaves the isoelectric line to its deepest point.

QRS Interval. The QRS interval is measured from the beginning to the end of the QRS complex (see Fig. 4–9). Whichever waveform begins the QRS complex (whether it is a Q or an R) marks the beginning of the interval. Therefore, the *first* deflection, either positive or negative, that follows the P wave indicates the beginning of the interval. The QRS interval is measured from the point of first deflection to where the *final* deflection returns to baseline. The final deflection may be an R or an S wave.

The normal width of the QRS complex is 0.06 to 0.10 seconds. This figure equates to 1.5 to 2.5 small boxes in length. When the QRS interval is longer than normal, conduction of the impulse through the ventricle is delayed.

When the QRS width is greater than 0.10 seconds, the patient is said to have a bundle branch block (BBB), or as is sometimes noted, an intraventricular conduction delay. The delay in conduction is most commonly caused by coronary artery disease. Either or both of the bundle branches can be blocked. A BBB causes a change in the normal conduction of impulses through the ventricles, hence, the prolonged interval.

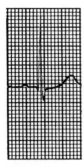

Normal Q wave

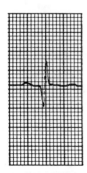

Pathological Q wave

Figure 4–11. Normal versus pathological Q wave. (From Davis, D. (1985). *How to quickly and accurately master ECG interpretation* (p. 175). Philadelphia: J. B. Lippincott Co.)

BBBs also result in a change in the QRS complex morphology.

A right BBB produces a QRS that has two distinct R waves in V_1 (Fig. 4–12). The second R wave results from delayed conduction through the right ventricle. Normally, the QRS complex is evidence of biventricular depolarization. However, in right BBB, the first R wave is evidence of left ventricular depolarization, and the second R wave is evidence of the delayed right ventricular depolarization.

A left BBB usually produces a wide, negative QRS complex in V_1. The widening of the QRS complex occurs as a result of delay of the impulse's entry into the left ventricle (see Fig. 4–12).

T Wave. The T wave represents ventricular repolarization (see Fig. 4–9). Note that a waveform indicating atrial repolarization has not been described in this chapter. Such a waveform probably exists, but it would be obscured by the large QRS complex.

Some beginning students of electrocardiography state that they have problems differentiating the P wave from the T wave. This differentiation should not be a problem, because the P wave immediately precedes the QRS, and the T wave immediately follows the QRS. Additionally, the T wave is usually of greater size and amplitude than the P wave. This is because the atria are smaller muscle masses and therefore produce smaller waveforms than do the larger ventricles. T-wave amplitude is measured at the center of the waveform and should be no greater than five small boxes, or 5 mm high. Changes in T wave amplitude can indicate electrical disturbances resulting from electrolyte imbalance or myocardial infarction. For instance, hyperkalemia can cause an increase in T-wave amplitude.

ST Segment. The ST segment connects the QRS complex to the T wave. Under normal conditions, the ST segment should be isoelectric, or flat. However, in some conditions, such as myocardial ischemia, injury, and infarction, the segment may be depressed, falling below baseline, or elevated, rising above baseline. The ST segment is not measured as a separate interval. However, its measurement is encompassed in a larger interval known as the QT interval (see Fig. 4–9).

The QT interval is measured from the beginning of the QRS complex to the end of the T wave. This interval measures the time taken for ventricular depolarization and repolarization. No standard QT interval exists. Normal QT intervals are based on heart rate. The slower the heart rate, the longer the normal QT, and the faster the rate, the shorter the normal QT. QT intervals are normally longer in females. A QT chart is used to determine the outer limits for normal intervals (Table 4–1).

A final waveform that might be noted on the ECG is the U wave. The U wave is a small waveform of unknown origin. If present, it immediately follows the T wave and is of the same deflection (see Fig. 4–9). In other words, if the T wave is positive, the U wave is also positive. U waves may be seen in patients with electrolyte imbalance, particularly hypokalemia, and in those who have had a myocardial infarction. However, the U wave is sometimes a normal finding; therefore, diagnosis of pathology should be dependent on more specific indicators.

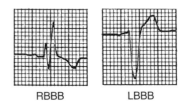

RBBB   LBBB

Figure 4–12. Right and left bundle branch blocks. (From Davis, D. (1985). *How to quickly and accurately master ECG interpretation* (pp. 152, 154). Philadelphia: J. B. Lippincott Co.)

Table 4–1. UPPER LIMITS OF THE QT INTERVAL, CORRECTED FOR HEART RATE

Rate (bpm)	QT Interval (sec)
40	0.49–0.50
50	0.45–0.46
60	0.42–0.43
70	0.39–0.40
80	0.37–0.38
90	0.35–0.36
100	0.33–0.34
110	0.32–0.33
120	0.31–0.32

From Abedin, Z., & Conner, R., (1989). *Twelve-lead ECG interpretation*. Philadelphia, W. B. Saunders Co.
bpm = beats per minute.

Systematic Interpretation of Dysrhythmias

This section proposes a systematic approach for the analysis and interpretation of dysrhythmias. Systematic analysis focuses attention on the following areas:

- Assessment of rhythmicity, both atrial and ventricular
- Assessment of rate, both atrial and ventricular
- Assessment of waveform configuration and location
- Assessment of intervals

RHYTHMICITY

Rhythmicity refers to the regularity or pattern of the heart beats. P waves are used to establish atrial rhythmicity, and R waves establish ventricular rhythmicity. When an atrial rhythm is perfectly regular, each P wave is an equal distance from the next P wave. When a ventricular rhythm is perfectly regular, each R wave is an equal distance from the next R wave. Systematic interpretation of rhythm strips requires looking at both atrial and ventricular rhythmicities.

Rhythmicity can be established through the use of calipers or paper and pencil and must be analyzed in both the atria and the ventricle. Establishing atrial rhythmicity requires placing one caliper point on one P wave and the other caliper point on the next consecutive P wave. The second point is left stationary, and the calipers are flipped over. If the first caliper point lands exactly on the next P wave, the atrial rhythm is perfectly regular. If the point lands one small box or less away from the next P or R wave, the rhythm is essentially regular. If the point lands more than one small box away, the rhythm is considered irregular.

The same process is followed for assessing ventricular rhythmicity *except* that the caliper points are placed on R waves. For establishment of ventricular rhythmicity, one caliper point is placed on one R wave and the other caliper point on the next consecutive R wave. The second point is left stationary, and the calipers are flipped over. If the first caliper point lands exactly on the next R wave, the ventricular rhythm is perfectly regular (Fig. 4–13).

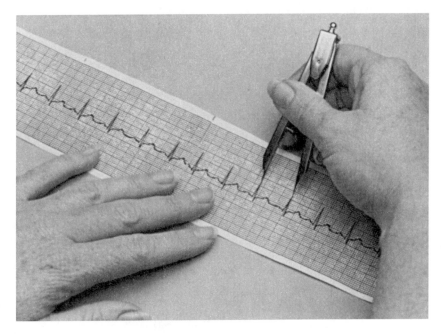

Figure 4–13. Establishing ventricular rhythmicity with calipers.

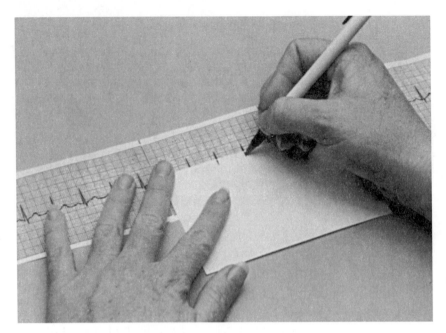

Figure 4–14. Establishing ventricular rhythmicity with paper and pencil.

Rhythmicity can also be established by use of paper and pencil. A piece of blank paper is slid over the rhythm strip, and the straight edge is placed along the peak of the P wave to assess atrial rhythmicity, or along the peak of the R wave to assess ventricular rhythmicity. With the pencil, the peak of either the P or the R wave is marked on the paper. Without movement of the paper, another mark is made on the next P or R wave. The paper is then slid over to the next P or R waveform. If the pencil mark lands exactly on the next P or R wave, the rhythm is perfectly regular. If the pencil mark is one small box or less away from the next P or R wave, the rhythm is essentially regular. If the pencil mark lands more than one small box away from the next P or R wave, the rhythm is irregular (Fig. 4–14).

Irregular rhythms can be regularly irregular or irregularly irregular. Regularly irregular rhythms have a pattern. In other words, the irregularity occurs in a predictable fashion, for instance, every second beat (Fig. 4–15). Irregularly irregular rhythms have no pattern and no predictability (Fig. 4–16).

RATE

Obviously, rate equals how fast the heart is depolarizing. Under normal conditions, the atria and the ventricles depolarize at the same rate. However, each can depolarize at a different rate. An important part of systematic analysis is calculation of both the atrial and the ventricular rates. P waves are used for calculation

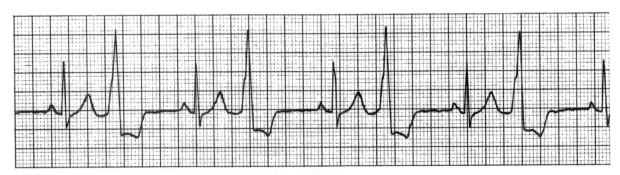

Figure 4–15. Note that the irregularity in rhythm is predictable. The abnormal complexes occur every other beat. (From Patel, J., McGowan, S., & Moody, L. (1989). *Arrhythmias: Detection, treatment, and cardiac drugs* (p. 67). Philadelphia: W. B. Saunders Co.)

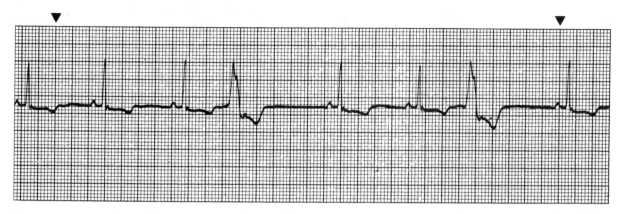

Figure 4–16. Note that the irregularity in rhythm is unpredictable. The abnormal complexes occur randomly, without pattern. (From Huff, J., Doembach, D., & White, R. (1985). *ECG workout: Exercises in arrhythmia interpretation.* Philadelphia: J. B. Lippincott Co.)

of the atrial rate, and R waves are used for calculation of the ventricular rate.

Rate can be assessed in various ways. This text addresses two popular methods:

1. The rule of 1500 is used to calculate the *exact* rate of a *regular* rhythm. In this method, two consecutive P or R waves are located. P waves are used if the atrial rate is to be calculated, and R waves are used if the ventricular rate is to be calculated. The tallest point of either the P wave or the R wave is located. The number of small boxes between the highest points of two consecutive P or R waves are counted, and that number of small boxes is divided into 1500 to determine the exact heart rate in beats per minute. For example, if 16 small boxes are between two consecutive R waves, 16 is divided into 1500, for a rate of 94 ventricular beats per minute (Fig. 4–17). This method is reserved for use with regular rhythms. If the rule of 1500 is used for irregular rhythms, the calculated rate

is accurate only between the two consecutive beats chosen. Charts are available for the calculation of heart rate based on the rule of 1500.

2. The rule of 10 is a popular method for calculating the *approximate* rate. This method can be used for either regular or irregular rhythms. The rule of 10 is accomplished by counting the number of P or R waves in a 6-second strip and then multiplying that number by 10. This equation yields an approximate heart rate for 60 seconds, or 1 minute. For example, if six R waves are found on one 6-second strip, those six complexes are multiplied by 10 for an approximate rate of 60 ventricular beats per minute. This method is used when a quick assessment of rate is needed or when a patient is having an irregular rhythm.

Cardiac monitors display heart rates, usually in a digital form. However, these monitor-calculated rates may be inaccurate and should *always* be verified by one of the aforementioned rate-calculation methods.

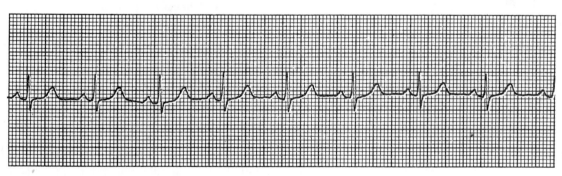

Figure 4–17. Calculating ventricular rate with the rule of 1500. Count the number of small boxes between two consecutive QRS complexes, then divide that number into 1500. In this rhythm strip there are 16 small boxes between QRS complexes. Sixteen boxes divided into 1500 gives a resultant rate of 94. (From Davis, D. (1989). *How to quickly and accurately master arrhythmia interpretation* (p. 38). Philadelphia: J. B. Lippincott Co.)

WAVEFORM CONFIGURATION AND LOCATION

In the systematic analysis of ECG rhythms, configuration and location of the normal P, Q, R, S, and T waveforms are very important.

Configuration

Each cardiac cell is capable of generating electrical impulses. This capability is referred to as *automaticity*. Each cardiac cell, once depolarized, creates a distinct waveform configuration that manifests on the ECG rhythm strip. Various waveforms can be recognized as originating from certain areas of the heart by their shape and appearance. For instance, small, slightly rounded waveforms known as P waves are associated with atrial depolarization; combinations of positive and negative waveforms known as QRS complexes, with ventricular depolarization; and larger, rounded waveforms known as T waves, with ventricular repolarization.

Under normal conditions, if all the P waves are originating from the SA node, then all P waves on a 6-second strip should look the same. If all impulses travel through the ventricle in the same way, then all QRS complexes in a 6-second strip should look the same. Also, if ventricular repolarization is always accomplished in the same way, all T waves in a 6-second strip should look the same. It also follows that if a waveform is coming from an abnormal place, that waveform does not look like the normal waveforms.

The configuration, or the shape and appearance, of a waveform is often the first clue in the assessment of dysrhythmias. Once a clinician is knowledgeable regarding normal waveform configuration, he or she can easily discern abnormal waveforms. No systematic analysis and interpretation are complete without careful study and comparison of each waveform on the 6-second strip, in which both normal and abnormal configurations are sought.

Location

Location of waveforms is very important for a systematic analysis of dysrhythmias. The normal waveforms P, Q, R, S, and T should occur in their natural order. A P wave should precede each QRS. QRS complexes should be followed by T waves, and T waves should be followed by P waves.

In the analysis of rhythm strips, it is very important to note whether waveforms occur in this order. If not, the location should be closely reviewed. In the later discussion of the basic dysrhythmias, several rhythms are characterized by abnormal location or sequencing of waveforms (Fig. 4–18).

INTERVALS

A final important aspect of the systematic analysis of rhythm strips is the assessment of the intervals discussed previously in the section on analysis of the normal ECG tracing. No rhythm strip analysis is complete, and no interpretation is possible, without the assessment of the PR, QRS, and QT intervals.

The Basic Dysrhythmias

The word *dysrhythmia* means difficult or abnormal rhythm. In this case, dysrhythmia refers to abnormal cardiac rhythms. People also speak of cardiac arrhythmias. The word *arrhythmia* means no rhythm. Therefore, dysrhythmia is a more useful and descriptive term for the rhythms encountered in the clinical setting. The basic dysrhythmias can be grouped under the following anatomical areas:

- Dysrhythmias of the SA node
- Dysrhythmias of the atria
- Dysrhythmias of the AV node
- Dysrhythmias of the ventricles
- Atrioventricular blocks

A section has been developed for each anatomical

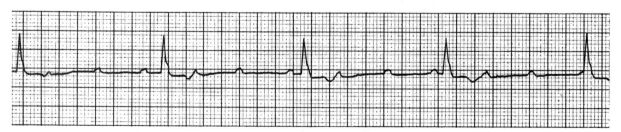

Figure 4–18. Note how P, Q, R, S, and T waves are out of normal sequence and location. (From Patel, J., McGowan, S., & Moody, L. (1989). *Arrhythmias: Detection, treatment, and cardiac drugs.* Philadelphia: W. B. Saunders Co.)

area and includes rhythm strip examples of common dysrhythmias associated with that anatomical area or structure. However, of more importance is the description of characteristics that make each dysrhythmia unique and recognizable to the practitioner. These characteristics are listed as the criteria for the diagnosis of that particular dysrhythmia. The most critical criteria for diagnosis are listed first and are designated with an asterisk.

These critical criteria eliminate the confusion surrounding dysrhythmia analysis and interpretation. Intuition has no place in such analysis; instead, the practitioner must learn the criteria for each rhythm and then makes a diagnosis based on the criteria.

Those beginning the study of basic electrocardiography should memorize these critical criteria or keep them in a notebook for easy referencing. Initially, the task seems overwhelming, and a great deal of information must be learned. Focusing on the critical criteria helps organize the information for easier analysis and interpretation.

The criteria become easier to use and remember as the clinician encounters patients with the dysrhythmia. Dysrhythmia analysis and interpretation are skills that develop through practice.

Each dysrhythmia discussed has an impact on the body's ability to maintain a normal hemodynamic status. Normal hemodynamic status is defined as an adequate cardiac output, as evidenced by a normal arterial blood pressure. The hemodynamic effects of each dysrhythmia are discussed. The treatments for the dysrhythmias are discussed at the end of the chapter.

NORMAL SINUS RHYTHM

The most important rhythm of this chapter, normal sinus rhythm is the rhythm against which all others are compared. Without a thorough understanding of what is normal, abnormal cannot be understood. Initial analysis of a rhythm strip should determine whether the rhythm is normal sinus rhythm or a dysrhythmia that requires further analysis.

The SA node is the master pacemaker of the heart. Under normal circumstances, this special group of cardiac cells generates an electrical impulse that is conducted down the normal conduction pathway, thereby depolarizing all cardiac cells (Fig. 4–19).

Critical Criteria for Diagnosis of Normal Sinus Rhythm

* 1. Upright, small, rounded P waves are present in lead II.
* 2. P waves precede each QRS complex.
* 3. Both the atrial rate and the ventricular rate are the same, and that rate is between 60 and 100 beats per minute.
* 4. Rhythm is regular or essentially regular.
  5. The PR interval is 0.12 to 0.20 seconds in duration.
  6. The QRS interval is 0.06 to 0.10 seconds in duration.

Hemodynamic Effects

The normal sinus rhythm is the optimal cardiac rhythm for the maintenance of adequate cardiac output and blood pressure.

DYSRHYTHMIAS OF THE SINOATRIAL NODE
Sinus Bradycardia

Bradycardia is defined as a slowed heart rate. Sinus bradycardia results when the SA node generates fewer than 60 beats per minute (Fig. 4–20). The following sections discuss several processes that can lead to sinus bradycardia.

Increased Vagal Stimulation. The parasympathetic nervous system influences the heart rate via the vagus nerve. When the vagus nerve is stimulated, an impulse is sent to the heart, and the heart rate is decreased. The Valsalva maneuver, as well as coughing, gagging, suctioning, and vomiting, can stimulate the vagus nerve and cause sinus bradycardia.

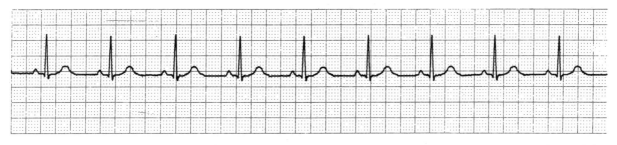

Figure 4–19. Normal sinus rhythm. Rhythm strip generated by the AA-700 Rhythm Simulator. (Reproduced with permission from Armstrong Medical Industries, Lincolnshire, IL: *DataSim*, Fig. O.)

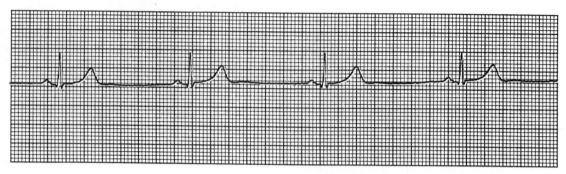

Figure 4–20. Sinus bradycardia. (From Davis, D. (1985). *ECG workout: Exercises in arrhythmia interpretation* (p. 38). Philadelphia: J. B. Lippincott Co.)

Drug Effects. Many of the drugs administered to patients with cardiac disease decrease heart rate. This slowing in heart rate is often a desired result of treatment. When a patient's heart beats at a slower rate, oxygen demands are lessened. When bradycardia occurs as a side effect of a drug, the drug is said to have a negative chronotropic effect. Drugs with positive chronotropic effects increase heart rate.

Sinoatrial Node Ischemia. When the patient has myocardial ischemia, injury, or infarction in the area surrounding the SA node, the node may become less able to generate impulses. Bradycardia can result.

Effects of Hypoxia. Sinus bradycardia can occur during episodes of hypoxia. Hypoxia may result from both acute and chronic conditions.

Bradycardia as a Normal Finding. Athletes and others who are physically fit may have a slower than normal heart rate. Physical conditioning leads to increased strength of the cardiac muscle, and, therefore, increased effectiveness of the heart as a pump. An effective pump can deliver adequate amounts of blood to the body at a slower heart rate.

Increased Intracranial Pressure. Cushing's reflex is a hemodynamic response to increased intracranial pressure. Blood pressure increases and heart rate decreases and often becomes irregular (Wright and Shelton, 1993).

Critical Criteria for Diagnosis of Sinus Bradycardia

The criteria are the same as for normal sinus rhythm *except* that the heart rate is less than 60 beats per minute.

Hemodynamic Effects

Patients demonstrate various hemodynamic responses to sinus bradycardia. Many patients continue to maintain an adequate cardiac output and blood pressure, despite a lowered heart rate. This ability to compensate is better in patients with a healthy heart. Other patients experience a decrease in cardiac output and blood pressure as their pulse slows.

Sinus Tachycardia

Tachycardia is defined as a rapid heart rate. Sinus tachycardia results when the SA node generates more than 100, but fewer than 150, beats per minute (Fig. 4–21). Sinus tachycardia is a normal response to stimulation of the sympathetic nervous system. Sinus tachycardia is also a normal finding in children under the age of 6 years. Several other processes can lead to sinus tachycardia, including exercise, use of stimulants, increased body temperature, and alterations in fluid status.

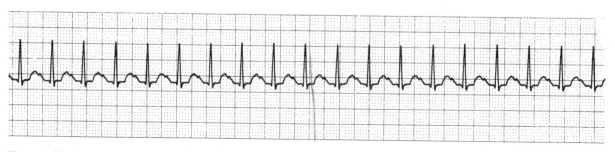

Figure 4–21. Sinus tachycardia. Rhythm strip generated by the AA-700 Rhythm Simulator. (Reproduced with permission from Armstrong Medical Industries, Lincolnshire, IL: *DataSim*, Fig. 1.)

Exercise. Exercise is a natural stimulant to the heart. Heart rate increases as the body's oxygen demand and consumption increase.

Stimulants. Many types of stimulants can increase the heart rate. Commonly used and abused drugs, like caffeine and nicotine, stimulate heart rate. Additionally, drugs such as decongestants and appetite suppressants can markedly increase heart rate. Stress and pain stimulate the sympathetic nervous system, resulting in a faster heart rate.

Increased Body Temperature. Elevation in body temperature causes an increase in heart rate.

Alterations in Fluid Status. Both hypovolemia and hypervolemia can result in increased heart rate. When the circulating blood volume is low, such as in dehydration or after hemorrhage, the heart must beat faster to maintain an adequate cardiac output and blood pressure. When the circulating blood volume is increased, such as in fluid overload, the heart must beat faster to compensate for the increased blood coming into the heart.

Critical Criteria for Diagnosis of Sinus Tachycardia

The criteria are the same as for normal sinus rhythm *except* that the heart rate is greater than 100 beats per minute.

Hemodynamic Effects

Sinus tachycardia leads to a decrease in ventricular filling time. A decrease in ventricular filling time leads to less blood volume in the ventricle for the next systole and consequently a lower cardiac output and arterial blood pressure. Another, possibly severe, consequence of sinus tachycardia is increased myocardial oxygen consumption. This condition is especially det-

rimental in the patient with inadequate coronary artery perfusion.

Sinus Dysrhythmia

Sinus dysrhythmia is a cardiac rhythm disturbance that is associated with normal respiration. During inspiration, air is brought into the lungs by a negative intrathoracic pressure. Because the heart lies within the thoracic cavity, this negative intrathoracic pressure associated with breathing causes more blood to be brought into the right atrium from the superior and inferior venae cavae. As compensation for this increased amount of blood coming to the heart, heart rate is increased.

With expiration, the pressure in the thoracic cavity is changed to positive, and air is forced from the lungs. During expiration, the flow of blood into the heart returns to normal, as does the heart rate.

The ECG tracing demonstrates an alternating pattern of faster heart rate, which is associated with inspiration, then slower heart rate, which is associated with expiration (Fig. 4–22). This rhythm is considered a normal phenomenon; however, certain conditions, such as increased intracranial pressure, increased vagal tone, and myocardial ischemia, injury, and infarction, can cause the rhythm changes.

Critical Criteria for Diagnosis of Sinus Dysrhythmia

* 1. The criteria are the same as for normal sinus rhythm *except* for a phasic increasing and decreasing of heart rate.

* 2. Changes in heart rate are associated with respiration.

* 3. Rhythm is usually regularly irregular.

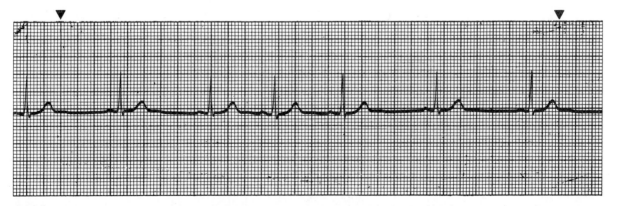

Figure 4–22. Sinus dysrhythmia. Note decreased rate at beginning and ending of strip. Slowing of rate is associated with expiration. Increased rate in the middle of strip is associated with inspiration. (Adapted from Huff, J., Doembach, D., & White, R. (1985). *ECG workout: Exercises in arrhythmia interpretation.* Philadelphia: J. B. Lippincott Co.)

Hemodynamic Effects

Significant changes in cardiac output and blood pressure rarely occur with this rhythm. It is normally tolerated well unless the heart rate decreases to less than 60 beats per minute or increases to greater than 100 beats per minute.

Sinus Arrest/Sinus Exit Block

Occasionally, the sinus node temporarily fails as the dominant pacemaker. This failure may be caused by an inability of the sinus node to generate an electrical impulse (sinus arrest), or the impulse may be generated but blocked from exiting the SA node (sinus exit block). The end result is that no atrial or ventricular depolarization occurs. In this situation, the normal cardiac waveforms are completely absent. In other words, for one heart beat or more, no P, Q, R, S, and T waves are present (Fig. 4–23).

This loss of the normal waveforms creates a pause of varying length on the ECG tracing. A pause is a long flat line between two beats that exceeds the normal amount of space found between other beats. If this pause is long enough to drop the heart rate to less than 60 beats per minute, then the AV node or the Purkinje fibers may be used as a back-up pacemaker and generate an escape beat or escape rhythm. The escape beat is so named because it allows the patient to escape the slowed heart rate, thus preventing further compromise.

Sinus arrest or sinus exit block may be caused by enhanced vagal tone, coronary artery disease, or use of certain drugs (Huszar, 1994).

Enhanced Vagal Tone. The Valsalva maneuver, coughing, gagging, or vomiting may temporarily suppress impulse generation in, or conduction from, the SA node.

Coronary Artery Disease. Coronary artery disease can lead to decreased perfusion of the SA node, resulting in impaired performance.

Effects of Drugs. Administration of various cardiac drugs that slow heart rate can lead to episodes of sinus arrest and exit block.

Critical Criteria for Diagnosis of Sinus Arrest/Sinus Exit Block

* 1. Heart rate can be normal (60 to 100 beats per minute) or slower than normal.
* 2. Pauses caused by missed beats are noted on the ECG.
* 3. Rhythm is irregular as the result of missed beats.
 4. Pauses may be interrupted by an escape beat from the AV node or the Purkinje fibers.

Hemodynamic Effects

The hemodynamic effects of sinus arrest and/or exit block depend on the number of sinus beats that are arrested or blocked and the length of the resulting pause. When occasional beats are arrested or blocked, the hemodynamic effects are the same as for sinus bradycardia. Changes in cardiac output and blood pressure dependent on how low the heart rate falls.

When multiple beats are arrested or blocked, asystole results. The patient ceases to have any cardiac output and adequate blood pressure.

DYSRHYTHMIAS OF THE ATRIA

Increased automaticity in the right, the left, or both atria can result in abnormal cardiac rhythms. These dysrhythmias are most often caused by in-

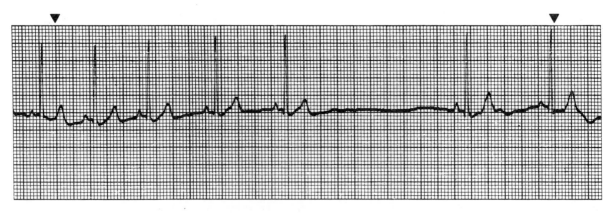

Figure 4–23. Sinus arrest/sinus exit block. (From Huff, J., Doembach, D., & White, R. (1985). *ECG workout: Exercises in arrhythmia interpretation.* Philadelphia: J. B. Lippincott Co.)

creased automaticity. Increased automaticity can result from a wide variety of processes that are outlined in the following sections (Guzzetta and Dossey, 1992).

Stress. The stress response causes the liberation of epinephrine and norepinephrine. This phenomenon can cause increased automaticity in the atria. Drugs that stimulate the sympathetic nervous system, such as amphetamines, cocaine, and decongestants, can also cause atrial dysrhythmias (American Heart Association, 1994).

Electrolyte Imbalances. Electrolyte imbalances, particularly hypokalemia, can result in increased automaticity in the atria.

Hypoxia. The atria become irritable when they are deprived of oxygen. Patients with chronic obstructive pulmonary disease are at high risk for atrial dysrhythmias.

Injury to the Atria. When the atria are injured, such as with trauma related to cardiac surgery, they are more prone to generation of ectopic beats.

Digitalis Toxicity. Administration of digitalis in toxic doses can be stimulating to the myocardium, particularly to the atria. Digitalis may convert atrial dysrhythmias to sinus rhythm, or it may only slow the ventricular response to atrial tachycardias.

Hypothermia. Lowered body temperature predisposes a patient to atrial dysrhythmias.

Hyperthyroidism. Hyperthyroidism places a patient in a metabolic state that is very similar to the stress response. The hormones produced by the thyroid gland have a stimulating effect on the heart.

Alcohol Intoxication. Alcohol is a cardiac stimulant that has an irritating effect on the heart.

Pericarditis. When the pericardial lining surrounding the heart is inflamed or infected, the atria become more irritable. Indeed, atrial dysrhythmias may be one of the first signs of pericarditis.

Premature Atrial Contractions

Premature atrial contractions (PACs) are common dysrhythmias and are usually seen in the setting of normal sinus rhythm. Like the premature junctional contractions/premature nodal contractions discussed later, PACs are generated very near the SA node. This frequently leads to depolarization of the tissue surrounding the SA node and causes a pause on the ECG. This pause is usually noncompensatory (Fig. 4–24).

Critical Criteria for Diagnosis of Premature Atrial Contractions

* 1. The ectopic beats are premature.
* 2. The PR interval is usually normal but often differs from the PR interval seen during normal sinus rhythm.
* 3. PACs are *usually* followed by a noncompensatory pause.
* 4. P wave of the premature beat may be found in the T wave just before the premature beat. When this occurs, the T wave of the preceding beat is distorted. The T wave of the beat preceding the premature beat can be compared with other, normal, T waves on the ECG strip.

Occasionally, a premature atrial contraction is generated and conducted down to the AV node just after a normal impulse has been conducted. The PAC arrives at the AV node when the bundle of His and its branches are refractory to, or unable to conduct, the premature impulse. The impulse is blocked and is not allowed to enter the ventricle. This blocked PAC can be detected as a pause on the ECG. Before the pause, a different-looking T wave can usually be noted. The

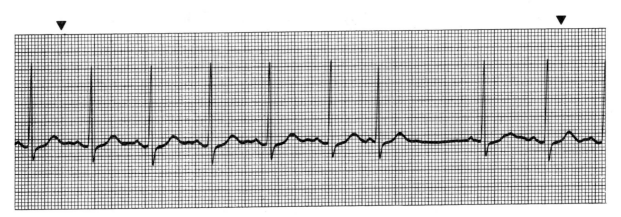

Figure 4–24. Premature atrial contraction. Note noncompensatory pause. (From Huff, J., Doembach, D., & White, R. (1985). *ECG workout: Exercises in arrhythmia interpretation.* Philadelphia: J. B. Lippincott Co.)

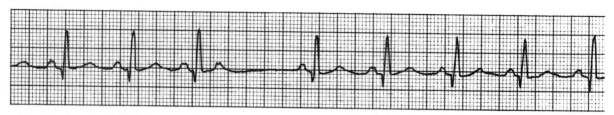

Figure 4–25. Blocked premature atrial contraction (PAC). Note unusual looking T wave following the PAC. (Adapted from Patel, J., McGowan, S., & Moody, L. (1989). *Arrhythmias: Detection, treatment, and cardiac drugs.* Philadelphia: W. B. Saunders Co.)

unusual T wave is caused by the PAC's premature P wave imposed on the normal T wave (Fig. 4–25).

Critical Criteria for Diagnosis of Blocked Premature Atrial Contraction

* 1. A pause is noted on the ECG tracing.
* 2. A premature P wave, which differs from the normal P wave, is found in the T wave, or just after the T wave, of the last normal beat before the pause.

Hemodynamic Effects

Premature atrial contractions do not usually alter the cardiac output or blood pressure in a significant way. However, many patients do report having palpitations. Increasing numbers of PACs may herald the development of atrial fibrillation or flutter.

Wandering Atrial Pacemaker

A wandering atrial pacemaker is a rhythm most often seen in a patient with chronic obstructive pulmonary disease and is caused by hypoxia (Wright and Shelton, 1993). This dysrhythmia is characterized by a wandering of pacemaking activity throughout the atria. For the criteria for this rhythm to be met, at least three sites of atrial pacemaking must be documented.

When impulses are generated from different pace-making sites, different waveforms manifest. Therefore, if at least three different atrial cell groups are generating impulses, then at least three different P-wave morphologies are present on the ECG. Use of the term *varying waveform morphology* is another way of saying that the P waves look different in shape, slope, or orientation. P waves in wandering atrial pacemaker can be upright, inverted, flat, pointed, notched, and/or slanted in different directions.

The PR interval varies because the impulses are originating from different locations within the atria. The length of the PR interval depends on how far the impulse is generated from the ventricle (Fig. 4–26).

Critical Criteria for Diagnosis of Wandering Atrial Pacemaker

1. *At least* three different-looking P waves must be seen.
2. The heart rate must not be greater than 100 beats per minute.
3. The PR intervals vary.
4. The rhythm is usually irregular.

Hemodynamic Effects

As in the nodal rhythms, atrial depolarization may be less effective in wandering atrial pacemaker.

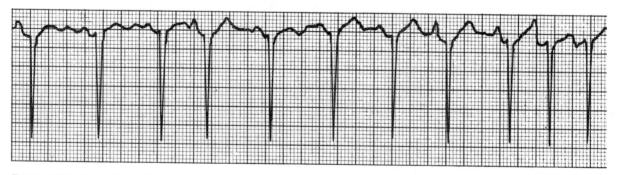

Figure 4–26. Wandering atrial pacemaker. Note the varying P wave morphologies. (From Patel, J., McGowan, S., & Moody, L. (1989). *Arrhythmias: Detection, treatment, and cardiac drugs.* Philadelphia: W. B. Saunders Co.)

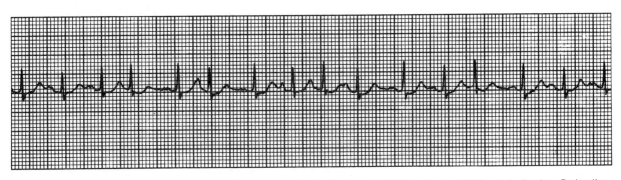

Figure 4-27. Multifocal atrial tachycardia. (From Patel, J., McGowan, S., & Moody, L. (1989). *Arrhythmias: Detection, treatment, and cardiac drugs.* Philadelphia: W. B. Saunders Co.)

Therefore, ventricular filling may be affected, and a consequent decrease in cardiac output and blood pressure may occur.

Multifocal Atrial Tachycardia

Multifocal atrial tachycardia is essentially the same as wandering atrial pacemaker except that in multifocal atrial tachycardia, the heart rate exceeds 100 beats per minute. It is almost exclusively found in the patients with chronic obstructive pulmonary disease. The cause of the dysrhythmia is thought to be right atrial dilation secondary to increased pulmonary pressures (Guzzetta and Dossey, 1992) (Fig. 4-27).

Critical Criteria for Diagnosis of Multifocal Atrial Tachycardia

The criteria are the same as for wandering atrial pacemaker *except* that the heart rate is greater than 100 beats per minute.

Hemodynamic Effects

The hemodynamic effects of multifocal atrial tachycardia are the same as those for wandering atrial pacemaker. The faster the rate, the more pronounced

the hemodynamic effects, primarily lowered cardiac output and blood pressure.

Paroxysmal Atrial Tachycardia

Paroxysmal atrial tachycardia is a rapid rhythm that arises from the atria without warning. Because of the fast rate, paroxysmal atrial tachycardia can be a life-threatening dysrhythmia. It is usually seen in patients with cardiac disease; however, it may also occur in healthy patients. In some instances, increased numbers of PACs precede the onset of paroxysmal atrial tachycardia.

When the atria generate impulses more rapidly than the AV node can conduct, varying degrees of block may result. Blocking of impulses by the AV node is indicated by P waves that are not followed by QRS complexes. P waves may merge with T waves. Sometimes, the AV node blocks impulses in a set pattern, such as every third or fourth beat. When the AV node conducts every second atrial impulse, a two-to-one block exists. In other words, for every two atrial impulses, or every two P waves, only one is conducted (Fig. 4-28).

The degree of block may be fixed or varied. Varied means that the number of P waves being con-

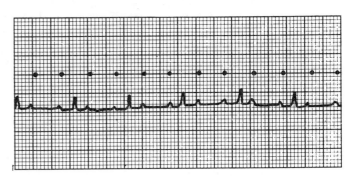

Figure 4-28. Paroxysmal atrial tachycardia with fixed degree of block. Note every second P wave is conducted. (Reproduced with permission. © *Textbook of Advanced Cardiac Life Support,* 1987, 1990 Copyright American Heart Association.)

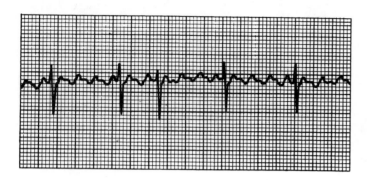

Figure 4–29. Paroxysmal atrial tachycardia with varying degrees of block. (Reproduced with permission. ©*Textbook of advanced cardiac life support,* 1987, 1990. Copyright American Heart Association).

ducted through to the ventricles is unpredictable (Fig. 4–29).

Critical Criteria for Diagnosis of Paroxysmal Atrial Tachycardia

* 1. Occurs suddenly, usually without warning.
* 2. Heart rate is usually 150 to 250 beats per minute.
* 3. Rhythm is absolutely regular.
4. P waves, if present, usually merge with the preceding T waves, thereby altering the appearance of the T wave.
5. AV block that may be of a fixed or varying degree is present.
6. Width of QRS is usually normal.

Hemodynamic Effects

The hemodynamic effects of paroxysmal atrial tachycardia can vary from none to shock. The faster the rate, the less time exists for ventricular filling. At faster rates, cardiac output and blood pressure can be severely compromised.

Atrial Flutter

Atrial flutter is a dysrhythmia that arises from a single irritable focus in the atria. Atrial flutter is most commonly seen in patients with heart disease. Patients who have valvular disease seem particularly susceptible to its development (Guzzetta and Dossey, 1992).

The waveforms associated with atrial flutter are flutter, or "F," waves. Flutter waves have a sawtooth configuration and are best seen in leads II, III, and aVF. They are biphasic: the first component of the waveform is inverted, or negative, followed by an upright, or positive, waveform (Fig. 4–30). In the calculation of rates, measuring between the negative points of the flutter waves is easiest.

Flutter waves occur incessantly and with perfect regularity. The irritable focus in the atria never stops firing. This means that the flutter waves continue throughout the ECG strip, often altering the appearance of the QRS complex and the T wave (see Fig. 4–30).

Flutter waves are usually generated at a rate of 250 to 350 beats per minute. However, the AV node is physiologically unable to conduct all of these impulses. Therefore, as in paroxysmal atrial tachycardia, the AV node selectively conducts a given number of flutter waves down to the ventricle. If, for example, the atrial focus generates 300 beats per minute, the AV node might be able to conduct every third beat. This would be a 3:1 ratio of conduction, and the resultant ventricular rate would be 100 beats per minute (300 ÷ 3 = 100) (Figure 4–31).

As in paroxysmal atrial tachycardia, the degree of

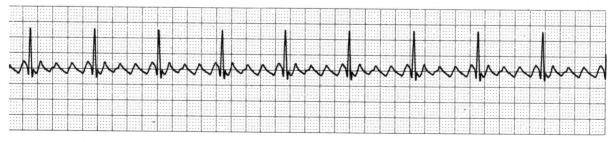

Figure 4–30. Atrial flutter. Note sawtooth configuration and negative orientation of the flutter waves. Rhythm generated by the AA-700 Rhythm Simulator. (Reproduced with permission from Armstrong Medical Industries, Lincolnshire, IL: *DataSim,* Fig. 4.)

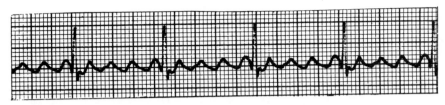

Figure 4–31. Atrial flutter with fixed degree of block (3:1). Atrial rate is 300 beats per minute (bpm), and ventricular rate is 100 bpm. Note a QRS occurs only after every third flutter wave. (Adapted from Fenstermacher, K. (1989). *Dysrhythmia recognition and management* (p. 32). Philadelphia: W. B. Saunders Co.)

block may be fixed and predictable (2:1, 3:1, 4:1), or unpredictable and varied (Fig. 4–32).

Critical Criteria for Diagnosis of Atrial Flutter

* 1. Negative flutter waves are present in leads II, III, and aVF.

* 2. Atrial rate is usually 250 to 350 beats per minute. Ventricular rate varies with the degree of AV block.

3. Onset is usually rapid.

Hemodynamic Effects

The hemodynamic effects of atrial flutter are completely dependent on the ventricular rate, sometimes called the ventricular response. In patients who are conducting high numbers of atrial impulses through the AV node, compromise of the cardiac output and blood pressure is likely.

Patients whose AV nodes are blocking greater numbers of the atrial impulses and who maintain a heart rate between 60 and 100 beats per minute tend to maintain a more normal cardiac output and blood pressure.

Atrial Fibrillation

Atrial fibrillation is a dysrhythmia that is characterized by erratic impulse formation throughout the atria. Widespread irritability and increased automaticity lead to a chaotic state of impulse formation (Fig. 4–33).

Atrial fibrillation produces a wavy baseline with no discernible P waves (Fig. 4–34). As the AV node is bombarded with rapidly fired atrial impulses, it conducts impulses to the ventricles in an unpredictable fashion. This erratic conduction results in an irregularly irregular ventricular rhythm.

As the AV node attempts to regulate the movement of impulses into the ventricle, it may conduct an impulse before the bundle and the branches are able to conduct. In particular, the right bundle branch requires a longer time to repolarize after depolarization than the left one does. Premature impulses are more likely to be conducted successfully down the left bundle branch. However, the right bundle branch is often found to be refractory, or unable to conduct. When an impulse is unable to be conducted via the right bundle branch, it must cross the ventricular septum and move down the left bundle branch first, and then cross back over the septum and depolarize the right ventricle.

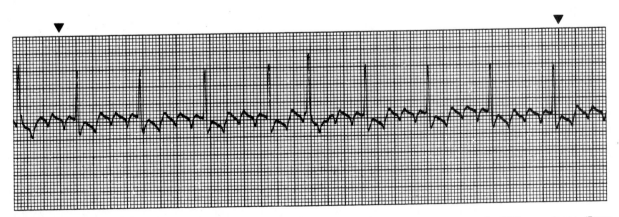

Figure 4–32. Atrial flutter with varying degree of block. There are varying ratios of flutter waves to QRS complexes. (From Huff, J., Doembach, D., & White, R. (1985). *ECG Workout: Exercises in arrhythmia interpretation.* Philadelphia: J. B. Lippincott Co.)

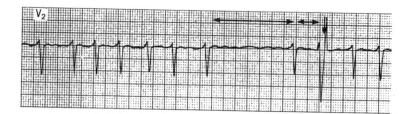

Figure 4–33. Atrial fibrillation. Note Ashman's beat, following a long, short cycle. (From Laver, J. (1992). Electrical activity of the heart and dysrhythmias. In C. Guzzetta, & B. Dossey (Eds.), *Cardiovascular nursing: Bodymind tapestry.* St. Louis: C. V. Mosby Co.)

When this event occurs, the impulse is said to be aberrantly conducted.

Aberrant conduction refers to the abnormal, or roundabout, way in which the impulse travels through the ventricles. When an impulse takes an aberrant pathway, depolarization takes longer. This situation results in a widened time interval for the QRS complex. In atrial fibrillation, aberrantly conducted beats are referred to as Ashman's beats. Aberrantly conducted Ashman's beats are more likely to occur when an atrial impulse arrives at the AV node just shortly after a previously conducted impulse (see Fig. 4–33) (Huszar, 1994).

The blood that collects in the atria is agitated by fibrillation, and normal clotting is accelerated. Small thrombi begin to form along the walls of the atria. These clots are called mural thrombi. If the patient converts back to a normal sinus rhythm and the atria begin to contract normally, these clots could be dislodged and sent out to the lungs and the body.

For this reason, if a patient has been in atrial fibrillation for an unknown amount of time, and if the blood pressure is stable, the patient should receive anticoagulation therapy before any attempt is made to convert atrial fibrillation to normal sinus rhythm. Intravenous heparin is the drug of choice for anticoagulation.

If the atrial fibrillation persists or is recurrent, long-term warfarin (Coumadin) therapy is usually prescribed to diminish the risk of thromboembolism (Shlafer, 1994).

Critical Criteria for Diagnosis of Atrial Fibrillation

* 1. Wavy baseline with no discernible P waves exists.

* 2. Irregularly irregular ventricular rhythm exists.

3. QRS width may vary between normal and slightly widened.

4. Ashman's beats are present.

Hemodynamic Effects

Fibrillation results in an ineffective quivering of the atria. The atria are never fully depolarized and therefore do not contract. This loss of atrial systole, or kick, diminishes the effectiveness of ventricular filling. The hemodynamic effects of atrial fibrillation also relate to the rate at which atrial impulses are conducted down through the ventricles. Patients who conduct 60 to 100 atrial impulses per minute tend to better tolerate the rhythm. Those who conduct at markedly slower or faster rates are more likely to experience a decrease in cardiac output and blood pressure.

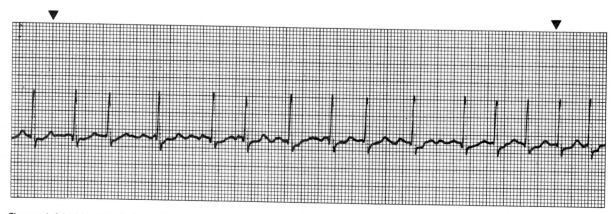

Figure 4–34. Atrial fibrillation. (From Huff, J., Doembach, D., & White, R. (1985). *ECG Workout: Exercises in arrhythmia interpretation.* Philadelphia: J. B. Lippincott Co.)

DYSRHYTHMIAS OF THE ATRIOVENTRICULAR NODE

Junctional Rhythm

Dysrhythmias of the AV node are called junctional rhythms. However, in the literature and in clinical practice, the term *nodal rhythms* is also used. The AV node is located in the middle of the heart between the atria and the ventricles. The tissue immediately surrounding the AV node is referred to as junctional tissue. Both the AV node itself and the junctional tissue surrounding it are capable of generating cardiac rhythms. In this text, the terms *nodal* and *junctional* will be used interchangeably.

There are two primary causes of junctional rhythms:

1. Dysrhythmias can originate in the AV node or the junctional tissue surrounding it. When a singular beat, or ongoing rhythm, originates in an area other than the sinus node, that beat or rhythm is considered *ectopic*. Ectopic means out of the normal place. Ectopic rhythms are usually caused by increased automaticity. Increased automaticity is commonly caused by stress or the use of nicotine or caffeine. However, it can also result from myocardial ischemia, injury, or infarction. Digitalis toxicity can produce all forms of junctional rhythms. At toxic levels, digitalis can suppress heart rate or act as a myocardial stimulant (Shlafer, 1994).

2. Escape rhythms can be generated from the AV node should the sinus node fail. The AV node is capable of generating 40 to 60 beats per minute as a back-up pacemaker.

Several ECG changes are common to all the junctional dysrhythmias. These changes include P-wave abnormalities and PR-interval changes.

Electrocardiographic Changes

P-Wave Changes

Because of the location of the AV node, in the center of the heart, impulses generated may be conducted forward, backward, or both. Like waves from a rock thrown into a pool of water, the impulse can radiate both forward and backward. With the potential of forward, backward, or bidirectional impulse conduction, three different P waveforms may be associated with junctional rhythms:

1. When forward conduction occurs, *P waves are absent* because the impulse enters the ventricle first. The atria do not receive the wave of depolarization; therefore, no P wave exists. Without depolarization, the atria do not contract (Fig. 4–35).

2. When the impulse is conducted in a backward motion, an *inverted P wave* is produced. Backward, or retrograde, conduction moves back toward the atria, allowing for at least partial depolarization of the atria. When depolarization occurs in a backward fashion, an inverted P wave is created. Once the atria have been depolarized, the impulse then moves down the bundle of His and depolarizes both ventricles normally (Fig. 4–36).

3. When the impulse is conducted in both a forward and a backward fashion, *P waves may be present after the QRS*. In this type of conduction, the impulse first moves into the ventricles, depolarizing them and creating a QRS complex. Because the impulse is also conducted backward, some atrial depolarization occurs, and a late P wave is noted after the QRS complex (Fig. 4–37).

PR-Interval Changes

The length of the PR interval in junctional rhythms depends on where the impulse originates.

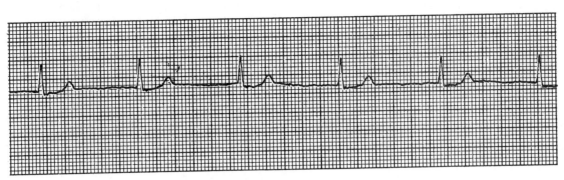

Figure 4–35. Junctional/nodal rhythm. Note absence of P waves. (From Davis, D. (1985). *How to quickly and accurately master ECG interpretation* (p. 288). Philadelphia: J. B. Lippincott Co.)

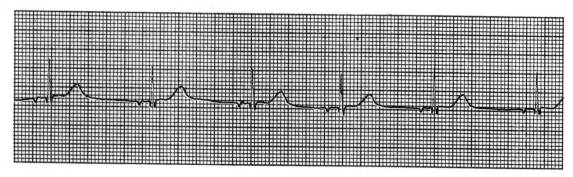

Figure 4–36. Junctional (nodal) rhythm. Note inverted P waves prior to the QRS. (From Davis, D. (1985). *How to quickly and accurately master ECG interpretation* (p. 288). Philadelphia: J. B. Lippincott Co.)

When the impulse is generated high in the AV node or junctional tissue, near the atria, the PR interval is slightly shorter than normal. If the impulse is generated low in the AV node or junctional tissue, nearer the ventricle, the PR interval is also shorter than normal. If the P wave is absent, the PR interval cannot be measured.

Critical Criteria for Diagnosis of Junctional Rhythm

* 1. P waves may be absent or inverted or may follow the QRS complex.
* 2. The heart rate is 40 to 60 beats per minute.
* 3. The PR interval is at the low end of normal or shorter than normal.
4. The rhythm is usually regular.
5. The QRS complex is of normal width.

Hemodynamic Effects

In junctional rhythms, atrial depolarization is usually less effective or absent. With ineffective or absent depolarization of the atria, the amount of ventricular filling is less than normal. The net effect is diminished cardiac output and blood pressure. This effect may go unnoticed in some patients, whereas it may cause significant hypotension in others.

Junctional Tachycardia/Accelerated Nodal Rhythm

The normal intrinsic rate for the AV node and junctional tissue is 40 to 60 beats per minute, but rates can accelerate higher. Any rate higher than the normal upper limit of 60 beats per minute is considered junctional tachycardia. The upper rate capability for the AV node is considered to be 150 beats per minute (Fig. 4–38).

Critical Criteria for Diagnosis of Junctional/Nodal Tachycardia

Same as for junctional rhythm except that the heart rate is greater than 60 beats per minute.

Hemodynamic Effects

The hemodynamic effects of junctional tachycardia are the same as for a junctional rhythm. However, ventricular filling may be further compromised by the more rapid heart rate. On the other hand, the acceleration in heart rate may actually improve cardiac output. Cardiac output is affected by both the amount of blood available for pumping from the ventricles and the heart rate. Improvement in cardiac output, secondary

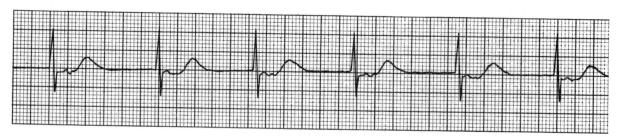

Figure 4–37. Junctional (nodal) rhythm. Note P waves after the QRS. (From Patel, J., McGowan, S., & Moody, L. (1989). *Arrhythmias: Detection, treatment, and cardiac drugs.* Philadelphia: W. B. Saunders Co.)

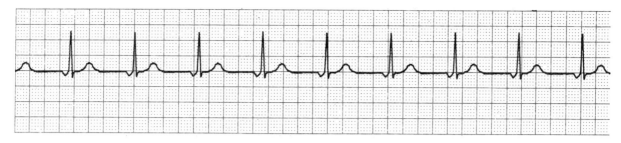

Figure 4–38. Junctional tachycardia (accelerated nodal rhythm). Rhythm generated by the AA-700 Rhythm Simulator. (Reproduced with permission from Armstrong Medical Industries, Lincolnshire, IL: *DataSim,* Fig. 22.)

to increased heart rate, is dependent on the health of the heart.

Premature Junctional Contractions

Irritable areas in the AV node and junctional tissue can generate beats that are premature, or earlier than the next expected beat. These premature beats most often occur in the setting of normal sinus rhythm and temporarily upset the rhythmicity. The SA node response to premature beats is important in the analysis and interpretation of dysrhythmias. The SA node either compensates for the one premature beat and continues the normal rhythm or it does not compensate and the normal rhythm is upset.

The closer the site of premature impulse generation to the sinus node, the less likely it is that the SA node will compensate. When a premature impulse fires close to the SA node, a wave of depolarization moves backward toward the sinus and excites the tissue of the SA node. After depolarization has occurred, the sinus requires time for repolarization before generating the next beat. This situation creates a pause on the ECG called a *noncompensatory pause* (Fig. 4–39).

For a determination of whether a pause is com-

pensatory or noncompensatory, a rhythm strip with a premature beat is analyzed. Calipers or paper and pencil are needed for this analysis. Two consecutive normal beats are located just before the premature beat, and the caliper points or pencil marks are placed on the R wave of each normal beat. The calipers are flipped over, or the paper is slid over, to where the next normal beat should have occurred. The premature beat occurs early.

Now, with care being taken not to lose placement, the calipers are flipped, or the paper is slid over, one more time. If the point of the calipers or the mark on the paper lands exactly on the next normal beat's R wave, the sinus node *compensated* for the one premature beat and kept its normal rhythm (Fig. 4–40). If the caliper point or pencil mark does not land on the next normal beat's R wave, then the sinus did *not compensate* and had to establish a new rhythm.

Critical Criteria for Diagnosis of Premature Junctional Contractions

* 1. The ectopic beats are premature.
* 2. If a P wave is present before the QRS, the PR interval is usually shorter than normal.

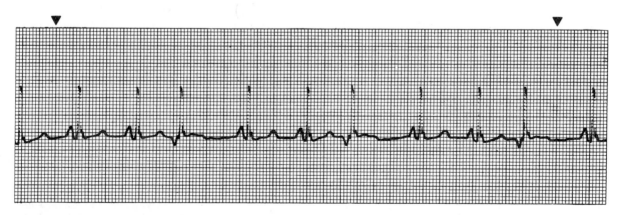

Figure 4–39. Premature junctional (nodal) contractions. Note noncompensatory pause. (From Huff, J., Doembach, D., & White, R. (1985). *ECG workout: Exercises in arrhythmia interpretation.* Philadelphia: J. B. Lippincott Co.)

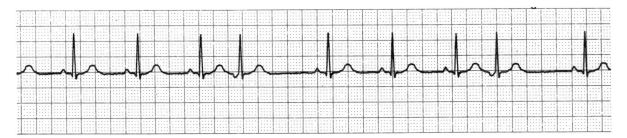

Figure 4–40. Premature junctional (nodal) contraction with a compensatory pause. Rhythm generated by the AA-700 Rhythm Simulator. (Reproduced with permission from Armstrong Medical Industries, Lincolnshire, IL: *DataSim*, Fig. 24.)

* 3. Premature junctional contractions are *usually* followed by a noncompensatory pause.

* 4. P waves may be absent or inverted or may occur after the QRS complex.

Hemodynamic Effects

Premature junctional contractions do not usually alter the cardiac output or blood pressure in a significant way. However, many patients do report having palpitations. Increasing numbers of premature junctional contractions may herald the development of nodal tachycardia.

DYSRHYTHMIAS OF THE VENTRICLE

Ventricular dysrhythmias are ectopic or escape rhythms that originate in the ventricles. Because impulses for ventricular dysrhythmias are generated in the lower portion of the heart, depolarization occurs in an abnormal way. Depending on where the impulse originates, it must travel in a backward or sideways fashion to depolarize the ventricles. This abnormal flow of electricity lengthens the normal time interval in which depolarization of the ventricles occurs. The result is a widened QRS complex. The QRS interval extends beyond the normal of 0.06 to 0.10 seconds.

Depolarization after an abnormal ventricular beat rarely moves as far backward as the atria. Therefore, most ventricular dysrhythmias have no evident P waves. However, if a P wave is present, it is usually seen in the T wave of the previous beat. Two types of ventricular dysrhythmias exist: ectopic and escape:

1. The ectopic rhythms are abnormal and disturb or override the normal sinus rhythm. These ectopic rhythms are capable of firing at fast rates and may be life threatening.

2. The Purkinje fibers, which are deep in the ventricles, can act as a site for back-up pacemaking should the SA and AV nodes fail. The Purkinje fibers can generate an escape rhythm of 15 to 40 beats per minute under normal circumstances. Although this is a very slow intrinsic rate, some patients are able to maintain an adequate cardiac output and blood pressure with rates that are close to 40 beats per minute. However, most patients are compromised (Guzzetta and Dossey, 1992).

Generation of ventricular dysrhythmias can be secondary to myocardial ischemia, injury, or infarction; hypokalemia; hypomagnesemia; hypoxia; or acid-base imbalances (American Heart Association, 1994).

Myocardial Ischemia, Injury, and Infarction. When blood supply is decreased to an area of the ventricle, the blood-deprived area becomes irritable and is more likely to have increased automaticity. Prolonged ischemia can lead to permanent injury to the area, creating an even greater potential for ectopic impulse formation. Ultimately, the area deprived of blood supply infarcts or dies. Once cellular death has occurred, *no* electrical activity is generated.

Hypokalemia. Low serum potassium levels can facilitate the development of ventricular dysrhythmias. As discussed earlier, potassium plays an important role in the normal depolarization/repolarization process.

Hypomagnesemia. Low serum magnesium levels have been correlated with the development of ventricular dysrhythmias, and in particular torsades de pointes (American Heart Association, 1994). Torsades de pointes is a type of ventricular tachycardia in which the QRS complex changes polarity from negative to positive.

Hypoxia. Inadequate amounts of oxygen are irritating to the ventricles and often stimulate ectopic beats, dysrhythmia formation, or both.

Acid-Base Imbalances. Both alkalosis and acidosis can stimulate ventricular ectopy.

Premature Ventricular Contractions

Premature ventricular contractions (PVCs) are a common ventricular dysrhythmia. The beats can be generated anywhere in the ventricles. When only one

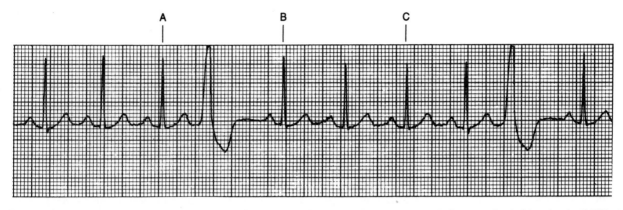

Figure 4–41. *A–C,* Unifocal premature ventricular contractions. (From Patel, J., McGowan, S., & Moody, L. (1989). *Arrhythmias: Detection, treatment, and cardiac drugs.* Philadelphia: W. B. Saunders Co.)

focus of ventricular irritability exists, all of the ectopic beats appear the same. Ventricular beats coming from one area are called *unifocal* PVCs (Fig. 4–41).

There can also be multiple areas, or foci, of ventricular irritability. When multiple areas are generating abnormal impulses, waveform configuration varies. Ventricular beats coming from more than one area are called *multifocal* PVCs (Fig. 4–42).

Because PVCs are generated in the ventricles, a considerable distance from the SA node, the SA node is usually able to compensate for the premature beat. This compensation is noted on the ECG tracing as a compensatory pause that follows the PVC (see Fig. 4–42).

Premature ventricular contractions may also occur in a predictable pattern. For example, PVCs may occur every other beat, every third beat, or every fourth beat. When PVCs occur every other beat, the pattern is referred to as bigeminy (Fig. 4–43). When the PVCs occur every third beat, the pattern is called trigeminy, and every fourth beat, quadrigeminy. Premature ven-

tricular contractions can also occur sequentially. Two PVCs in a row are termed a *couplet* (Fig. 4–44). Three PVCs in a row are termed a *triplet,* or *salvo* (Fig. 4–45).

The downslope of the T wave is called the vulnerable period. If a ventricular ectopic impulse (PVC) is generated during this time, ventricular fibrillation may occur. This is referred to as *R on T phenomenon.* In R on T phenomenon, the R wave of a PVC falls on the T wave of a normal beat (Fig. 4–46). R on T phenomenon occurs frequently in the clinical setting, often without significant consequence (Conover, 1993).

Isolated or rare PVCs are rarely treated. Rather, PVCs are considered signs of underlying pathology that requires attention, for instance, hypoxia, ischemia, injury, or infarction. PVCs in the myocardial infarction patient are treated when associated with such symptoms as angina or hypotension (American Heart Association, 1994). The larger the infarct size, the greater the chance for ventricular dysrhythmias (Guzzetta and Dossey, 1992).

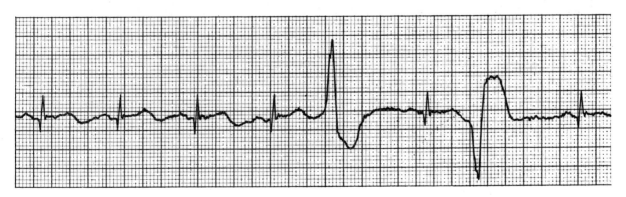

Figure 4–42. Multifocal premature ventricular contractions. (From Patel, J., McGowan, S., & Moody, L. (1989). *Arrhythmias: Detection, treatment, and cardiac drugs.* Philadelphia: W. B. Saunders Co.)

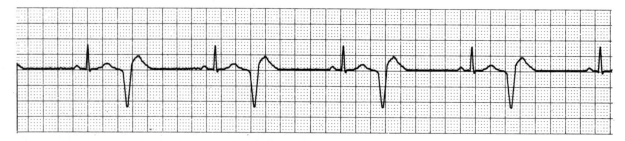

Figure 4–43. Premature ventricular contractions in a bigeminal pattern. Rhythm strip generated by the AA-700 Rhythm Simulator. (Reproduced with permission from Armstrong Medical Industries, Lincolnshire, IL: *DataSim,* Fig. 27.)

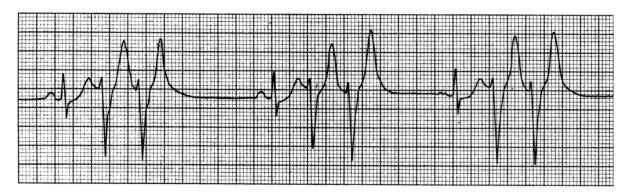

Figure 4–44. Two premature ventricular contractions in a row (couplet). (From Patel, J., McGowan, S., & Moody, L. (1989). *Arrhythmias: Detection, treatment, and cardiac drugs.* Philadelphia: W. B. Saunders Co.)

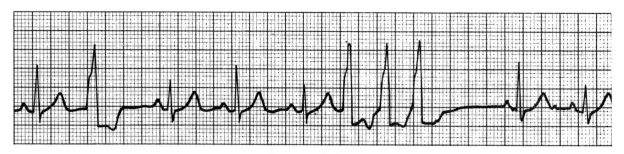

Figure 4–45. Three premature ventricular contractions in a row (triplet). (From Patel, J., McGowan, S., & Moody, L. (1989). *Arrhythmias: Detection, treatment, and cardiac drugs.* Philadelphia: W. B. Saunders Co.)

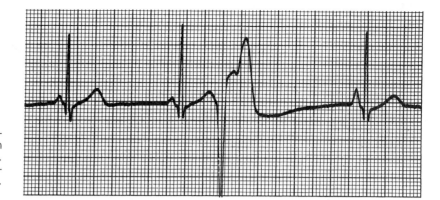

Figure 4–46. R on T premature ventricular contraction. (Adapted from Huff, J., Doenbach, D., & White, R. (1993). *ECG workout: Exercises in arrhythmia interpretation* (2nd ed.). Philadelphia: J. B. Lippincott Co.)

Previously, PVCs were thought to serve as a warning for ventricular tachycardia and ventricular fibrillation. However, studies have shown that ventricular fibrillation occurs without warning in 40 to 84% of patients (Pasternak et al., 1988). PVCs, couplets, R on T phenomenon, and multifocal ventricular ectopy should be considered as warning dysrhythmias; however, other clinical data should also be included in the decision to treat (American Heart Association, 1994).

Critical Criteria for Diagnosis of Premature Ventricular Contractions

* 1. Ectopic beat occurs prematurely, before the next anticipated sinus beat.
* 2. The QRS complex of the premature beat is wider than 0.10 seconds.
* 3. The rhythm is irregular as a result of the premature beats. However, the premature beats may occur in a regular pattern.
* 4. The premature beat is usually followed with a compensatory pause.
* 5. The ST segment of the PVC slopes away from, or is in the opposite direction of, the QRS of the PVC. In other words, if the QRS complex of the PVC is upright, or positive, then the ST segment is downward, or negative (see Fig. 4–44).
  6. P waves are usually absent before the ectopic beat.
  7. Premature ventricular contractions may be unifocal or multifocal.

Hemodynamic Effects

The hemodynamic effects associated with PVCs are varied. Some patients may be asymptomatic, whereas others report having palpitations and lightheadedness. Symptoms usually worsen with an increase in the number of ectopic beats. An increasing number of PVCs may serve as a warning for the potential development of ventricular tachycardia.

Ventricular Tachycardia

Ventricular tachycardia is a rapid life-threatening dysrhythmia that originates in the ventricles. It is characterized by at least three premature ventricular complexes in a row. Ventricular tachycardia occurs at a rate greater than 100 beats per minute. This is a life-threatening dysrhythmia. The site of irritability in the ventricle is unifocal; therefore, all waveforms produced appear the same. Because ventricular tachycardia is considered to be an ectopic rhythm, depolarization of the ventricles occurs in an abnormal way. Abnormal depolarization of the ventricles produces a widened QRS (Fig. 4–47).

The wave of depolarization associated with ventricular tachycardia rarely reaches the atria. Therefore, P waves are not usually evident on the ECG. However, if P waves are present, they have no association with the QRS. This dissociation between the P waves and the QRS complexes is the result of the distance between the sinus node and the ectopic focus in the ventricles. The ventricular tachycardia focus is so far away from the sinus node that the sinus node may be unaware and unaffected by the ectopic beats. Therefore, the sinus node continues to depolarize at its normal rate, unaware that the ventricle is being depolarized abnormally by an ectopic pacer. P waves appear to be randomly scattered throughout the rhythm, but the P waves are actually being fired at a consistent rate from the sinus node.

Critical Criteria for Diagnosis of Ventricular Tachycardia

* 1. The occurrence of greater than three PVCs in a row is considered ventricular tachycardia.

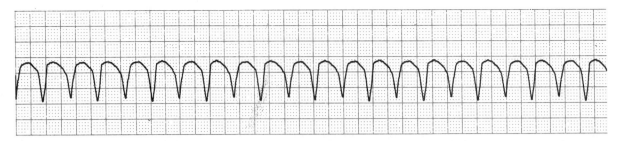

Figure 4–47. Ventricular tachycardia. Rhythm strip generated by the AA-700 Rhythm Simulator. (Reproduced with permission from Armstrong Medical Industries, Lincolnshire, IL: *DataSim*, Fig. 13.)

* 2. Heart rate is greater than 100 beats per minute.

* 3. QRS complex width is greater than 0.10 second.

4. P waves may or may not be visible. If visible, P waves appear to be scattered throughout the rhythm and have no relationship to the QRS.

Hemodynamic Effects

Hemodynamic effects associated with ventricular tachycardia may vary. Most patients have a significant loss of cardiac output, with a resultant low blood pressure. Many patients become pulseless, with no obtainable blood pressure.

However, in rare instances, some patients maintain a pulse and a blood pressure while experiencing ventricular tachycardia. Treatment of the dysrhythmia is dependent on the presence or absence of a pulse and a blood pressure (American Heart Association, 1994).

Ventricular Fibrillation

Ventricular fibrillation is a chaotic rhythm that is characterized by a quivering of the ventricles that results in a total loss of cardiac output. Patients experiencing ventricular fibrillation are in a state of clinical death. Clinical death means that the patient's heart has stopped contracting; therefore, there is no blood flow to the vital organs.

Ventricular fibrillation can occur without a known cause. Fibrillation without the presence of cardiac dis-

ease is considered primary ventricular fibrillation. More commonly, however, fibrillation occurs secondary to the processes listed under the discussion of PVCs.

The electrical energy created by ventricular fibrillation varies in amplitude. When voltage is low in the fibrillating ventricle, the result is a small-amplitude waveform. This form of ventricular fibrillation is referred to as *fine* (Fig. 4–48).

When voltage is greater in the fibrillating ventricle, the result is a larger-amplitude waveform. This form of ventricular fibrillation is referred to as *coarse* (Fig. 4–49). Coarse ventricular fibrillation responds better to defibrillation than does fine ventricular fibrillation (American Heart Association, 1994). It is always important to confirm ventricular fibrillation in at least two leads.

Critical Criteria for Diagnosis of Ventricular Fibrillation

* 1. Fluctuating, jagged baseline exists. No discernible P, Q, R, S, and T waves are present.

2. Ventricular fibrillation may be coarse or fine.

Hemodynamic Effects

Hemodynamic effects are profound in ventricular fibrillation. All atrial and ventricular contractions cease, leading to total loss of cardiac output. No palpable pulse is present, and no blood pressure can be obtained. Brain death occurs within 4 to 6 minutes if

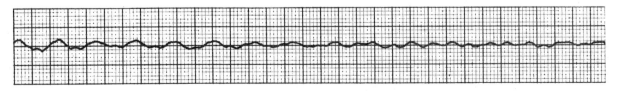

Figure 4–48. Fine ventricular fibrillation. (From Patel, J., McGowan, S., & Moody, L. (1989). *Arrhythmias: Detection, treatment, and cardiac drugs.* Philadelphia: W. B. Saunders Co.)

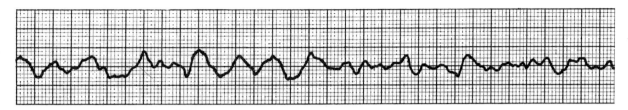

Figure 4–49. Coarse ventricular fibrillation. (From Patel, J., McGowan, S., & Moody, L. (1989). *Arrhythmias: Detection, treatment, and cardiac drugs.* Philadelphia: W. B. Saunders Co.)

life support is not instituted (American Heart Association, 1994).

Idioventricular Rhythm

Idioventricular rhythm is an escape rhythm that is generated by the Purkinje fibers. This rhythm emerges only when the SA and AV nodes have failed. The Purkinje fibers are capable of an intrinsic rate of 15 to 40 beats per minute. Because this rhythm originates in the deepest portion of the ventricles, normal depolarization is impossible. Aberrant conduction results. Therefore, the QRS of the idioventricular rhythm is wider than normal. Because of the distance of the impulse formation from the atria, atrial depolarization is not likely to occur. Usually, no evidence of P waves is present on the ECG strip (Fig. 4–50).

Some patients with cardiac disease may experience idioventricular rhythm while sleeping. During deep sleep, the metabolic demands of the body are diminished. The number of sinus depolarizations per minute, or the heart rate, normally decreases with the decrease in metabolic demands. If the patient is in sinus bradycardia to begin with, this further slowing can encourage competition between the SA node and the Purkinje fibers.

The group of cardiac cells that is capable of beating the fastest paces the heart. For example, if the sinus rate falls to 39 beats per minute and the Purkinje fibers can beat at 40 beats per minute, an idioventricular rhythm may emerge. This occurrence is more common in patients with severe coronary artery disease and in those whose SA and AV nodes are suppressed by drugs.

Critical Criteria for Diagnosis of Idioventricular Rhythm

* 1. Heart rate is 15 to 40 beats per minute and regular.
* 2. Widened QRS interval is present, usually 0.12 seconds or greater.
  3. P waves are not usually visible.

Hemodynamic Effects

Hemodynamic effects vary with the idioventricular rhythm. Some patients are able to maintain an adequate cardiac output and blood pressure, whereas others become hypotensive.

When the rhythm occurs during sleep, it is often difficult to impossible to obtain the blood pressure

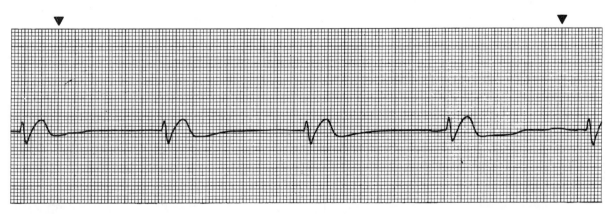

Figure 4–50. Idioventricular rhythm. (From Huff, J., Doembach, D., & White, R. (1985). *ECG workout: Exercises in arrhythmia interpretation.* Philadelphia: J. B. Lippincott Co.)

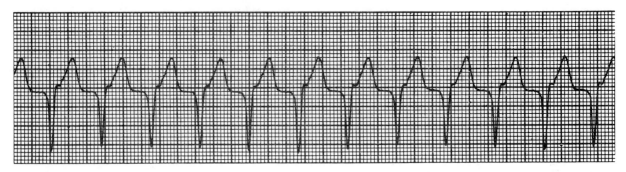

Figure 4–51. Accelerated idioventricular rhythm. (From Patel, J., McGowan, S., & Moody, L. (1989). *Arrhythmias: Detection, treatment, and cardiac drugs.* Philadelphia: W. B. Saunders Co.)

while the rhythm is present. Because the patient is usually awakened suddenly for the taking of vital signs, his or her sympathetic nervous system is stimulated. This situation liberates epinephrine and norepinephrine into the bloodstream and stimulates the SA node to increase its rate and regain pacemaking function.

Accelerated Idioventricular Rhythm

Accelerated idioventricular rhythm is the same as that discussed for idioventricular rhythm except that the rate exceeds 40 beats per minute. The faster rate is the result of increased automaticity in the Purkinje fibers. This effect is most often caused by myocardial ischemia, injury, or infarction, but it can also be caused by hypokalemia, digitalis toxicity, or various forms of heart disease (Fig. 4–51).

Critical Criteria for Diagnosis of Accelerated Idioventricular Rhythm

Same as for idioventricular rhythm except that heart rate is greater than 40 beats per minute but less than 100 beats per minute (Patel et al., 1989).

Hemodynamic Effects

The hemodynamic effects of accelerated idioventricular rhythm correspond to the heart rate. Patients with heart rates of less than 60 beats per minute tolerate this rhythm best.

Ventricular Standstill (Asystole)

Ventricular standstill is characterized by complete cessation of all electrical activity. A flat baseline is seen, without any evidence of P, Q, R, S, or T waveforms. Ventricular standstill is also called asystole because all contraction of the heart muscle stops.

Asystole may occur as the end result of a severe bradycardia or sinus arrest. In the evaluation of asystole, the nurse should *always* remember to check that the patient's electrodes and ECG monitor patches are intact. If an electrode or patch is loose, the ECG pattern may be lost, creating a flat line that appears to be asystole or fine ventricular fibrillation (Fig. 4–52). Asystole should be confirmed in two leads.

Critical Criteria for Diagnosis of Ventricular Standstill (Asystole)

Flat baseline is observed, with no evidence of P, Q, R, S, or T waveforms.

Hemodynamic Effects

The hemodynamic effects are the same as for ventricular fibrillation. The patient loses all perfusion, and death occurs without intervention.

ATRIOVENTRICULAR BLOCKS

Atrioventricular block refers to an impairment in the conduction of impulses from the atria to the ventricles. This impairment may cause slowed conduction

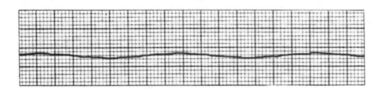

Figure 4–52. Ventricular standstill or asystole. (From Fenstermacher, K. (1989). *Dysrhythmia recognition and management* (p. 54). Philadelphia: W. B. Saunders Co.)

of impulses, intermittent blockage of impulses, or complete blockage of impulse conduction from the atria to the ventricles.

The following section discusses most common processes related to impairment of impulse conduction (Guzzetta and Dossey, 1992).

Coronary Artery Disease. Both acute and chronic coronary artery disease can lead to impairment of impulse conduction. Coronary artery disease robs the conduction pathway of its normal blood supply, thereby impairing impulse generation and conduction.

Infectious and Inflammatory Processes. Infectious and inflammatory processes can damage the conduction pathway, leading to impairment or blockage of impulses. These processes include systemic lupus erythematosus and myocarditis.

Enhanced Vagal Tone. When the vagus nerve is stimulated, heart rate decreases, and a transient impairment in impulse conduction may occur.

Effects of Drugs. Many cardiac drugs have a negative dromotropic effect; that is, they slow down conduction of impulses from the atria to the ventricles. This is a desired effect, in that a slower heart rate decreases the myocardial oxygen demand. In patients with a bradycardiac rhythm, this effect may cause compromise.

Four types of atrioventricular blocks exist, each categorized in terms of degree. The four types are first-degree, second-degree type I, second-degree type II, and third-degree block. The higher the degree of block, the more severe the consequences. First-degree block has minimal consequences, whereas third-degree block may have life-threatening consequences.

Each form of AV block is distinctly different from the others. However, the critical criteria for diagnosis of each type of block are related to the PR interval. The PR interval measures the amount of time it takes for an impulse to be generated in the atria, travel down to the AV node, and then be delayed there before entering the ventricles. When the impulse is delayed for longer than usual, the PR interval lengthens.

First-Degree Block

First-degree block is a common dysrhythmia in the elderly and in patients with cardiac disease. As the normal conduction pathway ages or becomes diseased, impulse conduction becomes slower than normal. First-degree block often occurs in the setting of normal sinus rhythm or sinus bradycardia (Fig. 4–53).

Critical Criteria for Diagnosis of First-Degree Block

* 1. The underlying rhythm is usually normal sinus rhythm.
* 2. The PR interval is longer than 0.20 seconds.
* 3. The PR interval of each beat is the same.
    4. First-degree block is often accompanied by sinus bradycardia.

Hemodynamic Effects

Usually, no hemodynamic changes are associated with first-degree block. Changes in blood pressure are more likely to occur if first-degree block is associated with bradycardia.

Second-Degree Block

Two types of second-degree block exist. Both types are characterized by distinctive criteria for diagnosis.

Second-Degree Block Type I: Mobitz I (Wenckebach's Phenomenon)

Second-degree AV block type I usually occurs at the level of the AV node and is characterized by progressive delay of impulse conduction. The normal conduction tissue becomes progressively unable to conduct impulses from the atria to the ventricles. This inability is demonstrated by a steadily progressive lengthening PR interval from one beat to the next.

The conduction tissue finally becomes unable to

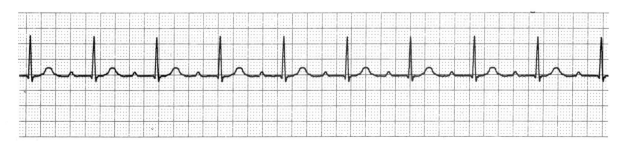

Figure 4–53. First-degree block. Rhythm strip generated by the AA-700 Rhythm Simulator. (Reproduced with permission from Armstrong Medical Industries, Lincolnshire, IL: *DataSim*, Fig. 19.)

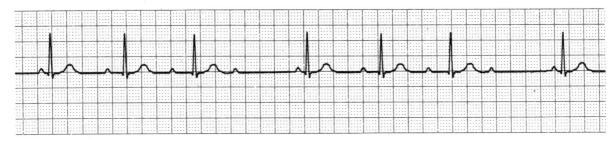

Figure 4–54. Second-degree block, Mobitz type I, or Wenckebach's phenomenon. Note steadily lengthening PR interval. Rhythm strip generated by the AA-700 Rhythm Simulator. (Reproduced with permission from Armstrong Medical Industries, Lincolnshire, IL: *DataSim,* Fig. 6.)

conduct the next sinus beat. Therefore, a P wave is seen on the ECG that is not followed by a QRS complex. By not conducting this one beat, the AV node is able to recover and then conduct the next atrial impulse (Fig. 4–54).

Critical Criteria for Diagnosis of Second-Degree Block Type I

* 1. PR interval progressively lengthens on a beat-by-beat basis until a P wave is not conducted. The lengthening of the PR may occur over three to four beats, or it may occur over fewer beats.

* 2. Pauses are noted on the ECG after the unconducted P waves.

3. A patterning or grouping of beats appears before each missed beat.

4. P to P intervals are usually regular.

5. R to R intervals are usually irregular.

6. QRS width is usually normal.

Hemodynamic Effects

Second-degree block type I is considered a self-limiting rhythm. In other words, it rarely progresses to a higher or more severe degree of block (American Heart Association, 1994). If the patient experiences any hemodynamic effects, they are related to the

pauses seen on the ECG. If the patient is already bradycardiac, these pauses cause a further decrease in heart rate and a more pronounced effect on the cardiac output and the patient's blood pressure.

Second-Degree Block Type II: Mobitz II

Second-degree block type II is a more severe form of AV block. As in type I, atrial impulses are blocked from entering the ventricle. Unlike type I, however, these blocked beats are not preceded by a steadily lengthening PR interval. Instead, the PR interval remains constant. Despite the fact that the PR interval remains unchanged, a P wave occasionally, and without warning, is not conducted down to the ventricles.

In some instances, the nonconducted beats occur in a pattern, such as every other beat or every third beat. At other times, the nonconducted beats occur randomly, without a pattern (Fig. 4–55). Second-degree type II block may progress to the more clinically significant third-degree block.

Critical Criteria for Diagnosis of Second-Degree Block Type II

* 1. Occasional P waves are not followed by a QRS complex. These unconducted P waves may occur in a regular pattern, such as every other beat, or they may occur randomly, without a pattern.

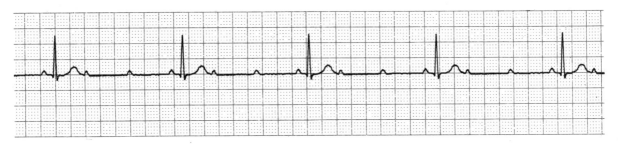

Figure 4–55. Second-degree block, Mobitz type II. Note fixed PR interval. Rhythm strip generated by the AA-700 Rhythm Simulator. (Reproduced with permission from Armstrong Medical Industries, Lincolnshire, IL: *DataSim,* Fig. 7.)

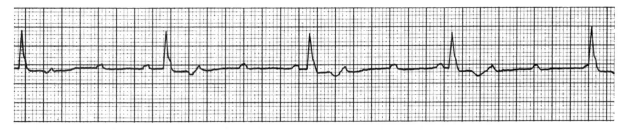

Figure 4–56. Third-degree block with nodal escape. (From Patel, J., McGowan, S., & Moody, L. (1989). *Arrhythmias: Detection, treatment, and cardiac drugs.* Philadelphia: W. B. Saunders Co.)

* 2. The PR interval of conducted beats is consistently the same, or fixed.
* 3. The P to P interval is regular.

Hemodynamic Effects

The hemodynamic effects of second-degree block type II correspond to the decrease in rate caused by the nonconducted beats. Essentially, missed beats create a bradycardia. The greater the number of unconducted beats, the greater the impact on the cardiac output and blood pressure. Patients with second-degree block type II may require transvenous or permanent pacemaking.

Third-Degree Block (Complete Heart Block)

Third-degree block is often called complete heart block because no atrial impulses are conducted down to the ventricles. The block in conduction can occur at the level of the AV node, the bundle of His, or the bundle branches (Patel et al., 1989).

When a complete block exists between the atria and the ventricles, the rhythm of the heart beat becomes uncoordinated. The atria beat at one rate, and the ventricles beat at a different rate. No communication exists between the two. For this reason, third-degree block is sometimes called AV dissociation.

In third-degree block, the atria are paced by the SA node, usually at a rate of 60 to 100 beats per minute. However, the atrial impulses are blocked from entering the ventricles. When the ventricles do not receive an impulse from the atria, either the AV node or the Purkinje fibers can generate an escape rhythm. If the AV node acts as the back-up pacemaker, the rate is 40 to 60 beats per minute, and this rhythm is referred to as a nodal or a junctional escape (Fig. 4–56). Because AV impulses are formed above the level of the ventricle, they proceed down the normal ventricular conduction pathway. This phenomenon produces a QRS complex of normal width. If the Purkinje fibers act as the back-up pacemaker, the rate is 15 to 40 beats per minute, and this rhythm is referred to as a ventricular escape (Fig. 4–57). Impulses generated in the ventricles must depolarize the heart in an abnormal way, resulting in a widened QRS complex.

Third-degree block that occurs at the level of the AV node is often transient and is associated with a junctional escape rhythm. The junction is a more dependable pacemaker than the Purkinje fibers. Third-degree block at the bundle branch level is more often permanent and is associated with a ventricular escape rhythm (American Heart Association, 1994).

In third-degree block, the ECG waveforms do not occur in normal sequence. Because the atrial rate is usually faster than the ventricular rate, more P waves than R waves are noted on the ECG. This effect produces a very unusual looking ECG. The P waves

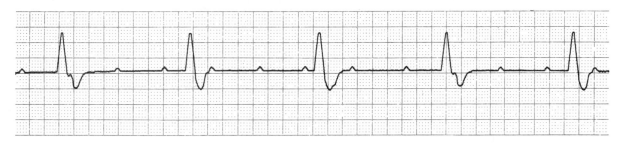

Figure 4–57. Third-degree block with ventricular escape. Rhythm strip generated by the AA-700 Rhythm Simulator. (Reproduced with permission from Armstrong Medical Industries, Lincolnshire, IL: *DataSim*, Fig. 8.)

are regularly spaced throughout the strip. The R waves are also regularly spaced but occur at a slower rate.

Even if P waves appear before QRS complexes, the P waves are not related to the QRS complex. They cannot be related, because a block in conduction exists between the atria and the ventricles. This lack of communication between the P waves and the QRS complexes can be further demonstrated by what appears to be a widely varying PR interval. Because no conduction exists between the atria and the ventricles, no PR interval can exist (see Fig. 4–57). Whenever a strip appears to have no consistent, predictable relationship between P waves and QRS complexes, third-degree block should be considered.

Critical Criteria for Diagnosis of Third-Degree Block (Complete Heart Block)

* 1. A difference exists in the atrial and ventricular heart rates. The atrial rate is usually greater than the ventricular rate.
* 2. The P to P intervals are regular.
* 3. The R to R intervals are regular.
* 4. The PR interval varies constantly from beat to beat.
* 5. Waveforms occur in an abnormal sequence and are dissociated from one another.
* 6. Either a junctional or a ventricular escape rhythm is present.

Hemodynamic Effects

The hemodynamic effects of third-degree block depend on the adequacy of the ventricular rate in maintaining cardiac output and blood pressure. Cardiac output and blood pressure are usually improved with nodal escape rhythms owing to the faster rate.

Interventions for Dysrhythmias

Dysrhythmia interpretation is a required skill for the nurse working with the critically ill patient. However, interpreting a rhythm correctly is only part of an important task. The nurse must be able to respond appropriately to patients experiencing cardiac dysrhythmias.

Learning the criteria for each rhythm is a difficult enough challenge, and attempting to learn the treatment for each dysrhythmia may seem overwhelming. As a means of simplifying this process, the treatments for dysrhythmias discussed in this chapter are organized into the three following categories: tachycardias, bradycardias, and pulseless rhythms.

Treatments discussed under each category are based on recommendations presented in the third edition of the *Textbook of Advanced Cardiac Life Support*, published by the American Heart Association in 1994. Advanced cardiac life support (ACLS) combines basic life support and dysrhythmia recognition with more aggressive techniques, including intubation, drugs, and pacemaking.

The ACLS textbook details the standards commonly accepted by health care professionals for the care of patients who require advanced life-saving techniques and interventions. These standards are presented, in an abbreviated form, in a decision tree known as an algorithm. This discussion of treatments is an elaboration of the ACLS algorithms. Additional information on code management is included in Chapter 7 of this text.

TACHYCARDIA

Premature atrial, nodal, and ventricular contractions are discussed under the heading of tachycardias because they may warn of the development of tachy-dysrhythmias.

Premature Beats

Premature beats are caused by increased irritability or automaticity in the atria, AV node, or ventricles. Treatment of premature beats is based on the patient's symptoms and the risk of further dysrhythmia development. If the patient is asymptomatic and not at high risk for further dysrhythmia development, no treatment is necessary. However, if the patient reports palpitations, light-headedness, or syncope, treatment may be required. Premature beats in the setting of myocardial infarction are usually treated.

If treatment is required, it usually includes modification of known risk factors and use of appropriate cardiac drugs. Patients experiencing premature beats often have known risk factors for dysrhythmia development. Reduction of stress, withdrawal from caffeine and nicotine, and correction of hypoxia may be sufficient to control or suppress the irritable areas that produce the premature beats.

Differentiating Between Supraventricular and Ventricular Tachycardias

Two types of tachycardias exist: supraventricular tachycardia (SVT) and ventricular tachycardia (VT). Tachycardias that originate above the level of the ventricles are referred to as SVTs. Tachycardias originating in the SA node, atria, or AV node are supraventricular. SVT is a generic and nonspecific term that clarifies that the tachycardiac rhythm is *not* from the ventricles and therefore does not require or respond to many of the treatments used for VT. VT originates in the ventricles.

Of the dysrhythmias covered in this chapter, several are characterized by rapid rates: sinus tachycardia; atrial tachycardia, fibrillation, and flutter; nodal tachycardia; and VT. The American Heart Association (1994) defines tachycardia as a heart rate greater than 100 beats per minute. In both SVT and VT, when the ventricular rate exceeds 150 and is associated with significant signs and symptoms, immediate cardioversion is recommended. In addition to heart rate, serious signs or symptoms, including chest pain, shortness of breath, decreased level of consciousness, low blood pressure, shock, pulmonary congestion, congestive heart failure, or acute myocardial infarction associated with tachycardia, require immediate treatment.

Treatment of rapid-rate dysrhythmias may include the following:

1. Mediating the effects of the parasympathetic and sympathetic nervous systems
2. Intervening with appropriate cardiac drugs
3. Using electrical energy to convert the rapid rhythm to a slower, more normal rhythm

Successful treatment of these dysrhythmias may include one or all of these approaches. The severity of the patient's symptoms also dictates the treatment choice and timing. When a tachycardiac patient does not have serious signs and symptoms, less aggressive means of treatment, such as those discussed under mediation of the nervous system effects, can be employed. When a tachycardiac patient is experiencing one or more serious signs or symptoms, intervention is more aggressive and includes the use of cardiac drugs, electrical energy, or both.

Mediating the Effects on the Nervous System

When the sympathetic nervous system is stimulated by pain or anxiety, it releases epinephrine and norepinephrine. Epinephrine increases automaticity in the heart and predisposes the patient to tachycardias.

If a patient is hemodynamically stable while experiencing one of the rapid-rate dysrhythmias, a noninvasive maneuver can be used to decrease the stimulating effect of norepinephrine. These maneuvers include relaxation techniques, pain and anxiety relief, and vagal maneuvers.

Relaxation Techniques

Relaxation techniques are used to diminish the stress response. Guided imagery, biofeedback, and au-diotapes may be useful for some patients who experience rapid-rate dysrhythmias that are stress related (Guzzetta and Dossey, 1992). Often, patients have recurrent episodes of these dysrhythmias. The patient can be taught various relaxation techniques to slow the heart rate as well as to prevent recurrences.

Pain and Anxiety Relief

Pain and anxiety relief should be a nursing goal for any patient who has, or is at risk for, dysrhythmias. In addition to providing the aforementioned relaxation therapies, the nurse must remember to keep the patient and family informed of all procedures. Knowledge deficit can lead to increased anxiety, which may manifest in the form of dysrhythmias. Therefore, patient education is an important part of the patient care plan.

Additionally, the use of mild sedatives may be indicated in some patients. Drugs such as diazepam (Valium) and alprazolam (Xanax) may be ordered on schedule or as required for patients at high risk for anxiety-related dysrhythmias. Diazepam is often the drug of choice because it can be given both orally and intravenously. The drugs lorazepam (Ativan) and propotol (Diprivan) can be given as a continuous drip for patients requiring consistent and ongoing sedation.

Pain relief should also be a primary goal that is included in the patient care plan. Any source of pain, whether acute or chronic, can lead to stimulation of the sympathetic nervous system and can increase the heart rate. Although chest pain is of ultimate concern to the nurse caring for the patient with cardiac disease, other sources of pain should not be ignored or remain untreated.

Appropriate drugs should be ordered for the treatment of both acute and chronic pain. Morphine sulfate is often the drug of choice for acute pain. It is administered intravenously in 1- to 2-mg increments. Meperidine hydrochloride (Demerol) may also be used in patients who are allergic to morphine. Any medication that the patient has been taking for chronic pain before hospitalization should also be administered to the patient during hospitalization.

Vagal Maneuvers

Vagal maneuvers are used to stimulate the vagus nerve of the parasympathetic nervous system. Vagus stimulation slows the heart rate. The parasympathetic nervous system acts as a counterbalance for the sympathetic nervous system. The vagus nerve is usually stimulated in one of two following ways:

1. When a patient is experiencing a rapid-rate dysrhythmia, carotid massage can be used to stimulate

the vagus nerve. Gentle, downward pressure on *one* carotid artery, just beneath the mandible, can lead to increased vagal tone, resulting in a slowing of the heart rate. This effect is caused by suppression of automaticity in the SA node as well as decreased conduction through the AV node. This maneuver is usually performed by the physician. The patient must be closely observed for changes in mental status as the carotid artery is massaged. If a patient has poor blood flow through the carotid arteries, this maneuver may lead to inadequate cerebral perfusion.

2. The Valsalva maneuver also elicits strong vagal tone. The patient is asked to tense the abdominal muscles briefly. This bearing down causes increased vagal stimulation. This maneuver should not be used in patients with increased intracranial pressure (Wright and Shelton, 1993).

As vagal maneuvers are performed, the bedside ECG is closely monitored. If the maneuver is successful, the heart rate begins to return to normal. If the patient is experiencing paroxysmal atrial tachycardia, fibrillation, or flutter, fewer of the rapid atrial impulses may be conducted to the ventricles.

Intervening with Cardiac Drugs

Many classes of cardiac drugs are used to control or decrease heart rate. These agents include antidysrhythmics, beta-blockers, calcium channel blockers, and cardiac glycosides.

Antidysrhythmics

Adenosine is a quick-acting antidysrhythmic used for supraventricular tachycardia. Adenosine is given by rapid intravenous (IV) push. If the agent is effective, a 5- to 10-second asystole is induced. The half-life of the drug is 10 seconds, and then the drug is cleared from the body. After the brief period of asystole, a more normal rhythm should emerge. If the tachycardia resumes, adenosine can be repeated every 1 to 2 minutes. Adenosine is suitable only for emergency treatment of tachycardia. If the tachycardia is recurrent, other oral or IV drugs are used (Grauer and Cavallero, 1993).

Lidocaine is the drug of choice for VT occurring with a pulse. IV access is established, and the patient is given a bolus dose of 1 mg/kg of lidocaine. The usual bolus is between 50 and 100 mg IV push. Lidocaine can be repeated at half the original dose every 8 minutes until the rhythm converts or until a total dose of 3 mg/kg has been given (American Heart Association, 1994).

Lidocaine comes in a variety of packaging. Pre-filled syringes containing 100 mg, 1 g, and 2 g are available. The nurse must select and administer the correct dosage. The 100-mg syringe is appropriate for IV boluses. Erroneous administration of the 1- or 2-g syringe can result in patient death. The nurse must *always* check and double check that the correct syringe is in hand before the drug is administered. If a patient is allergic to lidocaine, procainamide (Pronestyl) or bretylium can be used instead. These drugs are discussed in greater detail in Chapter 7.

Beta-Blockers

The sympathetic nervous system exerts two types of effects, alpha and beta. The alpha effects of the sympathetic nervous system primarily relate to vasoconstriction and the resultant increase in blood pressure. The beta effects of the sympathetic nervous system are increased heart rate, increased strength of cardiac contraction, and bronchodilation. Beta-blocking drugs block or diminish the beta effects of the sympathetic nervous system (Shlafer, 1994).

In the setting of myocardial infarction, beta-blockers are particularly useful for preventing and treating tachycardiac rhythms. In addition to suppressing automaticity in the SA node, beta-blockers also effectively suppress automaticity in irritable areas surrounding the infarct area. The beta-blockers are particularly useful in slowing down the rate of sinus tachycardia, atrial tachycardia, fibrillation, and flutter. A secondary benefit in the use of beta-blockade in myocardial infarction is the decreased oxygen consumption associated with decreasing heart rate (American Heart Association, 1994). Propranolol (Inderal) and labetalol (Normodyne) are two beta-blocking drugs that can be given intravenously or orally.

In addition to monitoring the effects of slowed heart rate, the nurse must also watch for decreased strength of contractility. Blocking of the beta effect of increased contractile strength can lead to a less effective cardiac contraction. This situation can result in decreased cardiac output and lowered blood pressure. Patients who are known to have a history of congestive heart failure or myocardial infarction should be monitored closely for signs of decreased contractility while they are taking beta-blockers (Shlafer, 1994). Beta-blockers block the beta effect of bronchodilation. Beta-blockers should be used with extreme caution in chronic obstructive pulmonary disease.

Calcium Channel Blockers

The calcium channel–blocking drugs are useful for the slowing of rapid heart rates. Calcium is involved in the cardiac cycle; it moves across the cardiac cell membrane during depolarization. Blocking some of calcium's movement causes the rate of depolarization to be slowed. When depolarizations are slowed, heart rate and oxygen consumption are decreased.

The calcium channel blocker diltiazem is used in patients with paroxysmal atrial tachycardia, atrial fibrillation, and atrial flutter. It is available in intravenous form. Verapamil can be used if the patient is normotensive or hypertensive.

Cardiac Glycosides

The drugs digoxin (Lanoxin) and digitoxin are cardiac glycosides, or cardiotonics. They are known for their ability to increase the strength of contraction; however, they are also very useful in suppressing sinus depolarization and atrial irritability and slowing conduction through the AV node. Available in oral and intravenous forms, these drugs are used for sinus and nodal tachycardia and acute or chronic atrial dysrhythmias (Shlafer, 1994).

For adequate drug levels and effectiveness to be ensured, the patient must undergo digitalization over a period of time. Intravenous digitalization is accomplished by administration of 0.5 mg of digitalis in divided doses over 24 hours. This can also be accomplished by oral doses. For oral digitalization, up to 1 mg is given as a loading dose and is then followed by 0.125 to 0.5 mg daily.

When a patient's hemodynamic status is compromised secondary to a rapid atrial dysrhythmia, the route of choice is IV. The ECG is monitored closely as the initial dose is given. Effects may not occur until 30 minutes to 2 hours after the initial dose (Skidmore-Roth, 1995).

One sign of digitalis or digitoxin toxicity is the development of dysrhythmias. The toxic patient may present with the same dysrhythmias that he or she was taking the cardiotonic to treat. In addition to atrial dysrhythmias, the patient may also develop bradycardia or AV block. A serum digoxin level is drawn to determine if the patient is toxic.

Using Electrical Energy to Treat Supraventricular and Ventricular Tachycardias

When patients experience tachycardias exceeding 150 beats per minute that are associated with significant signs and symptoms, it is often necessary to use electrical energy to convert the rapid rate to a more normal one. Synchronized cardioversion, the implantable cardioverter-defibrillator, and radiofrequency ablation are useful treatment modalities for tachycardias.

Synchronized Cardioversion

Synchronized cardioversion involves the use of varying amounts of electrical energy delivered strategically on the R wave to convert tachycardic rhythms into more normal ones. Delivery of energy on the R wave prevents accidental shock-induced ventricular fibrillation during the vulnerable period of the T-wave downslope. Fifty to 360 joules (J) may be used. Rhythms such as atrial flutter usually require low initial doses of electricity (50 J). Ventricular, atrial, and nodal tachycardia and atrial fibrillation usually require 100 J initially. Up to 360 J may be used if necessary (American Heart Association, 1994). Care of the patient before, during, and after cardioversion is outlined in detail in Chapter 7, in which code management is discussed.

The defibrillator is used for synchronized cardioversion. It is set so that the electrical energy is delivered directly on top of one of the patient's R waves. In other words, it is synchronized with the patient's QRS complex. Synchronizing the electricity with the patient's own ventricular depolarization allows for a better chance of halting the rapid-rate dysrhythmia.

It is hoped that when the shock is delivered directly on the QRS, the irritable area creating the dysrhythmia will be depolarized. Repolarization always follows depolarization. During this resting phase, the SA node has the opportunity to emerge as the dominant pacemaker. Sometimes, multiple shocks are necessary to convert the abnormal rhythm to normal sinus rhythm. The amount of electricity is increased with each sequential shock until the rapid-rate dysrhythmia is converted.

Defibrillation

If the patient's ECG does not demonstrate a clear R wave, delivery of a synchronized dose of electricity on the R wave is inaccurate, if not impossible. In this case, defibrillation may be required. If a patient with rapid-rate dysrhythmia has no pulse, defibrillation is also required (American Heart Association, 1994).

Implantable Cardioverter-Defibrillator

Patients who have experienced and survived sudden cardiac death, patients with tachycardias that are unresponsive to medical treatment, and patients with unexplained syncope are candidates for an implantable cardioverter-defibrillator (ICD). The ICD is an implantable device that is slightly larger than a standard pacemaker and is capable of assessing tachycardias and responding with electrical therapies appropriate for the tachydysrhythmia. Depending on the sophistication and programming of the device, ICDs are capable of cardioversion, defibrillation, and back-up ventricular pacing.

First-generation and second-generation ICDs were implanted in the operating room. Depending on the generator used and patient's needs, electrodes were positioned transvenously or epicardial patches were used. Because of the larger-sized generator, ICDs were usually implanted in the abdomen, and their wires were tunneled under the skin to the heart. Third-generation ICDs are now implanted in the shoulder area, and leads are advanced transvenously as with other pacemakers. ICDs are now placed in the cardiac catheterization laboratory; this method results in less risk and trauma for the patient.

The ICD can be programmed to detect and respond to SVT and VT as well as ventricular fibrillation. The device monitors the patient's electrographically, by use of an internally derived ECG. The device assesses the dysrhythmia based on programmed criteria. For instance, the device may be programmed to respond to eight wide QRS beats with a heart rate exceeding 175. These beats are called *events* in ICD terminology. The device charges and delivers the programmed therapy. Depending on the patient's dysrhythmia, the device can use synchronized cardioversion or defibrillation to convert the rhythm. Because the energy is delivered directly to the heart, without the impedence created by skin, muscle, and bone, *much* less energy is required. Typically 10 J or less is required.

Devices can be programmed to deliver multiple therapies. The more frequently the device is called on to charge and fire, the shorter the life of the generator's battery. Most devices have a battery half-life of 3 years. Additionally, the newer ICDs have back-up ventricular pacing capability. Often, after cardioversion or defibrillation, the patient may return to a bradycardiac rhythm. The new ICDs are programmed to provide back-up pacing, most typically at 60 to 70 beats per minute, until the patient's normal sinus rhythm returns.

The activities of patients with ICDs have historically been curtailed in terms of driving, swimming, and operating heavy machinery. However, some physicians allow patients to engage in more activity if their device has not fired for 3 to 6 months. There is no risk to people near the patient should the device fire. Patients often report "feeling the shock," but there should be no risk to people who are near or touching the patient. Despite the presence of the ICD, if a patient experiences a tachydysrhythmia or ventricular fibrillation, critical care nurses must be prepared to respond appropriately.

The ICD should scan, charge, and deliver the appropriate therapy in 30 seconds or less. Should the ICD not fire, nurses should be prepared to use external cardioversion or defibrillation as necessary (American Heart Association, 1994).

Radiofrequency Ablation

For patients with recurrent tachycardias, either SVTs or VTs, radiofrequency ablation is a treatment option. Radiofrequency ablation uses electrical energy to destroy abnormal sites of pacemaking and conduction. The patient is taken to the electrophysiology laboratory, and areas of ectopic pacemaking are located by use of sophisticated pacing catheters. Once the ectopic site is located, it can be destroyed by heat created via the ablation catheter (Guzzetta and Dossey, 1992). Radiofrequency ablation is now considered to be a cure for many tachycardias (Porterfield and Porterfield, 1993).

BRADYCARDIA

Many of the dysrhythmias discussed in this chapter have the overall effect of slowing the heart rate. Slowing of the heart rate, regardless of whether it results from decreased automaticity, blocking of impulses, or the emergence of a lower-rate pacemaker creates the same hemodynamic response and requires the same basic treatment. Slow-rate dysrhythmias include sinus bradycardia, dysrhythmia, and arrest/exit block; nodal rhythm; atrioventricular blocks; and idioventricular rhythm.

Treatment of slow heart rates may include the following:

1. Suppression of the parasympathetic nervous system effects
2. Use of appropriate cardiac drugs
3. Use of electrical energy to increase heart rate

Treatment of the slow dysrhythmias should be based on the presence of significant signs and symptoms, *not* on heart rate alone. Significant signs and symptoms include hypotension, shortness of breath, chest pain, decreased level of consciousness, congestive heart failure, pulmonary congestion, and myocardial infarction (American Heart Association, 1994).

Suppression of the Parasympathetic Nervous System Effects

Stimulation of the parasympathetic nervous system via the vagus nerve results in a slowing of heart rate. The nurse must be aware of processes that can increase vagal tone, such as vomiting, gagging, carotid massage, and the Valsalva maneuver.

Nausea and vomiting should be controlled with antiemetics or nasogastric suctioning, if necessary. Palpation of the carotid arteries should be performed cautiously and avoided, if possible. Prevention of constipation through the administration of stool softeners and laxatives keeps the patient from straining at stool (e.g., performing the Valsalva maneuver).

Hypoxia can also lead to slowing of the heart rate. In the critical care setting, endotracheal suctioning is a common cause of hypoxia and vagal stimulation and often results in bradycardia. Endotracheal suctioning should be based on breath sounds and should not be performed on an arbitrary schedule. Patients should be hyperoxygenated via ventilator or a bag-valve device before they undergo suctioning. The bedside monitor should be watched as the patient undergoes this procedure.

Use of Appropriate Cardiac Drugs

The drugs atropine, dopamine, epinephrine, and isoproterenol (Isuprel) are commonly used to increase heart rate in the symptomatic patient. Atropine is classified as a vagolytic drug because it blocks the effect of the vagus nerve and increases heart rate. Atropine is given in 0.5- to 1.0-mg doses by IV push. This dose may be repeated to a *total dose* of 0.04 mg/kg of body weight. Dopamine, 5 to 20 μg/kg/min, and/or epinephrine, 2 to 10 μg/min, can be given in an IV drip form to stimulate heart rate and increase blood pressure.

Isoproterenol has a chemical composition that is similar to that of norepinephrine. It causes an increase in heart rate via stimulation of the beta effects of the sympathetic nervous system. Isoproterenol is given in an IV drip. Four milligrams of isoproterenol is mixed in a 250-ml bag of 5% dextrose in water and then titrated until the heart rate and blood pressure begin to increase. Isoproterenol can lead to worsening of dysrhythmias, especially ventricular tachycardia, and should be used with caution and only if other drugs of choice are ineffective (American Heart Association, 1994).

Both atropine and isoproterenol must be used cautiously and appropriately. Increased heart rate results in increased myocardial oxygen consumption. In the patient with cardiac disease, this increased rate and oxygen consumption may lead to ischemia, injury, and ultimately infarction (American Heart Association, 1994). Therefore, these drugs should be reserved for use *only* when bradycardia is accompanied by significant signs and symptoms.

Use of Electrical Energy/Pacemakers

In severe cases of bradycardia, use of electrical energy is necessary for pacing of the heart. This energy is delivered in the form of a temporary cardiac pacemaker. A pacemaker is required when the SA node fails and when the AV node and the Purkinje fibers prove inadequate or fail to act as back-up pacemakers (Guzzetta and Dossey, 1992).

Cardiac pacemakers can deliver varying amounts of electrical energy at varying rates. The pacemaker is set at a rate and electrical output that maintains an adequate cardiac output and blood pressure. Second-degree type II block and third-degree block often require the use of a pacemaker. The need for the pacemaker may be temporary or permanent.

Temporary Pacemakers

Two types of temporary pacemakers are used for slow heart rates in the clinical setting. They are discussed in the order in which they appear in the ACLS algorithm for bradycardia: external and transvenous (American Heart Association, 1994).

Pacemaking generators have five basic controls:

1. On/off switch.
2. Rate control—usually varies between 30 and 180 beats per minute.
3. Electrical output—registered in milliamperes (mA). Electrical output can be varied between 0.1 and 20 mA.
4. Sensitivity control—registered in milliamperes. Sensitivity can be varied between 0.5 and 20 mA.
5. Mode—the pacemaker can function in either a demand or an asynchronous mode.

External Pacemaking. The external pacemaker, also called the external noninvasive pacemaker, may be a free-standing piece of equipment or a part of the defibrillator (see Chapter 7, Fig. 7–14).

The external pacemaker delivers electrical current directly to the skin via two electrodes. External pacing is accomplished by positioning of two large monitor patches. One patch is placed on the anterior chest, over the heart. The other patch is placed on the patient's back, over the posterior surface of the heart (see Chapter 7, Fig. 7–15). An electrode is attached to each monitor patch and then connected to the external pacemaker. Electricity conducts through the skin, the skeletal muscle, and then through the heart muscle, causing depolarization.

The external pacemaker has two modes: demand and asynchronous. The demand mode paces the heart based on need. For instance, a heart rate is set at 60 beats per minute, and if the patient's heart rate decreases to less than 60, the pacemaker generates an impulse to pace the heart. The asynchronous mode paces the heart at a set rate, independent of any activity

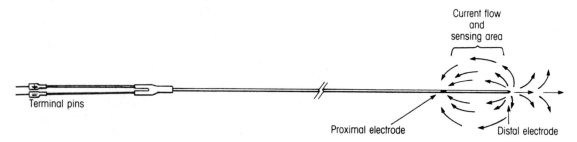

Figure 4–58. A bipolar pacing catheter. (From Sager, D. (1992). The person requiring cardiac pacing. In C. Guzzetta, & B. Dossey (Eds.), *Cardiovascular nursing: Bodymind tapestry.* St. Louis: C. V. Mosby Co.)

the patient's heart generates. The demand mode is safer for the patient and is therefore the mode of choice.

Once the mode is set, the electrical output is adjusted until the patient is 100% paced. Heart rate is then adjusted until an adequate blood pressure is obtained. A more thorough discussion of pacing follows under the discussion of transvenous pacemaking.

External pacemaking can be instituted within seconds of the event. It does not require a physician and can be initiated by a nurse. However, this means of pacing is *temporary.* External pacing is a bridge to transvenous or permanent pacemaker insertion. The direct application of electrical current to the skin is uncomfortable, and sedation may be necessary. If the patient's situation requires ongoing support for pacemaking, a transvenous pacemaker should be inserted as soon as possible.

Transvenous Pacemaking. In transvenous pacemaking, a large-bore catheter is introduced into a large vein, such as the subclavian, brachial, femoral, or jugular vein, by use of sterile technique. A special pacing catheter can then be threaded via the introducer into the appropriate chamber for pacing. The atria, the ventricles, or both, can be paced. If atrial pacing is needed, the flexible catheter is threaded via the introducer through the superior or inferior vena cava and into the right atrium. If ventricular pacing is needed, the catheter is threaded into the right ventricle. An

ideal position is achieved when the catheter tip touches the wall of the heart and stabilizes in the folds of the endocardium (Guzzetta and Dossey, 1992).

Most pacing catheters use a bipolar lead. *Bipolar* means that two electrodes are encased within the pacing catheter. One electrode terminates at the end of the pacing catheter; it is designated the distal electrode. The second electrode terminates above the level of the distal electrode; it is designated the proximal electrode (Fig. 4–58). Electrical energy flows between these two electrodes and causes depolarization.

Temporary pacing catheters are available for atrial, ventricular, and AV pacing. Straight tips, J-shaped tips, and balloon-tipped catheters exist in a range of sizes from 3 to 7 French.

Once the pacemaking catheter is in contact with the wall of the heart, a pacemaking generator is attached to the ends of the pacemaking wire left outside of the patient's body. Generators are used for accomplishing AV pacing and for accomplishing simpler ventricular pacing.

When the atria alone or both the atria and ventricles require pacing, an AV sequential pacemaking generator is usually used. The generator has dual controls for setting electrical output and heart rate for both the atria and the ventricles. For beginning the temporary pacing, the generator is turned on. Generators are battery powered. If the unit fails to come on, the battery

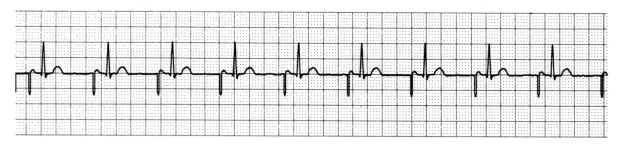

Figure 4–59. Paced rhythm: atrial. Note spike in front of the P wave. Rhythm strip generated by the AA-700 Rhythm Simulator. (Reproduced with permission from Armstrong Medical Industries, Lincolnshire, IL: *DataSim*, Fig. 32.)

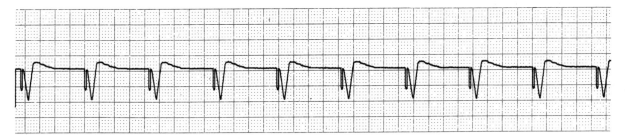

Figure 4–60. Paced rhythm: ventricular. Note spike in front of the QRS. Rhythm strip generated by the AA-700 Rhythm Simulator. (Reproduced with permission from Armstrong Medical Industries, Lincolnshire, IL: *DataSim*, Fig. 36.)

may be dead. Most pacemakers have a safety lock for the on/off switch that prevents the generator from being accidentally turned off.

Once the generator is turned on, the rate control is usually set at 60 to 70 beats per minute. Then, the electrical output is turned up until the patient's heart is 100% paced by the pacemaker. When the patient's heart is paced, the ECG strip demonstrates an electrical artifact called the pacer spike. If the atria are paced, the spike appears before the P wave (Fig. 4–59). If the ventricles are paced, the spike appears before the QRS (Fig. 4–60). If both the atria and the ventricles are paced, spikes appear before the P wave and the QRS (Fig. 4–61).

This thin, vertical spike is typically followed by a larger-than-normal P wave or a wider QRS complex. Because the heart is paced in an artificial or abnormal fashion, the path of depolarization is altered, and, consequently, waveforms and intervals are altered.

Depolarization of the atria or ventricle, as evidenced by a pacer spike and the enlarged P wave or widened QRS complex, is called *capture*. The minimum amount of electrical energy required for capture to be achieved is called *threshold*. Usually, less than 1 mA is required for capture to be achieved (American Heart Association, 1994). For the maintenance of capture, the electrical output is set at two to three times threshold.

Once capture has been assured, the pacer rate can be set so that an adequate blood pressure results. The lowest-paced rate possible is used so that myocardial oxygen demands and consumption are diminished.

The generator has an asynchronous mode and a demand mode. Again, asynchronous means that the pacer does not synchronize its pacemaking with the patient's own intrinsic pacemaking. Demand mode means that the pacemaker generates an impulse only when the patient is unable to generate his or her own. As in external pacemaking, demand is the mode of choice.

The final control to be set on the generator is sensitivity. Sensitivity relates to the generator's ability to "sense" that the patient is having his or her own heart beat. A sense/pace indicator light or needle is at the top of every generator. When the generator delivers a paced beat, the pace light comes on or the needle indicates "paced." If the patient generates his or her own beat, the sense indicator should register. Sensitivity is adjusted until the indicator registers all intrinsic beats.

After all controls have been set, the pacemaker generator should be secured. In addition, precautions should be taken to protect the patient from microshock. For safety, the generator should be secured with a cloth fastening strap to the patient's chest or arm for a subclavian, jugular, or brachial insertion and to the thigh for a femoral insertion. The generator should

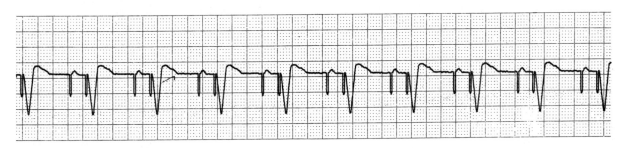

Figure 4–61. Paced rhythm: atrioventricular sequential. Note spikes prior to the P wave and the QRS. Rhythm strip generated by the AA-700 Rhythm Simulator. (Reproduced with permission from Armstrong Medical Industries, Lincolnshire, IL: *DataSim*, Fig. 33.)

never be secured to the patient's gown, bed, or IV pole (Guzzetta and Dossey, 1992). The patient should be taught how to turn and move in bed so as not to dislodge pacing wire placement.

In the older generators, the connection between the pacing wire and the generator is exposed. These generators should be covered by a rubber glove. Insulating the generator with the rubber glove protects the patient and the nurse from any leakage of electricity. Newer generators conceal the terminal connections within the generator. However, for safety, the nurse should still wear rubber gloves when working with the generator.

Other electrical safety precautions include limiting the use of line-powered electrical devices, such as volume infusion pumps, lamps, and ECG machines. These machines may cause electrical interference with the pacemaker. If these devices are used, they should not be allowed to touch the metal bed frame. The patient should not use an electrical razor.

Troubleshooting for the Transvenous Pacemaker. In addition to the usual risks of bleeding and infection associated with invasive techniques, two primary problems can occur with a temporary pacemaker. The first is failure to capture and the second is failure to sense.

Failure to Capture. When the pacemaker generates an electrical impulse and no cardiac muscular response occurs, failure to capture occurs. On the ECG, a pacer spike occurs with no evidence of depolarization. If an atrial pacer fails to capture, the atrial pacer spike is not followed by a P wave. If a ventricular pacer fails to capture, the ventricular pacer spike is not followed by a QRS (Fig. 4–62). Failure to capture can be caused by pacing wire displacement or fracture and battery failure. If the battery is not the problem, the pacing wire can be repositioned to ensure that it is in close contact with the wall of the heart.

If failure to capture still occurs, a chest x-ray study should be obtained to check for lead fracture. The pacing catheter is radiopaque, and therefore interruption in the wire can sometimes be seen on x-ray study. If lead fracture has occurred and the patient continues to need pacing, a new pacing catheter must be inserted.

If all of the aforementioned problems are ruled out and failure to capture still occurs, the electrical output can be increased. If the pacing catheter has drifted into an area of muscular injury or infarct, higher milliamperes may be required for capture to be obtained.

Failure to Sense. The pacemaker generator must be able to sense when the patient's heart is generating an intrinsic beat. Otherwise, the pacemaker generator could deliver an electrical impulse on top of the patient's own heart beat. When a pacemaker impulse falls on the T wave, a life-threatening dysrhythmia, such as ventricular fibrillation, may be stimulated (Conover, 1993).

Failure to sense manifests as inappropriate pacer spikes on the ECG tracing, inappropriate in that the spikes fall on or near the patient's own beats (Fig. 4–63). This problem can occur when the catheter has become dislodged or fractured. The first intervention should be to increase the sensitivity. If that does not correct the problem, the physician can attempt to reposition the pacing catheter and can obtain a chest x-ray study to check for dislodgement or fracture.

If the inappropriate pacer spikes are falling on the patient's T wave, or if ectopic beats are being generated, the nurse can turn the pacemaker off. If the pacemaker is turned off, the patient must be closely monitored. If the patient does have an irregular rhythm, the ECG and blood pressure should be monitored closely. The situation can then be evaluated, and pacing can be discontinued or a new pacing wire can

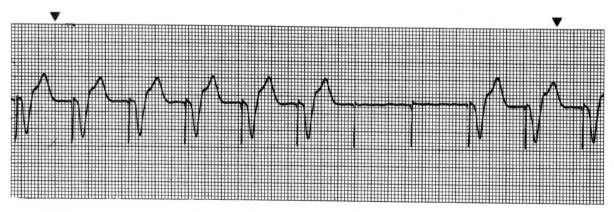

Figure 4–62. Paced rhythm with failure to capture. (From Huff, J., Doembach, D., & White, R. (1985). *ECG workout: Exercises in arrhythmia interpretation.* Philadelphia: J. B. Lippincott Co.)

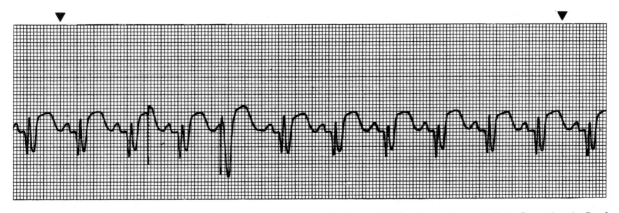

Figure 4–63. Paced rhythm with failure to sense. Note spike without a QRS to follow. (From Huff, J., Doembach, D., & White, R. (1985). *ECG workout: Exercises in arrhythmia interpretation.* Philadelphia: J. B. Lippincott Co.)

be inserted. If the patient is unable to generate a heart rate, or if that heart rate is inadequate to sustain a normal blood pressure, external pacing may be required.

Insertion of a transvenous pacemaker can be time consuming and requires an adept physician. When time is limited, the patient is compromised, or no physician is available to place the transvenous pacemaking catheter, external temporary pacing should be used.

PULSELESS RHYTHMS

Ventricular fibrillation and asystole are rhythms that cause a cessation of cardiac output and blood pressure. Therefore, patients experiencing these rhythms are pulseless. Additionally, patients with VT can also present without a pulse. When VT occurs *without* a pulse, it is treated exactly like ventricular fibrillation. Treatments of ventricular fibrillation/VT without a pulse and asystole are discussed separately, and ACLS guidelines are followed. Further information is available in Chapter 7.

Ventricular Fibrillation/Ventricular Tachycardia Without A Pulse

Ventricular fibrillation and VT without a pulse are life-threatening dysrhythmias. Survival depends on rapid detection and immediate intervention. The rhythm must be correctly assessed.

The amplitude of ventricular fibrillation can be very low, producing a fine, wavy baseline. Because of this, asystole can be diagnosed in error. Coarse ventricular fibrillation can be mistaken for VT. For these reasons, at least two leads should be reviewed before ventricular fibrillation is diagnosed.

The primary treatment for ventricular fibrillation

is defibrillation. If a defibrillator is not immediately available, cardiopulmonary resuscitation is initiated in the interim. As soon as a defibrillator is accessible, immediate defibrillation should be accomplished.

The ACLS guidelines state that the initial defibrillation should be accomplished with 200 J. If the rhythm does not convert, defibrillation is repeated at 300 J. If the fibrillation continues, 360 J is used. After this initial series of 200, 300, and 360 J, cardiopulmonary resuscitation is continued. Intravenous access is established, and drugs, including epinephrine, lidocaine, bretylium, magnesium sulfate, and procainamide, are used. Concurrent with these activities, the patient is intubated, and respirations are supported.

Throughout the rest of the arrest, defibrillation at 360 J follows the administration of the various drugs. A sequence of drugs, then defibrillation, is repeated until the patient is successfully resuscitated or the code is terminated. A thorough discussion of the drugs used to treat ventricular fibrillation is included in Chapter 7.

Asystole

Asystole carries a grave prognosis. Asystole is usually the result of end-stage cardiac disease. However, it can also be the end result of severe sinus bradycardia or sinus arrest/exit.

In the patient experiencing asystole, transcutaneous pacing should be the initial supporting treatment. If external pacing is not available, then cardiopulmonary resuscitation should be instituted. Epinephrine, 1.0 mg IV push, can be used to stimulate automaticity. Atropine, 1 mg, should also be used in case the asystole is the end result of bradycardia. Sodium bicarbonate may also be considered if the patient is acidotic.

RESEARCH APPLICATION
Article Reference
Bainger, E. and Fernsler, J. (1995). Perceived quality of life before and after implantation of an internal cardioverter defibrillator. *American Journal of Critical Care, 4*(1), 36–43.
Review of Methods and Findings
Seventy people with implanted cardioverter defibrillators (ICDs) were surveyed on their perceived quality of life. The responses of the ICD recipients were compared with those of a population of patients who have undergone percutaneous transluminal coronary angioplasty (PTCA) and a population of healthy persons. ICD recipients were asked to retrospectively self-report on their perceived quality of life before and after the implantation of the device. The Quality of Life (QOL) Index: Cardiac Version developed by Ferrans and Powers was used. No significant differences existed between the perceived overall quality of life of ICD recipients before and after implantation. ICD recipients reported an overall quality of life that was higher than that reported in the healthy population and comparable to that reported in the population that had undergone PTCA.
Critique
This study is limited in that it used retrospective self-reports in a convenience sample. Administering the QOL instrument before the implantation of the device versus asking patients to recall their QOL would have strengthened the study. Whether patients who have had PTCA are similar to patients who have had ICD implantation is unsubstantiated. However, the study was well performed, used a reliable and valid instrument, and generated useful information.
Implications
Implications for the study are primarily educational. Study results can be shared with patients and families undergoing ICD implantation. Sharing the study results of no significant change in QOL before and after implantation may help decrease the fear of living with an ICD.

Summary

The intention of this chapter is to demystify the analysis and interpretation of basic dysrhythmias. ECG interpretation is a basic skill that develops only through practice. For the beginning student, the critical criteria for diagnosis provide the structure by which rhythms are analyzed. Initial effort should be the memorization of these criteria.

It is hoped that this chapter will be a valuable reference in the delivery of high-quality care to patients with cardiac dysrhythmias and to their families.

CRITICAL THINKING QUESTIONS

1. You are working in the coronary intensive care unit and your patient's heart rate suddenly decreases from 88 to 52 beats per minute. Would you administer atropine? What data would guide your decision?

2. An implantable cardioverter-defibrillator unit will be implanted in a patient tomorrow. He asks, "How will this pacer limit my activities?" What would you tell him?

3. Discuss why patients with pulmonary disease are prone to atrial dysrhythmias.

4. You are working in the emergency department. Mrs. J. comes into the emergency department for the treatment of nausea and vomiting for 24 hours. She has a history of hypertension and coronary artery disease. When you connect her to the monitor you note a heart rate of 50 beats per minute.
   a. What assessment data will you collect related to the bradycardia?
   b. What questions will you ask Mrs. J. during your nursing history?

5. Why does tachycardia sometimes lead to heart failure?

REFERENCES

Abedin, Z., & Conner, R. (1989). *Twelve-lead ECG interpretation.* Philadelphia: W. B. Saunders Co.

Alspach, J. G. (1991). *Core curriculum for critical care nurses.* Philadelphia: W. B. Saunders Co.

American Heart Association. (1994). *Textbook of advanced cardiac life support.* Dallas: Author.

Conover, M. B. (1993). *Understanding electrocardiography: Arrhythmias and the 12-lead ECG.* St. Louis: C. V. Mosby Co.

Copstead, L. (1995). *Perspectives on pathophysiology.* Philadelphia: W. B. Saunders Co.

Drew, B. (1993). Bedside electrocardiographic monitoring. *AACN Clinical Issues, 4*(1), 25–32.

Drew, B. (1991). Bedside electrocardiographic monitoring: State of the art for the 1990's. *Heart and Lung, 20*(6), 610–623.

Fenstermacher, K. (1989). *Dysrhythmia recognition and management*. Philadelphia: W. B. Saunders Co.

Grauer, K., & Cavallaro, D. (1993). *ACLS certification preparation*. St. Louis: C. V. Mosby Co.

Guzzetta, C., & Dossey, B. (Eds.) (1992). *Cardiovascular nursing: Bodymind tapestry*. St. Louis: C. V. Mosby Co.

Huszar, R. (1994). *Basic dysrhythmia interpretation and management*. St. Louis: C. V. Mosby Co.

Patel, J., McGowan, S., & Moody, L. (1989). *Arrhythmias: Detection, treatment, and cardiac drugs*. Philadelphia: W. B. Saunders Co.

Pasternak, R., Braunwald, E., & Alper, J. (1988). Acute myocardial infarction. In E. Braunwald et al. (Eds.), *Harrison's principles of internal medicine* (3rd ed.). Philadelphia: W. B. Saunders Co.

Porterfield, L., & Porterfield, J. (1993). Radiofrequency ablation of a left-sided free wall accessory pathway: A case study. *Critical Care Nurse, 13*(2), 46–49.

Shlafer, M. (1993). *The nurse, pharmacology and drug therapy*. Redwood, CA: Addison-Wesley.

Skidmore-Roth, L. (1995). *Mosby's 1995 nursing drug reference*. St. Louis: C. V. Mosby Co.

Wright, J., & Shelton, B. (1993). *Desk reference for critical care nursing*. Boston: Jones & Bartlett Publishers.

RECOMMENDED READINGS

Fenstermacher, K. (1991). *Basic cardiac rhythm interpretation*. Baltimore: Medi-Sim/Williams & Wilkins.

Lipman, B., & Cascio, T. (1994). *ECG: Assessment and interpretation*. Philadelphia: F. A. Davis Co.

Robinson, B., Anisman, P., & Eshaghpour, E. (1994). A primer on pediatric ECGs. *Dimensions of Critical Care Nursing, 11*(4), 69–72.

Speers, A. (1994). Crossword puzzles: A teaching strategy for critical care nursing. *Dimensions of Critical Care Nursing, 13*(1), 52–55.

CHAPTER

5

Hemodynamic Monitoring

Joan M. Vitello-Cicciu, M.S.N., R.N., CCRN, C.S., FAAN
Cynthia Kline O'Sullivan, M.S.N., R.N.

OBJECTIVES

- Identify the physiological basis for hemodynamic monitoring in critically ill patients.
- Describe the indications, measurement, complications, and nursing implications associated with monitoring of central venous pressure, left atrial pressure, pulmonary artery pressure, and intra-arterial pressure.

- Identify the normal values of the aforementioned pressures.
- Analyze the conditions that alter hemodynamic values.
- Explain the clinical relevance of, and the methods for, measuring cardiac output.
- Discuss the rationale and methods for continuous monitoring of mixed venous oxygen saturation.

Introduction

A person's initial exposure to the critical care environment may be rather mystifying. Comprehending the complicated equipment, such as digital readouts, waveforms, and alarms, and the tangle of wires, tubings, and cables may at first seem impossible. However, even when the technical equipment and data obtained are well understood, this technology serves only to augment patient care and should not detract from a holistic perspective. Furthermore, viewing the patient as a person first and using the equipment as merely an adjunct should be the focus in critical care, no matter how much the clinical practice is influenced by technology.

Much of the equipment used in the critical care setting is for the purpose of hemodynamic monitoring. The term *hemodynamics* refers to the interrelationship

of the various physical forces that affect the blood's circulation through the body. Development of a working knowledge of the concepts known as pressure, flow, and resistance provides the foundation for this understanding. Insight into the factors affecting the heart's ability to pump effectively is also essential. Thus, this chapter discusses the basic principles of hemodynamics, the role of the heart as a pump, and hemodynamic monitoring. Essential nursing considerations for patients being hemodynamically monitored are also introduced.

Physiology

PRESSURE, FLOW, AND RESISTANCE

One of the basic laws of physics can be explained by the following equation:

$$\text{Pressure} = \text{Flow} \times \text{Resistance}$$

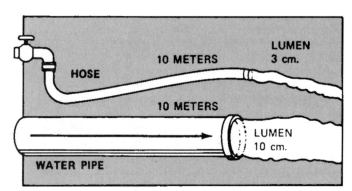

Figure 5–1. Schematic drawing illustrating the flow of fluid through a garden hose and a water pipe. Blood flow is decreased through the narrower lumen (hose) as compared to the wider lumen (pipe). (From Jackle, M., & Halligan, M. (1980). *Cardiovascular problems: A critical care nursing focus.* Bowie, MD: Robert J. Brady.)

This principle can be illustrated with a water pipe (Fig. 5–1); altering either the flow or the resistance of the pipe affects the water pressure inside it. For example, turning the faucet increases the flow of water through the pipe, thereby increasing the pressure. Similarly, partially occluding the pipe with sand or leaves and narrowing the opening causes the flow of water to be met with increased resistance, and pressure builds up within the pipe.

Another law of physics is that a natural tendency exists for liquids to flow from an area of higher pressure to an area of lower pressure. This phenomenon occurs frequently in the body and is exemplified by the movement of blood through the cardiac chambers. These concepts may be better understood when the aforementioned equation is applied to blood pressure, such that

Blood Pressure = Cardiac Output (Flow)
 × Peripheral (Systemic) Vascular Resistance

In this equation, blood pressure is affected by both cardiac output (CO) and peripheral (systemic) vascular resistance. CO is defined as the volume of blood that circulates through the body per minute and therefore represents flow. Peripheral (systemic) vascular resistance is the opposition to blood flow exerted by the blood vessels and is affected by blood viscosity, vascular tone, and friction imposed by the inner lining of the blood vessels. In the clinical setting, a patient's blood pressure may decrease from 136/70 mm Hg to 80/50 mm Hg. The decrease in blood pressure has occurred because either the flow (CO) has been reduced or the resistance has decreased. Conversely, if this patient's blood pressure increases to 190/90 mm Hg, either the CO or the resistance has increased.

A major factor that influences peripheral (systemic) vascular resistance is the lumen size (diameter) of the vessel. For example, if the lumen size narrows, the resistance increases, and vice versa. In the critical care setting, vasoactive drugs are often used to alter the lumen size of the peripheral vessels (predominantly the arterioles), with the aim of either decreasing or increasing blood pressure.

Many factors can influence the CO, as is illustrated by the following equation:

$$CO = Heart\ Rate \times Stroke\ Volume$$

Stroke volume (SV) may be defined as the volume of blood ejected by the heart per contraction. Therefore, a change in either the SV or the heart rate (HR) affects the CO. This concept is expanded later in this chapter.

THE BLOOD AND CIRCULATORY SYSTEM

The complex network of the veins, the arteries, and the heart that comprises circulation is in many ways analogous to the water pipe illustration. However, the human circulatory system is unique for many reasons. Blood itself possesses characteristics that make it unlike any other bodily substance, in that it is a viscous liquid with both cellular and fluid components. The cells of the blood vary in shape, size, structure, and function. For example, neutrophils, monocytes, macrophages, and eosinophils are collectively known as white blood cells, or leukocytes. Leukocytes are found in relatively small numbers within the circulating blood and perform immunological functions. Conversely, red blood cells, or erythrocytes, make up a much larger portion, contributing to approximately 99% of the total number of cells. The major function of erythrocytes is the transport of oxygen, in the form of hemoglobin, from the lungs to the tissues. Because most of the blood's cellular component is made up of erythrocytes, they provide the blood with many of its physical properties.

Typically, approximately 40% of the total blood volume is cellular, and the remainder is plasma. Environmental factors, certain disease states, and gender all affect the number of circulating blood cells. An increase in blood cells causes the blood to become more viscous. This increased viscosity results in greater friction and therefore makes the flow of blood through small vessels more difficult. However, blood is able to flow freely through the tiny capillaries by the alignment of erythrocytes within these vessels. Thus, blood moves through the capillaries as a "plug" of erythrocytes rather than randomly, as occurs in the larger vessels. This is an important feature because tissue oxygenation occurs at the capillary level, and the erythrocytes provide this valuable function.

The human circulatory system is actually one continuous circuit (Fig. 5–2). Under normal conditions, the system contains a volume of blood that remains relatively constant. Therefore, when the body's metabolic demands increase, blood needs to be circulated more quickly through the circuit to meet those demands. Likewise, when the body is at rest and its demands are reduced, some of the blood volume is essentially stored (in veins) within the circulatory system itself.

The body uses several mechanisms to regulate the flow of blood through the blood vessels in order to meet metabolic demands (Fig. 5–3). The first mechanism involves the ability of blood vessels to change their diameter or lumen size, as was discussed earlier. Unlike the water pipe, the walls of the vessels, particularly the veins, have the ability to constrict or dilate according to need. For example, in response to increased demands, the veins constrict. As a result, more blood is forced back to the heart. It then passes through the lungs, where it is reoxygenated, and it is returned to the heart to be pumped out to the tissues. Likewise, when the body is at rest and demands are reduced, the veins become dilated. As their diameter increases, the veins are able to accommodate a larger volume of blood. In this way, they serve as a reservoir, so that a smaller volume of blood is returned to the heart. Circulation is therefore accomplished efficiently, thereby reducing the cardiac workload, because only the amount of blood required to meet the demand is being pumped by the heart.

Two other mechanisms that control blood flow involve the heart's ability to control heart rate (HR) and strength of contraction (contractility). These mechanisms are regulated by a complex interaction between the autonomic and central nervous systems in conjunction with input from the circulatory and endocrine systems. The kidneys also play a role in regulating circulation through mechanisms that adjust blood pressure and blood volume via the renin-angiotensin system.

THE CARDIAC CYCLE

A knowledge of the cardiac cycle is necessary for a full understanding of hemodynamics. The cardiac cycle occurs in two phases: diastole, during which the left and right ventricles receive blood from the atria, and systole, during which the ventricles contract, thereby squeezing blood out of the heart through the aorta and the pulmonary artery (PA). Diastole occurs simultaneously between the left and right sides of the heart, as does systole. The flow of blood through the circulatory system is illustrated by a description of the entire sequence, from the right side of the heart to the left side.

After supplying oxygen to the tissues, deoxygenated blood is collected by the systemic veins. Venous blood from the peripheral circulation enters the right atrium of the heart via the superior and inferior venae cavae. During diastole, as the right atrium begins to fill with blood, the tricuspid valve is closed (Fig. 5–4). As the right atrium fills more completely, right atrial pressure becomes higher than right ventricular pressure. This pressure difference forces the tricuspid valve to open. Blood then rushes from the right atrium into the right ventricle.

As the right ventricle fills with blood from the right atrium, pressure within the atrium drops, whereas it rises within the ventricle. Simultaneously, the right atrium contracts, ejecting enough blood into the right ventricle to fill it completely (Fig. 5–5). As this occurs, right ventricular pressure surpasses right atrial pressure, causing the tricuspid valve to snap closed, thereby preventing blood from entering the right ventricle.

During systole, the right ventricle begins to contract, thereby increasing intraventricular pressure (Fig. 5–6). When the pressure rises sufficiently to overcome the pressure exerted on the pulmonic valve, the valve then opens. Blood is therefore ejected out of the right ventricle into the PA. In turn, blood travels through the pulmonary circulation and is oxygenated at the level of the capillaries and alveoli. Oxygenated blood is then transported back to the heart via the pulmonary vein.

Oxygenated blood from the pulmonary circulation enters the left atrium during diastole. At this time, the mitral valve is closed. As the left atrium fills, left atrial pressure (LAP) exceeds left ventricular pressure. The pressure difference forces the mitral valve to open, and blood then rushes into the left ventricle. As the left ventricle fills, the left atrium contracts, ejecting enough blood to fill the left ventricle (Fig. 5–7).

Left ventricular pressure now transcends LAP, causing the mitral valve to snap closed and preventing additional blood from entering the left ventricle. The amount of blood in the left ventricle at this phase in the cardiac cycle is known as the *left ventricular end-diastolic volume*. This volume is significant because it determines the amount of blood that is ejected into the

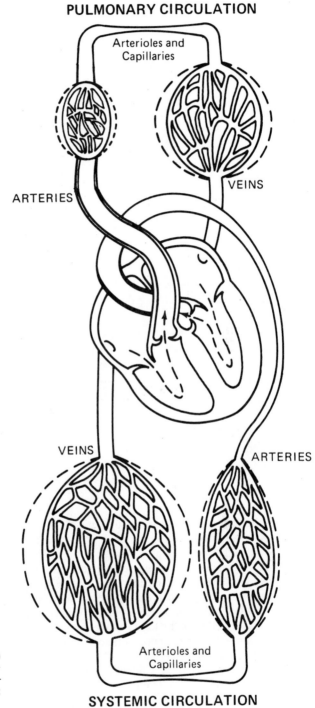

PULMONARY CIRCULATION

Arterioles and Capillaries

ARTERIES

VEINS

VEINS

ARTERIES

Arterioles and Capillaries

SYSTEMIC CIRCULATION

Figure 5–2. Illustration depicting the closed circuit, which is composed of the systemic and the pulmonary circulation. (From Jackle, M., & Halligan, M. (1980). *Cardiovascular problems: A critical care nursing focus.* Bowie, MD: Robert J. Brady.)

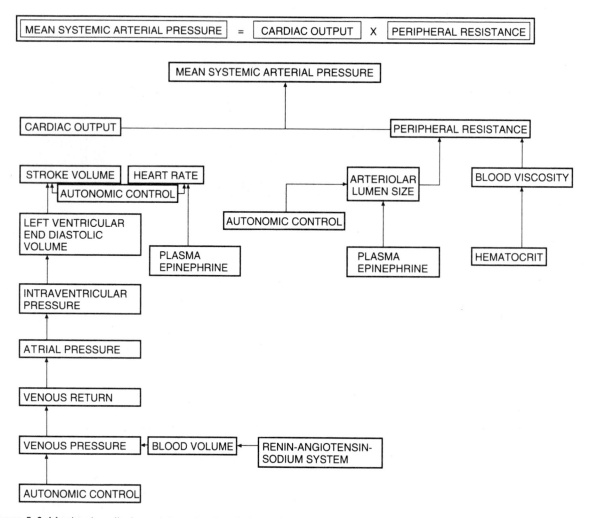

Figure 5–3. Mechanisms that regulate systemic arterial pressure. (From Vander, A., Sherman, J. H., & Luciano, D. S. (1980). *Human physiology* (3rd ed.) (pp. 304-305). New York: McGraw-Hill. Reproduced with the permission of McGraw-Hill.)

systemic circulation. The left ventricular end-diastolic volume is commonly referred to as preload and is described in further detail in a later section.

During systole, the left ventricle contracts, elevating the left ventricular pressure to such a degree that it overcomes the pressure exerted on the aortic valve from the systemic circulation (Fig. 5–8). Oxygenated blood is then ejected from the left ventricle through the aorta into the systemic circulation, where it ultimately supplies the tissues with oxygen.

As previously stated, the volume of blood that is ejected during systole is referred to as the SV. The volume that remains in the left ventricle at the end of systole is the *left ventricular end-systolic volume*. The left ventricle never ejects its entire end-diastolic volume. It merely ejects a fraction of this volume, known as the ejection fraction, which is normally 60 to 70% of the total end-diastolic volume.

CARDIAC OUTPUT/STROKE VOLUME

The CO is the amount of blood ejected from the heart per minute and is essentially equal to the amount of venous blood that is returned to the right atrium from the peripheral circulation. Physiologically, the CO is equal to the SV times the HR. Therefore, anything that can affect the HR, the SV, or both, affects the CO. Moreover, SV is influenced by three variables: (1) preload, (2) afterload, and (3) contractility (Fig. 5–9).

Preload may be defined as the amount of muscle fiber stretched before the next contraction. This muscle fiber stretch (also known as the presystolic fiber length) is directly affected by the end-diastolic volume in the ventricles. The end-diastolic volume actually stretches the muscle fibers before contraction (during diastole). Thus, preload can also be defined clinically

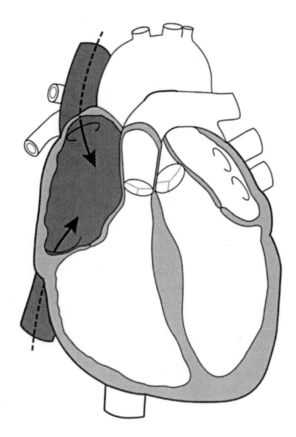

Figure 5–4. Illustration depicting blood flow into the right atrium during diastole.

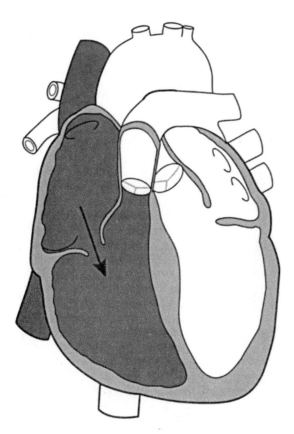

Figure 5–5. As blood continues to flow into the right atrium, the resulting pressure causes the tricuspid valve to open. Blood is then able to enter the right ventricle.

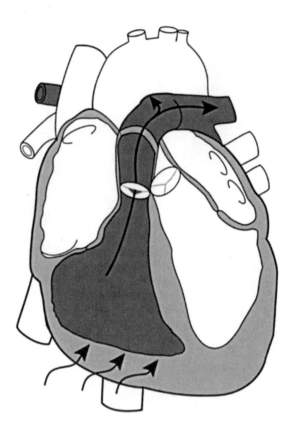

Figure 5–6. During systole, the right ventricle contracts, squeezing its contents through the pulmonic valve and into the pulmonary circulation.

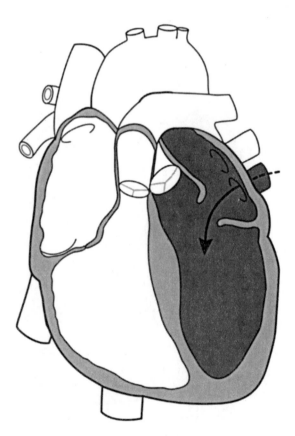

Figure 5–7. Oxygenated blood from the lungs now enters the left atrium. As atrial pressure builds, the mitral valve is forced open so that blood may pass into the left ventricle (not shown).

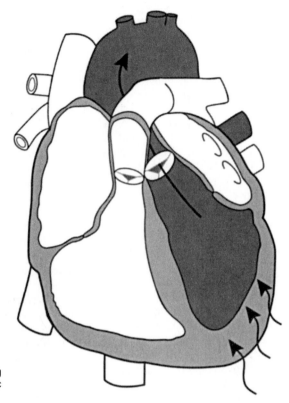

Figure 5–8. During systole, the left ventricle contracts, squeezing its contents through the aortic valve and into the systemic circulation to oxygenate the tissues.

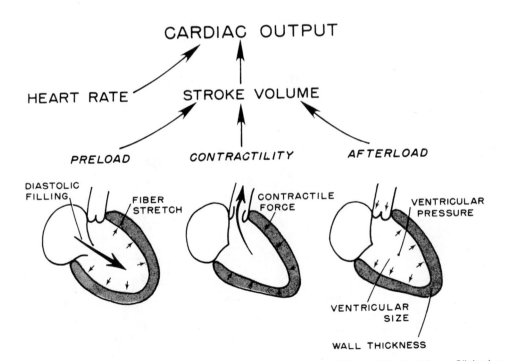

Figure 5–9. Factors affecting cardiac output (From Price, S., & Wilson, L. (1986). *Pathophysiology: Clinical concepts of disease processes* (3rd ed.) (p. 351). New York: McGraw-Hill Book Co. Copyrighted by The C. V. Mosby Co., St. Louis.)

as either the ventricular end-diastolic volume or pressure. Another important factor that influences SV is that within physiological limits, ventricular contraction is stronger as the muscle fiber stretch (preload) increases. This phenomenon is often referred to as the Frank-Starling principle insofar as CO or SV is related to the presystolic fiber length. Clinically, this principle means that a decrease in preload (decrease in end-diastolic volume) for a patient often results in a decrease in the force of contraction.

Afterload is defined as the pressure or resistance to blood flow out of the ventricle. This pressure or resistance must be overcome for the ventricle to eject its SV. The principal factor that offers resistance to this blood flow out of the ventricles is the arterial blood pressure. Thus, if the arterial blood pressure is high, the left ventricle must exert more force to effectively pump blood out of its chamber. Moreover, additional energy is required to generate enough pressure or force to eject this blood; the oxygen requirements of the heart increase in order to generate sufficient energy to accomplish this ejection. Clinically, an increase in afterload may cause a decrease in SV, especially if the left ventricle is unable to generate enough force to overcome this resistance.

Contractility, the third variable affecting SV, is defined as a measure of how forcefully the ventricle contracts to eject its SV. Contractility is the intrinsic ability of the muscle fibers to shorten. How much (extent) and how fast (velocity) these fibers shorten also affect SV. For example, if the ventricular fibers can shorten effectively and rapidly, the rate of pressure rise in the ventricle during systole is able to exceed the arterial blood pressure, resulting in a rapid forceful ejection of SV. Conversely, if the ventricular fibers lose their strength of contraction, the SV decreases. Thus, contractility directly affects SV, as do preload and afterload, as previously discussed.

Essential Components of Hemodynamic Monitoring

All hemodynamic monitoring equipment contains the following basic components: (1) transducer, (2) amplifier, (3) display instrument, (4) fluid-filled catheter, tubing, and flush system (Fig. 5–10).

The *transducer* is an instrument that is used to sense physiological events and transform them into electrical signals. Transducers come in many shapes

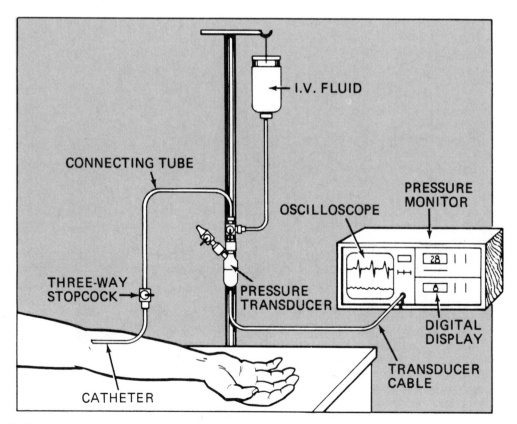

Figure 5–10. Essential components for invasive monitoring, using the brachial approach. (From Jackle, M., & Halligan, M. (1980). *Cardiovascular problems: A critical care nursing focus*. Bowie, MD: Robert J. Brady.)

and sizes and can be disposable or nondisposable. Some of the physiological events commonly measured by a transducer are (1) pressure, (2) flow, (3) temperature, (4) light intensity, and (5) sound. Housed within the pressure monitor are the amplifier and the display instrument. The *amplifier* connects to the transducer by an electrical cable. It functions by picking up the electrical event from the transducer and amplifying it while also filtering out interference signals. The improved signal is then transmitted to an instrument where it can be displayed.

Display instruments may be used to record or provide a quantifiable display of the original signal. The signal may be seen as a waveform, a digital readout, or a fluctuation on a meter. The method generally used to monitor hemodynamic pressures is to display a pressure waveform on an oscilloscope (a screen) and a digital reading of the pressure values on the pressure monitor.

The fourth component necessary for the performance of hemodynamic monitoring is the *catheter, tubing, flush system*. This system is composed of a blood-compatible catheter that may be inserted into an artery, a vein, or a heart chamber, depending on the type of hemodynamic monitoring required for the care of a critically ill patient. The catheter is then attached to rigid, noncompliant tubing that is ideally less than 48 inches long, which is then attached to some type of flush device that can control flow of solution through the tubing. A flush solution (e.g., lactate Ringer's solution, normal saline) that often contains heparin is used to keep the tubing and catheter patent and free of blood clots. A continuous flow of 3 to 5 ml/h of this flush solution is often required to keep the system patent. This heparinized solution is delivered from a compressible bag that is pressurized by either a pressure bag or an inflatable cuff. The pressure bag is necessary to provide enough pressure to the flush solution to drive the continuous flow of fluid through the tubing and catheter.

The use of heparin to avoid clot formation and to promote catheter patency was investigated by the American Association of Critical-Care Nurses (AACN) in the Thunder Project I, a national multicenter nursing research study that was designed to evaluate the effect of heparinized and nonheparinized flush solutions on the patency of arterial pressure lines. The results of this study showed that heparin significantly affects the patency of arterial pressure lines. Variables that were found to promote patency in this study included (1) heparinized flush solutions, (2) arterial catheters longer than 2 inches, (3) femoral placement of arterial catheters, (4) anticoagulant or thrombolytic therapy, (5) and male gender (AACN, 1993).

The equipment must first be standardized for reliable measurements to be obtained. For this purpose, the transducers used for monitoring hemodynamic pressures must be leveled, balanced, and calibrated.

To level a transducer, the nurse positions the air-fluid interface of the stopcock at approximately the level of the patient's right atrium. This area is known as the phlebostatic axis and is located at the fourth intercostal space, midway between the anterior and posterior aspects of the chest (often referred to as midaxillary position; Fig. 5–11). The transducer may be placed directly on the patient's chest, or it may be attached to an intravenous line pole positioned near the patient. A leveling instrument may be used for ensuring the proper height of the transducer when it is mounted on a pole rather than placed directly on the patient's body.

Balancing, or "zero referencing," is an operation performed to eliminate the influence of surrounding air pressure on the monitoring system. In order to control for this, the stopcock on the flush system is turned so that the patient's pressure is no longer being displayed, and only environmental pressures are sensed by the equipment. The straight line that appears on the display screen and the corresponding digital readouts are then adjusted to read "zero." In this manner,

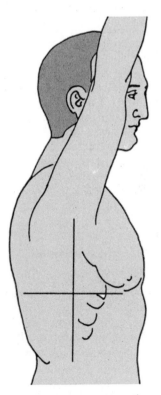

Figure 5–11. Locating the phlebostatic axis. (From Taylor, T. (1986). Monitoring left atrial pressure in the open-heart surgical patient. *Critical Care Nurse, 6*(2),64.)

atmospheric pressure is negated, even though it actually measures about 760 mm Hg at sea level.

Calibration is performed to ensure numerical accuracy within the electrical system. Most monitors are designed with a specific mechanism to accomplish this, such that a specific pressure reading is displayed when a button is pushed. Comparison of the value indicated on the display screen, the digital readout, and the monitor's specific calibration factor enables the accuracy of the system to be assessed.

CENTRAL VENOUS PRESSURE MONITORING

The central venous pressure (CVP), or the right atrial pressure, is a direct measurement of the pressure of the right atrium, but it may also be measured from the superior and inferior venae cavae. Because no valves are present between the right atrium and the venae cavae, the pressures within these areas are essentially equal. However, the clinical importance of CVP measurement lies in its ability to also reflect right ventricular pressure. During diastole, the heart's tricuspid valve is open, thereby allowing a clear passage for blood to flow from the right atrium to the right ventricle. Because of this, the CVP measurement is a reliable reflection of right ventricular preload, or right ventricular end-diastolic pressure.

The CVP measurement is particularly valuable for helping to reflect right ventricular pressure and right ventricular end-diastolic pressure. Generally, fluctuations in CVP affect either circulatory volume status or right ventricular function. For example, a patient with a low CVP may be experiencing hypovolemia, vasodilation, or any other condition that reduces venous return to the heart. On the other hand, a high CVP may be indicative of any condition that reduces the right ventricle's ability to eject blood, thereby increasing right ventricular pressure and hence right atrial pressure. These conditions include hypervolemia, vasoconstriction, right-sided heart failure, and pulmonary hypertension.

Methods of Measuring Central Venous Pressure

Catheters used for CVP measurement are generally stiff and radiopaque. They may vary in length and diameter depending on the vein that is used: shorter catheters are generally used for subclavian insertion, and longer catheters are used for upper extremity vein insertion.

Several sites may be used for CVP line insertion. The internal jugular site is often preferable because it allows the patient a high degree of mobility, and the risks of infection and thrombophlebitis are relatively

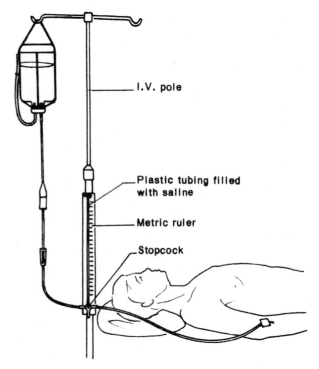

Figure 5–12. Measuring central venous pressure using a water manometer. I.V. = intravenous. (Adapted from Cyginski, J., & Tardieu, B. (1980). *The essentials in pressure monitoring: Blood and other body fluids. An illustrated guide* (p. 85). The Hague, Netherlands: Martinus-Nijhoff Publishing.)

low. The subclavian artery is another commonly used site, but it subjects the patient to an additional risk of pneumothorax during insertion. Other veins that may be suitable include the cephalic, femoral, antecubital, and occasionally the basilic and saphenous veins.

The insertion procedure for central lines is analogous to that for the PA. However, the design of the CVP catheter is different in that it contains only a single lumen (see section on PA catheters for a description of this procedure). CVP may be measured by use of either a conventional pressure transducer system or a device called a water manometer (Fig. 5–12). The latter is a quick, simple method that requires little equipment to use. It functions by the principle that fluids move from an area of higher pressure to an area of lower pressure. A fluid-filled tube called a manometer is the measuring device that relays the patient's pressure reading without the use of electrical equipment. The manometer is connected to the patient's intravenous infusion system that in turn connects to the central venous catheter. When the stopcock is turned so that the infusion is turned off, fluid from the manometer flows into the patient's vein and levels off when the patient's CVP and the pressure exerted by the fluid in the manometer equalize. After the measurement is recorded, the stopcock may again be turned so that the infusion may resume. Measurements taken from a water manometer are recorded in centimeters of water (cm H_2O).

Measurement of CVP by use of a pressure transducer is analogous to most other types of pressure monitoring. It requires all the standard equipment illustrated in Figure 5–10. Measurements taken from a pressure transducer are recorded in millimeters of mercury.

The typical CVP tracing consists of three upwardly deflected waves that correspond to various phases in the cardiac cycle. The "a" wave is produced by atrial contraction, and the "c" wave is produced by tricuspid valve closure. The "v" wave depicts the cumulative effect that occurs when the right ventricle contracts as the right atrium fills with blood, causing the tricuspid valve to bulge upward into the right atrium. Figure 5–13 illustrates a typical CVP tracing. Figure 5–14 denotes normal pressures and oxygen saturation in the various locations in the heart.

The normal value for CVP measurement is zero to 8 mm Hg, or 3 to 8 cm H_2O (water manometric value). The two measurements are not interchangeable; for conversion of a reading from one form to another, the following equation may be used:

$$\text{CVP in cm } H_2O/1.36 = \text{CVP in mm Hg}$$

Abnormalities in CVP measurement, as discussed earlier, are generally caused by any condition that alters venous tone, blood volume, or right ventricular contractility. Because the right ventricle does not generate significant pressure during atrial contraction, the atrial pressure is recorded as a mean pressure rather than as a systolic and a diastolic pressure. Mean pressures may be obtained directly from the monitor display with most conventional systems.

Complications of Central Venous Pressure Insertion and Monitoring

Because insertion of a CVP catheter involves a disruption of skin integrity, a risk of infection exists. However, this risk is greatly reduced if attention to hand washing and sterile technique during insertion and site care is observed.

Other complications may occur during the insertion itself. These include carotid puncture, pneumothorax, hemothorax, perforation of the right atrium or ventricle, and disturbances in cardiac rhythm, generally either atrial or ventricular dysrhythmias.

Nursing Implications

For accurate CVP measurements to be obtained, the air-fluid interface of the transducer must be properly placed at the phlebostatic axis (described previously). Measurements should be taken when the patient is in the supine position, either flat or with the head of the bed slightly elevated (< 30°). In a recent nursing study, CVP measurements taken in cardiac

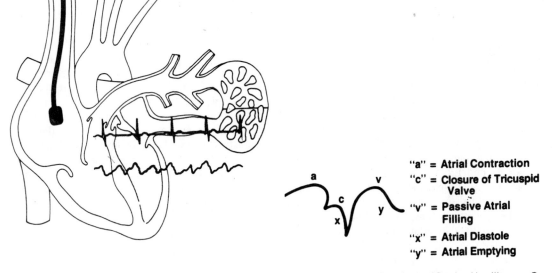

"a" = **Atrial Contraction**
"c" = **Closure of Tricuspid Valve**
"v" = **Passive Atrial Filling**
"x" = **Atrial Diastole**
"y" = **Atrial Emptying**

Figure 5–13. Right atrial pressure waveform correlating with electrocardiogram. (Courtesy of Baxter Healthcare Corporation, Baxter Edwards Critical-Care Division, Irvine, CA.)

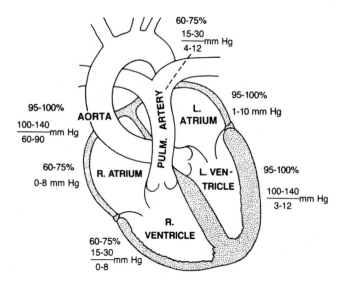

Figure 5–14. Schematic illustration of heart model depicting the pressure and oxygen saturation measurements in the various chambers of the heart. L. = left; Pulm. = pulmonary; R. = right. (Adapted from Gardner, P. E., & Woods, S. L. (1989). Hemodynamic monitoring. In S. L. Underhill, S. L. Woods, E. S. Sivarajan-Froelicher, & C. J. Halpenny (Eds.), *Cardiac nursing* (2nd ed.) (p. 452). Philadelphia, J. B. Lippincott Co.)

surgical patients lying on their side were significantly different than those taken in patients in supine positions (Emerson and Banasik, 1994). Changes in body position may be corrected for by adjusting the level of the transducer. These adjustments are also described in the next section.

Another method of recording CVP is analysis of the CVP waveform from a printout on a bedside or central station recorder that has been calibrated to an oscilloscope. Information derived from this method is more precise than the numerical display or the waveform from the oscilloscope, both of which may be misleading because of respiratory variation. These printout recordings need to be examined whenever serious alterations in values occur. These recordings permit the clinician to take into account the influence of the respiratory cycle. All hemodynamic waveforms can be obtained by printout recording.

Respiratory variation is a second consideration that must be addressed in CVP monitoring. Any situation that alters intrathoracic pressure, such as spontaneous inspiration and mechanical ventilation, affects the CVP waveform. For this reason, the CVP measurement should be read at the end of expiration for the most accurate information to be obtained.

Another important nursing consideration in the care of patients undergoing CVP monitoring is close observation for any complications. The complications that may occur are discussed in further detail in the section on PA catheters. Infection, although uncommon, is a potentially dangerous situation for any patient, particularly one who is critically ill. Therefore, daily observation of the insertion site is of utmost importance. Signs of infection include an elevated body temperature and pain, warmth, redness, and puru-

lent drainage at the insertion site. Any of these signs should be reported to the patient's physician immediately.

Finally, one nursing consideration that is paramount in CVP monitoring is accurate interpretation of the data. Measurements of CVP are most valuable when compared with other physiological parameters. A careful physical assessment can help to identify false readings, and a comparison of several hemodynamic values in conjunction with a thorough physical assessment generally provides the most accurate interpretation of the patient's condition.

LEFT ATRIAL PRESSURE MONITORING

Left atrial pressure is the pressure of the blood as it returns to the left side of the heart. The LAP is a reflection of the left ventricular preload. As discussed earlier, preload is defined as the volume or pressure in the ventricle at the end of diastole (left ventricular end-diastolic volume or left ventricular end-diastolic pressure). On the left side of the heart during diastole, the mitral valve is opened, allowing for communication between the left atrium and the left ventricle. Thus, at the end of diastolic filling under normal circumstances, the LAP is nearly identical to the left ventricular end-diastolic pressure. The normal LAP is 1 to 10 mm Hg (see Fig. 5–14). Because the left atrium does not generate significant pressure during atrial contraction, the atrial pressure is recorded as an average (mean) pressure rather than as a systolic or diastolic pressure.

Catheter Insertion

The left atrial catheter is inserted during cardiac surgery. The catheter itself is composed of a polyvinyl material and is approximately 6 inches long. The surgeon may insert this catheter in one of two ways. The most common technique is through a needle puncture of the right superior pulmonary vein, which empties into the left atrium, followed by insertion of the catheter into the left atrium (Taylor, 1986).

The second method is through direct insertion via a needle puncture into the intra-atrial groove into the left atrium, just above the mitral valve (Fig. 5–15) (Taylor, 1986). The catheter is then sutured into place and brought out through an incision into the chest wall, usually toward the right inferior end of the patient's sternal incision. Then the catheter is connected to a pressurized tubing system as previously described. The LAP waveform is then displayed on the oscilloscope. A sterile dressing is usually placed over the insertion site of the catheter and is changed daily. The LAP catheter is normally used for 24 to 72 hours and then is removed by a physician or other

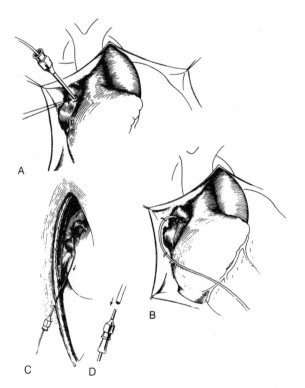

Figure 5–15. Left atrial line placement. Method of inserting left atrial pressure monitoring line. *(A)* A polytetrafluoroethylene (Teflon) catheter is inserted through purse-string suture into right upper pulmonary vein through large needle. *(B)* It is then secured to pericardium to prevent accidental dislodgment. *(C)* Catheter is passed through chest wall with large needle. *(D)* Blunt needle adapter is used to connect catheter to extension tubing for measurement of pressure. (Adapted from Behrendt, D. M., & Austen, G.(1985). *Patient care in cardiac surgery* (p. 50). Boston, Little, Brown & Co.)

designated person, depending on the policies of the institution.

Complications of Left Atrial Pressure Monitoring

The danger of introducing air or debris into the LAP catheter system is of paramount importance because of the peril of causing an embolism into the coronary or cerebral circulation. The nurse must ensure that all connections are tightly fitted and that all stopcocks have been capped. Medications or fluids should not be routinely administered through this catheter so that the danger of introducing any air into the system is not increased.

Another complication of the LAP catheter is clot formation. Small clots can pose the same danger as air bubbles. If a clot is suspected, the nurse should manually try to aspirate the clot back into the syringe. However, if this attempt is unsuccessful, the physician should be notified, and the catheter should be removed.

The third potential complication is infection. The LAP catheter is a direct line into the heart, and any microorganism that invades the cardiac tissue may directly affect the heart's performance. Thus, constant surveillance of the insertion site is mandatory, and adherence to dressing changes per hospital policy should be maintained.

Nursing Implications

For accurate LAP recordings to be obtained, the air-fluid interface of the transducer must be positioned at the phlebostatic axis when the patient is in the supine position (see Fig. 5–11). If the patient assumes the lateral position facing the transducer, the air-filled interface of the transducer must be leveled as shown in Figure 5–16. An imaginary line is drawn at the fourth intercostal space along the chest wall, and another line is drawn at midsternum. The point where the lines intersect is the approximate position of the left atrium and is where the air-fluid interface of the transducer should be leveled.

If the patient's back is facing the transducer, then another reference point for leveling of the air-fluid interface of the transducer is necessary (Fig. 5–17). This point is obtained by drawing an imaginary line along the fourth intercostal space at approximately the T4–T6 level and by drawing a second line along the midline of the spinal column. The transducer is then leveled at the point of intersection of both lines.

Another consideration for the obtaining of accurate LAP readings is the effect of the respiratory cycle. Again, LAP is ideally obtained at the end of expiration, regardless of whether a patient is undergoing mechani-

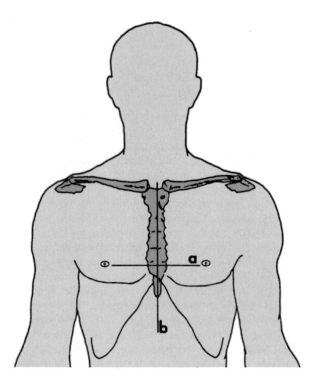

Figure 5–16. Site for leveling the transducer in the anterior lateral position. (From Taylor, T. (1986). Monitoring left atrial pressure in the open-heart surgical patient. *Critical Care Nurse*, 6(2),65.)

cal ventilation. The rationale for this is that the end-expiratory pleural pressure usually remains at a relatively constant level and allows for a stable pressure waveform that facilitates accurate measurements.

A third consideration in obtaining accurate LAP measurements is the use of positive end-expiratory pressure (PEEP). The patient may receive PEEP for the correction of hypoxemia (low partial pressure of arterial carbon dioxide). In this case, the LAP reading should be obtained while the patient is undergoing mechanical ventilation using PEEP regardless of the level of PEEP because removing the PEEP to obtain any parameter has been found to be detrimental to the patient's oxygen level and may actually cause hypoxia. While the patient is undergoing PEEP, the readings should be assessed for any trends that may indicate that another intervention is required. It is also important to note that strip/chart recording can be used to ascertain the LAP.

Variables Influencing Left Atrial Pressure

The LAP can be either increased or decreased, depending on the clinical condition of the patient. A lowering of the normal LAP is found in the following

conditions: hypovolemia, massive vasodilation, and excessive PEEP (10 cm H_2O). Increases in LAP may be found in the following conditions: hypervolemia, massive vasoconstriction, pulmonary congestion, mitral stenosis, mitral regurgitation, cardiac tamponade, constrictive pericarditis, and depressed contractile states, such as in myocardial infarction, cardiomyopathy, and hypothermia.

A series of LAP readings depicting trends is more informative than a single reading that deviates from the normal baseline range. Like any other hemodynamic parameter, the LAP should be correlated with other assessment data before any changes in therapy are instituted.

PULMONARY ARTERY MONITORING

The introduction of the PA catheter in 1970 by Swan and Ganz represented a major breakthrough in hemodynamic monitoring. Before this time, the central venous catheter was the only method by which cardiac function could be monitored. No matter how important the CVP is in the monitoring of right-sided parameters, it is of little help in detecting left-sided problems.

The PA catheter allows the clinician to indirectly

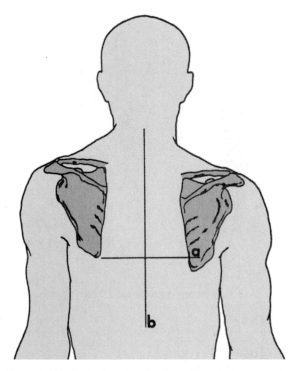

Figure 5–17. Site for leveling the transducer in the posterior lateral position. (From Taylor, T. (1986). Monitoring left atrial pressure in the open-heart surgical patient. *Critical Care Nurse*, 6(2), 65.)

monitor valuable information regarding left ventricular function. As was discussed earlier, through the contraction of the left ventricle, blood is ejected systemically to the tissues, where oxygen and nutrients are then made available to the cells. Any alterations in left ventricular function can severely compromise blood flow to the tissues. Because left ventricular SV is influenced by the blood volume and contractility of the left ventricle during systole, the PA catheter is helpful in identifying conditions that contribute to abnormalities in both of these indices.

Types of Catheters

The PA catheter is a long, hollow, pliable catheter that is radiopaque and is constructed with a variable number of lumens, or sections, that extend to several points (measured in centimeters) along the length of the catheter. Distal and proximal lumens are for pressure monitoring, and these are filled with fluid. Medications or fluids should not be routinely administered through the distal lumen of the PA catheter. A thermistor lumen is used during CO monitoring, and it houses temperature-sensitive wires. The balloon inflation lumen is equipped with a valve that enables a tiny balloon on the tip of the catheter to be inflated with a syringe. This balloon is inflated during insertion of the catheter to allow the catheter tip to flow through the various cardiac structures without causing damage to the cardiac tissue.

Several types of PA catheters are available with varying numbers of lumens and features. *Two-lumen* PA catheters are the simplest type; these are rarely used (Fig. 5–18). They contain one lumen, which is referred to as the distal hub or port, for PA pressure monitoring and a second lumen for inflation of the balloon during insertion.

Three-lumen catheters contain one proximal hub for positioning in the right atrium, one distal hub for

the positioning in the PA, and one balloon-inflation valve (Fig. 5–19). The right atrial (proximal) lumen functions identically to the CVP catheter, or right atrial catheter, discussed previously. The proximal hub may therefore be used for monitoring purposes as well as for intravenous administration of solutions.

Four-lumen catheters contain, in addition to the two hubs and valve found in the triple-lumen catheter, a thermistor wire connector is used for obtaining CO measurements (Fig. 5–20).

Five-lumen catheters (Fig. 5–21) contain, in addition to the four ports described earlier, a fifth port called the proximal infusion lumen hub, which is situated high in the right atrium. It is used solely for infusion purposes and is sometimes referred to as the venous infusion port. Five-lumen catheters have several advantages over four-lumen catheters. First, they provide a mechanism for continuous monitoring of CVP pressure without interruption of the intravenous infusion. Second, because blood flows through the right atrium at a high velocity, two medications can be infused simultaneously, one through the right atrial lumen and another through the fifth lumen, without fear of drug incompatibility.

Some PA catheters are also designed for the purpose of transvenous pacing. This technique involves the insertion of pacemaker electrodes through the PA catheter in order to provide temporary ventricular pacing capabilities when other methods are not readily available. This modality is used in situations in which the patient's own natural pacemaker is functioning ineffectively, and dysrhythmias or absence of cardiac rhythm (asystole) result. Figure 5–22 illustrates a typical transvenous pacemaker system, which is inserted into a specially designed PA catheter. An external generator is used to "fire" the pacing impulse. For more information regarding pacemakers, see Chapter 4.

A recent technological advancement has been in

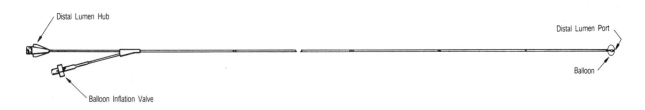

Double Lumen Catheter

Figure 5–18. Two-lumen pulmonary artery catheter, which has the balloon inflation valve (to obtain wedge pressure) and distal lumen hub (to obtain pulmonary artery pressure). (Courtesy of Baxter Healthcare Corporation, Baxter Edwards Critical-Care Division, Irvine, CA.)

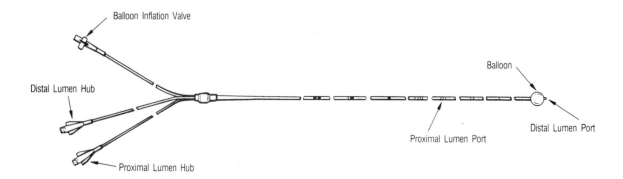

Triple Lumen Catheter

Figure 5–19. Triple-lumen pulmonary artery catheter with balloon inflation valve, proximal injection hub (to obtain right atrial pressure), and distal injection hub. (Courtesy of Baxter Healthcare Corporation, Baxter Edwards Critical-Care Division, Irvine, CA.)

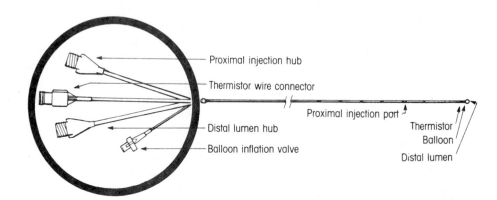

Figure 5–20. Quadruple-lumen pulmonary artery catheter containing the balloon inflation valve, proximal and distal injection hubs, and a thermistor lumen for obtaining cardiac output measurements. (From Davis, S. G., & Silverman, B. (1984). Hemodynamic monitoring. In C. G. Guzetta & B. M. Dossey (Eds.), *Cardiovascular nursing: Bodymind tapestry* (p. 260). St. Louis: C. V. Mosby Co.)

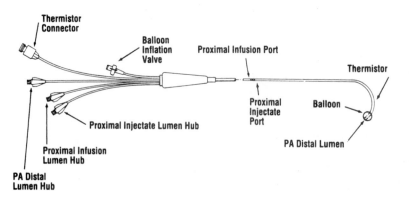

Figure 5–21. Five-lumen pulmonary artery catheter containing the quadruple-lumen components in addition to a second proximal lumen for infusion of fluid or medications. PA = pulmonary artery. (Courtesy of Baxter Healthcare Corporation, Baxter Edwards Critical-Care Division, Irvine, CA.)

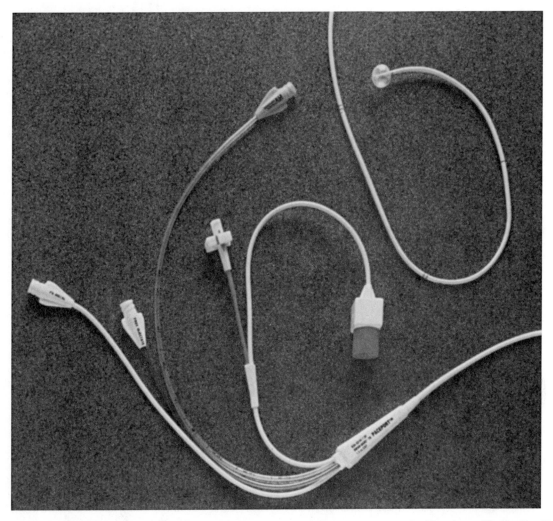

Figure 5–22. Thermodilution pacing catheter, consisting of quadruple-lumen components. (Courtesy of Baxter Healthcare Corporation, Baxter Edwards Critical-Care Division, Irvine, CA.)

the development of the continuous CO catheter. This new catheter uses a heat filament that is positioned in the right ventricle to raise the temperature of the blood; the raised temperature is then detected by a thermistor at the catheter tip. In addition to the five standard lumens as described earlier, these catheters have a continuous CO heat filament port and a mixed venous oxygen saturation ($S\bar{v}O_2$) port. Continuous monitoring of $S\bar{v}O_2$ is through a fiberoptic network housed inside a conventional PA catheter. For measurement of $S\bar{v}O_2$, a tiny beam of light is transmitted through the catheter and into the patient's PA circulation. Blood flowing through the PA is illuminated by this light. The patient's cardiac function and oxygenation determine how much the blood reflects the light, and a tiny microchip located within the catheter quantifies this

amount. These results are ultimately converted to a numerical value, which is displayed on a monitoring screen for continuous assessment. The concept of continuous CO and $S\bar{v}O_2$ is further discussed in a later section.

Nursing Responsibilities Before Insertion

Despite the differences in the types of PA catheters available, the nursing responsibilities before the catheter is inserted are relatively similar. The differences depend on the patient's individual condition as well as on the personal preference of the physician and the brand of equipment used.

Of primary importance is the need for patient teaching before the catheter is inserted. Patients are often anxious and uncertain about this procedure and can benefit from simple, straightforward explanations. The following is a sample of the information that should be presented to the patient when the decision has been made to insert a PA catheter. Informed consent may be required by an institution. The physician should explain the procedure briefly, along with the risks and benefits of the procedure, but the critical care nurse must be able to reinforce necessary information while providing emotional support.

Hello, Mrs. Smith. The doctor has discussed the pulmonary artery catheter with you. I can help to clarify some points with you if you like.

The pulmonary artery catheter will give us valuable information about how your heart is working and will help us to decide the best possible treatment.

The procedure will probably take about 30 minutes. It won't be too painful, but it will involve the insertion of a small catheter through your skin and up into your heart. The skin will be numbed with a local anesthetic. It will be important for you to remain still while the catheter is being passed, but I'll be with you during the entire procedure to make sure you'll be as comfortable as possible.

As the physician continues the procedure, the nurse provides additional reinforcement to help decrease the patient's anxiety. Special attention by the nurse regarding the patient's comfort level and need for emotional support contributes to the well-being of the patient, especially if the procedure is taking longer than usual.

Equipment

The equipment required for PA monitoring is similar to the pressure transducer system discussed in the section on CVP monitoring: a transducer, an amplifier, and a display instrument with a tubing system for continuous flushing of the line. Variations from this method are possible when catheters contain both a right atrial port (proximal port) and PA port (distal port). Two sections of tubing are needed for continuous flushing of both ports of the catheter, and two transducers are necessary for simultaneous monitoring of right atrial and PA pressures.

Because of certain risks involved in this proce-

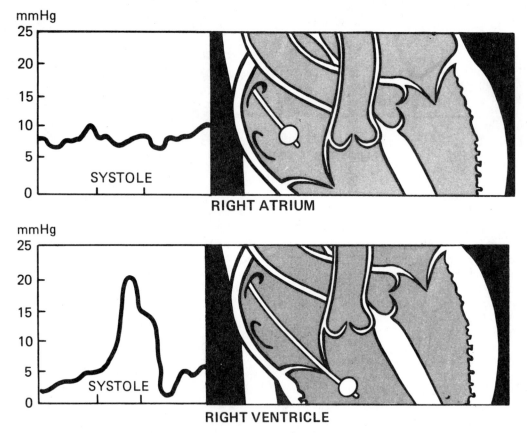

Figure 5–23. Pulmonary artery catheter as it floats into the right atrium *(top)*, crossing the tricuspid valve, and then passing into the right ventricle *(bottom)*. (Adapted from Jackle, M., & Halligan, M. (1980). *Cardiovascular problems: A critical care nursing focus.* Bowie, MD: Robert J. Brady.)

dure, emergency medications and equipment must be readily available. Complications include hemothorax, pneumothorax, perforation of the vein or cardiac chamber, and cardiac rhythm disturbances. The PA catheter passes through the right ventricle before it comes to the PA. As it passes through the ventricle, it can irritate it, causing ventricular rhythm disturbances, such as premature ventricular contraction and ventricular tachycardia. For this reason, a prefilled syringe of 50 to 100 mg of intravenous lidocaine must be kept available to be infused emergently should these rhythm disturbances become hemodynamically significant.

Insertion Method

Brachial Site

The site is cleaned and draped. A tourniquet is applied to the upper arm. A local anesthetic may be injected into the skin. The vein is punctured with a needle, and needle placement in the vein is confirmed by a free flow of blood into the catheter. After the tourniquet is removed, the catheter is advanced.

Subclavian, Internal Jugular, or External Jugular Site

The patient's bed is placed in the Trendelenburg position to promote venous filling in the upper body for easier insertion of the catheter. This position can also prevent air embolism during insertion. If the Trendelenburg position is contraindicated, such as in a patient with pulmonary edema, a blanket roll can be placed between the shoulder blades to facilitate insertion. The skin is cleaned and draped, and the skin is injected with a local anesthetic. A needled syringe is used to puncture the vessel and confirm placement by backward flow of blood into the syringe. The syringe is removed, and a guide wire is threaded through the

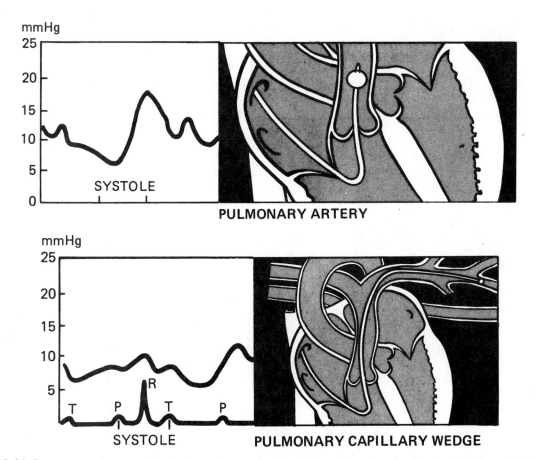

Figure 5–24. Pulmonary artery catheter being advanced through the pulmonic valve from the right ventricle to the pulmonary artery *(top)*. Catheter is then floated into a smaller pulmonary arteriole in order to obtain the wedge pressure *(bottom)*. (From Jackle, M., & Halligan, M. (1980). *Cardiovascular problems: A critical care nursing focus.* Bowie, MD: Robert J. Brady.)

needle into the vessel. The needle is then removed so that a hollow tube, called an introducer, may be passed over the guide wire. The wire is then removed and the PA catheter passed freely into the vessel through the hollow introducer. Several variations of this method of insertion exist, and physicians may have their own preferences. Technique may also vary according to the brand of equipment used and the patient's anatomy. A chest x-ray study is often obtained after the procedure to verify catheter placement if fluoroscopy was not used during the insertion.

Surgical Cutdown

Occasionally, a surgical cutdown approach may be necessary for PA catheter insertion because of the lack of suitable veins. In this method, the skin and surrounding muscle are surgically excised in order to expose the underlying vein. Once this is accomplished, the catheter may be placed similarly to the method described for sublcavian, internal jugular, or external jugular veins.

Nursing Responsibilities During Insertion

As the catheter is passed through the cardiac chambers, the nurse must pay particular attention to HR, rhythm, and blood pressure. Therefore, vital signs should be recorded frequently. Any dysrhythmias that occur during the procedure should be documented, and the usual emergency equipment and medications should be made available.

As the tip of the catheter passes through each chamber, the waveform changes, and the pressures displayed need to be recorded. These waveforms ap-

pear as follows: right atrial, right ventricular, PA systolic and diastolic, and PA wedge pressure (Figs. 5–23 and 5–24). The last waveform signals the end of insertion, at which time the physician deflates the balloon. Once the balloon is deflated, the tip of the catheter falls back in position in the PA.

The nurse reinflates the balloon in order to monitor PA wedge pressures as ordered or according to unit protocol. The balloon should not be inflated for more than a few seconds, so that ischemia is not caused by obstruction of blood flow. After the PA catheter is inserted, the centimeters measuring depth of insertion should be noted to provide the clinician with an assessment clue should the catheter be accidentally pulled out or advanced.

Clinical Significance of Pulmonary Artery Catheter Values

The PA pressure consists of a systolic, a diastolic, and a mean pressure (Fig. 5–25). The systolic pressure is the peak pressure attained as the right ventricle ejects out its SV. The diastolic pressure is the lowest pressure on the waveform that reflects of the movement of blood from the PA out into the lung capillaries. The third parameter, the mean pressure, is the average pressure exerted on the pulmonary vasculature. The normal PA pressure is approximately 25/10 mm Hg, and the mean pressure is 15 mm Hg (see Fig. 5–14).

The fourth parameter, known as the PA wedge pressure or pulmonary capillary wedge pressure (PCWP) (Fig. 5–26), is a mean pressure with a normal value of 6 to 12 mm Hg (see Fig. 5–14). When the balloon is inflated, the PCWP reflects the pressure

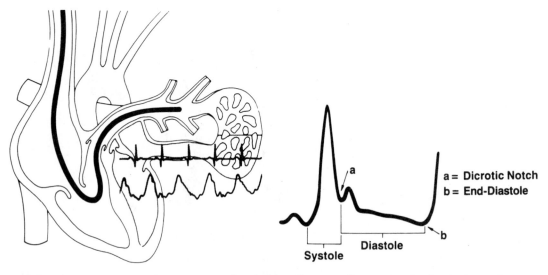

Figure 5–25. Pulmonary artery waveform corresponding to PA catheter position and patient's electrocardiogram. (Courtesy of Baxter Healthcare Corporation, Baxter Edwards Critical-Care Division, Irvine, CA.)

ahead of the catheter, which is both the LAP and the left ventricular end-diastolic pressure. Thus, the PCWP is a reliable indirect measurement of left ventricular function. In the absence of valvular disease and pulmonary vascular congestion, the PA diastolic pressure (PADP) also closely approximates the pressure in the left atrium and left ventricle just before contraction (end diastole) as well as the mean pressure in the pulmonary capillaries (pulmonary wedge pressure). These pressures are equal because the mitral valve is open during end diastole, therefore providing an open circuit for the free movement of blood from the PA to the lungs and back to the left atrium and the left ventricle.

An understanding of the PADP and its relationship to left ventricular end-diastolic pressure is a valuable guide to therapy. In patients with normal left ventricles, an increase in left ventricular end-diastolic pressure (and, hence, PADP) indicates an increase in left ventricular blood volume that will be ejected with the next systole. Likewise, a decrease in left ventricular end-diastolic pressure (and a subsequently low PADP) signals a reduction in left ventricular blood volume that will be available for the next contraction. Increased PADP may occur in patients who have been overhydrated with intravenous fluid as well as in those with renal disease who cannot produce adequate urine output. Conditions causing a low PADP include dehydration, excessive diuretic therapy, and hemorrhage.

An increase in PADP can also provide the clinician with early information about impending left ventricular failure, as may be seen with myocardial infarction. An increased PADP may be the first observable change in the patient's condition before any other physical signs are apparent. Through monitoring of changes and trends, the PADP can be invaluable in determining the most appropriate therapy as well as the effectiveness of that therapy.

The PCWP, being comparable to the PADP for most patients, can also be used as a physiological indicator of left ventricular failure and blood volume alterations. However, because the balloon of the catheter cannot be inflated for more than a few seconds at a time, the PCWP cannot be used for continuous monitoring. Furthermore, frequent inflation of the balloon should be avoided in order to prevent the possibility of the balloon's rupturing and causing air embolization, as is discussed later. Also, the nurse should never try to force balloon inflation if resistance is met and should make sure that the balloon is deflated if resistance is met on deflation. Periodic comparison of the PADP and PCWP is helpful in assessing the accuracy of the PADP measurement, especially in patients experiencing acute hemodynamic changes.

Complications of Pulmonary Artery Monitoring

Complications that may occur with PA monitoring are uncommon. Table 5–1 lists the most common complications as well as implications for the nurse in these situations.

Nursing Implications for Patient Positioning

It has been assumed that the patient must be flat and supine for reproducible measurements to be

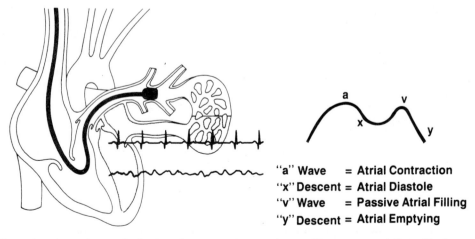

"a" Wave = Atrial Contraction
"x" Descent = Atrial Diastole
"v" Wave = Passive Atrial Filling
"y" Descent = Atrial Emptying

Figure 5–26. The pulmonary artery catheter in pulmonary artery wedge position measures left ventricular pressure. During diastole, the mitral valve is open, creating an open column of blood from the pulmonary arteries to the left atrium and left ventricle. When the balloon is inflated, blood flow from behind the catheter is obstructed so that the catheter tip reflects the pressure in front of the catheter (left heart pressure). (Courtesy of Baxter Healthcare Corporation, Baxter Edwards Critical-Care Division, Irvine, CA.)

Table 5–1. COMPLICATIONS OF PULMONARY ARTERY CATHETERS

Complication	Cause	Clinical Presentation	Nursing Implications
Infection	Violation of aseptic technique.	Redness, pain, irritation, warmth, purulent drainage at insertion site; elevated body temperature.	Daily observation for clinical signs of infection
	Catheter not secured to the surrounding skin.	As above; the nonsterile section of the catheter can slip forward into the vessel.	Adherence to aseptic technique during dressing changes
Dysrhythmias	Irritation to the endocardium caused when the balloon is deflated at the catheter tip. It can also occur when the catheter tip migrates back into the right ventricle.	Premature ventricular contractions, ventricular tachycardia visible on monitor. Reduced perfusion with ventricular dysrhythmias may cause hypotension, mental status changes, decreased cardiac output, and other problems.	Have lidocaine available to treat lethal dysrhythmias. Never advance the catheter without inflating the balloon. Continuous ECG monitoring
Air embolization	Balloon rupture. Poor technique during insertion. Disconnected infusion line.	Signs of shock ($\downarrow$ BP, $\uparrow$ HR). Patient may appear to have had a CVA (change in level of consciousness, possibly seizures, motor weakness).	If embolization occurs, position the patient with head down (20°) and on left side. During catheter insertion, the patient needs to be positioned head down (Trendelenburg's position). Notify physician immediately—this is an emergency situation
Pulmonary thromboembolism (PTE)	Thrombus formation on the catheter caused by inadequate flushing, using nonheparinized flush solution.	Sudden onset of dyspnea, chest pain, tachycardia, may lead to pulmonary infarction (see below).	Notify physician immediately of suspected PTE. Maintain anticoagulant therapy (heparin infusion) as ordered. Monitor partial thromboplastin time (PTT) while patient receives heparin. Optimize ventilation. Administer inotropic medications as indicated. Preventive measures: use heparinized flush solution, ensure adequate flushing of lines, be alert for PA lines left in over 72 h
Pulmonary artery rupture	Overinflation of the balloon. Deflated balloon tip passed during insertion of the catheter, causing perforation. Frequent inflation of balloon.	Signs of hemorrhage— $\downarrow$ BP, $\downarrow$ CO, $\uparrow$ HR. Decreased pulmonary blood flow.	Use no more than 1.5 ml of air to inflate balloon. Never flush catheter when it is in the wedge position. If the waveform appears dampened, never force flush the line; instead, aspirate the clot
Pulmonary infarction	Catheter movement into the wedged position. Balloon left inflated. Thrombus formation around the catheter, causing occlusion.	Cough, hemoptysis (bloody sputum), pleuritic pain, high fever, bronchial breathing, and pleural friction rub. Hypoxemia, hypocardia, and respiratory alkalosis.	Inflate the balloon with no more than 1.5 ml of air, and deflate it immediately after wedge tracing appears on monitor. If tracing appears to be wedged, and balloon is deflated, notify physician. A chest x-ray study may be necessary to confirm position

Data from Woods, S. L., & Grose, B. L. (1989). Hemodynamic monitoring in patients with acute myocardial infarction. In S. L. Underhill, S. L. Woods, E. S. Sivarajan-Froelicher, & C. J. Halpenny (Eds.), *Cardiac nursing* (pp. 293–294). Philadelphia: J. B. Lippincott Co.

CVA = cerebrovascular accident; ECG = electrocardiogram; BP = blood pressure; HR = heart rate; CO = cardiac output; PA = pulmonary artery.

obtained. However, several studies have determined the effects of varying backrest positions up to 60° on PA pressure, PCWP, and LAP. These studies have found little effect on these hemodynamic measurements, provided that the phlebostatic axis and proper leveling to the air-fluid interface of the stopcock are used as the zero reference level (Chulay and Miller, 1984; Retailliau et al., 1985; Dobbin et al, 1992).

One study evaluating the effect of the side-lying position found that reliable PA pressure and PCWP can be obtained when the patient is in the 90° lateral decubitus position, provided that the fourth intercostal space and midsternum are used as the reference level (Kennedy et al., 1984). The zero reference level for various degrees of lateral positioning are unknown; thus, PA pressure and PCWP may not be reliable if they are obtained in other lateral positions of less than 90° (Whitman et al., 1982; Wild, 1984; Osika, 1989). Moreover, Kennedy et al. (1984) recommended that baseline measurements be performed and compared in the supine, right lateral, and left lateral decubitus positions before measurements in either of the lateral positions are used.

CARDIAC OUTPUT MONITORING

As was previously discussed, CO is the amount of blood that has been pumped out of each ventricle (SV) each minute. CO can be calculated by multiplying the SV (amount of blood pumped out of each ventricle during each contraction) by the HR (the number of ventricular contractions per minute). Thus, the formula is

$$CO = SV \times HR$$

In the critical care setting, CO is an important hemodynamic parameter. It is used to assess whether the heart is pumping enough blood to supply oxygen to all of the body tissues. Although CO may now be measured continuously, the intermittent thermodilution method remains in conventional use. The intermittent thermodilution method involves injecting a known amount of solution at a known temperature (iced or room temperature) via the proximal port (CVP port or right atrial) of a quadruple-lumen PA catheter and then measuring the resultant drop in temperature downstream (by use of the thermistor of the PA catheter) (Fig. 5–27). The CO for the right side of the heart is calculated via a computer. Although this CO is a reflection of right ventricular blood flow, the CO of the left ventricle closely equals that of the right side.

Equipment for Intermittent Thermodilution

The equipment needed for intermittent thermodilution CO includes (1) a four- or five-lumen PA cathe-

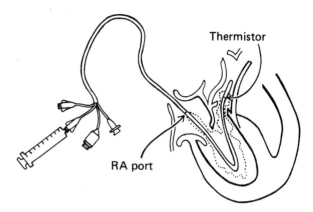

Figure 5–27. Illustration depicting injection into right atrium (RA) for cardiac output measurement. (Adapted from Gardner, P. E., & Woods, S. L. (1989). Hemodynamic monitoring. In S. L. Underhill, S. L. Woods, E. S. Sivarajan-Froelicher, & C. J. Halpenny (Eds.), *Cardiac nursing* (2nd ed.) (p. 464). Philadelphia, J. B. Lippincott Co.)

ter with thermistor, (2) an injectate (3, 5, or 10 ml of 5% dextrose in water or saline solution), and (3) a CO computer. Two methods of injecting the solution into the proximal port exist. The first method is referred to as the *open injectate delivery system.* This method involves preparing prefilled syringes (usually 10 ml of dextrose or saline solutions) and then putting these syringes in a sterile bath of ice chips and water (Fig. 5–28). (Prefilled syringes are available from certain

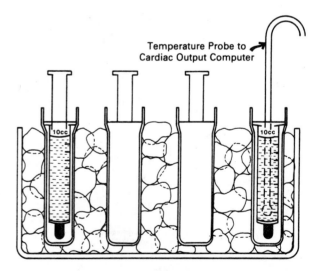

Figure 5–28. Illustration depicting iced injectate preparation. Preloaded syringes are placed in plastic or metal tubes, or in resealable bags that are suspended in an ice bath. (From Gardner, P. E., & Woods, S. L. (1989). Hemodynamic monitoring. In S. L. Underhill, S. L. Woods, E. S. Sivarajan-Froelicher, & C. J. Halpenny (Eds.), *Cardiac nursing* (2nd ed.) (p. 465). Philadelphia, J. B. Lippincott Co.)

manufacturers.) Maintaining the sterility of the ice bath is a major concern. One nursing study that investigated the ice bath encasing the syringes found bacterial growth after 8 to 24 hours (Grose et al., 1981). It is, therefore, recommended that this ice bath be changed every 8 hours. Another consideration is that these syringes need to be chilled to the range of zero to 5°C. In addition, it takes approximately 12 to 60 minutes for this temperature to be reached before these syringes can be used (Grose et al., 1981). Erroneous variations in CO can occur if these syringes are not properly chilled.

The second method is known as the *closed injectate delivery system*. This method involves use of a completely closed set-up of a sterile injectate solution, tubing coils, and a syringe attached near the proximal injectate port for the instillation of the predetermined amount of solution (Fig. 5–29). The advantages of this method include elimination of the need to prepare prefilled syringes, reduction in nursing preparation time, and reduction in the risk of infections by avoiding multiple entries into a sterile system.

Measuring Cardiac Output

Care must be exercised in obtaining accurate COs. Table 5–2 depicts causes of incorrect COs. The following points are important for the accurate obtaining of this information:

1. The correct position of the PA catheter should be verified by the waveform because malposition of the catheter causes erroneous CO values.

2. The appropriate computation or calibration constant (per manufacturer's instruction) must be displayed on the computer to obtain accurate cardiac output. Catheter size and type, and the volume and temperature of the injectate are factors that will determine which constant is required. Refer to the manufacturer's operation manual.

3. When chilled prefilled syringes are used, they should be placed in the ice bath solution for at least 12 to 60 minutes. The temperature of syringes should not exceed 5°C when the iced-injectate method is used (Levett and Replogle, 1979; Runciman et al., 1981).

4. Handling of the barrel of the syringe should be avoided because heat gained during handling distorts the value.

5. When a prefilled syringe is used, injection should occur within 30 seconds of removal of the syringe from the ice bath (Gardner and Woods, 1989). When either the prefilled or the manually closed injectate (5- or 10-ml) syringe is used, the manner of injection should be smooth and rapid (within 4 sec-

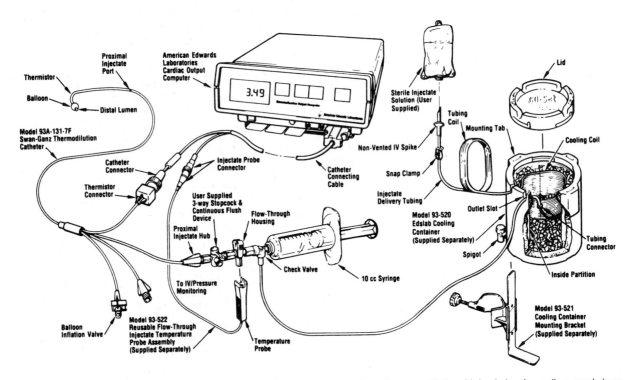

Figure 5–29. Schematic illustration of the closed injectate delivery system for use with iced injectate. A cooling container is not used for room-temperature injectate. (Courtesy of Baxter Healthcare Corporation, Baxter Edwards Critical-Care Division, Irvine, CA.)

onds) (Ganz and Swan, 1972), preferably at the end of expiration (Gardner, 1989).

6. The proximal port should be assessed for the patency and type of intravenous fluid infusing through this line during CO injectates. Vasoactive drugs should not be routinely administered through this line, because harmful effects could result from rapid CO instillations.

7. The patient should ideally be positioned in the supine position in a backrest elevation of zero to 20° (Doering and Dracup, 1988).

8. Three CO measurements should be obtained, and an average CO should be calculated. The first CO may be erroneous, especially if the catheter is filled with room-temperature fluid and ice injectate is used. If a 10% difference exists between these readings, the first value should be discarded and not used in averaging the CO.

A high correlation has been found when iced-temperature COs and room-temperature injectates have been compared. In some pathophysiological conditions resulting in high- or low-output states, investigators have recommended using 10 ml of iced injectate to allow for a more reliable reading (Gardner and Woods, 1989).

Continuous Cardiac Output

A distinctive PA catheter and monitor developed by Baxter-Edwards Co. now allows clinicians to obtain continuous CO readings (Fig. 5–30). This catheter has a specialized filament that delivers pulses of energy every 30 to 60 seconds. The filament warms the blood in the right ventricle, and the temperature change is detected by the thermistor at the tip of the PA catheter. The monitor in turn interprets the temperature change and averages the CO over a 3- to 6-minute period. No boluses are infused; thus, all the controversy in the research regarding the method of injectate or the temperature of the bolus infusion is not an issue with continuous COs. Furthermore, there are no delays between readings, no need to change the computation constant, and no extra fluid to be given to patients. The latest version of the Baxter-Edwards system combines continuous CO and S$\bar{v}$O$_2$ so that both parameters can be obtained simultaneously.

Recent research has indicated that the accuracy of continuous CO is similar to that of the intermittent thermodilution technique (Lichtenthal and Wade, 1993; Appavu et al., 1994) and may even affect patient outcomes by allowing clinicians to intervene in a more timely manner (Lichtenthal and Wade, 1994).

Table 5–2. CAUSES OF ERRORS IN CARDIAC OUTPUT

Faulty technique
Slow injection (>4 sec)
Injectate too warm (when using iced injectate method)
Incorrect computation constant set on computer
Incorrect position of PA catheter
Faulty thermistor
Catheter not properly connected to computer
Patient changes in position or movement
Dysrhythmias
Ventilators with positive end-expiratory pressure
Intracardiac shunts (atrial/ventricular septal defect)

Clinical Relevance

In the critically ill patient, the thermodilution method has gained widespread acceptance because of its accuracy, ease of use, safety, and ability to obtain repeated COs. The normal CO value is in the range of 4 to 6 L/min. CO varies with body size; for this reason, the cardiac index (CI) is used because this parameter takes into account the body size of a patient and is considered to be a more precise measurement of CO. The normal CI is 2.5 to 4.0 L/min/m^2. The formula is as follows:

$$CI = \frac{CO \text{ (L/min)}}{BSA}$$

where BSA = body surface area.

The body surface area in square meters can be calculated based on the patient's height and weight. The DuBois Body Surface Chart enables quick calculation of a patient's body surface area. CO computers automatically calculate the body surface area based on the height and weight of the patient that has been entered and also automatically calculate the CI.

The ability to obtain the CI enables health care personnel to assess patients' responses to pharmacological agents or fluid administration because changes in CO may occur soon after therapy has begun. Another use for the CI is assessment of ventricular pump performance. For example, if the left ventricle of a patient should begin to fail, one would expect a gradual decline to occur in the CI. This decline in turn has implications regarding the patient's prognosis (Table 5–3).

Alterations in the CI result from variations in SV or HR. Moreover, as was discussed earlier, three factors affect SV: preload, afterload, and contractility.

Causes of a low CI include the following:

1. Abnormally fast or slow HR that causes poor filling of the left ventricle

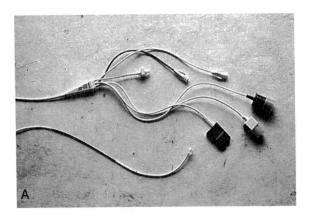

A

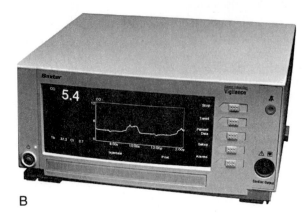

B

Figure 5–30. Continuous cardiac output catheter and monitor (Courtesy of Baxter Healthcare Corporation, Baxter Edwards Critical-Care Division, Irvine, CA.)

2. Low SV resulting from a decrease in preload that is caused by
    a. Diuresis
    b. Dehydration
    c. Third space shift
    d. Hypovolemia
    e. Vasodilation (septic shock)
3. Low SV caused by an increase in afterload as a result of
    a. Vasoconstriction due to hypothermia or low-flow states
    b. Left ventricular failure
    c. Increased blood viscosity
4. Low SV caused by a decrease in contractility (decreased cardiac function) as a result of
    a. Myocardial ischemia or infarction
    b. Cardiomyopathies
    c. Cardiogenic shock
    d. Cardiac tamponade
5. Valvular disorders, such as stenosis or regurgitation (insufficiency)

    Causes of a high CI can result from the following:

    1. Increased physical activity (exercise)

2. Increased anxiety
3. Pulmonary edema
4. Increased metabolic states (e.g., hyperthyroid, fever, tachycardia, adrenal disorders)
5. Anemia
6. Sepsis (initial stages)
7. Mild hypertension with a wide pulse pressure

Treatment of a low CI in the critical care patient is often aimed at correcting the underlying problem. Thus, the following therapies may be instituted:

1. Correct the abnormal HR by use of a pacemaker, pharmacological agents (beta-blockers, calcium

Table 5–3. CLINICAL STATES OF DECREASED CARDIAC INDEX (CI)

CI	Clinical States
2.0–2.2 L/min/m²	Onset of cardiac failure
1.5–2.0 L/min/m²	Cardiogenic shock
<1.5 L/min/m²	Irreversible stage of shock

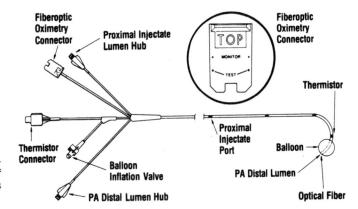

Figure 5–31. Mixed venous oxygen saturation fiberoptic pulmonary artery catheter. (Courtesy of Baxter Healthcare Corporation, Baxter Edwards Critical-Care Division, Irvine, CA.)

channel blockers, antidysrhythmic drugs) or elective cardioversion.

2. Increase the SV by increasing the preload via fluid administration (either crystalloid or colloid solutions) and by avoiding diuretics.

3. Increase the SV by decreasing afterload through the use of diuretics or afterload-reducing drugs, such as sodium nitroprusside (Nipride) or nitroglycerin.

4. Increase the SV by increasing contractility through the use of a positive inotropic agent, such as digitalis preparations, dobutamine, dopamine, epinephrine, isoproterenol (Isuprel), milrinone, and amrinone.

5. Replace a severely diseased cardiac valve that is causing the problem.

MIXED VENOUS OXYGEN SATURATION

Monitoring System

Mixed venous oxygen saturation is another hemodynamic parameter that can be monitored on a continuous basis or obtained intermittently via blood sampling. The advent of the fiberoptic PA catheter has enabled clinicians to obtain continuous $S\bar{v}O_2$ measurements. Intermittent measurements can be obtained by the drawing of blood from the PA distal port.

This blood is known as mixed venous blood because blood returns to the PA from various organs that have different oxygen needs. This venous blood is then "mixed" in the PA and therefore reflects an overall picture (represented by a percentage) of the oxygen used by the various tissues and organs.

After the mixed venous sample is drawn, it is sent to the laboratory for blood gas analysis. This analysis includes an $S\bar{v}O_2$ measurement as well as measurement of other mixed venous blood gas parameters.

The fiberoptic PA catheter (Fig. 5–31) is inserted in the same manner previously described in the section

on PA catheters. However, three distinct components exist that enable continuous $S\bar{v}O_2$ monitoring: (1) a fiberoptic catheter, which transmits and receives light waves; (2) an optical module, which sends and receives light to the end of the catheter via a fiberoptic channel; and (3) a microprocessor, which interprets $S\bar{v}O_2$ values by changing the light signal into an electrical signal that is then displayed as a digital numerical display (Fig. 5–32).

Clinical Significance of Mixed Venous Oxygen Saturation Value

The $S\bar{v}O_2$ is a measurement that reflects the degree to which the tissues of the body are using oxygen (demand) as well as the adequacy of the oxygen supply at the tissue level. In other words, it helps evaluate whether or not the oxygen supply can meet the oxygen demands of the tissues of the body. Oxygen supply is determined by several variables, such as the content of oxygen in the arterial blood (assessed by the hemoglobin), the partial pressure of arterial oxygen, the arterial oxygen saturation, and the delivery of this oxygen-rich blood to the tissues of the body (assessed by the CO). Oxygen demand is determined by the patient's condition. Factors that increase the oxygen demand include shivering, exercise, fever, pain, anxiety, increased work of breathing, turning activity, bathing or showering activity, back care, vasoactive drug therapy, and endotracheal suctioning. Therefore, if the oxygen supply cannot meet the increase in the oxygen demand, this condition is reflected in the $S\bar{v}O_2$ measurement.

The normal $S\bar{v}O_2$ measurement is 60 to 80%, and the mean $S\bar{v}O_2$ is 75%. Whenever the oxygen supply fails to meet the oxygen demand, the $S\bar{v}O_2$ decreases to less than 60%, a value that alerts the nurse that either the oxygen supply is too low or the oxygen demand is too high. Interventions are then aimed either at increasing the oxygen supply (increasing CO or increasing oxygen saturation via blood transfusion) or

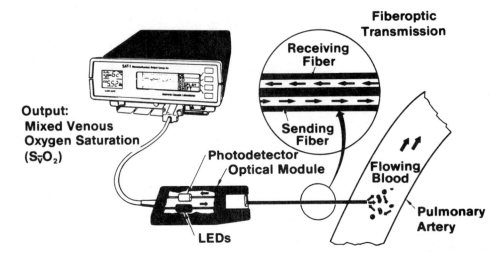

Figure 5–32. Illustration depicting the SAT-1 fiberoptic oximetry system from American Edwards Laboratories. LED = light-emitting diode. (Courtesy of Baxter Health Care Corporation, Baxter Edwards Critical-Care Division, Irvine, CA.)

at decreasing the oxygen demand (determining the factor that is increasing the demand and then alleviating or decreasing it).

Increases in $S\bar{v}O_2$ may occur when the oxygen delivery (supply) exceeds the oxygen demand or when a decrease in demand occurs. This increase may occur with the following conditions: hypothermia, anesthesia, early stages of septic shock, wedged PA catheter, or deposits of fibrin on the tip of the catheter. Table 5–4 summarizes many of the factors that increase or decrease the $S\bar{v}O_2$.

INTRA-ARTERIAL MONITORING

Intra-arterial monitoring is an invasive technique of monitoring arterial blood pressure. This method, as opposed to the noninvasive cuff technique, allows for continuous and accurate measurement of arterial pressure.

Although the sphygmomanometer method of determining arterial pressure is simple and accessible, for the critically ill patient, it is not always the most accurate. As the patient's SV falls, the Korotkoff sounds become more difficult to auscultate. This is why the intra-arterial method is preferred in unstable patients.

The most common noninvasive method of measuring blood pressure is sphygmomanometry, but blood pressure measurement can also be obtained noninvasively with electronic indirect blood pressure devices. With a sphygmomanometer, an inflatable cuff

Table 5–4. ALTERATIONS IN MIXED VENOUS OXYGEN SATURATION (SvO₂)

Alteration	Cause	Possible Cause
Low $S\bar{v}O_2$ (<60%)	↓ O_2 supply	Hypoxia or hemorrhage, anemic states, hypovolemia, cardiogenic shock, dysrhythmias, myocardial infarction, congestive heart failure, cardiac tamponade, massive transfusions of stored blood, restrictive lung disease, ventilation/perfusion abnormalities
	↑ O_2 demand	Strenuous exercise, hyperthermia, pain, anxiety or stress, hormonal imbalances, increased work of breathing, bathing, pheochromocytoma, thiamine/vitamin deficiency, septic shock, seizures, shivering
High $S\bar{v}O_2$ (>80%)	↑ O_2 supply	Increase in FiO_2, hyperoxia
	↓ O_2 demand	Hypothermia, anesthesia, hypothyroidism, pharmacological paralysis (pancuronium bromide or vecuronium bromide), early stages of sepsis, cirrhosis
High $S\bar{v}O_2$ (>80%)	Technical error	PA catheter in wedged position, fibrin clot at end of catheter, noncalibrated monitor

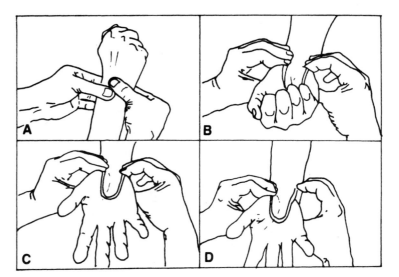

Figure 5–33. Modified Allen's test. When the patient's hand is held above the head with the fist clenched, both the radial and ulnar arteries are compressed (A). The hand is lowered (B) and opened (C). Pressure is then released over the ulnar artery (D). Color should return to the hand within 6 seconds, indicating a patent ulnar artery and an intact superficial palmar arch. (From Kaye, W (1983). Invasive monitoring techniques: Arterial cannulation, bedside pulmonary artery catheterization, and arterial puncture. *Heart and Lung, 12*(4), 400.)

attached to a mercury manometer is placed over an artery, generally at the brachial site. The cuff is then inflated with air until the artery is compressed against the underlying bones of the extremity. The pressure produced ultimately occludes the artery completely as the cuff pressure exceeds the systolic pressure of the extremity. A stethoscope is then placed below the cuff over the superficial artery. As the cuff is slowly deflated, blood is once again allowed to flow freely through the artery. As the first jets of blood pass through the artery, the sound produced is detected by the stethoscope. The corresponding pressure observed on the mercury manometer is recorded as systolic pressure, or the pressure generated by contraction of the ventricles. As the cuff continues to deflate, more blood is allowed to flow through the artery. When these sounds disappear, the corresponding measurement on the mercury manometer is recorded as diastolic pressure. Diastolic pressure is the pressure exerted on the arteries between cardiac contractions. The characteristic sounds auscultated with sphygmomanometry are called Korotkoff's sounds.

Equipment

The following components are required for the monitoring of intra-arterial pressure:

1. A catheter is placed into a radial, brachial, or femoral artery, either percutaneously or via surgical cutdown. If the catheter is placed into the radial artery, an Allen test should be performed to assess the patency of the radial and ulnar arteries (Fig. 5–33). In patients whose radial ulnar arch is not patent, a radial line should not be placed, because any thrombosis could

result in circulatory compromise to the hand, leading to possible limb loss.

2. A pressurized heparinized fluid source is attached to the arterial catheter in order to keep the catheter patent. The intravenous fluid should be pressurized to 300 mm Hg by use of an inflatable bag to prevent backflow of arterial blood into the tubing-catheter system. Sufficient pressure needs to be exerted to force the heparinized solution to flow against the patient's systolic pressure.

3. The transducer is attached to the hub of the catheter (see Fig. 5–10) via the connecting tubing. Once the transducer is attached to the monitor, it should be balanced, set to zero, and calibrated (see previous section on essential components of hemodynamic monitoring).

4. The bedside monitor amplifies the signal from the transducer and displays the arterial waveform on an oscilloscope. This arterial waveform is displayed continuously along with numerical values.

Arterial Pressure Waveform/Measurements

The normal arterial waveform consists of a steep ascent during systole, followed by a gradual descent during diastole. As the left ventricle contracts, the systolic pressure wave is transmitted to the transducer and is then depicted as a sharp rising wave. The systolic pressure is then measured at the peak of the waveform (Fig. 5–34). This pressure is considered to reflect the function of the left ventricle. Thus, if the left ventricle contracts poorly, the systolic pressure decreases in order to reflect this decrease in function.

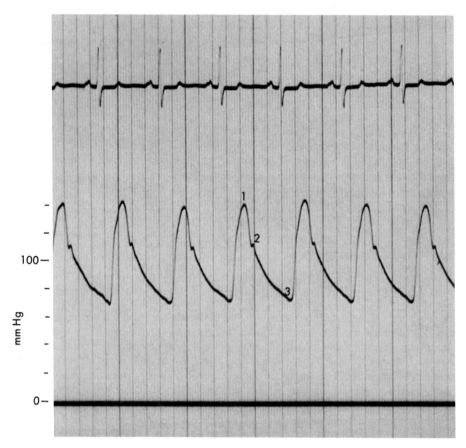

Figure 5–34. Normal arterial pressure tracing: (1) systole, (2) dicrotic notch, and (3) diastole. (From Daily, E. & Schroeder, J. S. (1990). *Hemodynamic waveforms* (2nd ed.) (p. 95). St. Louis, C. V. Mosby Co.)

The normal value of the systolic pressure is 90 to 140 mm Hg.

The diastolic pressure is shown as the lowest point on the arterial waveform (see Fig. 5–34). This pressure is a reflection of peripheral resistance. Therefore, if the resistance increases, the diastolic pressure also increases. The normal diastolic pressure is 60 to 80 mm Hg.

The dicrotic notch is a small notch on the downstroke of the waveform (see Fig. 5–34). It occurs as a result of the closure of the aortic valve. This closure is commonly considered the reference point between the systolic and the diastolic phases of the cardiac cycle.

The mean arterial pressure is a calculated pressure that closely estimates the perfusion pressure in the aorta and its major branches. It represents the average pressure in the peripheral arterial system during the entire cardiac cycle. However, it is not the average of the systolic and diastolic pressure but more closely approximates the diastolic pressure rather than the systolic pressure. It can be calculated by determining the area under the pulse-pressure curve, which is done by most patient monitoring systems. The mean arterial pressure (MAP) can be calculated by using the following formula:

$$\frac{\text{Systolic BP} + (2 \times \text{Diastolic BP})}{3}$$

The normal mean arterial pressure is 70 to 100 mm Hg. The mean arterial pressure must be maintained at greater than 60 mm Hg for the vital organs of the body to be perfused. The pulse pressure is defined as the arithmetic difference between the systolic and diastolic pressure.

Systolic pressure	=	140 mm Hg
Diastolic pressure	=	70 mm Hg
Pulse pressure	=	70 mm Hg

The pulse pressure widens when the systolic and diastolic pressures get farther apart. As these pressures become closer, the pulse pressure narrows.

Indications

Intra-arterial pressure monitoring is indicated for critically ill patients in whom continuous arterial pressure monitoring is essential. Ideally, any patient who is continuously receiving intravenous vasoactive drugs should undergo intra-arterial monitoring so that the response to therapy can be evaluated. Other populations that should undergo this monitoring include the following:

1. Patients in whom frequent arterial blood sampling is necessary
2. Patients in whom the rapid removal of blood (phlebotomy) is vital
3. Patients in low-flow states (shock) or who have hypotension
4. Patients who are severely hypertensive
5. Patients whose condition results in severe vasoconstriction or vasodilation

Complications

The major complications of arterial pressure monitoring include (1) thrombosis, (2) embolism, (3) blood loss, and (4) infection. Thrombosis (blood clot) may occur if a continuous flush solution with heparin is not used. Also, a greater incidence of thrombosis has been reported when the catheter used is very long (Kaye, 1983). In addition, radial artery catheters left in place longer than 48 hours increase the risk of thrombosis and infection (Kaye, 1983). Embolism may occur as a result of small clot formation around the tip of the catheter. In addition, air embolism may result from air's entering the closed tubing system, especially during intermittent flushing by hand.

Blood loss is usually a result of sudden dislodgment of the catheter from the artery in which it has been placed or from disconnection of the tubing. Rapid blood loss may occur (because this is in an artery not a vein) if either of these occurrences are not promptly recognized.

Infection is usually the result of a catheter's being left in place for a prolonged period of time. Most infections occur when catheters are in for more than 72 hours (Band and Maki, 1979). The incidence of infection is also increased when a catheter has been inserted via a surgical cutdown approach (Mandel and Dauchot, 1977). Good hand washing is also important for reducing the incidence of nosocomial infection.

Clinical Considerations

The invasive method of obtaining blood pressure is considered to be more accurate than noninvasive methods because it gives beat-by-beat information instead of measuring vibrations (Korotkoff's sounds) of the arterial wall over several beats. In patients who are hypotensive, a serious discrepancy may exist between the blood pressures obtained by invasive and noninvasive means, whereby the cuff pressure may be significantly lower, leading to dangerous mistakes in the treatment of such a patient. Under normal circumstances, a difference of 5 to 20 mm Hg between invasive and noninvasive blood pressure is expected, whereby the invasive blood pressure should be greater than the noninvasive value (Kaye, 1983).

When a difference between the invasive and noninvasive blood pressure is such that the noninvasive value is higher than the invasive number, one must become suspicious of equipment malfunction or technical error (Kaye, 1983). Table 5–5 lists the possible causes. One sign of a possible problem is a waveform that appears to decrease in amplitude, loses the dicrotic notch on the downslope (Fig. 5–35), and depicts low systolic pressure. This phenomenon is referred to as a *damped waveform*. This phenomenon indicates the presence of interference with the transmission of the pulse through the fluid-filled catheter to the transducer. A damped waveform could result from lodging of the catheter against the arterial wall, a clot at the catheter tip or in the stopcock, air in the transducer, or kinks in the tubing system. To make sure that this damped waveform does not indicate that the patient is becoming acutely hypotensive, the nurse should take a cuff pressure immediately and should compare that value to the intra-arterial value. If the noninvasive value is indeed higher, the nurse is then alerted to a possible technical problem and should investigate the system for one of the previously mentioned causes of damping. Damping caused by catheter obstruction may be

---

Table 5–5. CAUSES OF HIGHER NONINVASIVE VERSUS INVASIVE BLOOD PRESSURE

Air bubbles
Improper cuff size
Improper cuff placement
Incorrect calibration of sphygmomanometer
Improper calibration of transducer
Failure to zero the transducer
Blood in catheter system
Blood clot at catheter tip
Kinking of the tubing system
Loose or open connections
Dislodgment of catheter tip against arterial wall
Soft compliant tubing
Long tubing (>4 ft)
Too many stopcocks (>3)

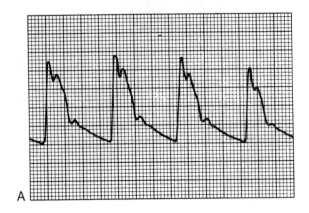

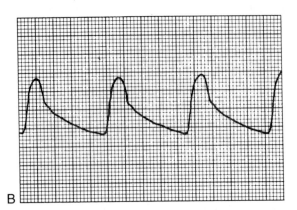

Figure 5–35. (A) Normal arterial waveform depicting sharp upstroke and clear dicrotic notch. (B) Damped waveform depicting slow upstroke, lower systolic pressure, and poor dicrotic notch. (From Jackle, M., & Halligan, M. (1980). *Cardiovascular problems: A critical care nursing focus.* Bowie, MD: Robert J. Brady.)

corrected by aspiration of any visible clots or by careful repositioning of the catheter if it seems to be lodged against the arterial wall.

Nursing Implications

Any nurse caring for a patient with an arterial line should try to prevent or reduce the incidence of complications. Thus, to prevent thrombosis, embolism, blood loss, and infection, the nurse must do the following:

1. Maintain a continuous heparinized flush solution through the catheter in order to prevent clot formation.

2. Document the insertion date of the catheter and keep the physician aware of placement time. The longer the catheter is in place, the greater the risk of clot formation is.

3. Keep the tubing free of kinks.

4. Maintain a pressure of 300 mm Hg on the flush solution.

5. Avoid intermittent flushing by hand so that the risk embolism is minimized.

6. Check the extremity frequently for color, temperature, sensation, and capillary refill.

7. Keep the patient's wrist in a neutral position and place it on an armboard.

8. Check for a damped waveform, and if noted, reposition catheter or aspirate for air or clots.

9. Tighten all connections and make sure that these connections remain tight so as to minimize possible blood loss.

10. Restrain an agitated patient to prevent sudden dislodgment of catheter or disconnection of tubing.

11. Set high and low alarms.

12. Ensure that adequate pressure is applied to the site of insertion for 10 minutes when the catheter is discontinued and withdrawn.

13. Keep sterile caps over the openings of stopcocks.

14. Change dressing by use of aseptic technique, according to recommendations outlined by the Centers for Disease Control and Prevention.

Summary

This chapter was designed as an introduction to the basic principles of hemodynamics and the technological aspects of hemodynamic monitoring. Discussion focused on the various types of hemodynamic monitoring used in the critical care setting, such as monitoring for CVP, LAP, PA pressure, PCWP, CO, $S\bar{v}O_2$, and arterial pressure. In addition, nursing considerations in the care of a patient undergoing each of these types of monitoring was highlighted.

Hemodynamic monitoring is an important physiological assessment tool in the care of critically ill patients. Data obtained from this modality should serve as a guide to the health care team in determining and evaluating interventions for such patients.

CRITICAL THINKING QUESTIONS

1. How does stroke volume affect cardiac output?
2. Describe how cardiac output affects the delivery of oxygen to tissues. What parameters would you monitor in a patient to assess this influence?
3. If a patient's mean arterial pressure continues to

RESEARCH APPLICATION

Article Reference

Driscoll, A., Shanahan, A., Crommy, L., & Gleeson, A. (1995). The effect of patient position on the reproducibility of cardiac output measurements. *Heart and Lung* 24(1), 38–44.

Review of Study Methods and Findings

This study was undertaken to determine the effect of patient position on the reproducibility of cardiac output measurements.

The design was a prospective study using a convenience sample of 30 patients who had a pulmonary artery catheter in place and were admitted to an intensive care unit. The subjects' age ranged from 39 to 80 years. They were assigned to one of two groups by the flip of a coin. Group A subjects were placed supine and after 5 minutes had cardiac outputs measured. They were then placed in the 45° upright position, and after an additional 5 minutes, cardiac outputs were measured. Group B underwent the reverse protocol: they were placed in the 45° upright position, underwent cardiac output measurement, then were placed in the supine position and underwent cardiac output measurement.

The results indicated that 70% ($n = 30$) of the sample population displayed a lower cardiac output in the 45° upright position than that obtained in the supine position, with the decrease ranging from 1 to 32% (mean decrease, 11%). Forty percent ($n = 30$) of cardiac output measurements obtained in the 45° upright position were greater than or equal to 10% less than those obtained in the supine flat position. The mean cardiac output was found to be statistically significantly higher ($P = 0.0083$) than the mean cardiac output at 45°. The effect of coexisting variables was analyzed with Kruskal-Wallis. The use of vasoconstrictive agents was the only variable in which a statistically significant change in cardiac output occurred that was associated with a change in position. The authors concluded that the results from this study indicated that cardiac output measurements are affected by alterations in patient position.

Brief Critique

This well-designed study had several limitations that were also noted by the researchers.

First, the sample population consisted mostly (80%) of cardiac surgical patients and thus was not representative of a group of intensive care unit patients and therefore the findings cannot be generalized to critically ill patients. Second, the cardiac index was not calculated for these patients. The cardiac index may not have been as statistically significant as the cardiac output, given the smaller parameter range. Third, the sample consisted mostly of elderly patients and was not normally distributed. Last, the most noted limitation was that these measurements were not performed over a long period of time; in time, the cardiac output measurements may have shown other variations.

Implications of the Study for Further Practice

The foremost implication, as noted by the researchers, was that the patient position in which the cardiac output measurements are obtained can be documented and that the cardiac output measurements can be obtained in the same position at which the previous measurement was obtained. It is hoped that this finding will ensure accurate comparisons between sequential readings. Further research is warranted in more diverse critically ill patients. Subsequent inquiry should be conducted that examines the cardiac index as well as the cardiac output.

The last implication is for patients with vasoconstrictive medications. They are more likely to have a decrease in cardiac output when cardiac output measurements are obtained in the upright position. Thus, it might be useful to compare these positions and find an optimal position for the patient.

rise significantly, indicating an increase in resistance and a diminished ability of the heart to eject blood, what parameters would also be altered as a result?

4. A patient who has undergone surgery has received a bed bath with back care and then undergoes suctioning and is turned. During these care activities, the patient experiences pain. What consequences does this have on the patient's hemodynamic status?

5. A patient is bleeding significantly and receives a transfusion of packed red blood cells. You note that the CVP remains low and that the CO drops again. What is the significance of these alterations? What additional interventions would you expect?

6. You are caring for a patient who requires CO measurements every 2 hours. What technical factors would you consider in obtaining an accurate intermittent CO reading?

REFERENCES

American Association of Critical Care Nurses (1993). Evaluation of the effects of heparinized and non-heparinized solutions on the patency of arterial pressure monitoring: The Thunder project. *American Journal of Critical Care, 2*(1), 3–15.

Appavu, S. K., Silver J., McKinney, G., Crosby, K., & Patel, S. (1994). Continuous cardiac output measurement. *International Journal of Critical Care Medicine, 5*(2), 13.

Band, J. D., & Maki, D. C. (1979). Infections caused by indwelling arterial catheters for hemodynamic monitoring. *American Journal of Medicine, 67*(5), 735–741.

Chulay, M., & Miller, T. (1984). The effect of backrest elevation on pulmonary artery and pulmonary capillary wedge pressures in patients after cardiac surgery. *Heart and Lung, 13*(2), 138–140.

Dobbin, K., Wallace, S., Ahlberg, J., & Chulay, M. (1992). Pulmonary artery measurement in patients with elevated pressures: Effect of back rest elevation and method of measurement. *American Journal of Critical Care, 1*(2), 61–69.

Doering, L., & Dracup, K. (1988). Comparisons of cardiac output in supine and lateral positions. *Nursing Research, 37*(2), 114–118.

Emerson, R. J., & Banasik, J. L. (1994). Effect of position on selected hemodynamic parameters in postoperative cardiac surgical patients. *American Journal of Critical Care, 3*(4), 289–299.

Ganz, W., & Swan, W. J. C. (1972). Measurement of blood flow by thermodilution. *American Journal of Cardiology, 29*, 241–245.

Gardner, P. E. (1989). Cardiac output: Theory, technique and troubleshooting. *Critical Care Nursing Clinics of North America, 1*(3), 577–587.

Gardner, P. E., & Woods, S. L. (1989). Hemodynamic monitoring. In S. L. Underhill, S. L. Woods, E. S. Sivarajan-Froelicher, & C. J. Halpenny (Eds.), *Cardiac nursing* (2nd ed.) (pp. 451–481). Philadelphia: J. B. Lippincott Co.

Grose, B. L., Adair, M., & Riem, M. (1981). Incidence of contamination of thermodilution cardiac output bath. *Circulation, 64*(Suppl. IV), 179.

Kaye, W. (1982). Catheter and infusion-related sepsis: The nature of the problem and its prevention. *Heart and Lung, 11*(3), 221–228.

Kaye, W. (1983). Invasive monitoring techniques: Arterial cannulation, bedside pulmonary artery catheterization, and arterial puncture. *Heart and Lung, 12*(4), 395–427.

Kennedy, G. T., Bryant, A., & Crawford, M. H. (1984). The effects

of lateral body positioning on measurements of pulmonary artery and pulmonary wedge pressures. *Heart and Lung, 13*(2), 155–158.

Levett, J. M., & Replogle, R. L. (1979). Thermodilution cardiac output: A critical analysis and review of the literature. *Journal of Surgical Research, 27*(6), 392–404.

Lichtenthal, P. R., & Wade, L. D. (1993). Accuracy of the Vigilance/Intellicath continuous cardiac output system during and after cardiac surgery. *Anesthesiology, 79*(3A), A474.

Lichtenthal, P. R., & Wade, L. D. (1994). Continuous cardiac output measurements. *Journal of Cardiothoracic and Vascular Anesthesia, 8*(6), 668–670.

Mandel, M. A., & Dauchot, P. J. (1977). Radial artery cannulation in 1,000 patients: Precautions and complications. *Journal of Hand Surgery, 2*(6), 482–485.

Osika, C. A. (1989). Measurement of pulmonary artery pressures: Supine versus side-lying head elevated positions [Abstract]. *Heart & Lung, 18*, 298–299.

Retailliau, M. A., Leding, M. M., & Woods, S. L. (1985). The effect of backrest position on the measurement of left atrial pressure in patients who have had cardiac surgery. *Heart and Lung, 14*(5), 477–483.

Runciman, W. B., Ilsley, A. H., & Robert, J. G. (1981). Thermodilution cardiac output: A systematic error. *Anesthesiology Intensive Care, 9*(2), 135–139.

Taylor, T. (1986). Monitoring left atrial pressures in the open heart surgical patient. *Critical Care Nurse, 6*, 62–68.

Whitman, G. R., Howaniak, D. L., & Verga, T. S. (1982). Comparison of pulmonary artery catheter measurements in 20° supine and 20° right and left lateral recumbent positions. *Heart and Lung, 11*(3), 256–257.

Wild, L. R. (1984). Effect of lateral recumbent positions on the measurement of pulmonary artery and pulmonary artery wedge pressures in critically ill adults. *Heart and Lung, 13*(3), 305.

RECOMMENDED READINGS

Briones, T. L. (1988). SvO$_2$ monitoring: Part 1. Clinical care application. *Dimensions of Critical Care Nursing, 7*(2), 70–72.

Cason, C. L., & Lambert, C. W. (1993). Positioning during hemodynamic monitoring: Evaluating the Research. *Dimensions of Critical Care Nursing, 12*(5), 226–232.

Cross, F. A., & Vargo, R. L. (1988). Cardiac output: Iced versus room temperature solution. *Dimensions of Critical Care Nursing, 7*(3), 146–149.

Daily, E. K., & Schroeder, J. S. (1994). *Techniques in bedside hemodynamic monitoring* (5th ed.). St. Louis: C. V. Mosby Co.

Enger, E. L. (1989). Pulmonary artery wedge pressure: When it's valid, when it's not. *Critical Care Nursing Clinics of North America, 1*(3), 603–618.

Gardner, P. E., & Laurent-Bopp, M. (1987). Continuous SvO$_2$ monitoring: Clinical application in critical care nursing. *Progress in Cardiovascular Nursing, 2*(1), 9–18.

Hardy, G. R. (1988). SvO$_2$ continuous monitoring techniques. *Dimensions of Critical Care Nursing, 7* 1),8–17.

Harper, J. (1992). Third level hemodynamics: Guiding clinical decisions. *Dimensions of Critical Care Nursing, 11*(3), 130–135.

Jackle, M., & Halligan, M. (1980). *Cardiovascular problems: A critical care nursing focus* (pp. 211–271). Bowie, MD: Robert J. Brady.

Kadota, L. (1985). Theory and application of thermodilution cardiac output measurement: A review. *Heart and Lung, 14*(6), 605–612.

Urban, N. (1993). Integrating the hemodynamic profile with clinical assessment. *AACN Clinical Issues in Critical Care Nursing, 4*(1), 161–179.

Urban, N. (1990). Hemodynamic clinical profiles. *AACN Clinical Issues in Critical Care Nursing, 1*(1), 119–130.

Verderber, A., & Gallagher, K. J. (1994). Effects of bathing, passive range of motion exercises, and turning on oxygen consumption in healthy men and women. *American Journal of Critical Care, 3*(5), 374–378.

Vitello-Cicciu, J. M., & Eagan, J. S. (1993). Data acquisition from the cardiovascular system. In M. R. Kinney, D. R. Packa, & S. B. Dunbar (Eds.), *AACN's clinical reference for critical care nursing* (pp. 471–507). St. Louis: C. V. Mosby Co.

Wadas, T. M. (1994). Pulmonary artery catheter removal. *Critical Care Nurse, 14*(3), 62–72.

6

Ventilatory Assistance

Mary Lou Sole, Ph.D., R.N., CCRN
Jacqueline Fowler Byers, Ph.D., R.N.

OBJECTIVES

- Review the anatomy and physiology of the respiratory system.
- Describe methods for assessing the respiratory system, including physical assessment, interpretation of arterial blood gases, and noninvasive techniques.
- Compare commonly used oxygen delivery devices.
- Discuss methods for maintaining an open airway.

- Identify indications for initiation of mechanical ventilation.
- Describe types and modes of mechanical ventilation.
- Relate complications associated with mechanical ventilation.
- Explain methods for weaning patients from mechanical ventilation.
- Formulate a plan of care for the mechanically ventilated patient.

Introduction

Maintaining an adequate airway and ensuring adequate breathing, or ventilation, are nursing interventions that are essential for all patients. These nursing interventions provide the framework for this chapter. Respiratory anatomy and physiology are reviewed in order to provide a basis for discussing ventilatory assistance. Assessment of the respiratory system is discussed, including physical assessment, arterial blood gas (ABG) assessment, and noninvasive methods for assessing gas exchange. Airway management and mechanical ventilation are also discussed.

Review of Respiratory Anatomy and Physiology

The primary function of the respiratory system is gas exchange. Oxygen and carbon dioxide are exchanged via the respiratory system to provide adequate oxygen to the cells and to remove excess carbon dioxide from the cells. The respiratory system can be divided into (1) the upper airway, (2) the lower airway, and (3) the lungs. The upper airway provides gas exchange to and from the lower airway, and the lower airway provides gas exchange to the alveoli. The anatomical structure of the respiratory system is shown in Figure 6–1.

UPPER AIRWAY

The upper airway consists of the nasal cavity and the pharynx. The bony structure of the nasal cavity is referred to as the nasal conchae. The nasal cavity conducts air, filters large foreign particles, and warms and humidifies air. The nasal cavity also is responsible for voice resonance, smell, and sneeze reflexes. The throat, or pharynx, transports both air and food. Air enters the superior part of the pharynx (the nasopharynx) and then passes behind the mouth through the oropharynx.

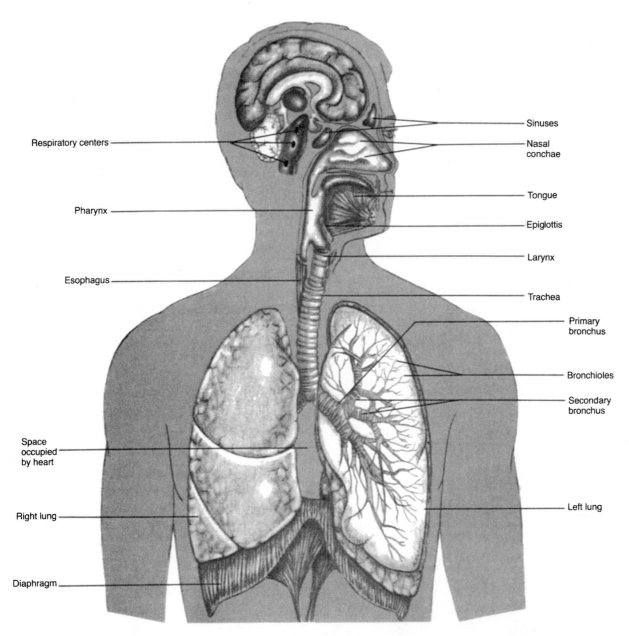

Figure 6–1. Anatomy of the respiratory system. The lungs are located in the thoracic cavity. The diaphragm forms the floor of the thoracic cavity, and separates it from the abdominal cavity. The internal view of one lung shows air passages. (From Solomon, E. P., & Phillips, G. A. (1987). *Understanding human anatomy and physiology* (p. 262). Philadelphia: W. B. Saunders Co.)

LOWER AIRWAY

The lower airway consists of the larynx, trachea, right and left mainstem bronchi, bronchioles, and alveoli. The larynx is the narrowest part of the conducting airways in adults. Also referred to as the voice box, the larynx contains the vocal cords. The larynx is partly covered by the epiglottis, which prevents aspiration of foods, liquids, or saliva into the lungs during swallowing. The passage through the vocal cords is called the glottis.

The windpipe, or trachea, warms, humidifies, and filters air. Cilia in the trachea propel mucus and foreign material upward through the airway. At about the level of the fifth thoracic vertebra (sternal angle, or angle of Louis), the trachea branches into the bronchi. This bifurcation is referred to as the carina.

The trachea divides into the right and left mainstem bronchi, which conduct air to the respective lungs. The right mainstem bronchus is shorter, wider, and straighter than the left. Mucosal cells in the bronchi trap foreign materials. The bronchi branch into the bronchioles, which in turn branch into the alveoli.

The alveoli are the distal airway structures and are responsible for gas exchange at the capillary level. More than 300 million of these tiny air sacs are present in the lungs. The alveoli consist of a single layer of epithelial cells and fibers that permit expansion and contraction. The alveoli are covered by a network of capillaries. Gas exchange occurs between the alveoli and these capillaries. The inner surface of the alveoli is coated with surfactant, which prevents them from collapsing. The structure of the alveolus is shown in Figure 6–2. The large combined surface area and single cell layer of the alveoli promote diffusion of gases.

LUNGS

The lungs consist of several lobes: the left lung has two lobes, and the right lung has three lobes. Each lobe consists of lobules, or segments, that are supplied by one bronchiole. The lungs are covered by the pleura, which consists of two layers. The visceral pleura is the inner layer that covers the lungs. The outer layer is referred to as the parietal pleura. The pleural space is the area between the parietal and visceral pleurae. The pressure in the pleural space, intrapleural pressure, is always negative (less than atmospheric) so that it can facilitate lung expansion on inspiration.

PHYSIOLOGY OF BREATHING

Changes in intrapleural pressure and intra-alveolar pressure (the pressure in the lungs) cause the act of breathing (Table 6–1; Fig. 6–3). At rest, intrapleural pressure is less than atmospheric (negative), whereas the intra-alveolar pressure equals atmospheric pressure. During inspiration, the diaphragm lowers and flattens, and the intercostal muscles contract, lifting the chest up and out to increase the size of the chest

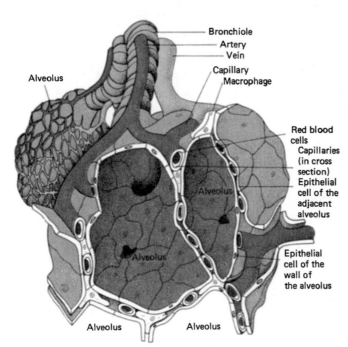

Figure 6–2. Structure and function of the alveolus. (From Solomon, E. P., & Phillips, G. A. (1987). *Understanding human anatomy and physiology* (p. 265). Philadelphia: W. B. Saunders Co.)

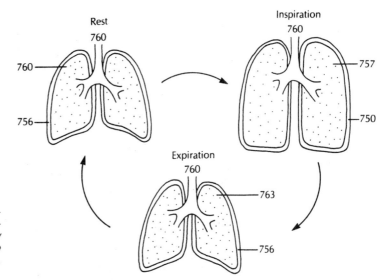

Figure 6–3. Changes in intra-alveolar and intrapleural pressures during inspiration and expiration. (From Harvey, M. A. (1992). *Study guide to the core curriculum for critical care nursing* (2nd ed.) (p. 5). Philadelphia: W. B. Saunders Co.)

cavity (Fig. 6–4). Subsequently, the intrapleural pressure becomes even more negative, and the intra-alveolar pressure becomes negative. Because atmospheric pressure is greater than both intra-alveolar and intrapleural pressure, air flows into the lungs. Expiration is considered a passive phenomenon. When intrapulmonary pressure in the lungs exceeds atmospheric pressure, expiration occurs; the diaphragm and intercostal muscles relax and the lungs recoil (see Fig. 6–4). This recoil generates positive alveolar pressure.

GAS EXCHANGE

The process of gas exchange (Fig. 6–5) consists of four steps: (1) ventilation, (2) diffusion at pulmonary capillaries, (3) perfusion (transportation), and (4) diffusion to the cells.

1. Ventilation is the movement of gases (oxygen and carbon dioxide) in and out of the alveoli.

2. Diffusion of oxygen (O_2) and carbon dioxide (CO_2) occurs at the pulmonary capillary level. Figure

6–6 illustrates diffusion of oxygen and carbon dioxide at the alveolar-capillary membrane. The alveoli contain higher levels of oxygen than exist in the capillaries, causing oxygen to diffuse from the alveoli into the capillaries. Carbon dioxide levels are higher in the capillaries, causing carbon dioxide to diffuse into the alveoli for elimination through the lungs.

3. The oxygenated blood in the pulmonary capillary is transported via the pulmonary vein to the left side of the heart. The oxygenated blood is perfused or transported to the tissues.

4. Diffusion of oxygen and carbon dioxide occurs at the cellular level based on concentration gradients. Oxygen enters the cells and carbon dioxide leaves the cells. Carbon dioxide is transported via the vena cava

Table 6–1. CHANGES IN INTRAPLEURAL AND INTRA-ALVEOLAR PRESSURES DURING INSPIRATION AND EXPIRATION

Pressures	At Rest (mm Hg)	Inspiration (mm/Hg)	Expiration (mm Hg)
Atmospheric	760	760	760
Intrapleural	756	750	756
Intra-alveolar	760	757	763

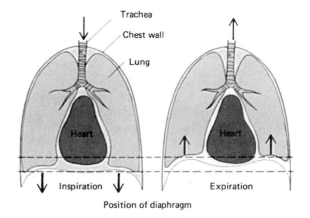

Figure 6–4. Changes in position of diaphragm during inspiration and expiration. (From Solomon, E. P., & Phillips, G. A. (1987). *Understanding human anatomy and physiology* (p. 265). Philadelphia: W. B. Saunders Co.)

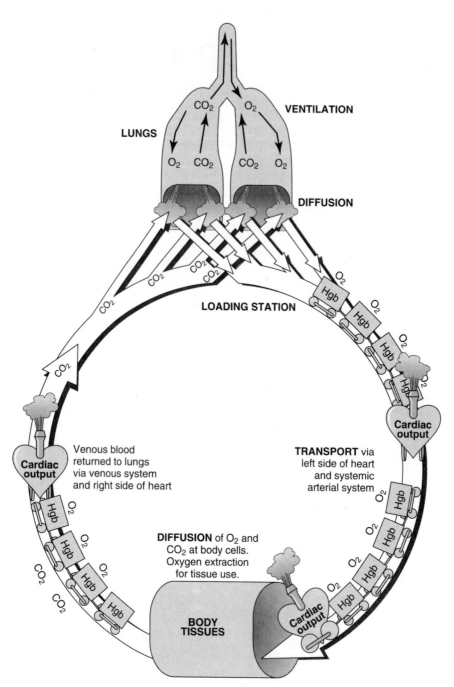

Figure 6–5. Schematic view of the process of gas exchange. Hgb = hemoglobin. (Adapted from Alspach, J. (1992). *AACN instructor's resource manual for the AACN core curriculum for critical care nursing* (Transparency 29). Philadelphia: W. B. Saunders Co.)

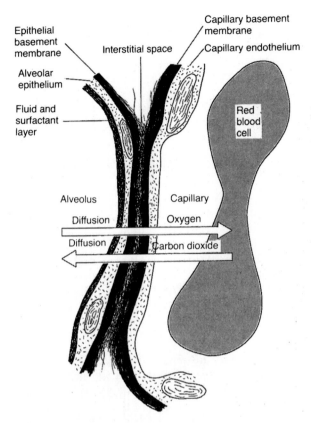

Figure 6–6. Diffusion of oxygen and carbon dioxide at the alveolar-capillary membrane. (From Guyton, A. (1991). *Textbook of human physiology* (8th ed.) (p. 429). Philadelphia: W. B. Saunders Co.)

to the right side of the heart for elimination through the lungs.

Numerous physiological features must be present for optimal gas exchange to occur. These include an intact nervous system, compliant lungs, a sufficient number of functioning alveoli, narrow alveolar-capillary membranes, an adequate hemoglobin level with normal shape, good cardiac output, and patent pulmonary vessels.

REGULATION OF BREATHING

The rate, depth, and rhythm of respirations are controlled by respiratory centers in the medulla and pons. When the carbon dioxide level is high or the oxygen level is low, receptors in the chemosensitive area of the respiratory center, carotid arteries, and aorta send messages to the medulla to regulate respiration. In individuals with normal lung function, respirations are stimulated by high levels of carbon dioxide. Many patients with long-term chronic obstructive pulmonary

disease (COPD) chronically have high levels of carbon dioxide, and they lose their ventilatory drive in response to these increased carbon dioxide levels. In these individuals, the stimulus to breathe is a low level of oxygen. These patients with chronically high levels of carbon dioxide should not be given high levels of supplemental oxygen, except in life-threatening situations, because it depresses their respiratory drive.

WORK OF BREATHING

The work of breathing is the amount of effort required for the maintenance of a given level of ventilation. The respiratory pattern changes automatically to assist in the work of breathing, depending on lung compliance and resistance. As the work of breathing increases, more energy is expended so that adequate ventilation can be obtained; this increased energy expenditure requires proportionately more oxygen and glucose.

Compliance

Compliance is a measure of the distensibility, or stretchability, of the lung and chest wall. It is defined as the change in volume per unit of pressure change.

Compliance = Change in Volume/Change in Pressure

Compliance is primarily determined by the amount of elastic recoil that must be overcome before lung inflation can occur. Elastic recoil, or elastance, refers to the ability of the lungs to return to a resting position after stretching during inspiration.

Elastic recoil and compliance are inversely related. For example, in pulmonary fibrosis, adult respiratory distress syndrome (ARDS), and pulmonary edema, lung tissue has greater elastic recoil that decreases distensibility. In these situations, compliance is low, and the lungs are stiff and difficult to distend. High pressures are required for inflation of the lungs. Severe obesity also decreases compliance because inflating the lungs in the presence of increased chest wall mass is more difficult.

In emphysema, destruction of lung tissue and enlarged air spaces cause the lungs to lose their elasticity. The decrease in elastic recoil causes compliance to be increased, or high. The lungs are more distensible in this situation and require lower pressures for ventilation.

Static compliance refers to compliance measured during a period of no airflow (e.g., while the patient holds his or her breath) and is an indicator of elastic recoil. An accurate measurement of static compliance is best performed in the pulmonary function laboratory.

The normal static compliance value is 200 ml/cm H_2O. In the mechanically ventilated patient with normal lung function, static compliance usually ranges from 70 to 100 ml/cm H_2O (Kersten, 1989).

Dynamic compliance is measured during breathing and is an indicator of both elastic recoil and airway resistance. Static compliance and dynamic compliance are usually equal in the normal adult. In the mechanically ventilated patient, dynamic compliance ranges from 50 to 100 ml/cm H_2O, or not more than 10 cm/H_2O greater than static compliance (Kersten, 1989).

Measurement of compliance in the mechanically ventilated patient is used for identifying trends in the patient's condition, not for diagnosing lung disease. Low compliance indicates increased lung elasticity, increased airway resistance, or both, and requires higher ventilatory pressures for adequate ventilation. Higher ventilatory pressures place the patient at increased risk for complications. Improved compliance reflects improved pulmonary status. The nurse or respiratory therapist routinely measures dynamic compliance and evaluates both the patient's pulmonary status and the appropriateness of current ventilator settings.

Resistance

Resistance refers to the opposition to gas flow in the airways. Resistance is increased with airway spasms (bronchoconstriction), mucus, and edema. Artificial airways, such as endotracheal tubes (ETTs), and ventilator tubing also increase airway resistance.

LUNG VOLUMES AND CAPACITIES

The lungs have several volumes and capacities that are important for determining adequate pulmonary function. Several of these terms are presented later in the chapter when methods and modes of mechanical ventilation are explained. Volumes are measured by a device called a spirometer. Lung volumes and capacities allow the practitioner to assess baseline pulmonary function (e.g., to determine surgical risk before surgery) and to monitor the improvement or progression of pulmonary diseases.

Volumes

Four different lung volumes can be measured. The total of these volumes equals the maximum volume that the lungs can expand. The volumes and capacities listed in this section are for healthy men; the values are approximately 20 to 25% less in women (Guyton, 1991). The lung volumes and capacities are shown graphically in Figure 6–7.

Tidal Volume (VT). The V_T is the volume of a normal breath. The average V_T is 500 ml, or 5 to 10 ml/kg.

Inspiratory Reserve Volume (IRV). The IRV is the maximum amount of gas that can be inspired at the end of a normal breath (over and above the V_T). The average IRV is 3000 ml.

Expiratory Reserve Volume (ERV). The ERV is the maximum amount of gas that can be forcefully expired at the end of a normal breath. The average ERV is 1100 ml.

Residual Volume (RV). The RV is the amount of air remaining in the lungs after maximum expiration. The average RV is 1200 ml.

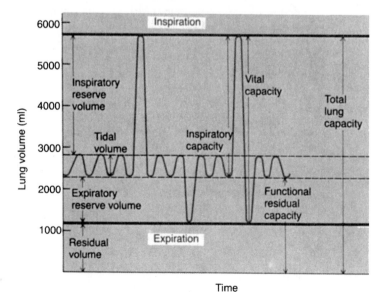

Figure 6–7. Lung volumes and capacities. (From Guyton, A. (1991). *Textbook of human physiology* (8th ed.) (p. 470). Philadelphia: W. B. Saunders Co.)

Capacities

Lung capacities consist of two or more lung volumes.

Inspiratory Capacity (IC). The IC is the maximum volume of gas that can be inspired at normal resting expiration. The IC distends the lungs to their maximum amount. The average IC is 3500 ml.

$$IC = V_T + IRV$$

Functional Residual Capacity (FRC). The FRC is the volume of gas remaining in the lungs at normal resting expiration. The average FRC is 2300 ml.

$$FRC = ERV + RV$$

Vital Capacity (VC). The VC is the maximum volume of gas that can be forcefully expired after maximum inspiration. The average VC is 4600 ml.

$$VC = V_T + IRV + ERV$$

Total Lung Capacity (TLC). The TLC is the volume of gas in the lungs at end of maximum inspiration. The average TLC is 5800 ml.

$$TLC = V_T + IRV + ERV + RV$$

Respiratory Assessment

Physical assessment of the respiratory system is an essential tool for the critical care nurse. Good assessment skills assist in identifying potential patient problems and evaluating patient response to interventions.

HEALTH HISTORY

Several questions should be asked when a patient's health history is obtained, including:

1. Tobacco use—type, amount and number of years used (or pack years)

$$\text{Pack years} = \text{Number of Packs of Cigarettes per Day} \times \text{Number of Years Smoked}$$

2. Occupational history, such as coal mining, asbestos work, farming
3. History of sputum production—type, amount, color, consistency, time of day, chronic or acute
4. History of shortness of breath, dyspnea, cough, anorexia, weight loss, or chest pain

5. Use of oral and inhalant respiratory medications, such as bronchodilators and steroids
6. Use of over-the-counter drugs
7. Allergies—medication and environmental
8. Date of last chest x-ray study and/or tuberculosis screening

PHYSICAL EXAMINATION

Inspection

Inspection provides an initial clue for potential acute and chronic respiratory problems. The head, neck, fingers, and chest are inspected for abnormalities.

Several assessments are made in the inspection of the head, neck, and fingers. Signs of acute respiratory distress include labored respirations with the use of accessory muscles, chest retraction, nasal flaring, asymmetrical chest movement, open-mouthed breathing, or gasping breaths. Cyanosis is a late sign of hypoxemia and should not be relied on as an early indicator of distress. Other indications of respiratory abnormalities include pallor or rubor, pursed lip breathing, jugular venous distention, prolonged expiratory phase of breaths, poor capillary refill, clubbing of fingers, or barrel-shaped chest.

The chest is observed for abnormal breathing patterns, use of chest and abdominal accessory muscles, asymmetrical chest wall movement, and abnormal chest excursions. The respiratory rate is noted, including the ratio of inspiration to expiration. The normal respiratory rate is 12 to 20 breaths per minute and expiration is usually twice as long as inspiration (inspiration to expiration ratio of 1:2). Alterations from normal should be documented and reported.

The normal breathing pattern is regular and even, with an occasional sigh. Normal breathing is referred to as *eupnea.* Alterations from this normal pattern should be noted. *Tachypnea* is defined as a respiratory rate of greater than 20 breaths per minute. Tachypnea may occur with anxiety, fever, pain, anemia, and blood gas abnormalities. *Bradypnea* is a respiratory rate of less than 10 breaths per minute. Bradypnea may occur in central nervous system disorders; it may also result from administration or ingestion of certain CNS depressant medications or alcohol, blood gas abnormalities, and fatigue.

Several abnormal breathing patterns (Fig. 6–8) are possible and should be reported to the physician if noted. *Cheyne-Stokes respirations* have a cyclical respiratory pattern. The patient has deep respirations that become increasingly shallow, followed by a period of apnea that lasts approximately 20 seconds. The cycle repeats after each apneic period. The apneic

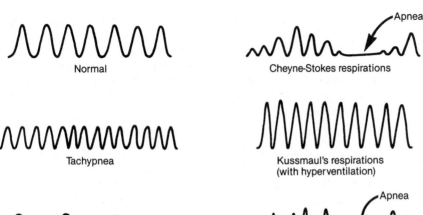

Figure 6–8. Breathing patterns. (Adapted from Kersten, L. D. (1989). *Comprehensive respiratory nursing* (p. 279). Philadelphia: W. B. Saunders Co.)

period may vary and progressively lengthen; therefore, the duration of the apneic period is timed for trending. Cheyne-Stokes respirations may occur in central nervous system disorders and congestive heart failure. *Kussmaul's respirations* are deep, regular, and rapid (usually more than 20 breaths per minute). Kussmaul's respirations commonly occur in diabetic ketoacidosis and other disorders that cause metabolic acidosis. *Biot's respirations*, or cluster breathing, are cycles of breaths that vary in depth and have varying periods of apnea. Biot's respirations are seen with some central nervous system disorders. *Apneustic respirations* are gasping inspirations followed by short, ineffective expirations. They are often associated with brain lesions.

The patient should also be observed for signs of COPD. Clues that might indicate COPD include wheezing, productive cough, pursed-lip breathing, barrel chest, and muscle wasting. The patient with COPD may also prefer to sit in a chair and lean forward rather than lie in bed.

Palpation

Palpation is frequently performed simultaneously with inspection. Palpation is used to evaluate chest wall and diaphragmatic excursion, tracheal deviation, chest wall tenderness, subcutaneous crepitus, and tactile fremitus.

During inspiration, chest wall excursion should be symmetrical. Asymmetrical excursion is usually associated with unilateral ventilation problems. The trachea is normally in a midline position; a tracheal shift may occur in tension pneumothorax. The chest wall should not be tender to palpation; tenderness is usually associated with inflammation or trauma. Subcutaneous crepitus, or subcutaneous emphysema,

is the presence of air beneath the skin surface. The fingertips are used to palpate for air under the skin. Subcutaneous crepitus may occur around chest tube and tracheostomy sites. It may also result from chest trauma, such as rib fractures, and from barotrauma.

Tactile fremitus is assessed by palpating the patient's chest wall with the palmar or ulnar surface of the hand and noting palpable vibrations transmitted through the chest wall while having the patient recite sounds that vibrate, such as "99." The intensity of vibrations is compared bilaterally. Tactile fremitus may be increased over consolidated areas of the lungs; vibrations may be decreased in pleural effusion and pneumothorax.

Percussion

The chest is percussed in order to identify respiratory disorders, such as hemothorax, pneumothorax, and consolidation. In percussion, the middle finger of one hand is tapped twice by the middle finger of the opposite hand. The vibrations produced by tapping produce different audible sounds, depending the densities of the area being percussed.

Five sounds may be audible on percussion: resonance, dullness, flatness, hyperresonance, and tympany. *Resonance* is the sound produced by percussion of normal lung tissue. Resonance is described as sounding like a muffled drum. *Dullness* is heard when tissue that is denser than normal is percussed and consists of a dull thud. Clinical conditions associated with dullness include pleural effusion, hemothorax, consolidation, atelectasis, tumors, and pulmonary fibrosis. *Flatness* is noted when air is absent in lung tissues. The sound heard with flatness is extreme dullness. Clinical conditions that may cause flatness include massive pleural effusion and lung collapse. *Hyperresonance* produces a slight musical sound, like a hollow drum, heard over tissue that has an increased amount of air. Clinical conditions associated with hyperresonance include emphysema, pneumothorax, and acute asthma. *Tympany* is a musical, drumlike sound produced by a large, air-filled area. Clinical conditions that produce tympany include tension pneumothorax or an air-filled cavity caused by an infection or abscess. Gastric distention may also produce tympany over the chest wall (Kersten, 1989).

Auscultation

Lung sounds are routinely assessed, often every 1 to 4 hours, in critically ill patients. Auscultation is performed for the assessment of quality of breath sounds, presence of adventitious lung sounds, and character of voice sounds.

A good stethoscope is essential for proper auscultation. The stethoscope should have both a diaphragm and a bell so that both high-pitched (diaphragm) and low-pitched (bell) sounds can be identified. Sounds are transmitted best through tubing that is thick and short; tubing that is too long decreases the transmission of sound. The ear pieces of the stethoscope should fit comfortably.

Several additional techniques facilitate auscultation. A quiet environment is essential. It may be necessary to turn off television, radios, and noise-producing equipment (e.g., hypothermia or hyperthermia units) during auscultation. The stethoscope should be placed directly on the chest; sounds are difficult to distinguish if they are auscultated through the patient's gown or clothing. When auscultation is performed over chest hair, the diaphragm should be held firmly against the skin in order to minimize a crackling sound that is produced by the hair. If auscultation must be performed over hairy areas, the chest hair should be wet with water before auscultation. Additionally, the stethoscope tubing should not rest against skin or objects such as sheets and bed rails during auscultation.

Auscultation is performed systematically. The anterior, posterior, and lateral aspects of the chest are auscultated (Fig. 6–9). Auscultation is best performed with the patient sitting in an upright position. The patient is asked to breathe deeply in and out through the mouth. Comparable pulmonary areas are auscultated on each side of the chest; the stethoscope is moved back and forth across the chest for comparison of sounds.

It may not be feasible for a critically ill patient to assume a sitting position for auscultation. In this circumstance, auscultation of the posterior and lateral chest is performed when the patient is turned to the side. Lung sounds must be evaluated both anteriorly and posteriorly so that all lobes are assessed.

Breath Sounds

Types of normal breath sounds include vesicular, bronchial, and bronchovesicular. *Vesicular* sounds are the breath sounds that are normally heard over the peripheral lung fields. They are heard throughout the chest, except over the central airways. Some texts classify vesicular sounds as "normal" breath sounds (Kersten, 1989). Vesicular breath sounds have a breezy quality, a moderate intensity, and a low pitch. Although the normal inspiration to expiration ratio is 1:2, vesicular breath sounds have an audible inspiration to expiration ratio of 3:1. This occurs because nearly all the air heard during expiration is expelled quickly, within the first third of the exhalation period.

Bronchial sounds are normally heard over the larger airways, that is, over the trachea and mainstem bronchus. They have a hollow, tubular quality; a loud intensity; and a high pitch. The audible inspiration to expiration ratio of bronchial sounds is 2:3. Bronchial lung sounds are not normally heard over the periphery; the presence of such sounds may reflect a disease process such as pneumonia.

Bronchovesicular sounds are normally heard over large central airways (e.g., over the sternum) and between the scapulae. They have a hollow, breezy quality; a moderate to low intensity; and a medium to high pitch. The audible inspiration to expiration ratio of bronchovesicular sounds is 1:1.

At times, breath sounds may be decreased. The presence of fluid, air, or increased tissue can cause decreased breath sounds. Some patients normally have decreased sounds in the left upper lobe related to differences in lung anatomy (Kersten, 1989). Shallow respirations can also mimic decreased breath sounds; therefore, the patient must take deep breaths during auscultation.

Table 6–2 reviews types of breath sounds.

Adventitious Breath Sounds

Adventitious, or abnormal, lung sounds include crackles, wheezing, and pleural friction rubs. Crackles (formerly called rales) are short, explosive, nonmusical, and discontinuous sounds. They are defined as fine to coarse, based on pitch. The presence of crackles usually indicates the presence of fluid in the alveoli and airways. Atelectasis is a frequent cause of crackles. Crackles are heard primarily in the inspiratory phase but may be noted during either inspiration or expiration. Crackles may also be audible when previously

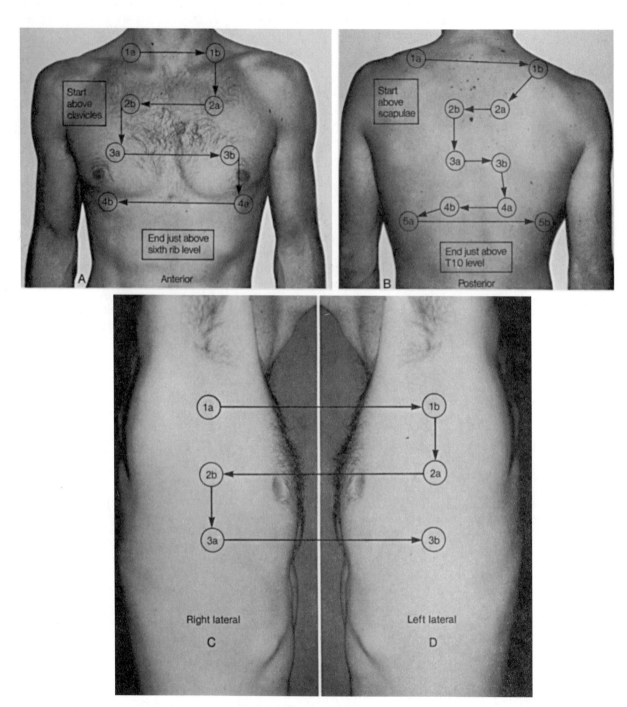

Figure 6–9. Systematic method for palpation, percussion, and auscultation of the lungs in *(A)* anterior, *(B)* posterior, and *(C* and *D)* lateral regions. The techniques should be performed systematically from a to b to compare right and left lung function. (From Kersten, L. D. (1989). *Comprehensive respiratory nursing* (p. 301). Philadelphia: W. B. Saunders Co.)

Table 6–2. TYPES OF BREATH SOUNDS

	Normal Location	Intensity	Pitch	Quality	I:E Ratio (Audible)	Graphic Representation
Normal	Throughout chest except over central airways	Moderate	Low	Breezy	3:1	
Decreased	Left upper lobe posteriorly in some people	Soft	Low	Breezy	3:1	
Bronchial	Over manubrium	Loud	High	Hollow, tubular	2:3	
Bronchovesicular	Over large, central airways: sternal area, between scapulae, right upper lobe posteriorly in some people	Moderate to loud	Medium to high	Hollow, breezy	1:1	
Tracheal	Over extrathoracic trachea (not usually auscultated)	Very loud	Very high	Hollow, harsh	5:6	

Adapted from Kersten, L. D. (1989). *Comprehensive respiratory nursing* (p. 302). Philadelphia, W. B. Saunders Co.
I:E = inspiration to expiration.

deflated airways are reinflated on inspiration; therefore, they sometimes disappear after coughing, suctioning, or taking of a deep breath.

Wheezes are continuous adventitious sounds resulting from rapid passage of air through narrow airways. They are high-pitched and musical when they originate in smaller airways, and low-pitched with a snoring sound when they originate in larger airways. Wheezes are more commonly heard on expiration, but the sounds may occur during both inspiration and expiration. Airway secretions sometimes produce wheezes; in this situation, wheezes should decrease after coughing or suctioning. (The American Thoracic Society has recommended that the term *wheezes* be used to classify all continuous adventitious sounds. However, some practitioners describe the musical sounds as wheezes and the snoring sounds as rhonchi. Both of these terms are used in Table 6–3 so that the learner better understands the associated problems and characteristics of the sounds.)

A pleural friction rub, or pleural rub, is a grating sound that occurs in the presence of inflammation of the pleura. Pleural rubs are usually heard during inspiration and expiration. If a rub is auscultated, a pleural rub must be distinguished from a pericardial rub because they sound similar. A pleural rub is audible during respirations, whereas a pericardial rub is audible with each heartbeat. A useful way to differentiate is to ask the patient to hold his or her breath; if the rub is no longer heard, it is a pleural friction rub. Adventitious lung sounds are reviewed in Table 6–3.

Voice Sounds

For the assessment of voice sounds, the chest is auscultated while the patient speaks. Voice sounds are transmitted from the larynx to the chest wall and are audible with a stethoscope. Voice sounds are normally muffled when auscultated because the vibrations are absorbed by the lung tissue.

Three abnormal voice sounds may be audible: bronchophony, egophony, and whispered pectoriloquy. Interpretation of abnormal voice sounds may be difficult and must be performed in relation to the entire pulmonary assessment. *Bronchophony* is an increase in the intensity of sounds heard when the patient says "99." Bronchophony may be present in lung consolidation. *Egophony* occurs when a loud-sounding "A" is heard when the patient says "E." Egophony may be present in lung consolidation. It is also commonly heard just above the fluid level in pleural effusion. *Whispered pectoriloquy* is an increase in intensity of the whispered voice when the patient says "99" or "1, 2, 3." It commonly occurs in consolidation.

Table 6–3. ADVENTITIOUS BREATH SOUNDS

Type	General Location	Associated Problem(s)	Characteristics	Graphic Illustration
Crackles (rales)	Peripheral airways and alveoli	Atelectasis Inflammation Excess fluid Excess mucus	Group of discrete crackles or popping sounds Discontinuous sound Usually inspiratory, may be inspiratory and expiratory	fine coarse
Rhonchi	Large airways	Inflammation Excess fluid Excess mucus	Coarse, low-pitched sonorous sounds Continuous sound Usually expiratory, may be inspiratory and expiratory	
Wheeze	Large and/or small airways	Bronchoconstriction (airway narrowing) from bronchospasm, fluid, mucus, inflammatory by-products, obstructive lesion Airway instability	High- (sometimes low-) pitched musical sound Continuous sound Usually expiratory, may be inspiratory and expiratory	
Pleural friction rub	Pleural surfaces	Inflamed or roughened pleural surfaces (pleuritis)	Grating sound with continuous and discontinuous qualities May appear intermittently Variable duration; usually inspiratory, may be inspiratory and expiratory Sounds the same or louder with coughing	

From Kersten, L. D. (1989). *Comprehensive respiratory nursing* (p. 310). Philadelphia, W. B. Saunders Co.

ARTERIAL BLOOD GAS INTERPRETATION

The ability to rapidly interpret ABG results is an essential critical care skill. ABG results reflect oxygenation, adequacy of gas exchange in the lungs, and acid-base status. Blood for ABG analysis is obtained either from a direct arterial puncture (radial, brachial, or femoral artery) or from an arterial line. Traditionally, ABGs are assessed periodically to aid in patient assessment. However, current technology allows continual ABG monitoring via fiberoptic sensors threaded through a catheter into the radial artery. Current continuous ABG monitoring systems are relatively accurate, particularly at a partial pressure of oxygen in the arterial plasma (PaO_2) of less than 150 mm Hg (Haller et al., 1994; Larson et al., 1994; Mahutte, et al., 1994; Venkatesh et al., 1994). They offer ongoing assessment of all ABG parameters in the critically ill patient without necessitating removal of blood for sampling. All blood gas findings should be interpreted in conjunction with the patient's clinical history and the physical assessment findings.

Oxygenation

The ABG values that reflect oxygenation include the PaO_2 and the arterial oxygen saturation of the hemoglobin (SaO_2). Oxygen is transported from the alveoli into the plasma. Approximately 3% of the available oxygen is dissolved in plasma. The remaining 97% of the oxygen attaches to hemoglobin in red blood cells, forming oxyhemoglobin.

PaO_2. The PaO_2 is the partial pressure of oxygen dissolved in arterial blood. The normal PaO_2 is 80 to 100 mm Hg at sea level. The PaO_2 decreases in the elderly; the value for individuals 60 to 80 years of age usually ranges from 60 to 80 mm Hg.

SaO_2. The SaO_2 refers to the amount of oxygen bound to hemoglobin. The normal saturation of hemoglobin ranges from 93 to 99%. The SaO_2 is very important because most oxygen supplied to the tissues is transported via hemoglobin.

Both the PaO_2 and the SaO_2 are used to assess oxygenation. Decreased oxygenation of arterial blood (PaO_2 < 80 mm Hg) is referred to as *hypoxemia*. Hypoxemia is different from hypoxia, which is a decrease in oxygen at the tissue level. Symptoms of hypoxemia are described in Table 6–4. A patient with a PaO_2 of less than 60 mm Hg requires immediate intervention, unless the patient has COPD and has adapted to lower oxygen levels. A PaO_2 of less than

Table 6–4. SIGNS AND SYMPTOMS OF HYPOXEMIA

Integumentary System
  Pallor
  Cool, dry
  Cyanosis (late)
  Diaphoresis (late)
Respiratory System
  Dyspnea
  Tachypnea
  Use of accessory muscles
  Respiratory arrest (late)
Cardiovascular System
  Tachycardia
  Dysrhythmias
  Chest pain
  Hypertension with increased heart rate
  Hypotension with decreased heart rate
Central Nervous System
  Anxiety
  Restlessness
  Confusion
  Fatigue
  Combativeness
  Coma

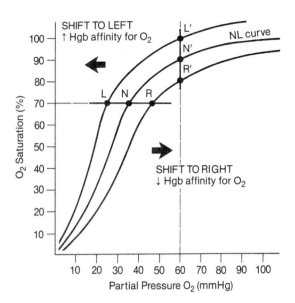

Figure 6–11. Shifts in the oxyhemoglobin curve. L = left shift; N = normal shift; R = right shift. (From Kersten, L. D. (1989). *Comprehensive respiratory nursing* (p. 48). Philadelphia: W. B. Saunders Co.)

40 mm Hg is life threatening because oxygen is not available for cellular metabolism, as is discussed later.

The relationship between the PaO_2 and the SaO_2 is shown in the S-shaped oxyhemoglobin dissociation

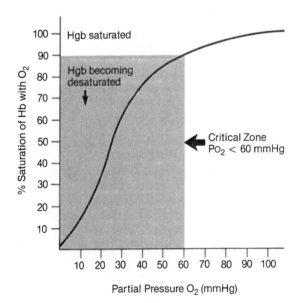

Figure 6–10. Oxyhemoglobin dissociation curve. The critical zone of the curve is noted. When the PaO_2 falls below 60 mm Hg, small changes in PaO_2 are reflected in large changes in oxygen saturation. (From Kersten, L. D. (1989). *Comprehensive respiratory nursing* (p. 48). Philadelphia: W. B. Saunders Co.)

curve (Fig. 6–10). Note that the upper portion of the curve ($PaO_2 > 60$ mm Hg) is flat. In this area of the curve, large changes in the PaO_2 result in only small changes in SaO_2. For example, the normal PaO_2 is 97 mm Hg and is associated with an SaO_2 of 97%. If the PaO_2 decreases to 80 mm Hg, the SaO_2 only decreases to 95%. Likewise, if the PaO_2 decreases from 80 to 60 mm Hg, the SaO_2 decreases from 95 to 90%. Although these examples reflect a drop in PaO_2, the patient is not immediately compromised, because the hemoglobin is still well saturated with oxygen.

The critical zone of the oxyhemoglobin dissociation curve occurs when the PaO_2 decreases below 60 mm Hg (see Fig. 6–10). At this point, the curve slopes sharply, and small changes in PaO_2 are reflected in large changes in the oxygen saturation. These changes in SaO_2 may cause a significant decrease in oxygen delivered to the tissues.

The oxyhemoglobin dissociation curve may shift in certain conditions (Fig. 6–11). When the curve shifts to the right, a decreased hemoglobin affinity for oxygen exists, resulting in the supply of increased oxygen to the tissues. Conditions that cause a right shift include acidemia, increased metabolism (e.g., fever), and increased levels of 2,3-diphosphoglycerate (2,3-DPG), which is a glucose metabolite that facilitates the release of oxygen from hemoglobin. Levels of 2,3-DPG are increased in anemia, chronic hypoxemia, and low cardiac output states.

When the curve shifts to the left, hemoglobin affinity for oxygen increases, and hemoglobin clings to oxygen. Conditions that cause a left shift include alkalemia, lowered metabolism, high altitude, carbon monoxide poisoning, and decreased 2,3-DPG level. Common causes of decreased 2,3-DPG level include administration of stored bank blood, septic shock, and hypophosphatemia.

Ventilation/Acid-Base Status

Blood gas values that reflect ventilation and acid-base include the pH, $PaCO_2$, HCO_3.

pH. The concentration of hydrogen ions (H^+) in the blood is referred to as the pH. The pH is the negative logarithm of the H^+ concentration. The normal pH is 7.40; the normal range for pH is 7.35 to 7.45. If the H^+ increases, the pH falls, resulting in acidemia. Conversely, a decrease in H^+ level results in a high pH and alkalemia. (The suffix "-emia" is used to refer to the alteration in pH. The suffix "-osis" is used to refer to the condition or process that causes the alteration in pH.) A pH of less than 7.11 is life threatening because vasodilation occurs.

$PaCO_2$. $PaCO_2$ is the partial pressure of carbon dioxide dissolved in arterial plasma. The normal $PaCO_2$ is 35 to 45 mm Hg. The $PaCO_2$ is regulated in the lungs. A $PaCO_2$ of greater than 45 mm Hg indicates respiratory acidosis, whereas a $PaCO_2$ of less than 35 mm Hg indicates respiratory alkalosis. If a patient hypoventilates, carbon dioxide is retained, leading to respiratory acidosis. Conversely, if a patient hyperventilates, excess carbon dioxide is excreted by the lungs, resulting in respiratory alkalosis. A helpful was to remember this concept is to think of carbon dioxide as an "acid" that is regulated by the lungs. Conditions that cause respiratory acidosis and alkalosis are noted in Table 6–5.

HCO_3. The HCO_3 is the concentration of sodium bicarbonate in the blood. The normal HCO_3 level is 22 to 26 mEq/L. HCO_3 is regulated by the kidneys. An HCO_3 level of greater than 26 mEq/L indicates metabolic alkalosis, whereas an HCO_3 level of less than 22 mEq/L indicates metabolic acidosis. It may be useful to think of HCO_3 as a substance that neutralizes acids. Therefore, a high HCO_3 value indicates the presence of metabolic alkalosis, and a low HCO_3 value indicates the presence of metabolic acidosis. Conditions that cause metabolic acidosis and alkalosis are noted in Table 6–5.

Buffer System

The body regulates acid-base balance through the buffer system. The buffer system can be described as a mechanism for the neutralization of acids. Three

Table 6–5. CAUSES OF COMMON ACID-BASE ABNORMALITIES

Respiratory Acidosis: Retention of carbon dioxide
  Central nervous system disorders
  Drug overdose
  Pneumonia
  Pulmonary edema
  Pneumothorax
  Restrictive lung diseases
Respiratory Alkalosis: Hyperventilation
  Anxiety, fear
  Pain
  Fever
  Pneumonia
  Atelectasis
  Asthma
  Adult respiratory distress syndrome (ARDS)
  Congestive heart failure, pulmonary edema
  Pulmonary embolus
  Central nervous system disorders
Metabolic Acidosis: Gain of metabolic acids or loss of base
  Increased acids
    Renal failure
    Diabetic ketoacidosis
    Anaerobic metabolism
    Drug overdose (salicylates, methanol)
  Loss of base
    Diarrhea
Metabolic Alkalosis: Gain of base or loss of metabolic acids
  Gain of base
    Excess ingestion of antacids
    Excess administration of sodium bicarbonate
  Loss of metabolic acids
    Vomiting
    Nasogastric suctioning/lavage
    Low potassium and/or chloride
    Increased levels of aldosterone
    Administration of steroids and/or diuretics

Adapted from Kersten, L. D. (1989). *Comprehensive respiratory nursing.* Philadelphia, W. B. Saunders Co.

buffer systems exist for maintaining acid-base status: the buffer system in the blood, that in the respiratory system, and that in the renal system (Fig. 6–12).

The blood buffer system is activated as the H^+ concentration changes. As H^+ level increases, the pH falls, resulting in acidosis. Bicarbonate (HCO_3) then combines with H^+ to form carbonic acid (H_2CO_3). Carbonic acid then breaks down into carbon dioxide (which is excreted through the lungs) and water (H_2O). The equation for this mechanism is as follows:

$$H^+ + HCO_3 \leftrightarrow H_2CO_3 \leftrightarrow H_2O + CO_2$$

The respiratory buffer system works by excreting excess carbon dioxide from the lungs. The respiratory buffer system begins to work immediately after an

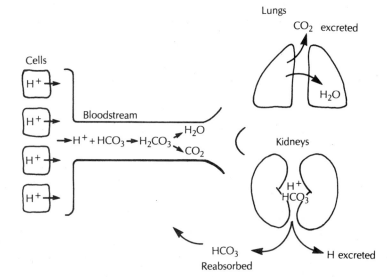

Figure 6-12. Buffer systems that regulate the body's acid-base balance. HCO_3^- = bicarbonate; H_2CO_3 = carbonic acid. (Adapted from Harvey, M. A. (1992). *Study guide to the core curriculum for critical care nursing* (2nd ed.) (p. 11). Philadelphia: W. B. Saunders Co.)

acid-base alteration is noted. The renal buffer system works by excreting excess H^+ and retaining bicarbonate. The renal buffer system activates more slowly and may take up to 2 days to regulate acid-base balance.

Steps in Arterial Blood Gas Interpretation

Arterial blood gas results should be interpreted systematically. The oxygenation is evaluated first. Second, the acid-base status is determined. Third, the primary imbalance is identified. Last, compensation, if any, is identified.

STEP 1. Evaluate Oxygenation

Oxygenation is analyzed by evaluation of the PaO_2 and the SaO_2. If the PaO_2 is less than the expected normal range, hypoxemia exists. PaO_2 is normally lower in the elderly and some patients with COPD.

STEP 2. Evaluate Acid-Base Status

For evaluation of acid-base status, the remainder of the ABG values are assessed individually.

1. Evaluate the pH. A pH of less than 7.35 indicates the presence of acidemia; a pH of greater than 7.45 indicates the presence of alkalemia.

2. Evaluate the $PaCO_2$. A $PaCO_2$ of less than 35 mm Hg indicates the presence of respiratory alkalosis or hyperventilation; a $PaCO_2$ of greater than 45 mm Hg indicates the presence of respiratory acidosis or hypoventilation.

3. Evaluate the HCO_3. An HCO_3 value of less than 22 mm Hg indicates the presence of metabolic acidosis; a HCO_3 of greater than 26 mm Hg indicates the presence of metabolic alkalosis.

STEP 3. Determine Primary Acid-Base Imbalance

The ABG results may reflect only one disorder. However, frequently, two acid-base disorders occur simultaneously (Table 6-6). Usually one is a *primary* disorder, whereas the other is a compensatory process aimed at restoring the acid-base balance. The *primary* cause of the acid-base imbalance is determined by evaluation of the pH. If the pH is less than 7.4, the primary disorder is acidosis. If the pH is greater than

Table 6-6. INTERPRETATION OF ARTERIAL BLOOD GAS RESULTS

	$PaCO_2 < 35$ mm Hg	$PaCO_2$ 35–45 mm Hg	$PaCO_2 > 45$ mm Hg
HCO_3 <22 mEq/L	Respiratory alkalosis Metabolic acidosis	Metabolic acidosis	Respiratory acidosis Metabolic acidosis
HCO_3 22–26 mEq/L	Respiratory alkalosis	Normal	Respiratory acidosis
HCO_3 >26 mEq/L	Respiratory alkalosis Metabolic alkalosis	Metabolic alkalosis	Respiratory acidosis Metabolic alkalosis

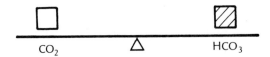

CO$_2$ △ HCO$_3$

An abnormal relationship creates an imbalance.

Acidosis   Alkalosis

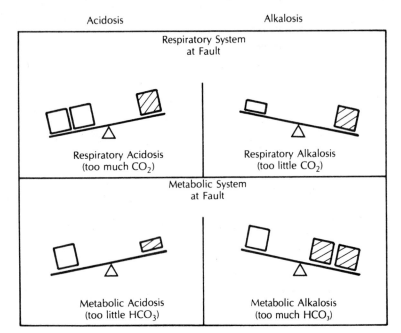

Figure 6–13. Acid-base imbalances. (From Harvey, M. A. (1992). *Study guide to the core curriculum for critical care nursing* (2nd ed.) (p. 11). Philadelphia: W. B. Saunders Co.)

7.4, the primary disorder is alkalosis. Occasionally, two primary disorders may occur simultaneously. For example, during cardiac arrest, both respiratory and metabolic acidosis commonly occur because of hypoventilation and lactic acidosis. Figure 6–13 illustrates the concepts of acid-base imbalances.

STEP 4. Determine Compensation

As previously noted, the body has three buffer systems that maintain a constant acid-base balance. If an abnormality is present, one or more buffer systems are activated in order to reverse the acid-base abnormality. For example, if a patient has respiratory acidosis, such as occurs in COPD (low pH, high PaCO$_2$), the kidneys respond by retaining more HCO$_3$ and excreting H$^+$ (metabolic alkalosis). Conversely, if a patient is in metabolic acidosis, such as occurs in severe vomiting or salicylate overdose (low pH, low HCO$_3$), the lungs respond by hyperventilation and excretion of carbon dioxide (respiratory alkalosis). A summary of compensatory mechanisms is shown in Table 6–7.

Compensation may be absent, partial, or complete. Compensation is absent if the usual compensatory mechanisms do not occur in response to a primary acid-base disturbance. If compensatory mechanisms are noted but the pH is still abnormal, compensation is partial. If compensatory mechanisms are present and the pH is within normal range, compensation is complete. Examples of ABGs and compensation are shown in Table 6–8.

NONINVASIVE ASSESSMENT OF GAS EXCHANGE

Arterial blood gas results have been the "gold standard" for the monitoring of gas exchange and acid-base status. In addition to invasive continuous ABG monitoring capability, several noninvasive tech-

Table 6–7. COMPENSATORY MECHANISMS IN ACID-BASE DISTURBANCES

Acid-Base Disturbance	Usual Compensatory Mechanism
Respiratory acidosis	Metabolic alkalosis
Respiratory alkalosis	Metabolic acidosis
Metabolic acidosis	Respiratory alkalosis
Metabolic alkalosis	Respiratory acidosis

Table 6–8. EXAMPLES OF ARTERIAL BLOOD GASES AND COMPENSATION

Example 1:
PaO_2	80 mm Hg (normal)
pH	7.30 (low; acidosis)
$PaCO_2$	50 mm Hg (high; respiratory acidosis)
HCO_3	22 mEq/L (normal)
Interpretation:	Respiratory acidosis; no compensation

Example 2:
PaO_2	80 mm Hg (normal)
pH	7.32 (low; acidosis)
$PaCO_2$	50 mm Hg (high; respiratory acidosis)
HCO_3	28 mEq/L (high; metabolic alkalosis)
Interpretation:	Partly compensated respiratory acidosis. The ABGs are only "partly compensated" because the pH is not yet within normal limits.

Example 3:
PaO_2	80 mm Hg (normal)
pH	7.36 (normal)
$PaCO_2$	50 mm Hg (high; respiratory acidosis)
HCO_3	29 mEq/L (high; metabolic alkalosis)
Interpretation:	Completely (fully) compensated respiratory acidosis. The pH is now within normal limits; therefore, complete compensation has occurred.

niques are available for the assessment of gas exchange: pulse oximetry, transcutaneous monitoring of oxygen and carbon dioxide, capnometry, and capnography.

Assessment of Oxygenation

Pulse Oximetry

The use of pulse oximeters has become commonplace in critical care units, the operating room, postanesthesia recovery units, and emergency departments. Pulse oximetry measures a value called SpO_2 and reflects the arterial oxygen saturation (SaO_2). Pulse oximetry uses light-emitting diodes to measure pulsatile flow and light absorption of the hemoglobin. A sensor that measures SpO_2 is placed on the finger, toe, ear, or forehead.

The oxyhemoglobin dissociation curve (see Fig. 6–10) shows the relationship between SaO_2 and PaO_2 and provides the basis for pulse oximetry. Note that an SaO_2 of 95% is equivalent to a PaO_2 of 80 mm Hg, whereas an SaO_2 of 90% is equivalent to a PaO_2 of 60 mm Hg, which is often considered the "critical zone." As previously discussed, when the PaO_2 decreases to less than 60 mm Hg, small changes in PaO_2 result in large changes in SaO_2. In general, SpO_2 values of

less than 90% require further assessment and rapid intervention.

Table 6–9 assists in interpretation of SpO_2 values. Factors that may shift the curve to the right or left must be considered in the interpretation of SpO_2 values. In addition to monitoring oxygenation, pulse oximetry may be used for weaning patients from mechanical ventilation and for monitoring patients' response to treatment (e.g., ventilator changes, pulmonary hygiene, suctioning). However, SpO_2 measures only oxygenation. Changes in ventilation (e.g., carbon dioxide retention or apnea) cannot be assessed with pulse oximetry.

Transcutaneous Monitoring of Partial Pressure of Arterial Oxygen

Transcutaneous PaO_2 ($tcPaO_2$) devices are primarily used in neonates to monitor oxygen levels. In $tcPaO_2$ monitoring, an electrode that records the oxygen level is attached to the skin. The device includes a heater that causes vasodilation under the electrode for the enhancement of oxygen diffusion. The $tcPaO_2$ reflects the PaO_2; however, the $tcPaO_2$ value is usually lower than the actual PaO_2, particularly if the electrode is placed on a poorly perfused area. Pulse oximetry is most commonly used to noninvasively assess arterial oxygenation; however, one potential use of $tcPaO_2$ is to detect peripheral hypoxia in the presence of trauma or wounds (Ahrens, 1993).

Assessment of Ventilation

Transcutaneous Monitoring of Carbon Dioxide

Transcutaneous monitoring of carbon dioxide ($tcPaCO_2$) is similar to transcutaneous measurement of oxygen. In fact, most transcutaneous monitoring electrodes measure both oxygen and carbon dioxide

Table 6–9. INTERPRETATION OF PULSE OXIMETRY VALUES (SpO_2)

Value on Pulse Oximeter (%)	Probable PaO_2
97	100
95	80
94	70
90	60
85	50
75	40
57	30
32	20
10	10

Table 6–10. OXYGEN DELIVERY DEVICES

Device	Oxygen Flow Rate (L/min)	Approximate FiO$_2$
Nasal cannula	1	0.24
	2	0.28
	3	0.32
	4	0.36
	5	0.40
	6	0.44
Face mask	5–6	0.40
	6–7	0.50
	7–8	0.60
Masks with reservoirs	6	0.60
	7	0.70
	8	0.80
	9	0.80–1.00
	10	0.80–1.00
Venturi mask	4	0.24
	5	0.28
	6	0.31
	7	0.35
	8	0.40
	10	0.50

(Hess and Kacmarek, 1993). Noninvasive measurement of tcPaCO$_2$ may be as much as one to two times higher than actual PaCO$_2$; therefore, it is best used to monitor patient *trends* rather than actual values (VonRueden, 1990).

End-Tidal Carbon Dioxide Monitoring

The measurement of expired carbon dioxide is referred to as capnometry, whereas capnography is the recording of carbon dioxide during the respiratory cycle. In end-tidal carbon dioxide monitoring, infrared light is used to measure carbon dioxide concentrations. The most common method of end-tidal carbon dioxide monitoring samples expired gas from an endotracheal tube (ETT), oral airway, or nasopharyngeal airway. The end-tidal carbon dioxide value correlates moderately with the PaCO$_2$ in patients with normal lung and cardiac function. Researchers have found end-tidal carbon dioxide values to consistently underestimate PaCO$_2$ and to move in the opposite direction of changes in PaCO$_2$ 22% of the time (Christensen et al., 1995). Therefore, end-tidal carbon dioxide values should be used for the evaluation of ventilation when precision is not essential. Uses of end-tidal carbon dioxide include monitoring the patient's response to ventilator changes and respiratory treatments, determining the proper position of the ETT, weaning the patient from mechanical ventilation, and detecting ventilator disconnection from the patient receiving neuromuscular blocking agents. It may also be useful in monitoring the effectiveness of cardiopulmonary resuscitation (VonRueden, 1990).

Oxygen Administration

Oxygen is frequently administered for the treatment or prevention of hypoxemia. Oxygen may be supplied by various sources: it may be piped into wall devices in hospital rooms, or it may be supplied by oxygen tanks or oxygen concentrators. Several devices are available for oxygen delivery to the patient. Oxygen is preferably humidified because administration can dry the mucous membranes.

COMMONLY USED OXYGEN DELIVERY DEVICES

Commonly used oxygen delivery devices include the nasal cannula, the face mask, the face mask with reservoir, and the Venturi mask. The oxygen delivery devices are summarized in Table 6–10. Generally, the least obtrusive method that provides adequate oxygenation is employed.

Nasal Cannula

A nasal cannula, or nasal prongs, are commonly used to deliver oxygen (Fig. 6–14). The device is relatively comfortable and is an inexpensive method of oxygen delivery. Oxygen delivered via a nasal cannula is usually administered at rates of 1 to 6 L/min. Oxygen administered at 1 L/min usually provides a fraction of inspired oxygen (FiO$_2$) of 0.24, depending on the patient's respiratory pattern. The FiO$_2$ increases by approximately 0.04 with each increase in liter of flow. Administration at greater than 6 L/min is not effective in increasing oxygenation.

Face Mask

The face mask delivers oxygen through a simple mask device (Fig. 6–15). A mask appropriate to the

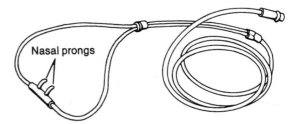

Figure 6–14. Nasal cannula. (From Kersten, L. D. (1989). *Comprehensive respiratory nursing* (p. 608). Philadelphia: W. B. Saunders Co.)

Nasal prongs

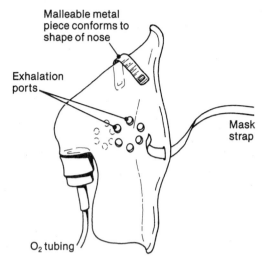

Malleable metal piece conforms to shape of nose

Exhalation ports

Mask strap

O_2 tubing

Figure 6–15. Simple face mask. (From Kersten, L. D. (1989). *Comprehensive respiratory nursing* (p. 609). Philadelphia: W. B. Saunders Co.)

size of the patient's face should be chosen for patient comfort. Oxygen is delivered at rates of 5 to 8 L/min, providing an FiO_2 of 0.40 to 0.60.

Face Masks With Reservoirs

These types of masks (Fig. 6–16), the partial rebreathing mask and the nonrebreathing mask, are used to provide oxygen concentrations of 60% or more. A reservoir is attached to the face mask. The purpose of the reservoir is to increase the amount of oxygen delivered to the patient. The partial rebreather delivers an FiO_2 of up to 0.60 at flow rates between 6 and 10 L/min. The nonrebreather delivers an FiO_2 of 0.80 to 1.00 at flow rates of 9 to 10 L/min. Either mask may be used in the critically ill patient with severe hypoxemia in an effort to prevent the need for endotracheal intubation and mechanical ventilation.

Venturi Mask

The Venturi mask, or Venti-mask, is a device that can deliver a high flow of oxygen at a fixed concentration (Fig. 6–17). Venturi masks ensure the accurate delivery of oxygen. Oxygen delivery is controlled by adjusting an adapter which alters the flow of oxygen. Venturi masks are commonly used in the patient with pulmonary disease so that the level of oxygen can be closely regulated to prevent complications associated with oxygen administration.

Bag-Valve Devices

If a patient needs assistance in breathing as well as oxygenation, a bag-valve device is used (see Chapter 7). The bag-valve device is also referred to as a manual resuscitation bag, or Ambu bag. The bag-valve device can be used with a face mask to ventilate and oxygenate a patient who is not breathing. It can also be attached to an ETT to ventilate an intubated patient. The bag-valve device should have a reservoir bag attached in order to increase the delivery of oxygen, and it should be connected to an oxygen source delivering 100% oxygen (usually 15 L/min).

Airway Management

POSITIONING

A patent airway is essential to survival. A primary nursing intervention with any patient is the maintenance of an open airway. The first method for maintaining a patent airway is proper head position. The head-tilt/chin-lift method is recommended for the maintenance of an open airway (see Chapter 7).

ORAL AIRWAYS

Other methods for maintaining an open airway include oral and nasopharyngeal airways (Fig. 6–18). Oral airways are rigid tubes that prevent the tongue from falling into the pharynx (Fig. 6–19). Oral airways are used for many reasons: to facilitate secretion removal from the oropharynx, to maintain an open airway when it is necessary to ventilate a patient with a bag-valve device and face mask, to prevent a patient from biting on an ETT, and to maintain an open airway in patients prone to seizures.

Sizes of oral airways vary from small adult (80 mm long) to medium adult (90 mm) to large adult (100 mm). Several brands are available. Some oral airways are made of rigid plastic, whereas others are made of softer plastic. The configuration of the tubes also varies.

The technique for inserting an oral airway is described in Table 6–11. After insertion, the nurse looks, listens, and feels for air movement through the mouth while observing the chest rise and fall. Noises indicating upper airway obstruction should be absent. Complications of oral airways include airway obstruction if the airway is too long, accumulation of secretions, trauma to the lips and tongue, and gagging in a conscious patient.

NASOPHARYNGEAL AIRWAYS

Nasopharyngeal airways, also known as nasal airways or nasal trumpets, are soft rubber or latex tubes

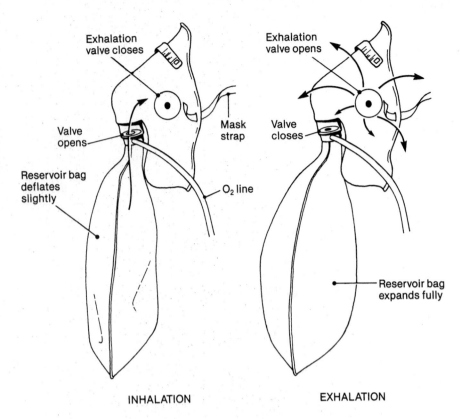

INHALATION

EXHALATION

Figure 6–16. Face mask with reservoir. (From Kersten, L. D. (1989). *Comprehensive respiratory nursing* (p. 611). Philadelphia: W. B. Saunders Co.)

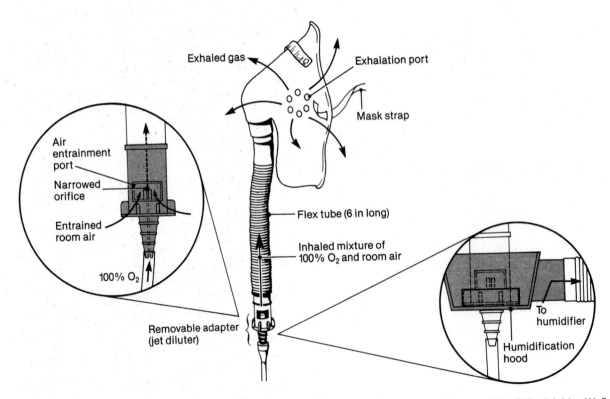

Figure 6–17. Venturi mask. (From Kersten, L. D. (1989). *Comprehensive respiratory nursing* (p. 611). Philadelphia: W. B. Saunders Co.)

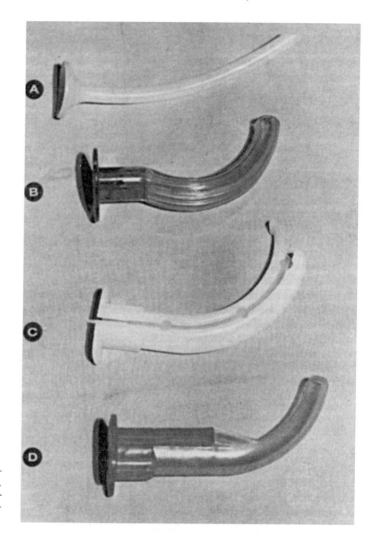

Figure 6–18. Airways: *(A)* nasopharyngeal; *(B)* oropharyngeal airway; *(C* and *D)* intubating airways. (From Chung, D. C., & Lamb, A. M. (1990). *Essentials of anesthesiology* (2nd ed.) (p. 128). Philadelphia: W. B. Saunders Co.)

inserted into the nares and nasopharynx (Fig. 6–20). Nasopharyngeal airways are better tolerated in the conscious patient, may be left in place for longer periods of time, and facilitate nasotracheal suctioning.

The procedure for inserting a nasotracheal airway is described in Table 6–12. Complications of nasopharyngeal airways include insertion into the esophagus if the airway is too long, nosebleeds, and ulceration of the nares. Sinusitis or otitis may occur if the airway is left in place for extended periods.

INTUBATION

Endotracheal Intubation

Intubation refers to the insertion of an endotracheal tube (ETT), into the trachea through either the mouth or the nose. Advantages of oral versus nasal endotracheal intubation are listed in Table 6–13. The ETT (Fig. 6–21) is a tube with a distal balloon, or cuff, that is inflated in order to facilitate ventilation of the patient. Most cuffs have high-volume, low-pressure capabilities. Most ETTs have cuffs that are inflated with air; however, some have foam cuffs that are passively inflated with air. (If a foam-cuff ETT is used, the manufacturer's instructions should be followed for the care and maintenance of the cuff.) The ETT also has a proximal adaptor that can be attached to a bag-valve device or to a mechanical ventilator.

Intubation may be performed to maintain an open airway, to assist in secretion removal, to prevent aspiration, and to provide mechanical ventilation. The procedure is performed by personnel who are trained and skilled in the procedure, such as anesthesiologists, nurse anesthetists, emergency department physicians, respiratory therapists, and some paramedics.

Frequently, intubation is performed as an emergency procedure during a cardiopulmonary arrest. Intu-

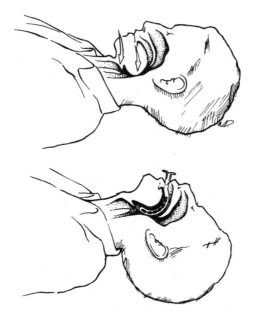

Figure 6–19. Maintaining an open airway with the use of an oral airway. (Reproduced with permission. American Heart Association (1994). *Textbook of advanced cardiac life support* (3rd ed.) (p. 2-2). Dallas: Author. Copyright American Heart Association.)

bation may also be performed as an elective procedure when a patient is having difficulty maintaining an adequate airway or is having difficulty maintaining ventilation or oxygenation. The goal of elective intubation is the prevention of cardiopulmonary arrest.

Nurses must be familiar with equipment used for intubation and must be able to gather equipment quickly before the procedure. Nurses also need to know how to assemble a laryngoscope (Fig. 6–22). Necessary equipment is frequently kept together on a

---

Table 6–11. INSERTION OF ORAL AIRWAY

1. Choose the proper size. The length is determined by measuring from the corner of the mouth to the ear lobe.
2. Suction mucus from mouth using a tonsil (Yankauer) tip catheter.
3. Turn airway upside down to facilitate insertion and open the mouth. (An alternate method is to use a tongue blade to depress the tongue while the airway is inserted in the proper position.)
4. When the posterior wall of the pharynx is reached, turn (rotate) the airway into the proper position.
5. After insertion, assess patency of airway: air movement through the airway, clear breath sounds, and chest movement.
6. Maintain proper head alignment after insertion.

Table 6–12. INSERTION OF NASAL AIRWAY

1. Choose the proper size. The length is determined by measuring from the nares to the ear lobe and adding 1 inch.
2. Lubricate the tip and sides of the nasal airway with a water-soluble lubricant.
3. If needed, lubricate the nasal passage with a topical anesthetic.
4. Insert the airway medially and downward. It may be necessary to rotate the airway slightly.
5. After insertion, assess patency of airway: air movement through the airway, clear breath sounds, and chest movement.

---

crash cart or tray in order to facilitate the intubation procedure (Table 6–14; Fig. 6–23).

Procedure for Oral Endotracheal Intubation

The patient is placed in a "sniffing" position to align the airway structures (Fig. 6–24). Placing a folded towel or bath blanket under the head may help achieve this position. If the procedure is performed electively, a topical anesthetic and/or premedication with a sedative or paralytic agent may be used so that the patient better tolerates the procedure.

Before the procedure is performed, the patient is hyperoxygenated and hyperventilated with 100% oxygen by use of a bag-valve device with a face mask. The proper-sized tube is chosen. All ETTs increase the work of breathing; however, a tube that is too small substantially increases the work of breathing and may make ventilation and weaning difficult. The average-sized ETT used for females ranges from 7.5 to 8.0 mm, whereas the average-sized ETT used for males ranges from 8.5 to 9.0 mm (Kersten, 1989). After the tube is selected, the cuff on the balloon is inflated to

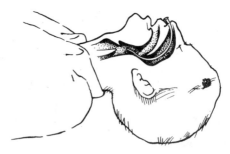

Figure 6–20. Maintaining an open airway with the use of a nasopharyngeal airway. (Reproduced with permission. American Heart Association (1994). *Textbook of advanced cardiac life support* (3rd ed.) (p. 2-2). Dallas: Author. Copyright American Heart Association.)

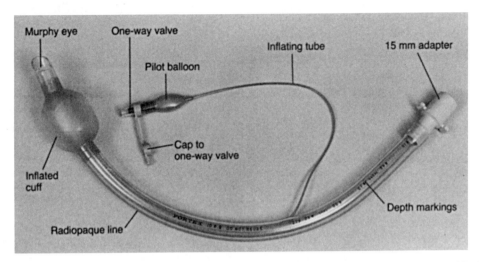

Figure 6–21. Endotracheal tube. (From Kersten, L. D. (1989). *Comprehensive respiratory nursing* (p. 637). Philadelphia: W. B. Saunders Co.)

check for proper functioning and/or any leaks. A stylet is used to stiffen the ETT and facilitate insertion. The ETT is lubricated with a water-soluble lubricant. The laryngoscope is attached to the appropriate size and

type of blade (straight or curved). The choice of blades varies. The straight blade elevates the epiglottis anteriorly to expose the vocal cords. The tip of the curved blade fits into the vallecula. When upward traction is placed on the laryngoscope, the epiglottis is displaced anteriorly. Use of the straight versus curved blade is shown in Figure 6–25.

The person doing the intubation inserts the laryngoscope into the mouth to visualize the vocal cords (see Fig. 6–24). Excess secretions and/or vomitus is suctioned to facilitate visualization of the vocal cords; the tonsil suction tip is very efficient in removing the secretions. The ETT is inserted 5 to 6 cm beyond the vocal cords, and the cuff is inflated.

Table 6–13. ORAL VERSUS NASOTRACHEAL INTUBATION

Oral Intubation
Advantages
    Easily and quickly performed
    Larger tube facilitates suction and procedures such
        as bronchoscopy
    Less kinking of tube
Disadvantages
    Not recommended in patients with suspected
        cervical injury
    Uncomfortable
    Mouth care more difficult to perform
    Impairs ability to gag and swallow
    May increase salivation
    May cause irritation and ulceration of the mouth

Nasotracheal Intubation
Advantages
    Greater patient comfort and better tolerance
    Better mouth care possible
    Fewer oral complications
    Less risk of accidental extubation
    Facilitates swallowing of secretions
    Can administer small amounts of oral liquids if
        patient able to swallow
Disadvantages
    More difficult to perform
    May cause nasal hemorrhage and sinusitis
    Secretion removal more difficult because of smaller
        tube diameter and longer tube length

Adapted from Kersten, L. D. (1989). *Comprehensive respiratory nursing*. Philadelphia, W. B. Saunders Co.

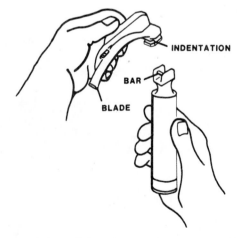

Figure 6–22. Assembly of a laryngoscope. The blade locks into place when assembled properly. (Reproduced with permission. American Heart Association (1994). *Textbook of advanced cardiac life support* (3rd ed.) (p. 2-3). Dallas: Author. Copyright American Heart Association.)

Table 6–14. EQUIPMENT FOR ENDOTRACHEAL INTUBATION

Endotracheal tube of proper size
  Average female size, 7.5–8.0 mm
  Average male size, 8.5–9.0 mm
Stylet
Laryngoscope and blade
  Straight blade (Miller)
  Curved blade (MacIntosh)
Suction
  Tonsil tip (Yankauer)
  Suction kit
Syringe to inflate balloon (usually 10 ml slip-tip)
Topical anesthetic
  Cetacaine spray, lidocaine jelly, or other agent
Water-soluble lubricant
Tape or device to secure tube
Stethoscope
Bag-valve device/manual resuscitation bag
  With reservoir
  Connected to oxygen at 15 L/min
Optional equipment
  Magill forceps
  Oropharyngeal airway

The procedure should be performed within 30 seconds. If the intubation is difficult, the patient should be manually ventilated between intubation attempts. Frequently, the patient requires endotracheal suctioning for removal of excess secretions immediately after intubation. If the patient needs assistance with breathing, ventilation is achieved with either the bag-valve device or a ventilator. (During cardiopulmonary resuscitation, ventilation is provided with a bag-valve device. If the patient is breathing spontaneously, supplemental oxygen is delivered through the ETT via a T-piece, or Briggs' device (Fig. 6–26).

Placement of the ETT is verified by the movement of air in and out of the tube, observation of bilateral chest expansion with inspiration, and auscultation of bilateral breath sounds while the patient is ventilated with a bag-valve device. Another method for verifying tube placement is end-tidal carbon dioxide monitoring. If the tube is in the trachea (versus the esophagus), carbon dioxide is detected in the exhaled air. After intubation, a portable chest x-ray study is always performed for verification of tube placement. The tip of the ETT should be approximately 2 to 5 cm above the carina.

Once proper tube placement is verified, the ETT is secured with tape or another device in order to prevent dislodging. A helpful way to document the depth of insertion is to mark the ETT with an indelible marker at the lip line. The length of the tube at the lip line (e.g., 23 cm) should also be documented in a readily available reference, such as the Kardex. These nursing measures facilitate frequent assessment of proper tube position.

Procedure for Nasotracheal Intubation

A nasotracheal ETT is usually better tolerated in an alert patient and may be easier to stabilize. In nasotracheal intubation, the ETT is usually inserted

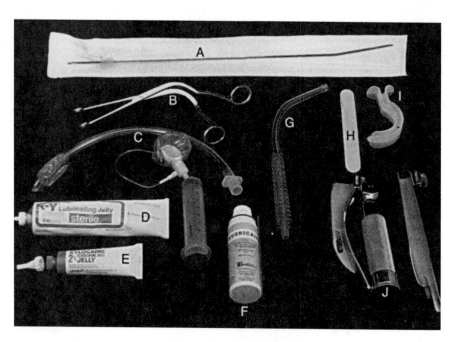

Figure 6–23. Equipment used for endotracheal intubation. (A) Stylet (disposable); (B) Magill forceps; (C) soft cuffed endotracheal tube with syringe for inflation; (D) water-soluble lubricant; (E) anesthetic jelly (optional); (F) topical anesthetic with spray stick attached to right side of canisters; (G) Yankauer pharyngeal suction tip (disposable); (H) tongue blade; (I) oral airway; (J) laryngoscope handle with a curved blade (attached) and straight blade (right). (From Kersten, L. D. (1989). Comprehensive respiratory nursing (p. 640). Philadelphia: W. B. Saunders Co.)

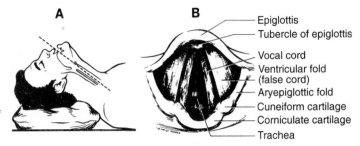

Figure 6–24. Patient positioning for endotracheal intubation. (A) Shows the correct position of the head and neck. (B) Shows the glottis as visualized through the laryngoscope. (Modified from Chung, D. C., & Lamb, A. M. (1990). *Essentials of anesthesiology* (2nd ed.) (p. 133). Philadelphia: W. B. Saunders Co.)

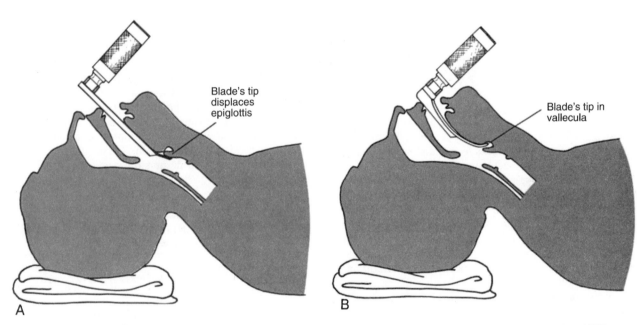

Figure 6–25. Use of a straight (A) versus curved (B) blade for endotracheal intubation. (From Kersten, L. D. (1989). *Comprehensive respiratory nursing* (p. 643). Philadelphia: W. B. Saunders Co.)

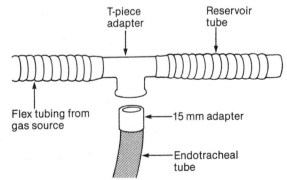

Figure 6–26. T-piece. The T-piece is used to provide supplemental oxygen through an endotracheal tube. (From Kersten, L. D. (1989). *Comprehensive respiratory nursing* (p. 672). Philadelphia: W. B. Saunders Co.)

through the nares and then passed "blindly" into the glottis during inspiration. The blind intubation method is performed in the alert patient who is capable of spontaneous respirations. The nose and pharynx are anesthetized before the procedure.

Nasotracheal intubation can also be performed through direct visualization. In this method, practitioners may use a laryngoscope and Magill forceps or fiberoptic bronchoscopy during the intubation.

Complications

Several complications may occur as a result of oral endotracheal or nasotracheal intubation. Complications include trauma to airway structures, hypoxemia, dysrhythmias, aspiration, intubation of esophagus, laryngospasm, bronchospasm, and intubation of the right mainstem bronchus.

TRACHEOSTOMY

A tracheostomy tube may be needed if the patient requires long-term (weeks to months) mechanical ventilation, frequent suctioning for the management of secretions, or bypassing of an airway obstruction (e.g., a tumor). The ETT can be left in place for up to 3 to 4 weeks; however, if it is known that the patient will require a tracheostomy for long-term ventilatory management, the ETT insertion should be performed within the first week (Rhodes, 1995).

The tracheostomy procedure has traditionally been a surgical technique performed in the operating room or by a surgical team at the bedside. However, a percutaneous tracheostomy technique can now be performed easily and safely at the bedside. Types of tracheostomy tubes include cuffed (low pressure or foam cuff), fenestrated, and cuffless.

Cuffed Tracheostomy Tube

A cuffed tracheostomy tube is inserted in the patient who requires long-term mechanical ventilation. This tube has a cuff that is similar to that in the ETT to ensure adequate ventilation and to prevent aspiration. The cuff may be a conventional low-pressure type or be constructed of foam. The foam cuff tube may prevent trauma to the airway because of the low pressure exerted. The foam cuff tube may also be used in patients who have difficulty maintaining a good seal with conventional cuffed tracheostomy tubes. Cuffed tubes may or may not have an inner cannula. Some tubes have disposable inner cannulas that facilitate tracheostomy care and may reduce the risk of infections.

FENESTRATED TRACHEOSTOMY TUBE

The fenestrated tracheostomy tube functions as a standard tracheostomy tube when the inner cannula is in place. When the inner cannula is removed, the fenestrated tracheostomy tube has one hole that allows air to flow above the larynx. This airflow assists in weaning the patients from the tracheostomy itself. Another advantage of the fenestrated tube is that the patient is able to emit vocal sounds, thereby facilitating communication. The inner cannula of the fenestrated tube has a universal adapter that must be used in order for the fenestrated tube to be attached to a mechanical ventilator or bag-valve device.

CUFFLESS TRACHEOSTOMY TUBE

A cuffless tracheostomy tube is used for long-term airway management in a patient who does not require mechanical ventilation and is at a low risk for aspiration. For example, some neurological patients need tracheostomies for secretion removal but do not require mechanical ventilation. These tubes are made from polyvinyl chloride material or metal.

Table 6–15. KEY POINTS FOR ENDOTRACHEAL SUCTIONING

1. Suction only as indicated by patient assessment.
2. Assemble equipment (suction kit with two gloves, sterile water or saline for rinsing the catheter).
3. Use sterile technique for the procedure.
4. Set suction vacuum at 80–150 mm Hg (Boggs, 1993).
5. Provide 3–5 quick hyperoxygenation breaths (100% oxygen) and hyperinflation (150% tidal volume) breaths to patient before, during, and after suctioning (Stone, 1990). These techniques can be performed via the ventilator circuit or by use of a bag-valve device.
   NOTE: If a bag-valve device is used, two personnel should participate in the procedure: one to suction and one to manually ventilate.
6. Gently insert suction catheter until resistance is met, then pull back 1 cm.
7. Suction patient no longer than 10–15 seconds while applying intermittent or constant suction.
8. Repeat endotracheal suctioning until airway is clear. Hyperoxygenate, hyperinflate, and hyperventilate between suction attempts.
9. After endotracheal suctioning is performed, rinse the catheter. Suction the mouth and oropharynx to remove excess saliva.
10. Adjust oxygen percentage to presuctioning level.
11. Auscultate the lungs to assess effectiveness of suctioning.
12. Document amount, color, and consistency of secretions.

ENDOTRACHEAL SUCTIONING

Patients with either an ETT or a tracheostomy tube frequently need to be suctioned in order to maintain a patent airway because they lose the normal protective ability to cough up secretions. Suctioning is performed according to a standard protocol in order to prevent complications. Complications associated with suctioning include hypoxemia, cardiac dysrhythmias, increased intracranial pressure, airway trauma, and infection. Suctioning also stimulates the cough reflex and stimulates increased mucus production.

Because suctioning is associated with complications as well as increased production of mucus, it should be performed only as indicated by physical assessment and *not* according to a predetermined schedule (e.g., every 2 hours). Indications for endotracheal suctioning include a change in vital signs (e.g., increased or decreased heart rate or respiratory rate), dyspnea, restlessness, visible secretions in the airway, high-pressure ventilator alarms, secretions audible on auscultation, or ineffective coughing.

Several techniques have been developed to reduce complications associated with suctioning. Key points related to endotracheal suctioning are discussed in Table 6–15. Hyperinflation, hyperventilation, and hyperoxygenation should be used before, during, and immediately after suctioning. The techniques are performed with either the ventilator or the bag-valve device. However, use of the ventilator is recommended because it is associated with fewer hemodynamic effects

of suctioning, such as increases in mean arterial pressure (Stone, 1990).

Hyperinflation involves the delivery of breaths 1.0 to 1.5 times the V_T. Hyperventilation is performed by giving the patient three to five quick breaths before and between suctioning attempts. Hyperoxygenation is the delivery of 100% oxygen before suctioning and between attempts. Newer ventilators have a built-in suction mode that delivers 100% oxygen for a short period of time (e.g., 2 minutes). However, many older ventilators have a "washout" time of up to 2 minutes that is required before 100% oxygen is delivered (Stone, 1990).

Alternatives to conventional suctioning include the use of suction catheters connected to an oxygen source (oxygen insufflation catheter), adapters, or closed tracheal suction devices. The oxygen insufflation catheter delivers oxygen to the patient via the suction catheter in order to prevent suction-induced hypoxemia. The use of adapters and closed tracheal suction devices permits suctioning without disconnecting the patient from the ventilator; therefore, they provide continuous oxygenation during suctioning and maintain positive end-expiratory pressure (PEEP) in the patient who requires this therapy. When an adapter (Fig. 6–27) is used, a conventional suction kit is used for suctioning the patient without removing the patient from the ventilator circuit.

The closed tracheal suction system consists of a suction catheter enclosed in a plastic sheath that is attached to the patient's ventilator circuit (Fig. 6–28).

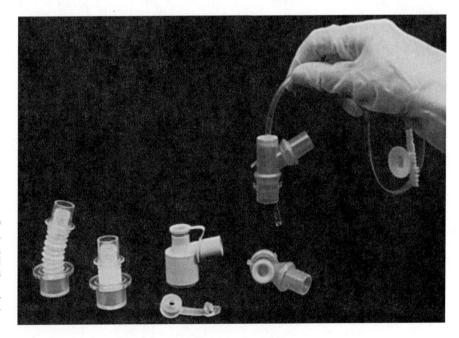

Figure 6–27. Suction adapters. Adapters permit suctioning of a patient without disconnecting mechanical ventilation. A suction catheter is introduced into one of the adapters shown. (From Kersten, L. D. (1989). *Comprehensive respiratory nursing* (p. 690). Philadelphia: W. B. Saunders Co.)

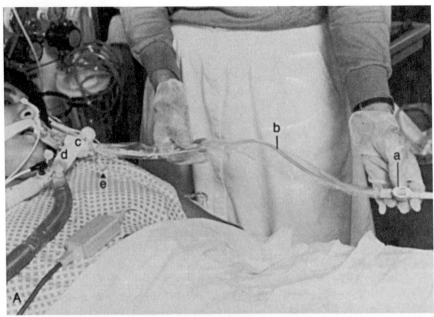

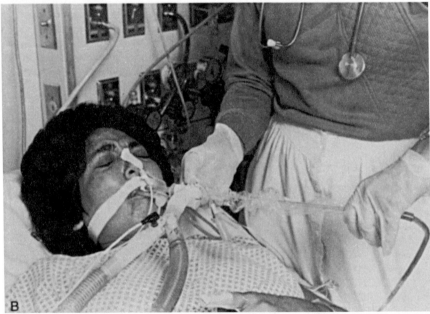

Figure 6–28. Closed tracheal suction device. *(A)* Shows the Ballard TrachCare closed suction system: (a) suction control; (b) suction catheter enclosed in sheath; (c) sealed T-piece, which connects to endotracheal tube; (d) flexible tubing, which connects to ventilator; and (e) irrigation port for tracheal lavage and rinsing suction catheter. *(B)* Demonstrates use of the closed suction device. (From Kersten, L. D. (1989). *Comprehensive respiratory nursing* (p. 688). Philadelphia: W. B. Saunders Co.)

The closed system can also be attached to a T-piece adapter. The closed tracheal suction system assists in maintaining oxygenation during suctioning, reduces symptoms associated with hypoxemia, maintains PEEP, permits administration of respiratory medications, protects staff from patient's secretions, and reduces patient anxiety; it is also usually cost effective (Noll et al., 1990; Johnson et al., 1994). Key points

for use of the closed tracheal suction system are discussed in Table 6–16.

Many practitioners routinely instill 3 to 5 ml of normal saline into the trachea during suctioning. The rationale for using the saline is that saline loosens secretions and facilitates airway clearance. However, limited studies do not support the routine use of saline. Adequate patient hydration and use of aerosolized mu-

Table 6–16. KEY POINTS FOR SUCTIONING WITH A CLOSED TRACHEAL SUCTION SYSTEM (CTSS)

1. Prior to using the CTSS, review the manufacturer's instructions for use.
2. Choose the proper-sized CTSS. The diameter of the suction catheter should be no more than half the diameter of the artificial airway.
3. Attach the CTSS to the ventilator circuit. (This step is frequently performed by a respiratory therapist.)
4. Set the suction regulator at 80 to 150 mm Hg *while depressing the suction control* on the CTSS.
5. Hyperoxygenate the patient via the ventilator circuit before, between, and after suctioning.
6. Using the thumb and forefinger of the dominant hand, insert the CTSS into the airway until resistance is met. At the same time, use the nondominant hand to stabilize the T-junction that connects the CTSS to the airway and ventilator. Withdraw the suction catheter, using a steady motion while applying intermittent or constant suction for no longer than 10 to 15 seconds.
7. Ensure that the catheter has been completely withdrawn from the airway. A marking is visible on the suction catheter when it is properly withdrawn.
8. Rinse the CTSS after each use. Connect a small vial or syringe of normal saline for tracheal instillation (without preservatives) to the irrigation port of the CTSS. Simultaneously instill the saline into the port while depressing the suction control of the CTSS.
9. If saline lavage is used (controversial), attach a vial of normal saline without preservatives to the irrigation port. Insert the suction catheter 4–6 inches into the airway. Instill 3 to 5 ml of normal saline into the CTSS. Suction the patient.
10. After the procedure is completed, ensure that the suction control knob on the CTSS is in the locked position to prevent inadvertent application of suction to the airway.
11. Change the system according to manufacturer's recommendations (usually every 24 hours).
12. Document effectiveness of suctioning. When CTSS is used, some patients may require periodic conventional suctioning to remove thick secretions. (Adequate humidification assists in loosening secretions.)
13. Keep the CTSS out of the patient's reach to avoid accidental self-extubation.
14. Suction the oropharynx with a tonsil or Yankauer device.

colytics are more effective than saline instillation in facilitating secretion removal (Connolly, 1995).

MECHANICAL VENTILATION

Indications

Mechanical ventilation is warranted for patients who have acute respiratory failure and are unable to maintain normal gas exchange. Respiratory failure oc-

curs from impaired alveolar ventilation or decreased pulmonary vascular perfusion. The outcome of respiratory failure is life-threatening hypoxemia. Respiratory failure may result from an acute process, such as airway obstruction or pulmonary embolus, or an exacerbation of a chronic pulmonary disease. An example of the latter is COPD in which superimposed pneumonia develops. Respiratory failure is discussed in Chapter 11.

Ongoing assessment is essential in determining the need for intubation and mechanical ventilation. Usually, progressive deterioration is noted. ABG results worsen, infiltrates and other abnormalities are noted on chest x-ray study, and the patient develops clinical signs of hypoxemia (see Table 6–4). Physiological parameters indicating the need for mechanical ventilation are presented in Table 6–17.

Types of Mechanical Ventilators

Mechanical ventilation is frequently used as a supportive therapy for the facilitation of gas exchange. Usually, an ETT or tracheostomy tube is needed for mechanical ventilation; however, noninvasive methods may occasionally be used. Categories of mechanical ventilation include negative pressure and positive pressure types.

Noninvasive Methods of Ventilation

Noninvasive techniques, that is, those that do not require the use of an ETT or tracheostomy, may be used to provide ventilation to the patient. Negative pressure ventilation and noninvasive positive pressure ventilation are two of the techniques.

Table 6–17. INDICATIONS FOR MECHANICAL VENTILATION

Parameter	Normal	Ventilation
ABGs		
PaO_2 (mm Hg)	>80	<60
$PaCO_2$ (mm Hg)	35–45	>50
pH	7.35–7.45	<7.25
$PaO_2 = PaCO_2$		
Other		
Respiratory rate/min	12–16	>35
Tidal volume (ml/kg)	6–8	<3.5
Vital capacity (ml/kg)	50–60	<10–15
NIF cm/H_2O*	>−25	<−20

*Negative inspiratory force (NIF) is the amount of negative pressure that a patient is able to generate to initiate spontaneous respirations. Normally NIF is −25 cm of H_2O or greater: e.g., −30 cm, −40 cm.

ABG = arterial blood gas.

Negative Pressure Ventilation

When negative pressure ventilation is used, the patient is placed in a device that applies negative pressure to the trunk or body. The negative pressure causes the chest wall to be pulled outward, causing inspiration to occur as a result of pressure changes in the pleural space. Examples of negative pressure ventilators include the iron lung, cuirass, poncho, and body wrap devices. Negative pressure devices are usually used in patients with chronic diseases who require assisted ventilation, frequently only during the night (Sonesso, 1990).

Noninvasive Positive Pressure Ventilation

Noninvasive positive pressure ventilation provides ventilation via a nasal or oral mask, nasal pillow, or mouthpiece with a tight seal. It is used in conjunction with a portable ventilator that provides either volume-cycled or flow-cycled breaths (Bi-PAP). Noninvasive positive pressure ventilation is primarily used in home care settings to treat individuals with chronic respiratory failure, often only at night. Newer uses in acute care settings include weaning patients from mechanical ventilation, supporting patients after extubation, and providing comfort to patients with terminal respiratory failure (Burns, 1990; Dabbs and Olslund, 1994).

Positive Pressure Ventilation

Positive pressure ventilation is the most common method for providing ventilation in the acute care setting. This method of mechanical ventilation forces air into the lungs, usually through an ETT or tracheostomy tube, via positive pressure. Types of positive pressure ventilators include time-cycled, pressure-cycled, and volume-cycled ventilators.

Time-Cycled Ventilators

Time-cycled ventilators allow air to flow into the lungs until a preset amount of time has elapsed. Delivered VT, pressure, and flow vary according to the length of the inspiratory cycle. This type of ventilator is used most frequently with neonates and children.

Pressure-Cycled Ventilators

Pressure-cycled ventilators allow air to flow into the lungs until a preset pressure has been reached. Once the pressure is reached, a valve closes, and expiration begins. Delivered VT varies widely with pressure-cycled ventilators and may result in hypoven-

tilation and respiratory acidosis. These ventilators are best for short-term use, such as in the emergency department after a patient is intubated or in the immediate postoperative period in a patient who requires short-term ventilation.

Volume-Cycled Ventilators

Volume-cycled ventilators are the most commonly used type of positive pressure ventilators. They allow air to flow into the lungs until a preset volume has been reached. A major advantage of these ventilators is that they deliver the VT regardless of changes in compliance or resistance.

Ventilators with Flexible Capabilities

Newer ventilators offer flexibility in the types of ventilation they provide. Built-in microprocessors provide a wide range of ventilatory support to facilitate work of breathing and to maximize oxygenation and gas exchange. These ventilators can provide advanced modes of ventilation (Table 6–18).

Modes of Mechanical Ventilation

Various modes of mechanical ventilation may be used to ensure adequate ventilation and optimum oxygenation of the patient. These modes include controlled ventilation, assist/control ventilation, intermittent mandatory ventilation (IMV), and synchronized IMV (SIMV). Waveforms depicting these various modes are shown in Figure 6–29.

Controlled Ventilation

The control mode of mechanical ventilation delivers a preset VT at a preset respiratory rate. It ventilates the patient regardless of the patient's respiratory effort. It is used in patients who have no inspiratory effort, such as those with high cervical spine injuries, or to decrease the work of breathing in patients with chest and/or head injuries. If controlled mechanical ventilation is ordered for a patient who initiates spontaneous breaths, the patient is medicated with sedatives and/or a neuromuscular blocking agent to prevent him or her from attempting to breathe in competition with the ventilator. Medications are discussed later in the chapter.

Assist/Control Ventilation

The assist/control mode of mechanical ventilation delivers a preset VT whenever the patient exerts a negative inspiratory effort. A preset respiratory rate ensures that the patient receives adequate ventilation,

Table 6–18. ADVANCED TECHNIQUES FOR MECHANICAL VENTILATION*

Technique	Description
Airway pressure-release ventilation	The patient breathes spontaneously while receiving continuous positive airway pressure. A valve opens during exhalation, releasing the pressure. Used for maintaining FRC in patients with acute lung injury or with postoperative pulmonary insufficiency who have adequate respiratory strength and drive (Pierce, 1995).
Mandatory minute ventilation	Ensures a constant minute ventilation, regardless of respiratory rate or spontaneous tidal volume. Computer adjusts settings on a breath-to-breath basis, according to analysis of patient's expired gases (Witta, 1990; Pierce, 1995).
Permissive hypercapnia	Uses smaller tidal volumes (<10–15 ml/kg) to reduce peak airway pressures in patients at risk for barotrauma, such as those with ARDS. The $PaCO_2$ is allowed to increase to 50–100 mm Hg. Contraindicated in patients with head injury (Pierce, 1995).
Pressure-controlled–inverse ratio ventilation	Uses pressure-controlled ventilation for a prolonged inspiratory time. The increased inspiratory time assists in opening and stabilizing alveoli. May require the use of sedatives and/or neuromuscular blocking agents to increase patient tolerance and comfort (St. John & LeFrak, 1990).
Pressure-regulated volume control ventilation	Adjusts inspiratory pressure while ensuring a minimum tidal volume. Intended for patients without spontaneous breathing capacity (Siemens-Elema AB, 1994). Used to decrease the risk of barotrauma.
Volume support; volume-assured pressure support	Combines pressure support with a guarantee of a minimum tidal volume. Starts as a pressure breath and ends as a volume breath if needed (Amato et al., 1992). The patient triggers every breath (Pierce, 1995).
Differential lung ventilation or simultaneous independent lung ventilation	Permits independent ventilation of each lung. Used to treat unilateral lung disease, such as pneumonia, contusion, and atelectasis. Requires a dual-lumen endobronchial tube. A ventilator is attached to each lumen to permit individualized settings for each lung (Mays and Eckert, 1994; Pierce, 1995). The ventilators are connected to synchronize inspiration and expiration. The patient may require sedation and/or neuromuscular blockade.
High-frequency ventilation (HFV)	Works by using small tidal volumes at very high respiratory rates. Ventilation and oxygenation are achieved by gas diffusion and convection (Kersten, 1989). Several variations of HFV exist, e.g., jet ventilation and oscillatory ventilation (Curley and Molengraft, 1994). The major advantage of HFV is a reduction in complications, e.g., barotrauma, associated with high airway pressures in conventional mechanical ventilation. HFV is primarily used in neonates and children but can be used in adults who cannot be effectively ventilated with conventional and advanced techniques. Special jet ventilators are required.
Extracorporeal lung assist (ECLA)	Method of ventilation in which the patient is attached to a circuit containing a blood pump and artificial "membrane" lungs (special equipment). Types of ECLA include extracorporeal membrane oxygenation, which has been successful in the treatment of infants with respiratory distress syndrome. ECLA facilitates removal of carbon dioxide and promotes lung rest. It is used to treat respiratory failure that is unresponsive to conventional mechanical ventilation, such as in patients with severe ARDS (Cottingham and Habashi, 1995).

*Names may vary, depending on the brand of mechanical ventilator.
CPAP = continuous positive airway pressure; FRC = functional residual capacity; ARDS = adult respiratory distress syndrome.

regardless of spontaneous efforts. For example, the assist/control respiratory rate may be set at 10 breaths/min at a VT of 800 ml. If the patient initiates a negative inspiratory effort 16 times per minute, he or she receives 800 ml of air for each of the 16 efforts. If the patient does not initiate any inspiratory effort (e.g., during sleep), he or she receives 800 ml VT 10 times per minute. The assist/control mode is useful in

patients with normal respiratory drive who are unable to sustain a normal VT. It also helps preserve pulmonary muscle tone as patients use their respiratory muscles to initiate a breath (Bolton and Kline, 1994).

One complication of the assist/control mode is respiratory alkalosis, especially if the patient hyperventilates. If respiratory alkalosis occurs, the patient may need to be sedated, or his or her regimen may need to

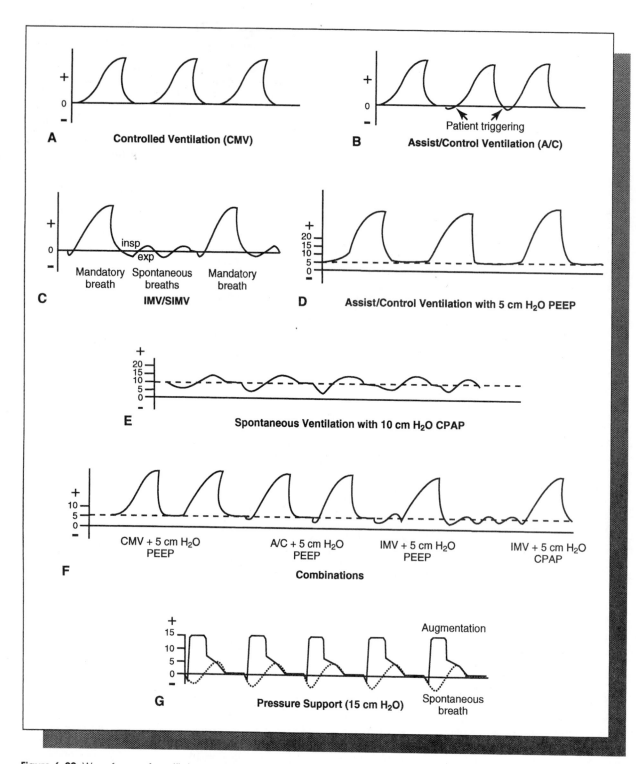

Figure 6–29. Waveforms of ventilator modes and adjuncts to ventilation. IMV/SIMV = intermittent mandatory ventilation/synchronized IMV; PEEP = positive end-expiratory pressure; CPAP = continuous positive airway pressure.

be changed to IMV. Another disadvantage of assist/control ventilation is that the effort needed to initiate a breath may be high if minute ventilation is high (Ashworth, 1990).

Intermittent Mandatory Ventilation/Synchronized Intermittent Mandatory Ventilation

The IMV and SIMV modes of mechanical ventilation deliver a preset VT at a preset respiratory rate and permit the patient to breathe spontaneously at his or her own respiratory rate and depth between the ventilator breaths. The IMV mode delivers the preset breaths, regardless of the patient's spontaneous effort, whereas the SIMV mode delivers preset breaths that are synchronized with the patient's spontaneous efforts. The SIMV mode prevents the patient from competing with the ventilator during spontaneous efforts. The IMV/SIMV modes are commonly used because they may prevent respiratory muscle weakness and the hyperventilation that commonly occurs in the assist/control mode. These modes are commonly used in weaning patients from mechanical ventilation; however, they may actually increase the workload of breathing for the patient because of muscle fatigue associated with spontaneous breathing efforts and the artificial airway (Boggs, 1993).

Adjuncts to Mechanical Ventilation

Several adjustments can be used in conjunction with the various modes of mechanical ventilation to enhance oxygenation and/or ventilation of the patient. Adjuncts to modes of mechanical ventilation include PEEP, continuous positive airway pressure (CPAP), and pressure support ventilation (PSV). They are shown in Figure 6–29.

Positive End-Expiratory Pressure

Positive end-expiratory pressure adds positive airway pressure to mechanically assisted breaths. Airway pressure remains higher than atmospheric pressure during both inspiration and expiration. PEEP keeps the patient's airway open at the end of expiration and increases the FRC. PEEP prevents the collapse of small airways, thereby maximizing the number of alveoli available for ventilation and resulting in increased oxygenation. Frequently, PEEP is used to decrease the FiO_2 needed for optimal oxygenation. For example, a patient may require an FiO_2 of 0.80 to maintain a PaO_2 of 85 mm Hg. If 10 cm of PEEP is added to the ventilator settings, the FiO_2 may be able to be de-

creased to 0.60, while still permitting the patient to have a PaO_2 of 85 mm Hg.

The range for PEEP is 5 to 20 cm H_2O, although levels up to 50 cm have been used in patients with severe respiratory distress and hypoxemia. Many patients routinely receive 3 to 5 cm H_2O of PEEP, a value often referred to as "physiological PEEP." This small amount helps to preserve a more normal FRC in patients with artificial airways who are usually kept supine (Pierce, 1995). Complications of PEEP include a decrease in cardiac output and an increased risk for barotrauma, such as a pneumothorax.

Continuous Positive Airway Pressure

Whereas PEEP is used to increase the FRC during mechanically-assisted breaths, CPAP is used to augment FRC during spontaneous ventilation and in combination with the spontaneous breaths of IMV and SIMV (Boggs, 1993). CPAP is also used as a method for weaning patients from mechanical ventilation.

Continuous positive airway pressure can be administered via face mask or mechanical ventilator. CPAP is delivered by face mask in spontaneously breathing patients to delay intubation while treatment, such as bronchodilators and chest physiotherapy, is initiated. It is also used at night by some patients who suffer from sleep apnea.

The mechanical ventilator is used to deliver CPAP to patients undergoing IMV/SIMV and as a weaning method. For example, a patient may be on a volume ventilator in the SIMV mode at a respiratory rate of 10 breaths/min and receive 8 cm H_2O of PEEP and 8 cm H_2O of CPAP. The PEEP is delivered with the 10 SIMV breaths. The CPAP is applied to the patient's spontaneous breaths.

Pressure Support Ventilation

In PSV, a preset level of positive pressure is used to augment or assist the spontaneous VT of the patient. It can be used with spontaneous ventilation and with IMV/SIMV. PSV provides sustained pressure during inspiration, allowing a more even distribution of inspired gas. During PSV, the decrease in airway pressure triggers a gas flow that increases the airway pressure to a preset level, resulting in an increased VT (Boggs, 1993). PSV facilitates the patient's ability to take a spontaneous breath by decreasing the workload associated with spontaneous breathing through an artificial airway, especially small ETTs. It may also increase patient comfort and provide conditioning of the diaphragm that facilitates weaning (Bolton and Kline, 1994).

Advanced Methods/Modes of Mechanical Ventilation

As noted earlier, the microprocessor ventilators offer a wide range of options for mechanical ventilation, often combining various conventional modes. These advanced techniques for ventilation (see Table 6–18) are usually used in patients with respiratory failure that is refractory to conventional treatment. Some of the techniques, such as jet ventilation and extracorporeal lung assist, require specialized machines.

Ventilator Settings

In most institutions, the ventilators are set up and managed by respiratory therapy personnel. All ventilators have numerous buttons and dials. The nurse should be familiar with the control panel so that the ventilator mode, adjuncts to ventilation, settings, and alarms can be verified at least once per shift.

Tidal Volume. The amount of air delivered with each preset breath is the VT. In ventilated patients, the VT is usually set at 10 to 15 ml/kg. Therefore, a patient who weighs 70 kg should have the VT set between 700 and 1050 ml. (If permissive hypercapnia is used, the VT is lower.)

Respiratory Rate. The respiratory rate is the frequency of breaths to be delivered by the ventilator.

Fraction of Inspired Oxygen. This is the fraction of inspired oxygen delivered to the patient by the ventilator. FiO_2 may be set from 0.21 (21% or room air) to 1.00 (100% oxygen).

Sigh. A sigh is a breath that has a greater volume than the preset VT, usually 1.5 to 2.0 times the VT. The rationale for using the sigh mechanism is to prevent atelectasis. However, the sigh mechanism may not be routinely used because higher than normal VT settings (10 to 15 ml/kg) eliminate the need for sighs.

Sensitivity. Sensitivity is used to determine the amount of patient effort needed to initiate an assisted breath. It is normally set at 2 cm H_2O less than baseline pressure. If the sensitivity is set too low (e.g. 4 cm H_2O less than baseline), the patient must generate more work in order to trigger gas flow. If it is set too high, auto-cycling of the ventilator and patient-ventilator dyssynchrony ("fighting the ventilator") may occur (Pierce, 1995).

Inspiratory to Expiratory Ratio. In normal respiration, inspiration is shorter than expiration. When a patient undergoes mechanical ventilation, the inspiration to expiration ratio is usually set at 1:2. It can be manipulated to facilitate gas exchange. Some newer methods of ventilation deliver inverse-ratio ventilation (see Table 6–18).

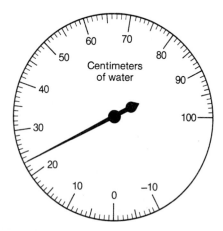

Figure 6–30. System pressure dial showing a peak inspiratory pressure of 23 cm H_2O. During expiration, the dial returns to zero cm H_2O unless the patient is receiving positive end-expiratory pressure. (Adapted from Kersten, L. D. (1989). *Comprehensive respiratory nursing* (p. 717). Philadelphia: W. B. Saunders Co.)

Peak Inspiratory Pressure. This pressure is the peak pressure registered on the airway pressure gauge during normal ventilation (Fig. 6–30). The value is used for setting high and low pressure alarm limits. The peak inspiratory pressure (PIP) increases when the pressure required to ventilate the patient increases, indicating a decrease in lung compliance or an increase in lung resistance.

Pressure Limits. The high pressure limit is the maximum pressure the ventilator can generate to deliver the preset VT. It is usually set 10 to 20 cm H_2O above the peak inspiratory pressure.

Respiratory Monitoring During Mechanical Ventilation

Several respiratory parameters are routinely obtained on mechanically ventilated patients by either nurses or respiratory therapists. These parameters include spontaneous VT and VC, negative inspiratory force, and compliance. The VT and VC are measured by a spirometer. The negative inspiratory force is measured by a specially designed meter.

Compliance is estimated by measuring peak inspiratory pressure and calculating static and dynamic values. In order to measure static compliance, a plateau pressure is measured at peak inspiration by use of the "inflationary hold" or "expiratory retard" dial on the ventilator. The formula for calculating static compliance is

$$\text{Static Compliance} = \frac{VT}{\text{Plateau Pressure} - \text{PEEP}}$$

Dynamic (or effective) compliance is estimated by the following formula:

$$\text{Dynamic Compliance} = \frac{V_T}{PIP - PEEP}$$

As previously noted, static compliance ranges from 70 to 100 ml/cm H_2O in the mechanically ventilated patient with normal lung function. Dynamic compliance ranges from 50 to 100 ml/cm H_2O, or not more than 10 cm/H_2O greater than static compliance (Kersten, 1989).

Compliance decreases with conditions such as ARDS, cardiogenic pulmonary edema, and pneumothorax. Examples of conditions resulting in increased compliance include recovery from ARDS, the addition of PEEP, and diuresis.

Complications of Mechanical Ventilation

Pulmonary System

Barotrauma. Barotrauma is the presence of extra-alveolar air. This air may escape into the pleura (pneumothorax), the mediastinum (pneumomediastinum), pericardium (pneumopericardium), or under the skin (subcutaneous emphysema, or crepitus). Barotrauma may occur when the alveoli are overdistended, such as with positive pressure ventilation, high V_T (>15 ml/kg), and PEEP. An increased incidence of barotrauma is likely if the patient is older, has a history of COPD, has an infection that destroys the alveoli, or has a high airway pressure. Signs and symptoms of barotrauma include high peak inspiratory pressure, decreased breath sounds, high mean airway pressures, tracheal shift, and symptoms associated with hypoxemia.

A life-threatening complication is tension pneumothorax. When tension pneumothorax occurs, pressurized air enters the pleural space. Air is unable to exit from the pleural space and continues to accumulate. Collapse of the cardiopulmonary system occurs rapidly. Treatment consists of immediate insertion of a chest tube. Whenever a pneumothorax is suspected in a patient receiving mechanical ventilation, the patient should be removed from the ventilator and should undergo manual ventilation with a bag-valve device until a chest tube is inserted.

Intubation of Right Mainstem Bronchus. The right mainstem bronchus is straighter than the left. If the ETT is manipulated, such as occurs during changing of the tapes or repositioning of the tube in the mouth, it may move into the right mainstem bronchus. Symptoms include absent or diminished breath sounds in the left lung. Whenever the ETT is moved or manipulated, the nurse must auscultate the chest for bilateral breath sounds after the procedure is completed.

Endotracheal Tube Out of Position/Unplanned Extubation. The ETT can become dislodged if it is not secured properly, if the patient moves, or during tape changes on the ETT. The ETT may end up in the back of the throat, in the esophagus, or completely removed. Auscultation of bilateral breath sounds and/or use of capnography can be used to verify that the ETT is in the airway. Strategies for preventing unplanned extubation are described in Table 6–19.

Tracheal Damage. Damage to the trachea can occur because of pressure from the cuff. However, the risk of tracheal damage has decreased since all ETTs and tracheostomy tubes have low pressure cuffs. An intervention for preventing tracheal damage is monitoring of cuff pressures on a routine basis; pressures should not exceed 30 cm H_2O. Various commercial devices that measure cuff pressures quickly and easily are available (see Nursing Care Plan).

Associated with Oxygen Administration. If 100% oxygen is administered, there is a lack of nitrogen in the distal air spaces. Nitrogen is needed in order to prevent collapse of the airway. Therefore, the patient is prone to absorption atelectasis. Other complications associated with oxygen administration include tracheobronchitis, acute lung injury (ARDS), and chronic pulmonary dysplasia. As a rule, an FiO_2 up to 1.0 can be tolerated for up to 48 hours. After that period, the goal is to lower the FiO_2 to less than 0.60 to prevent further lung damage (Dantzker, 1995).

Table 6–19. STRATEGIES FOR PREVENTING ACCIDENTAL OR UNPLANNED EXTUBATION

Provide adequate patient sedation and comfort.

Apply protective devices (e.g., wrist restraints).

Adequately secure the endotracheal tube with tape or commercially available devices.

Cut the end of the endotracheal tube to 2 inches beyond the fixation point.

Mark the lip line on endotracheal tube with an indelible marker; assess position.

Maintain adequate volume in the cuff of the artificial airway.

Provide support for the ventilator tubing and closed suction systems; keep these items away from patient's reach.

Use two staff members when repositioning endotracheal tube.

Educate the family.

Adapted from Boggs, R. L. (1993). Airway management. In R. L. Boggs, & M. Wooldridge-King, *AACN procedure manual for critical care* (3rd ed.). Philadelphia: W. B. Saunders Co.

Acid-Base Disturbances (Hypocapnia/Hypercapnia). If a ventilator is not set properly for the maintenance of adequate oxygenation and gas exchange, acid-base disturbances result. For example, if a patient is receiving assist/control ventilation and is breathing 30 times per minute, respiratory alkalosis usually occurs. If a patient is receiving IMV at a rate of six breaths per minute and is spontaneously breathing only six breaths per minute, respiratory acidosis may occur. (Sometimes ventilator adjustments are made in order to therapeutically alter acid-base status. For example, patients with increased intracranial pressure are routinely hyperventilated, which results in respiratory alkalosis and cerebral vasoconstriction.)

Aspiration. Most patients who require mechanical ventilation also require tube feedings. Gastric distention, impaired gastric emptying with large amounts of gastric residua, and esophageal reflux predispose patients to aspiration.

Infection. Patients with artificial airways are at an increased risk for pulmonary infection because normal defense mechanisms in the nose are bypassed. Additionally, procedures such as endotracheal suctioning also predispose the patient to an increased risk of infection. Bacteria that frequently cause nosocomial infections include *Streptococcus, Staphylococcus, Pseudomonas, Escherichia coli,* and *Serratia.* Because of their debilitated state, patients may also acquire fungal infections, such as from *Candida albicans.*

Ventilator Dependence/Inability to Wean. Patients who require long-term mechanical ventilation are usually very challenging to wean from the ventilator. Examples of patients in this category include those with underlying COPD and neuromuscular disease.

Cardiovascular System

A decreased cardiac output may be associated with mechanical ventilation, especially if PEEP therapy is used. Positive pressure ventilation and PEEP increase intrathoracic pressure, resulting in a decreased venous return to the heart and a decreased cardiac output.

Gastrointestinal System

Stress ulcers and gastrointestinal bleeding may occur in patients who undergo mechanical ventilation. Another possible complication is a paralytic ileus. Lastly, inadequate nutrition is common in patients who receive mechanical ventilation.

Endocrine System

Fluid retention may be associated with increased humidification provided by the ventilator. Another reason for fluid retention is that increased pressure on the baroreceptors in the thoracic aorta from positive pressure ventilation stimulates the release of antidiuretic hormone. This hormone causes water retention and stimulates the renin-angiotensin-aldosterone mechanism, which causes further fluid retention.

Psychosocial Complications

Several psychosocial hazards may occur as the result of mechanical ventilation. The patient may experience stress and anxiety because he or she requires a machine for breathing. If the ventilator is not set properly or if the patient resists breaths, "fighting" the ventilator may occur. Communication difficulties are common because the patient cannot communicate verbally with family members and caregivers. As a result of being a patient in the intensive care unit, the patient loses autonomy and control over care. Because of the noise of the ventilator as well as the need for frequent procedures, such as suctioning, alteration in sleep and wake patterns may occur. Lastly, the patient can become psychologically dependent on the ventilator, even when he or she is physically able to be weaned.

Nursing Care

Nursing care of the patient who requires mechanical ventilation is a challenge. The nurse must provide care in a holistic approach, despite the use of technology. A detailed plan of care is described in the Nursing Care Plan for the Mechanically Ventilated Patient.

Medications

Intubation, mechanical ventilation, advanced methods for ventilation (e.g., inverse ratio ventilation), and suctioning contribute to patient discomfort. Medication may be needed in order to minimize discomfort, reduce anxiety and agitation, facilitate mechanical ventilation, and improve oxygenation. Medications should be chosen based on the desired patient outcomes. Nonpharmacological methods, such as imagery or music therapy, may also be used. Commonly used medications include analgesics, sedatives, and neuromuscular blocking agents (Table 6–20). Patients often need a combination of drugs for therapeutic effects to be achieved (Luer, 1995). Many institutions use decision trees or algorithms to determine drug therapy. Medications are tapered or discontinued when the patient is ready to wean from mechanical ventilation.

Analgesics. Opioid analgesics are used for providing pain relief and sedation in patients who are hemodynamically stable. Agents include morphine sulfate and fentanyl.

Sedatives. Commonly used sedative agents include benzodiazepines, neuroleptics, and propofol. The benzodiazepines include diazepam (Valium), lorazepam (Ativan), and midazolam (Versed). They provide effective sedation with few side effects. Doses must be gradually tapered in order to prevent withdrawal symptoms. Neuroleptics provide efficient sedation with minimal respiratory depression. Haloperidol (Haldol) is a commonly used neuroleptic. Propofol (Diprivan) is a short-acting anesthetic agent given by constant infusion. It has an onset of less than 1 minute, and patients rapidly awaken when the drug is discontinued.

Neuromuscular Blocking Agents. Neuromuscular blocking agents are used when paralysis is desired, such as with patients who have acute lung injury or with those who require advanced mechanical ventilation modes. They are also often used in the management of head injuries to prevent increased intracranial pressure. Neuromuscular blocking agents provide paralysis; they have no anxiolytic, sedative, or analgesic properties. Commonly used neuromuscular blocking agents include pancuronium (Pavulon), atracurium (Tracrium), and vecuronium (Norcuron). Most institutions have protocols for monitoring patients receiving these agents. Patients receiving neuromuscular blocking agents require the administration of sedative agents and meticulous skin and eye care.

Monitoring the depth of paralysis is done via peripheral nerve stimulation. One method of peripheral nerve stimulation is the train-of-four technique. A nerve, usually the ulnar, is isolated, and electrodes are applied. The electrodes are connected to a peripheral nerve stimulator, which delivers four signals in rapid succession. The patient is monitored for a thumb twitch. One to two twitches (out of four) usually indicate adequate paralysis. The presence of four twitches usually indicates the need for a higher drug dose. An alternative to peripheral nerve stimulation is the use of respiratory waveform monitoring. The waveform indicates if a patient is initiating a spontaneous breath. Absence of spontaneous effort indicates adequate paralysis.

Troubleshooting

Individuals who care for patients receiving mechanical ventilation must be knowledgeable about the equipment and competent at troubleshooting. For the prevention of errors, *two important rules must be followed:*

1. *Never shut alarms off.* It is acceptable to silence alarms for a preset delay while working with a patient, such as during suctioning. However, alarms should *never* be shut off.

2. *Manually ventilate the patient with a bag-valve device if you are unable to troubleshoot alarms quickly or if you suspect equipment failure.*

Ventilator alarms vary from machine to machine; therefore, the nurse must be familiar with the ventilators used in the institution. Alarms can be categorized into two common causes: volume alarms and pressure alarms.

Volume Alarms. A low exhaled volume alarm sounds if the patient does not receive the preset VT. Causes of volume alarms include disconnection of the ventilator circuit from the artificial airway, a leak in the ETT or tracheostomy cuff, displacement of the ETT or tracheostomy tube, and disconnection of any part of the ventilator circuit.

Pressure Alarms. A high pressure alarm occurs if the amount of pressure needed for ventilating a patient exceeds a preset amount. Causes of pressure alarms include excess secretions; mucus plugs; patient's biting of the ETT; kinks in the ventilator circuit; patient's coughing, gagging, or attempting to talk; "fighting" the ventilator; ARDS or pulmonary edema; bronchospasm; pneumothorax or hemothorax; and pressure on the chest wall.

Weaning Patients From Mechanical Ventilation

Once the decision is made to mechanically ventilate a patient, caregivers should begin to plan for weaning the patient. Generally, patients who require short-term ventilatory support (e.g., in the immediate postoperative period) can be weaned quickly. Conversely, weaning is usually a slow, tedious process for patients who require long-term ventilatory support.

Assessment for Readiness to Wean

Patients who require mechanical ventilation require ongoing assessment for readiness to wean (Table 6–21). Several weaning indices that include these variables are available to assist in identifying when patients are ready to wean. The value of these indices in predicting successful weaning has not yet been shown; however, they are useful in assessing a patient's strengths and factors that may interfere with successful weaning (Burns et al., 1994).

Team Approach

A collaborative approach is essential for weaning patients from long-term mechanical ventilation. Team members include nurses, physicians, respiratory therapists, dietitian, physical therapist, occupational thera-

Table 6-20. MEDICATIONS COMMONLY USED TO FACILITATE MECHANICAL VENTILATION

Classification	Drug	Action/Uses	Dosage/Route	Common Side Effects	Nursing Implications
Analgesic	Morphine sulfate	Binds with opioid receptors within CNS, decreasing pain perception	1.0–5.0 mg IV push every 1–4 hours Dilute in sterile H_2O or NS, give over 4 to 5 minutes	Respiratory depression, hypotension, decreased cough reflex, nausea/vomiting, constipation, urinary retention	Assess level of pain and response to medication Monitor vital signs Monitor renal and bowel function Can be reversed with naloxone hydrochloride (Narcan)
Sedative (benzodiazepine)	Diazepam (Valium)	Potentiates action of gamma-aminobutyric acid (GABA), which inhibits neurotransmitters, resulting in CNS depression	2–10 mg IV push every 3–4 hours Do not dilute or mix with other drugs Give slowly, 5 mg/min	Drowsiness, CNS depression, respiratory depression, hypotension, antegrade amnesia, dependence	Assess level of sedation and response to medication Monitor vital signs Reduce dose in elderly, debilitated patients Assess IV site for phlebitis Can be reversed with flumazenil (Mazicon)
Sedative (benzodiazepine)	Lorazepam (Ativan)	See diazepam	1–4 mg IV push every 1–6 hours Dilute in equal amount of sterile H_2O or NS (NOTE: some institutions administer via continuous infusion)	See diazepam Excessive drowsiness, local IV irritation	See diazepam
Sedative (benzodiazepine)	Midazolam (Versed)	See diazepam	1–2.5 mg IV push every hour (give over 2 minutes) Additional doses up to 2.5 mg can be given after 2 minutes Infusion: 50–100 mg mixed in 100 ml NS or 5% D/W at 1–5 mg/h	See diazepam Local IV irritation, hiccoughs, nausea/vomiting, cough, headache	See diazepam
Sedative (neuroleptic)	Haloperidol (Haldol)	Blocks postsynaptic dopamine receptors, producing a tranquilizing effect	2–5 mg (up to 40 mg) IV push every 4–8 hours (can be given hourly if necessary)	Extrapyramidal symptoms, hypotension, dry mouth, blurred vision, urinary retention	Assess level of sedation and response to medication Monitor CNS effects Monitor vital signs Assess urine output Provide frequent mouth care

Classification	Drug	Action/Use	Dose	Adverse Effects	Nursing Implications
Sedative (anesthetic)	Propofol (Diprivan)	Action unknown; provides continuous sedation	Continuous infusion 5–75 µg/kg/min; average dose is 25–75 µg/kg/min. Dose can be titrated every 2 minutes. Premixed infusion: 500 mg/50 ml or 1 g/100 ml (10 mg/ml)	Involuntary muscle movement, apnea, hypotension, burning at site, bradycardia, hyperlipidemia	Assess level of sedation and response to medication; patients should awaken rapidly on discontinuation of the drug. Monitor vital signs. Contraindicated in patients with allergies to lipid emulsions
Neuromuscular blocking agent (NMBA)	Pancuronium bromide (Pavulon)	Blocks effects of acetylcholine at myoneural junction, preventing neuromuscular transmission. Used to chemically paralyze patients to facilitate mechanical ventilation and in patients with increased intracranial pressure	0.04–0.1 mg/kg IV push every 25–60 minutes	Tachycardia, prolonged apnea, bronchospasm	Assess level of paralysis with peripheral nerve stimulator or respiratory waveform monitoring. Drug has no effect on level of consciousness, anxiety, or pain; medicate patient with sedatives and/or analgesics. Provide total care (e.g., turning, eye care) because patient has no spontaneous movement. Explain procedures to patient. Reassure patient. Teach family about action and use of drug
NMBA	Atracurium (Tracrium)	See pancuronium bromide	Bolus dose of 0.4–0.5 mg/kg IV push followed by continuous infusion at 2–15 µg/kg/min. Infusion: 20–50 mg mixed in 100 ml of NS, 5% D/W, or 5% D/NS	Skin flushing, hypersensitivity, prolonged paralysis, hypotension, bradycardia/tachycardia	See pancuronium bromide
NMBA	Vecuronium (Norcuron)	See pancuronium bromide	Bolus dose of 80–100 µg/kg IV push followed by continuous infusion at 0.8–1.2 µg/kg/min. Infusion: 10–20 mg mixed in 100 ml of NS, 5%D/W, 5%D/NS, or lactated Ringer's solution	Hypersensitivity, prolonged paralysis, skeletal muscle weakness, atrophy	See pancuronium bromide

Adapted from Hodgson, B. B., Kizior, R. J., & Kingdon, R. T. (1995). *Nurse's drug handbook 1995.* Philadelphia: W. B. Saunders Co.; Lehne R. A. (1994). *Pharmacology for nursing care* (2nd ed.). Philadelphia: W. B. Saunders Co.; Vallerand, A. H., & Deglin, J. H. (1994). *Davis's guide to I.V. medications* (2nd ed.). Philadelphia: F. A. Davis Co.; *Physicians' desk reference* (50th ed). (1996). Montvale, NJ: Medical Economics.

CNS = central nervous system; IV = intravenous; NS = normal saline; D/W = dextrose in water; D/NS = dextrose in normal saline.

Table 6–21. ASSESSMENT PARAMETERS INDICATING READINESS TO WEAN

Underlying cause for mechanical ventilation resolved
  Improved chest x-ray findings
  Minimal secretions
  Normal breath sounds
Hemodynamic stability; adequate cardiac output
Adequate respiratory muscle strength
  Respiratory rate < 25 breaths/min
  Negative inspiratory force > −20 cm H_2O
  Spontaneous tidal volume 4–5 ml/kg
  Vital capacity 10–15 ml/kg
  Minute ventilation 5–10 L/min
Adequate ABG results without a high FiO_2 and/or a high
  PEEP
  PaO_2 > 60 mm Hg with FiO_2 <0.5
  $PaCO_2$ < 45 mm Hg
  PEEP ≤ 5 cm H_2O
Adequate level of consciousness
Good nutritional status and hydration
Absence of factors that impair weaning
  Infection
  Anemia
  Fever
  Fatigue
  Sleep deprivation
  Pain
  Abdominal distention
  Bowel abnormalities (diarrhea or constipation)
Mentally ready to wean
  Calm, relaxed
  Minimal or absent anxiety
  Motivated
Minimal need for sedatives and other medications that
  may cause respiratory depression

ABG = arterial blood gas.

pist, social worker, pastoral ministers, and family members. Each team member has a unique and important role in providing physical as well as psychological support during the weaning process. An advanced practice nurse, such as a clinical nurse specialist or a case manager, often coordinates the care delivered by the various team members. Periodic multidisciplinary patient care conferences are essential.

Methods for Weaning

Methods for weaning include the use of IMV/SIMV, T-piece (Briggs' device), pressure support, and CPAP. A combination of methods is frequently used.

Intermittent Mandatory Ventilation/Synchronized Intermittent Mandatory Ventilation. When IMV/SIMV is used for weaning, the respiratory rate is gradually decreased until the patient assumes all of the work of breathing. For example, the IMV/SIMV rate is decreased by two breaths per minute at designated

intervals as long as the patient tolerates the process. This method works exceptionally well in the weaning of patients from short-term mechanical ventilation, such as that used in patients who have undergone surgery. The respiratory rate is frequently decreased on an hourly basis until the patient is weaned and ready for extubation. In contrast, the patient who has been on the ventilator for an extended period of time may require the IMV rate to be decreased by one breath per minute each day. An advantage of using the IMV/SIMV method is that it is performed on a continuous basis. It can be used during the night as well as during the day. A disadvantage is that it may promote muscle fatigue when low IMV/SIMV rates are used in the patient who has required prolonged mechanical ventilation.

T-Piece. The T-piece, or Briggs device (see Fig. 6–26), requires that the patient be removed from mechanical ventilation for short periods of time, usually beginning with a 5-minute period. The ventilator is disconnected, and the T-piece is connected to the patient's artificial airway. Supplemental oxygen is provided through the device, often at an FiO_2 that is 10% higher than the ventilator setting. An option to the T-piece is to leave the patient connected to the ventilator with the respiratory rate set at zero.

The patient breathes spontaneously for a predetermined amount of time that is gradually increased. For example, initially, the patient may be weaned for 5 minutes every 6 hours. As the patient tolerates the procedure, the weaning may occur for 15 minutes every 4 hours. It is important to begin the procedure after the patient is well rested. It is also helpful to begin weaning after administration of a bronchodilator, followed by suctioning of secretions. The nurse should stay with the patient during the initial weaning attempts in order to adequately assess tolerance to the procedure and to relieve patient fear and anxiety. Ongoing assessment for patient fatigue is also essential. The T-piece method encourages respiratory muscle strengthening and may result in a shorter time on mechanical ventilation for patients receiving long-term ventilation.

Pressure Support. Pressure support is commonly used to assist in patient weaning. PSV decreases the workload of breathing and increases the patient's ability to initiate spontaneous breathing efforts. PSV is frequently used in conjunction with IMV/SIMV. For example, the IMV/SIMV rate can be gradually decreased to a rate of zero with 10 to 15 cm H_2O of PSV. Then, PSV is tapered; however, it is not necessary to reduce the PSV to zero in order to extubate the patient.

Continuous Positive Airway Pressure. Continuous positive airway pressure is another method used to facilitate weaning from mechanical ventilation. As

NURSING CARE PLAN FOR THE MECHANICALLY VENTILATED PATIENT

Nursing Diagnosis	Patient Outcomes	Nursing Interventions

Breathing pattern, ineffective, related to disease process, artificial airway, and mechanical ventilator.	The patient will breathe effectively while mechanically ventilated, maintain normal arterial blood gas values, and have absence of symptoms of hypoxemia.	1. Maintain endotracheal tube or tracheostomy:
		   a. Secure tubes with tape or other devices.
		   b. Restrain patient's wrists as necessary.
		 2. Assess respiratory status every 4 hours:
		   a. Auscultate breath sounds.
		   b. Assess chest excursion.
		   c. Assess patient's ability to initiate a spontaneous breath.
		   d. Assess for signs and symptoms of hypoxemia.
		 3. Monitor ventilator settings:
		   a. Tidal volume.
		   b. FiO_2.
		   c. Respiratory rate (machine and spontaneous).
		   d. Mode of ventilation.
		   e. Use of PEEP, CPAP, or pressure support.
		   f. Peak inspiratory pressure.
		   g. Alarms on.
		 4. Monitor cuff pressures of ETT or tracheostomy:
		   a. Cuff is usually inflated with the minimum amount of air in order to prevent leak of air around the cuff.
		   b. Several commercial devices are available to monitor cuff pressures. These devices attach to the pilot balloon of the ETT or tracheostomy tube and measure the pressure.
		   c. Notify the physician if cuff pressures exceed 30 cm H_2O.
		 5. Monitor oxygenation and ventilation. Notify the physician if parameters change:
		   a. Pulse oximetry.
		   b. ABGs.
		   c. End-tidal carbon dioxide measurements.
		   d. Transcutaneous oxygen and/or carbon dioxide monitoring.
		 6. Monitor serial chest x-ray studies:
		   a. Assess ETT or tracheostomy tube placement.
		   b. Assess improvement or worsening.
		 7. Maintain PEEP:
		   a. Avoid removing patient from the ventilator for suctioning or other procedures if PEEP is used.
		   b. Consider use of closed tracheal suction devices, or adapters.
		   c. Ensure that bag-valve device is equipped with a PEEP valve and is set appropriately.
		 8. Monitor for complications associated with positive pressure ventilation:
		   a. Barotrauma:
		     1. Assess for sudden increase in peak inspiratory pressure, decreased or absent breath sounds on affected side, tracheal deviation, extreme anxiety, symptoms of shock.
		     2. If symptoms occur, remove patient from ventilator and manually ventilate with bag-valve device.
		     3. Prepare for chest tube insertion.
		   b. Decreased cardiac output:
		     1. Measure CO at least every shift if pulmonary artery catheter is in place.

Continued on following page

NURSING CARE PLAN FOR THE MECHANICALLY VENTILATED PATIENT *Continued*

Nursing Diagnosis	Patient Outcomes	Nursing Interventions

		2. Assess for hypotension, tachycardia, dysrhythmias, decreased level of consciousness.
		9. Do not disconnect mechanical ventilation to perform tracheostomy care on a patient. To facilitate tracheostomy care:
		  a. Consider use of tracheostomy that does not require an inner cannula.
		  b. Consider use of tracheostomy tube with disposable inner cannula.
		10. Keep tubings free of moisture:
		  a. To avoid aspiration of moisture, empty tubings before repositioning patient.
		  b. Empty tubings as needed. Avoid draining water backward through the ventilator circuit where the tubing connects to the patient. Do not drain water into cascade.
		  c. Use devices (e.g., water traps) to facilitate drainage of moisture.
		11. Medicate the patient as needed (see Table 6–20).
		12. Monitor readiness to wean from ventilator (see Table 6–21):
		  a. Assess spontaneous respiratory efforts.
		  b. Assess tidal volume, vital capacity, negative inspiratory force.
		  c. Monitor vital signs.

Airway clearance ineffective, related to artificial airway, decreased ability to cough.	The patient will maintain an open airway free of secretions.	1. Assess need for suctioning: (pressure alarm on ventilator, audible secretions, harsh breath sounds). 2. Suction according to hospital protocol (see Tables 6–15 and 6–16). 3. Assess breath sounds after suctioning. 4. If tracheal secretions are thick, assess hydration of patient. 5. Reposition the patient frequently to mobilize secretions.

Communication impaired, verbal, related to artificial airway and mechanical ventilation.	Patient will be able to communicate needs to caregiver.	1. Establish method for communication:
		  a. Yes/no questions.
		  b. Clipboard with paper and pencil.
		  c. Magic slates.
		  d. Picture communication boards.
		  e. Computerized systems, if available.
		  f. Attempt lip reading if patient has nasotracheal tube or tracheostomy.
		2. Speak slowly and clearly to patient.
		3. Explain procedures.
		4. Use significant others to assist with communication.
		5. Consider use of "talking" tracheostomy tube.
		6. Expect frustration from both patient and nurse.

Oral mucous membranes, altered, related to artificial airway.	Moist oral mucous membranes; absence of ulceration or other lesions.	1. Assess oral mucous membranes for ulcerations or other lesions. 2. Carefully inspect the mouth around and under the devices, especially if commercial devices are used. Loosen the devices periodically as recommended by the manufacturers.

NURSING CARE PLAN FOR THE MECHANICALLY VENTILATED PATIENT *Continued*

Nursing Diagnosis	Patient Outcomes	Nursing Interventions

		3. Provide good mouth care at least once per shift:
		  a. Use oral swabs specifically designed for mouth care.
		  b. Brush teeth. Use syringe to rinse mouth and tonsil suction to remove secretions. A toothbrush that attaches to suction is also commercially available.
		  c. Lubricate lips with water-soluble ointment or emollients, such as Chapstick.
		  d. *Avoid* lemon-glycerine swabs (they dry the mouth).
		  e. Avoid mouthwashes that contain alcohol.
		4. Reposition endotracheal tube according to hospital protocol (usually once per day; may not be necessary if commercial device used):
		  a. Two personnel required for procedure: one to secure endotracheal tube and one for taping the tube.
		  b. Note marking of ETT at lip line.
		  c. Suction endotracheal tube prior to repositioning tube.
		  d. Move tube to opposite side of mouth and secure according to protocol.
		  e. If an ETT is repositioned, this is an excellent time to give mouth care.
		  f. After repositioning, assess tube position at lip line and auscultate for bilateral breath sounds

Anxiety and fear, related to need for mechanical ventilation, inability to communicate needs, psychological ventilator dependence.	Relief of anxiety and fear.	1. Talk to patient frequently. 2. Explain procedures. 3. Establish communication. 4. Reassure patient that needs are being met. 5. Keep call light within reach. 6. Encourage significant others to visit with patient.

Nutrition, altered, related to inability to take oral feedings, increased nutritional needs, impaired gastrointestinal function. Nutrition, altered: less than body requirement.	Patient will achieve adequate nutritional status.	1. Assess gastrointestinal function at least once per shift:
		  a. Assess bowel sounds.
		  b. Assess for gastric distention.
		2. Monitor bowel habits.
		3. Monitor daily weight.
		4. Obtain dietary consultation/nutritional evaluation.
		5. Administer parenteral or enteral feedings according to hospital protocol:
		  a. Add food color to enteral feedings to monitor for potential aspiration (controversial).
		  b. Check gastric residua every 4 hours.
		6. Observe ABG results for carbon dioxide retention.

Pulmonary infection, risk for, related to artificial airway.	Patient will remain infection free.	1. Monitor temperature every 4 hours. 2. Monitor amount, color, consistency, and odor of secretions.

Continued on following page

NURSING CARE PLAN FOR THE MECHANICALLY VENTILATED PATIENT *Continued*

Nursing Diagnosis	Patient Outcomes	Nursing Interventions
		3. Use good handwashing techniques. 4. Wear gloves for suctioning, oral care, and repositioning endotracheal tubes. 5. Use aseptic technique for suctioning. 6. Obtain tracheal aspirate for culture and sensitivity according to hospital protocol. 7. Administer antibiotics as ordered.
Injury, risk for, gastrointestinal bleeding related to positive pressure ventilation, stress of critical illness.	Patient will not experience bleeding.	1. Assess gastric contents and stools for presence of occult blood. 2. Observe for tarry and/or bloody stools. 3. Monitor serial hemoglobin and hematocrit values. 4. Monitor gastric pH. Administer antacids as ordered to decrease acidity of gastric contents. 5. Administer histamine antagonists as ordered, e.g., cimetidine (Tagamet) and ranitidine (Zantac).
Fluid volume excess, risk for, related to ventilator humidification, stimulation of renin-angiotensin-aldosterone mechanism.	Patient will not experience fluid overload.	1. Monitor intake and output every shift. 2. Monitor daily weight. 3. Assess breath sounds every 4 hours. 4. Assess vital signs every 2 to 4 hours.

previously noted, CPAP augments spontaneous breaths by increasing the FRC and prevents airway collapse. It is also commonly used with IMV/SIMV.

Steps for Weaning

During any weaning attempt, several steps should be followed. The procedure should be explained to the patient and family in a manner that reduces anxiety. The patient should be adequately rested and positioned comfortably. Baseline parameters, including vital signs, heart rhythm, and ABGs, should be obtained before any weaning attempt. The patient should be observed during the weaning process for tolerance or intolerance to the procedure.

When Weaning Should Be Discontinued

The weaning process should be stopped if physiological changes occur (Table 6–22). If a patient exhibits signs of not tolerating the weaning process, ABGs should be assessed, and the patient should resume ventilation at the previous settings.

Causes of Impaired Weaning

Weaning may be impaired owing to several causes: increased oxygen demand, decreased lung function, psychological factors, and equipment or tech-nique factors. Increased oxygen demands may be caused by anemia, fever, or pain. Decreased lung function may result from malnutrition, overuse of sedatives or hypnotics, and sleep deprivation. Psychological causes include apprehension and fear, helplessness, and depression. Equipment and technique problems include the time of day, inadequate weaning periods, and inability to tolerate the technique.

Weaning the Terminally Ill Patient

Occasionally, ventilatory support is gradually withdrawn from a terminally ill patient. This is referred

---

Table 6–22. CRITERIA FOR DISCONTINUING WEANING

Respiratory rate > 25–30 breaths per minute or < 8
Blood pressure increases > 30 mm Hg or decreases > 20 mm Hg
Heart rate increases > 30 beats/min
Dysrhythmias (e.g., premature ventricular contractions or bradycardia)
ST segment elevation
Significant decrease in spontaneous tidal volume
Use of accessory muscles
Labored respirations
Diaphoresis
Decreased level of consciousness
Restlessness
Anxiety

RESEARCH APPLICATION

Article Reference

Thomas, J., Kaelin, R. M., Joliet, P., & Chevrolet, J. (1995). Influence of the quality of nursing on the duration of weaning from mechanical ventilation in patients with chronic pulmonary disease. *Critical Care Medicine*, *23*, 1807-1815.

Study Overview

Six years of data were reviewed for an analysis of the influence of nursing care on patients with chronic obstructive pulmonary disease (COPD) in an intensive care unit in Switzerland. Nursing care was evaluated as a ratio of real versus ideal staffing based on patient acuity each year. Mathematical corrections were made for days off and number of novice and certified nurses. A ratio of 1.0 meant adequate staffing, whereas a ratio of less than 1.0 reflected inadequate staffing. Patient activity was tracked throughout the study period by one head nurse.

Patients had to meet specific inclusion criteria for the diagnosis of COPD in order to be included in this study. Throughout the 6-year period, the intensive care unit had the same medical director who followed all patients. This, in addition to intubation criteria and weaning protocols, promoted consistent approaches to care.

Numerous physiological parameters were averaged for patients admitted each year (year group). The number of patients reported for each year ranged from 8 to 18. Gender, age, pulmonary function test results, body weight, and serum protein levels were not different between each year group of patients. Differences between year groups of patients were reported for creatinine/height index, PaO_2, and mean ventilator days. The patients for each year group had similar demographic and physical status, except for the duration of mechanical ventilation.

When the pooled patient mechanical ventilation duration data were compared with the real/ideal (R/I) nursing index for each year by use of Spearman's rank coefficient test, a significant negative correlation was found ($P = 0.025$). When the real/ideal nursing ratio fell below 0.8 for a year, the duration of mechanical ventilation increased. In the years in which the R/I ratio was less than 0.8, the average duration of mechanical ventilation was 13.7 to 38.2 days. During the 2 years that the ratio exceeded 0.8, the average duration of mechanical ventilation was 7.3 to 10.1 days.

Critique

The strength of this study is that the investigators assessed for potential demographic or physiological differences between each year group of patients that might have skewed the findings. This study has two major weaknesses. First, the yearly averages of staffing patterns may or may not accurately reflect the adequacy of staffing for the days the patients with COPD were in the intensive care unit. Patients with COPD represented a small percentage of patients admitted to the intensive care unit. Second, the validity of the patient acuity system used by the head nurse was not reported, so it therefore cannot be assumed. A study design comparing nursing care hours and clinical outcomes including duration of mechanical ventilation for *individual* patients with COPD would be more reliable and valid.

Nursing Implications

Despite the weakness of this study design, the findings are logical. It makes sense that increased levels of nursing assessment and intervention would shorten the duration of mechanical ventilation. The findings support the important role that nurses can play in the treatment of acutely ill patients. Quantifying the impact of professional nursing practice on patient outcomes is a critical step in documenting the need for adequate professional nursing staff.

to as *terminal weaning*. During this period, it is important for the nurse to provide relief of symptoms and patient comfort. The patient may experience dyspnea, pain, anxiety, agitation, or excessive secretions during this time. Medications, such as morphine sulfate, lorazepam, haloperidol, and scopolamine, can be administered for the reduction of symptoms (Weatherill, 1995). Legal and ethical issues associated with terminal weaning must be addressed by the nurse caring for the patient.

Summary

Care of critically ill patients requires knowledge of normal anatomy and physiology and excellent assessment skills. Skills in establishing and maintaining an open airway and initiating mechanical ventilation are also essential. Care of the patient requiring mechanical ventilation is an everyday assignment in the critical care unit; therefore, it is essential that the nurse apply knowledge and skills in order to effectively care for these patients.

CRITICAL THINKING QUESTIONS

1. Based on your knowledge of clinical disorders, identify different clinical conditions that might cause problems with the following steps in gas exchange:
   a. Ventilation
   b. Diffusion
   c. Perfusion (transportation)
2. Your patient has the following ABG results: pH, 7.28; PaO_2, 52 mm Hg; SaO_2, 84%; $PaCO_2$, 55 mm Hg; HCO_3, 24 mEq/L.
   a. What is your interpretation of these ABGs?
   b. What clinical condition or conditions might cause the patient to have these ABG results?
3. Your patient undergoes mechanical ventilation for treatment. The pressure alarm keeps going off for a few seconds at a time, despite the fact that you have just suctioned the patient. What nursing actions are warranted at this time?
4. You are caring for a patient who has been mechanically ventilated for 2 weeks. Physically, she meets all of the criteria to begin weaning from mechanical ventilation. How can you assist her psychologically during the weaning process?
5. Many hospitals now care for mechanically ventilated patients outside of the intensive care unit. What special considerations are necessary for the care of these patients?

REFERENCES

Ahrens, T. (1993). Respiratory monitoring in critical care. *AACN Clinical Issues in Critical Care Nursing, 4,* 56–65.

Amato, M. B. P., Barbas, C. S. V., Bonassa, J., Saldiva, P. H. N., Zin, W. A., & Ribeiro De Carvalho, C. R. (1992). Volume-assured pressure support ventilation (VAPSV): A new approach for reducing muscle workload during acute respiratory failure. *Chest, 192,* 1225–1234.

American Heart Association (1994). *Textbook of advanced cardiac life support.* Dallas: Author.

Ashworth, L. J. (1990). Pressure support ventilation. *Critical Care Nurse, 10*(7), 20–25.

Boggs, R. L. (1993). Airway management. In R. L. Boggs, & M. Wooldridge-King (Eds.), *AACN Procedure manual for critical care* (3rd ed.) (pp. 1–65). Philadelphia: W. B. Saunders Co.

Bolton, P. J., & Kline, K. A. (1994). Understanding modes of mechanical ventilation. *American Journal of Nursing, 94*(6), 36–43.

Burns, S. M. (1990). Advances in ventilator therapy. *Focus on Critical Care, 17,* 227–237.

Burns, S. M., Burns, J. E., & Truwit, J. D. (1994). Comparison of five clinical weaning indices. *American Journal of Critical Care, 3,* 342–352.

Christensen, M. A., Bloom, J., & Sutton, K. R. (1995). Comparing arterial and end-tidal carbon dioxide values in hyperventilated neurosurgical patients. *American Journal of Critical Care, 4,* 116–121.

Chung, D. C., & Lamb, A. M. (1990). *Essentials of anesthesiology* (2nd ed.). Philadelphia: W. B. Saunders Co.

Connolly, M. (1995). Mucolytics and the critically ill patient: Help or hindrance? *AACN Clinical Issues: Advanced Practice in Acute and Critical Care, 6,* 307–315.

Cottingham, C. A., & Habashi, N. M. (1995). Extracorporeal lung assist in the adult trauma patient. *AACN Clinical Issues: Advanced Practice in Acute and Critical Care, 6,* 229–241.

Curley, M. A. Q., & Molengraft, J. (1994). Care of the child supported on high frequency oscillatory ventilation. *AACN Clinical Issues in Critical Care Nursing, 5,* 49–58.

Dabbs, A. D., & Olslund, L. (1994). The new alternative to intubation. *American Journal of Nursing, 94*(8), 42–45.

Dantzker, D. R. (1995). Respiratory failure. In D.R. Dantzker, N.R. MacIntyre, & E.D. Bakow (Eds.), *Comprehensive respiratory care.* Philadelphia: W. B. Saunders Co.

Guyton, A. C. (1991). *Textbook of medical physiology* (8th ed.). Philadelphia: W. B. Saunders Co.

Haller, M., Kilger, E., Briegel, J., Forst, H., & Peter, K. (1994). Continuous intra-arterial blood gas and pH monitoring in critically ill patients with severe respiratory failure: A prospective, criterion standard study. *Critical Care Medicine, 22,* 580–587.

Harvey, M. A. (1992). *Study guide to the core curriculum for critical care nursing* (2nd ed.). Philadelphia: W. B. Saunders Co.

Hess, D., & Kacmarek, R. M. (1993). Techniques and devices for monitoring oxygenation. *Respiratory Care, 38,* 646–669.

Hodgson, B. B., Kizior, R. J., & Kingdon, R. T. (1995). *Nurse's drug handbook 1995.* Philadelphia: W. B. Saunders Co.

Johnson, K. L., Kearney, P. A., Johnson, S. B., Niblett, J. B., MacMillan, N. L., & McClain, R. E. (1994). Closed versus open endotracheal suctioning: Costs and physiologic consequences. *Critical Care Medicine, 22,* 658–666.

Kersten, L. D. (1989). *Comprehensive respiratory nursing: A decision making approach.* Philadelphia: W. B. Saunders Co.

Larson, C. P., Jr., Vender, J., & Seiver, A. (1994). Multisite evaluation of a continuous intraarterial blood gas monitoring system. *Anesthesiology, 81,* 543–552.

Lehne, R. A. (1994). *Pharmacology for nursing care* (2nd ed.). Philadelphia: W. B. Saunders Co.

Luer, J. M. (1995). Sedation and chemical relaxation in critical pulmonary illness: Suggestions for patient assessment and drug monitoring. *AACN Clinical Issues: Advanced Practice in Acute and Critical Care, 6,* 333–343.

Mahutte, C. K., Sasse, S. A., Chen, P. A., & Holody, M. (1994). Performance of a patient-dedicated, on-demand blood gas monitor in medical ICU patients. *American Journal of Respiratory and Critical Care Medicine, 150,* 865–869.

Mays, L. C., & Eckert, S. (1994). Synchronous independent lung ventilation. *Dimensions of Critical Care Nursing, 13,* 249–255.

Noll, M. L., Hix, C. D., & Scott, G. (1990). Closed-tracheal suction systems: Effectiveness and nursing implications. *AACN Clinical Issues in Critical Care Nursing, 1,* 318–326.

Physicians' desk reference (50th ed.). (1996). Montvale, NJ: Medical Economics.

Pierce, L. N. B. (1995). *Guide to mechanical ventilation and intensive respiratory care.* Philadelphia: W. B. Saunders Co.

Rhodes, M. (1995). Trauma. In D. R. Dantzker, N. R. MacIntyre, & E. D. Bakow (Eds.), *Comprehensive respiratory care.* Philadelphia: W. B. Saunders Co.

Siemens-Elema A. B. (1994). *Servo ventilator 300: Operating manual 6.0.* Solna, Sweden: Siemens-Elema AB.

Solomon, E. P., & Phillips, G. A. (1987). *Understanding human anatomy and physiology.* Philadelphia: W. B. Saunders Co.

Sonesso, G. (1990). Negative pressure ventilation: New uses for an old technique. *AACN Clinical Issues in Critical Care Nursing, 1,* 313–317.

St. John, R. E., & LeFrak, S. S. (1990). Alternate modes of mechanical ventilation. *AACN Clinical Issues in Critical Care Nursing, 1,* 248–259.

Stone, K. S. (1990). Ventilator versus manual resuscitation bag as the method for delivering hyperoxygenation prior to endotracheal suctioning. *AACN Clinical Issues in Critical Care Nursing, 1,* 289–299.

Vallerand, A. H., & Deglin, J. H. (1994). *Davis's guide to I.V. medications* (2nd ed.). Philadelphia: F. A. Davis Co.

Venkatesh, B., Clutton Brock, T. H., & Hendry S. P. (1994). A multiparameter sensor for continuous intra-arterial blood gas monitoring: A prospective evaluation. *Critical Care Medicine, 22,* 588–594.

VonRueden, K. T. (1990). Noninvasive assessment of gas exchange in the critically ill. *AACN Clinical Issues in Critical Care Nursing, 1,* 239–247.

Weatherill, G. G. (1995). Pharmacologic symptom control during the withdrawal of life support: Lessons in palliative care. *AACN Clinical Issues: Advanced Practice in Acute and Critical Care, 6,* 344–351.

Witta, K. (1990). New techniques for weaning difficult patients from mechanical ventilation. *AACN Clinical Issues in Critical Care Nursing, 1,* 260–266.

RECOMMENDED READINGS

Anderson, S. (1990). Six easy steps to interpreting blood gases. *American Journal of Nursing, 90*(8), 42–45.

Burns, S. M., Clochesy, J. M., Hanneman, S. K. G., Ingersoll, G. E., Knebel, A. R., & Shekleton, M. E. (1995). Weaning from long-term mechanical ventilation. *American Journal of Critical Care, 4,* 4–22.

Chang, V. M. (1995). Protocol for prevention of complications of endotracheal intubation. *Critical Care Nurse, 15*(5), 19–27.

DePew, C. L., & Noll, M. L. (1994). Inline closed-system suctioning: A research analysis. *Dimensions of Critical Care Nursing, 13,* 73–83.

Dickson, S. L. (1995). Understanding the oxyhemoglobin dissociation curve. *Critical Care Nurse, 15*(5), 54–58.

Hanneman, S. K. G., Ingersoll, G. L., Knebel, A. R., Shekleton, M. E., Burns, S. M., & Clochesy, J. M. (1994). Weaning from short-term mechanical ventilation: A review. *American Journal of Critical Care, 3,* 421–443.

Henneman, E. A., Bellamy, P., & Togashi, C. (1995). Peripheral nerve stimulators in the critical care setting: A policy for monitoring neuromuscular blockade. *Critical Care Nurse, 15*(3), 82–88.

Hill, L. (1995). Peripheral electrical stimulation: Titrating neuromuscular blocking agent levels. *Dimensions of Critical Care Nursing, 14,* 305–314.

Jenson, D., & Justic, M. (1995). An algorithm to distinguish the need for sedative, anxiolytic, and analgesic agents. *Dimensions of Critical Care Nursing, 14,* 58–65.

Snider, B. S. (1993). Use of muscle relaxants in the ICU: Nursing implications. *Critical Care Nurse, 13*(6), 55–60.

Tasota, F. J., & Wesmiller, S. W. (1994). Assessing A.B.G.s: Maintaining the delicate balance. *American Journal of Nursing, 94*(5), 34–44.

Weilitz, P. B. (1993). Weaning a patient from mechanical ventilation. *Critical Care Nurse, 13*(4), 33–41.

Zavotsky, K. E., & D'Amelio, L. F. (1995). Bedside percutaneous tracheostomy: Implications for critical care nurses. *Critical Care Nurse, 15*(5), 37–43.

7

Code Management

Jacqueline Fowler Byers, Ph.D., R.N.
Marsha Martin, M.N., R.N., CCRN

OBJECTIVES

- Compare roles of caregivers in managing cardiopulmonary arrest situations.
- Identify equipment used during a code.
- Differentiate basic and advanced life support measures used during a code.
- Identify medications used in code management, including use, action, side effects, and nursing implications.
- Discuss treatment of special problems that can occur during a code.
- Identify information to be documented during a code.
- Describe care of patients after resuscitation.
- Identify psychosocial, legal, and ethical issues related to code management.

Introduction

Code, code blue, code 99, and *Dr. Heart* are terms frequently used in hospital settings to refer to emergency situations that require life-saving resuscitation and interventions. Codes are called when patients suffer a cardiac and/or respiratory arrest or a life-threatening cardiac dysrhythmia that has caused loss of consciousness. (The generic term *arrest* is used in this chapter to refer to these conditions.) Whatever the cause, patient survival and positive outcome depend on prompt recognition of the situation and immediate institution of basic and advanced life support measures. Code management refers to the initiation of a code and the life-saving interventions performed when a patient arrests.

This chapter discusses the roles of the personnel involved in a code and identifies the equipment that must be readily available during a code. Basic and advanced life support measures are presented, including drugs commonly used during a code. The chapter concludes with a brief discussion of psychosocial, legal, and ethical implications of code management. For

more in-depth information, the reader is referred to the following American Heart Association (AHA) publications:

Standards and guidelines for cardiopulmonary resuscitation and emergency cardiac care (1992). *Journal of the American Medical Association, 268,* 2135-2302; American Heart Association (1994). *Textbook of advanced cardiac life support.* Dallas: Author.

All personnel involved in hospital patient care should have basic cardiac life support (BCLS) certification, and this certification is also recommended for the lay public. Advanced cardiac life support (ACLS) provider training is available through the AHA and is strongly recommended for anyone working in critical care.

Roles of Caregivers in Code Management

Prompt recognition of patient arrest and rapid initiation of cardiopulmonary resuscitation (CPR) and advanced life support measures are essential for improved patient outcomes. The first person to recognize that a patient has suffered an arrest should call for help, instruct someone to "call a code," and begin CPR. One-person CPR is continued until additional help arrives.

CODE TEAM

Key personnel are notified to assist with code management. An overhead paging system or individual pagers may be used for contacting personnel, depending on hospital policies.

Most hospitals have code teams that are designated to respond to codes (Table 7–1). The code team usually consists of a physician, an intensive care unit or emergency department nurse, a nursing supervisor, an anesthetist or anesthesiologist, a respiratory therapist, a pharmacist or pharmacy technician, an electrocardiogram (ECG) technician, and a chaplain. The code team responds to the code and works in conjunction with the patient's nurse and primary physician, if present. If a code team does not exist, any available personnel usually respond.

DIRECTOR OF THE CODE

The person who directs, or "runs," the code is responsible for making diagnoses and treatment deci-

sions. The director is usually a physician who is preferably experienced in code management, such as an emergency department physician. However, the director may be the patient's primary physician or another physician who is available and qualified for the task. If several physicians are present, one should assume responsibility for being the code team leader and should be the only person giving orders for interventions so that confusion and conflict are avoided. In some small hospitals, codes may be directed by a nurse certified in ACLS. In this situation, standing physician orders are needed for guiding and supporting the nurse's decision making.

The director of the code needs as much information about the patient as possible in order to make treatment decisions. Necessary information includes the reason for the patient's hospitalization, the patient's current treatments and medications, and the events that occurred immediately before the code.

If possible, the code director should not be performing CPR or other tasks. The director should give full attention to assessment, diagnosis, and treatment decisions in order to direct resuscitative efforts.

CODE NURSES

Primary Nurse. The patient's primary nurse should be free to relate information to the person

Table 7–1. ROLES AND RESPONSIBILITIES OF CODE TEAM MEMBERS

Team Member	Primary Role
Director of the code (usually a physician)	Make diagnoses and treatment decisions
Primary nurse	Provide information to code director Contact attending physician Assist with medications and procedures
Nurse	Coordinate use of the crash cart Prepare medications Assemble equipment (intubation, suction) Defibrillate
Nursing supervisor	Control the crowd Assist with medications and procedures Ensure that a bed is available in intensive care unit Assist with transfer of patient to intensive care unit
Nurse or assistant	Record events
Anesthesiologist/nurse anesthetist/emergency physician	Intubate patient Manage airway and oxygenation
Respiratory therapist	Assist with ventilation Draw arterial blood gases Set up respiratory equipment
Code management pharmacist/technician	Assist with medication administration Prepare intravenous infusions
ECG technician	Obtain 12-lead ECG
Chaplain	Support family

directing the code. The primary nurse may also start intravenous (IV) lines, give emergency drugs, or defibrillate the patient as directed by the code director (if the primary nurse is qualified). In some cases, the primary nurse may need to leave the code situation in order to contact the patient's attending physician or to relate information to the family.

Second Nurse. An important task for the second nurse present is to coordinate the use of the crash cart. This nurse should be thoroughly familiar with the layout of the cart and the location of items. This nurse locates, prepares, and labels medications and IV fluids. He or she also assembles equipment for intubation, suctioning, and other procedures, such as central line insertion.

Nursing Supervisor. The nursing supervisor responds to the code in order to assist in whatever manner is needed. Frequently, more people respond to a code than are needed. One job of the supervisor is to limit the number of people in the code to only those necessary and those there for learning purposes. This measure decreases crowding and confusion. Other nursing supervisor responsibilities are maintenance of communication with staff and family and assistance with such procedures as IV insertion. If the patient needs to be transferred to the critical care unit, the supervisor can also coordinate the transfer and ensure that a critical care bed is available.

ANESTHESIOLOGIST/NURSE ANESTHETIST

The anesthesiologist or anesthetist assumes control of the patient's ventilation and oxygenation. This individual (or another trained person) intubates the patient to ensure an adequate airway and to facilitate ventilation. The primary or secondary nurse assists with the set-up and checking of intubation equipment.

RESPIRATORY THERAPIST

The respiratory therapist usually assists with manual ventilation of the patient before and after intubation. The therapist may also obtain a blood sample for arterial blood gas analysis, set up oxygen and ventilation equipment, and suction the patient. In some institutions, the respiratory therapist performs intubation.

PHARMACIST/PHARMACY TECHNICIAN

In some hospitals, a pharmacist or pharmacy technician responds to codes. This individual may prepare medications and mix IV infusions for administration during the code. The pharmacist may also calculate appropriate drug doses based on the patient's weight. Frequently, pharmacy staff are also responsible for bringing additional medications. At the termination of the code, pharmacy staff may replenish the crash cart

---

Table 7–2. TYPICAL CONTENTS OF A CRASH CART

Main Items	Specific Supplies
Back Cardiac board	
Side Portable suction machine, bag-valve device and oxygen tank	Suction canister and tubing, face mask and oxygen tubing
Top Monitor-defibrillator with recorder, clipboard with code record and drug calculation reference sheets	ECG leads, electrodes, conductive gel, or pads; possible transcutaneous pacemaker or combination unit
Airway supply drawer	Oral and nasal airways, endotracheal tubes, stylet, laryngoscope handle and curved and straight blades, Magill forceps, lubricating jelly, 5-ml syringes, and tape
IV supply drawer	IV catheters or various sizes, tape, syringes, needles and needleless adaptors, IV fluids (normal saline, Ringer's lactate solution and 5% dextrose in water), and IV tubing
Medication drawer	All IV push emergency medications in prefilled syringes if available, sterile water and normal saline for injection, and IV infusion emergency medications (see Table 7–8)
Miscellaneous supply drawer	Sterile and nonsterile gloves, suction catheters, nasogastric tubes, chest tubes, blood pressure cuff, blood collection tubes, sutures, pacemaker magnet, extra ECG recording paper
Procedure trays	Cut-down, tracheostomy, and central line insertion trays

supplies and make pharmacy charges to the patient's account.

ELECTROCARDIOGRAM TECHNICIAN

In some hospitals, an ECG technician responds to codes. This individual stands by to obtain 12-lead ECGs that may be ordered.

CHAPLAIN

Another person that may respond to a code is the hospital chaplain. The chaplain can be very helpful in comforting and waiting with the patient's family. If a chaplain is not available, the charge nurse or some other person should be available for this important task. The support person should take the family to a quiet, private area for waiting and should remain with them during the code. This individual may also be able to check on the patient periodically to give the family a progress report.

OTHER PERSONNEL

Other personnel should be available to run errands, such as taking blood samples to the lab or getting additional supplies. Meanwhile, other patients need monitoring and care. Only staff necessary for the code should remain; other staff should attend to the rest of the patients.

Equipment Used in Codes

While the first person to recognize a code calls for help and begins life support measures, another team member should immediately bring the crash cart to the patient's bedside (Fig. 7–1). Crash carts vary in organization and layout, but they all contain the same basic emergency equipment and medications. Many hospitals have standardized crash carts, so that anyone responding to the code is familiar with the location of the items on the cart. In other hospitals, the make-up and organization of the crash cart are unique to each unit. Whether carts are standardized or unique to an individual unit, nurses responding to codes must be familiar with the cart.

Most carts have equipment stored on top as well as in several drawers. Table 7–2 lists equipment on a typical crash cart. Equipment, such as back boards and portable suction machines, are frequently attached to the cart. Larger equipment is stored on the top of the cart or in a large drawer; smaller items, such as medications and IV equipment, are in the smaller drawers.

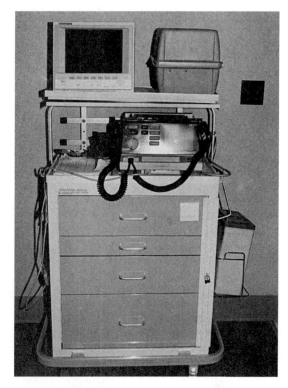

Figure 7–1. A typical crash cart.

A back, or "cardiac," board is usually located on the back or side of the cart. It should be placed under the patient as soon as possible in order to provide a hard, level surface for the performance of chest compressions. Alternatively, some hospital bed head boards are removable for use as a cardiac board. The patient is either lifted up or log rolled to one side for placement of the back board. Care should be taken to protect the patient's cervical spine if injury is suspected.

A monitor-defibrillator is usually located on top of the cart. The patient's cardiac rhythm is monitored via the leads and electrodes on this machine. Placing the defibrillation paddles on the chest by use of the "quick-look" method enables monitoring of cardiac rhythm. In the hospital setting, continuous monitoring via the electrodes is preferable to intermittent use of the defibrillation paddles for "quick looks." The monitor should have a recorder for documenting the patient's ECG rhythm for the cardiac arrest record.

A transcutaneous pacemaker may be stored on the crash cart. A combination monitor, defibrillator, and transcutaneous pacemaker is also available.

A bag-valve device (BVD) with an attached face mask and oxygen tubing is usually kept with the crash cart. The tubing should be connected either to a wall

Table 7–3. FLOW OF EVENTS DURING A CODE

Priorities	Equipment from Cart	Intervention
1. Recognition of arrest		1. Initiate CPR and call for help.
2. Arrival of resuscitation team, emergency cart, monitor-defibrillator	2.a. Cardiac board b. Mouth-to-mask or bag-valve-mask unit with oxygen tubing c. Oral airway d. Oxygen and regulator if not already at bedside	2.a. Place patient on cardiac board. b. Ventilate with 100% oxygen with oral airway and mouth-to-mask or bag-valve-mask device. c. Continue chest compressions.
3. Identification of team leader		3.a. Assess patient. b. Direct and supervise team members. c. Solve problems. d. Obtain patient history and information about events leading up to the code.
4. Rhythm diagnosis	4. Cardiac monitor with quick-look paddles—defibrillator (limb leads, 12-lead ECG machine)	4.a. Apply quick-look paddles first. b. Attach limb leads, but do not interrupt CPR.
5. Prompt defibrillation if indicated	5. Defibrillator	5. Use correct algorithm.
6. Venous access	6. Peripheral or central IV materials IV tubing, infusion fluid (normal saline)	6.a. Insert peripheral IV into antecubital sites. b. Central line may be inserted by MD.
7. Drug administration	7. Drugs as ordered (and in anticipation, based on algorithms) for bolus and continuous infusion	7. Use correct algorithm.
8. Intubation	8.a. Suction equipment b. Laryngoscope c. Endotracheal tube and other intubation equipment d. Stethoscope	8.a. Connect suction equipment. b. Intubate patient (interrupt CPR no more than 30 seconds). c. Check tube position (listen over epigastrium and bilateral lung fields). d. Secure tube. e. Hyperventilate and oxygenate.
9. Ongoing assessment of the patient's response to therapy during resuscitation		9. Assess frequently: a. Pulse generated with CPR (is there a pulse?). b. Adequacy of artificial ventilation. c. Arterial blood gases or other laboratory work. d. Spontaneous pulse after any intervention/rhythm change (is there a pulse?). e. Spontaneous breathing with return of pulse (is there breathing?). f. Blood pressure, if pulse is present. g. Decision to stop, if no response to therapy.
10. Drawing arterial and venous blood specimens	10. Arterial puncture and venipuncture equipment	10.a. Draw specimens. b. Treat as needed, based on results.
11. Documentation	11. Resuscitation record	11.a. Accurately record events while resuscitation is in progress. b. Record rhythm strips during the code.
12. Controlling or limiting crowd		12. Dismiss those not required for bedside tasks.
13. Family notification		13. Keep family informed of patient's condition Notify outcome with sensitivity
14. Transfer of patient to critical care unit		14. Get bed assigned for patient. Transfer with adequate personal emergency equipment.
15. Critique		15. Evaluate events of code and express feelings.

Adapted from American Heart Association (1987, 1990, 1994). *Textbook of advanced cardiac life support* (2nd and 3rd eds.). Dallas: Author.
CPR = cardiopulmonary resuscitation.

oxygen inlet or to a portable oxygen tank on the crash cart. Supplemental oxygen should always be used with the BVD.

Airway supplies are located in one of the drawers. Some institutions have a separate box or kit containing airway management supplies.

Another drawer contains IV supplies and IV solutions. Normal saline and Ringer's lactated solution are the IV fluids most often used. Five percent dextrose in 250-ml and 500-ml bags is used for preparing vasoactive infusions.

Emergency medications fill another drawer. These include IV push drugs as well as medications that must be added to IV fluids for continuous infusions. Most IV push drugs are available in prefilled syringes. Several drugs that are given via a constant infusion (e.g., lidocaine, dopamine) are also available as premixed infusions. Drugs are discussed in more depth in the segment on pharmacological intervention.

Other important items on the cart include a suction set-up and suction catheters, nasogastric tubes, and blood pressure cuff. Various trays, such as for venous cut-down, tracheotomy, and central line insertion, are also frequently kept on the crash cart.

The crash cart is usually checked by nursing staff every shift to ensure that all equipment and drugs are present and functional. Once the cart is fully stocked, it should be kept locked in order to avoid borrowing of supplies and equipment.

The nurse can become familiar with the location of items on the cart by being responsible for checking it. Management of the code is more efficient when the nurse knows where items are located on the crash cart as well as how to use them.

Resuscitation Efforts

The flow of events during a code is the result of a concentrated team effort. BCLS is provided until the code team arrives to provide advanced life support measures. Once help has arrived, CPR is continued by use of the two-person technique. Other tasks, such as connecting the patient to an ECG monitor, starting IVs, attaching an oxygen source to the BVD, and setting up suction, should be carried out by available personnel as soon as possible. The activities that occur during the code are summarized in Table 7–3. Often, several activities are performed simultaneously.

BASIC CARDIAC LIFE SUPPORT

The purposes of BCLS are (1) to prevent respiratory and/or cardiac arrest through prompt assessment and intervention and (2) to support respiration and circulation through CPR (AHA, 1994a). CPR must be initiated immediately in the event of an arrest in order to prevent brain damage and improve patient outcomes. Brain damage may occur after 4 to 6 minutes without adequate oxygen.

The ABCs of CPR are: *airway, breathing,* and *circulation.* Assessment is a part of each step, and the steps are performed in order (Table 7–4). The following summary is adapted from the AHA standards for BCLS (AHA, 1994a).

Airway

An open airway is essential. The first intervention is to assess unresponsiveness by tapping or shaking a patient and shouting, "Are you OK?" If the patient is unresponsive, the nurse calls for help by shouting to fellow caregivers or by using the nurse-call system. The patient is positioned on his or her back, and the airway is opened by use of the head-tilt/chin-lift method (Fig. 7–2). If the patient needs to be turned to the supine position, he or she is turned as a unit in order to prevent possible injury.

Breathing

The second step of CPR is to assess breathing and to initiate rescue breathing if necessary. Early initiation of rescue breathing may prevent a cardiac arrest in a patient who stops breathing but still has a pulse (e.g., a patient with hypercapnia). In order to assess breathing, the nurse *looks, listens,* and *feels* for

---

Table 7–4. STEPS IN BASIC CARDIAC LIFE SUPPORT

1. **Airway**
   Determine unresponsiveness.
   Call for help.
   Position patient on back.
   Open airway using head-tilt/chin-lift technique.

2. **Breathing**
   Assess breathing.
   If breathing present, maintain airway.
   If breathing absent, give two breaths.
   Activate the cardiac arrest team, if possible.

3. **Circulation**
   Determine pulselessness.
   Activate cardiac arrest team, if not previously done.
   If pulse present, perform rescue breathing at 12 breaths/min.
   If pulse absent, perform chest compressions at rate of 80 to 100 beats/min.
   Alternate compressions and breaths at a rate of 15:2.

Adapted from American Heart Association (1994). *Textbook of basic life support for healthcare providers.* Dallas: Author.

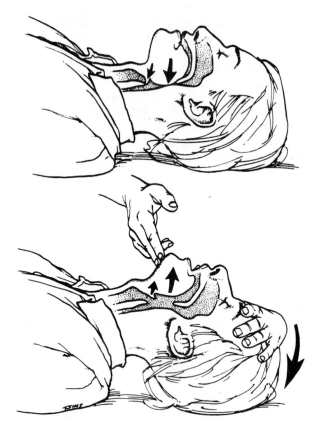

Figure 7–2. Head-tilt/chin-lift technique for opening the airway. *Top:* Airway obstruction produced by the tongue and epiglottis. *Bottom:* Relief by head-tilt/chin-lift. (Reproduced with permission. American Heart Association (1994). *Textbook of basic life support for healthcare providers* (p. 4–4). Dallas: Author. Copyright American Heart Association.)

breathing while maintaining an open airway. The nurse *looks* at the chest wall to see if it is moving up and down, *listens* for air movement, and *feels* for exhaled air. Rescue breathing, or ventilation, is initiated if the patient is not breathing.

If possible, the code team should be notified of the arrest at this time. The first person who arrives to help should "call the code." Some critical care units and emergency departments have an emergency call system that can be activated from the patient's room by the pressing of a button. If this type of system is not available and the nurse is alone, he or she presses the nurse-call system and begins rescue breathing. When the call is answered, the nurse states, "Call a code!"

In mouth-to-mouth resuscitation, the open airway is maintained, and the nurse seals his or her mouth over the patient's mouth, pinches off the patient's nose, and gives two slow breaths to the patient (Fig. 7–3).

If the nurse experiences difficulty in ventilating the patient, the patient's head should be repositioned because improper head position is the most common cause of inability to ventilate.

If the patient has a mouth injury or the nurse has difficulty maintaining a good seal, mouth-to-nose ventilation can be performed. Mouth-to-stoma ventilation is performed when the patient has a tracheostomy or laryngectomy.

Alternatives to mouth-to-mouth resuscitation include mouth-to-mask techniques and ventilation with a BVD and face mask. Both of these techniques are frequently used in the hospital setting. Many hospitals have a pocket mask at every patient's bedside. Additionally, most critical care units have a BVD in every patient's room.

The mouth-to-mask technique involves placing a pocket mask over the patient's mouth and breathing through a mouthpiece connected to the mask (Fig. 7–4). Pocket masks have a one-way valve that protects the nurse from the patient's exhalation.

Ventilation of the patient with a BVD and face mask requires that an open airway must be maintained. Frequently, an oral airway is used for keeping the airway patent and for facilitating ventilation. The BVD is connected to an oxygen source set at 15 L/min. The face mask is positioned over the patient's mouth and nose. While maintaining a good seal with the mask, the nurse manually ventilates the patient with the BVD (Fig. 7–5). Personnel should be properly trained to use the BVD effectively (see Chapter 6).

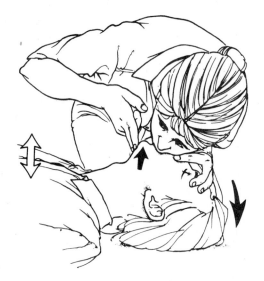

Figure 7–3. Mouth-to-mouth technique for rescue breathing (Reproduced with permission. American Heart Association (1994). *Textbook of basic life support for healthcare providers* (p. 4–7). Dallas: Author. Copyright American Heart Association.)

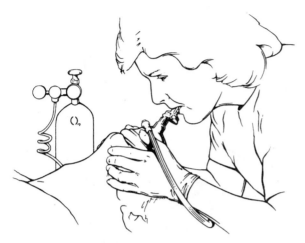

Figure 7–4. Mouth-to-mask technique for rescue breathing. (Reproduced with permission. American Heart Association (1994). *Textbook of basic life support for healthcare providers* (p. 2–8). Dallas: Author. Copyright American Heart Association.)

Circulation

The third step of CPR is to ensure adequate circulation. After the initial two breaths are given, the nurse assesses the patient to determine the presence or absence of a pulse. The pulse is assessed even if the patient is attached to a cardiac monitor because artifact or a loose lead may mimic a cardiac dysrhythmia. The nurse checks the patient's carotid pulse on the side nearest the nurse. The pulse is assessed for 5 to 10 seconds in order to detect bradycardia.

If a pulse is *present,* the nurse continues to perform rescue breathing at a rate of 12 breaths per minute, or 1 breath every 5 seconds. The pulse should be assessed periodically.

If the pulse is *absent,* the nurse begins cardiac compressions. If the code team has not yet been notified, they are notified now. The patient is placed supine, on a firm surface. Proper hand position is essential for performing compressions (Fig. 7–6). The location for compressions is the lower sternum above the xiphoid process. To locate the proper area, the nurse runs his or her fingers up the rib cage to the notch where the ribs and sternum meet. The middle finger is placed on the notch, and the index finger is aligned next to the middle finger. The heel of the opposite hand is placed next to the index finger. The first hand is then positioned on top of the hand on the sternum. Using both hands, the nurse begins compressions by depressing the sternum 1.5 to 2.0 inches for the average adult (Fig. 7–7). For the prevention of injury, care must be taken to ensure that fingers are raised off of the patient's chest wall. Compressions are performed at a rate of 80 to 100 per minute at a ratio of 15 compressions to two breaths (15:2). The carotid pulse is checked after 1 minute of CPR. If the pulse is absent, CPR is continued until additional help arrives. When there is adequate personnel to perform two-

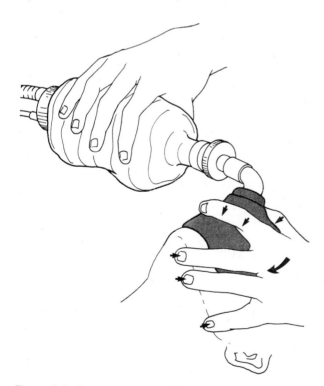

Figure 7–5. Rescue breathing with bag-valve device. (Adapted from Kersten, L. D. (1989). *Comprehensive respiratory nursing* (p. 629). Philadelphia: W. B. Saunders Co.)

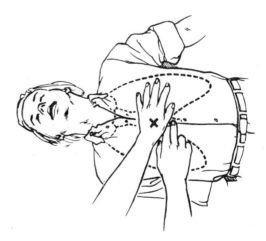

Figure 7–6. Proper hand placement for cardiac compressions during cardiopulmonary resuscitation. (Reproduced with permission. American Heart Association (1994). *Textbook of basic life support for healthcare providers* (p. 4–10). Dallas: Author. Copyright American Heart Association.)

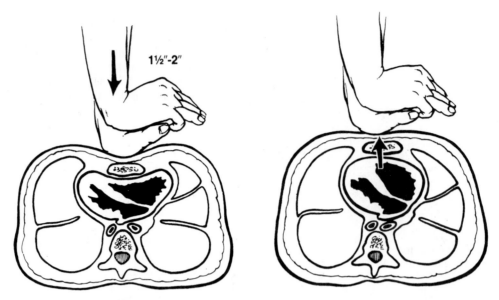

Figure 7–7. Technique for cardiac compressions. (Reproduced with permission. American Heart Association (1988). *Healthcare provider's manual for basic life support* (p. 43). Dallas: Author. Copyright American Heart Association.)

person CPR, one person maintains the airway and does rescue breathing while the other person performs compressions. During two-person CPR, the rate of compressions to breaths is 5:1.

ADVANCED CARDIAC LIFE SUPPORT

For cardiac or respiratory emergencies, many institutions follow the AHA standards for ACLS. The conceptual tools of management are the primary survey followed by the secondary survey (AHA, 1994b).

Primary Survey

The ABCDs of the primary survey focus on CPR and defibrillation. The ABCs of ACLS are the same as for BCLS: *airway, breathing, and circulation.* "D" refers to early *defibrillation* that can be accomplished with an automatic external defibrillator (AED) or a conventional defibrillator. It is now becoming a requirement that BCLS providers be trained in the use of AEDs. The AED is discussed in more detail in the section on electrical therapy.

The Secondary Survey

At defibrillation, the secondary survey is initiated. The ABCD (airway, breathing, circulation, differential diagnosis) in the secondary survey involves the performance of more in-depth assessments and interventions.

Airway

Airway management involves reassessment of original techniques established in BCLS. Endotracheal intubation is advised as soon as possible for several reasons during resuscitation:

1. It isolates the airway and keeps it patent.
2. It protects the patient from gastric distention and aspiration of stomach contents.
3. It permits suctioning.
4. It facilitates the administration of a high concentration of oxygen.
5. It provides a route for administration of certain medications.

During a cardiopulmonary arrest, CPR should not be disrupted for longer than 30 seconds while intubation is attempted. Techniques of endotracheal intubation are discussed in Chapter 6. Once the patient is intubated, the patient is manually ventilated with a BVD attached to the endotracheal tube (ETT) (Fig. 7–8). The BVD should have a reservoir and be connected to an oxygen source to deliver 100% oxygen while providing a tidal volume of 10 to 15 ml/kg. Ventilation of the intubated patient should not be synchronized to chest compressions but should instead be performed asynchronously at 12 to 15 ventilations per minute.

Breathing

Breathing assessment determines whether the ventilatory efforts are causing the chest to rise. After

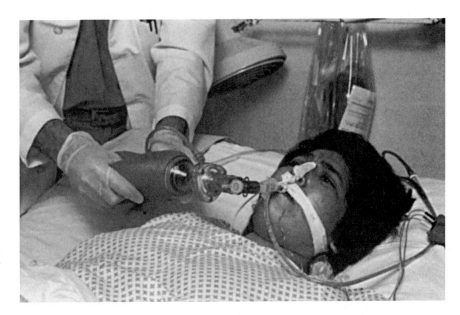

Figure 7–8. Ventilation with bag-valve device connected to endotracheal tube. (From Kersten, L. D. (1989). *Comprehensive respiratory nursing* (p. 630). Philadelphia: W. B. Saunders Co.)

intubation, the nurse first auscultates the epigastrium. If air is heard in this area, the ETT has mistakenly been placed in the stomach and should be removed immediately. ETT placement should be confirmed by bilateral breath sounds, end-tidal carbon dioxide indicators, and chest x-ray study.

Circulation

Circulation focuses on IV access, attachment of monitor electrodes and leads, rhythm identification, blood pressure measurement, and medication administration. A patent IV is necessary during an arrest for the adminstration of fluids, medications, or both. Drugs that can be administered through the ETT until an IV access is established are epinephrine, lidocaine, and atropine (AHA, 1994b).

Most critically ill patients already have IV access with an ongoing IV infusion or intermittent access device. If the patient does not have IV access, or needs additional IV access, a large-bore IV should be inserted. The antecubital vein should be the first target for IV access (AHA, 1994b). Other areas for IV insertion include the dorsum of the hands and the wrist. If a peripheral IV cannot be started, the physician inserts a central line for IV access.

Normal saline is the preferred IV fluid because it expands intravascular volume better than dextrose (AHA, 1994b). When any medication is administered by the IV route, it is best followed with a 20- to 30-ml bolus of IV fluid in order to enhance delivery to the central circulation.

Differential Diagnosis

Differential diagnosis involves investigation into the cause of the arrest. If a reversible cause is identified, a specific therapy can be initiated. Cardiac dysrhythmias that result in cardiac arrests have many possible causes. The lethal dysrhythmias include ventricular fibrillation/ventricular tachycardia (VF/VT), asystole, and pulseless electrical activity. Other dysrhythmias that may lead to a cardiopulmonary arrest include symptomatic bradycardias and symptomatic tachycardias. Algorithms for treating these rhythm disorders have been established by the AHA (1994b). Critical actions in the management of these dysrhythmias are summarized.

RECOGNITION AND TREATMENT OF DYSRHYTHMIAS

Ventricular Fibrillation and Pulseless Ventricular Tachycardia

The treatment for VF and pulseless VT is the same. If the arrest is witnessed, the patient has no pulse, and a defibrillator is not immediately available, a precordial thump may be administered.

Critical Actions

- Initiate the ABCD in the primary survey. Initiate CPR until a defibrillator is available. Defibrillate as soon as possible because early defibrillation increases the chance of survival.
- Defibrillate up to three times in rapid succession, if needed for persistent VF/VT (200 joules

[J], 200 to 300 J, 360 J). Assess the pulse and rhythm after the third defibrillation attempt if no change has occurred in the rhythm to this point.

- If VF/VT persists, continue CPR, intubate at once, and obtain IV access. Intubation optimizes airway management and provides a route for some medication administration.
- Administer epinephrine, 1 mg IV push every 3 to 5 minutes. If this dosing regimen is unsuccessful, intermediate-, escalating-, or high-dose epinephrine may be considered.

Intermediate—2 to 5 mg IV push every 3 to 5 minutes
Escalating—1 mg, 3 mg, 5 mg IV push 3 minutes apart
High—0.1 mg/kg IV push every 3 to 5 minutes

- Defibrillate at 360 J, within 30 to 60 seconds of each epinephrine dose. Defibrillation should continue after each dose of medication if VF persists. The pattern should be "drug-shock, drug-shock" (AHA, 1994b).
- Administer medications that are probably of benefit in persistent VF/VT. These medications include lidocaine, bretylium, magnesium sulfate, and procainamide. Sodium bicarbonate is considered only if there is a preexisting acidosis or tricyclic antidepressant drug overdose, or if other recommended interventions within a lengthy arrest have proved ineffective. Dosages and administration are discussed in the section on pharmacological intervention.
- Reassess the patient frequently. Check for return of pulse, spontaneous respirations, and blood pressure. Resume CPR if appropriate.

Pulseless Electrical Activity

The goal in treating any rhythm without a pulse is to determine and treat the probable underlying cause of this condition. This treatment algorithm applies to any rhythm that occurs in the absence of a pulse. Pulseless electrical activity is often associated with clinical conditions that can be reversed if they are identified early and treated appropriately (AHA, 1994b).

Critical Actions

- Initiate ABCD of the secondary survey. The patient is intubated, and IV access is obtained.
- Consider possible causes. Some of the causes of pulseless electrical activity include hypovolemia, hypoxia, cardiac tamponade, tension pneumothorax, drug overdose, pulmonary embolism, acidosis, and massive myocardial infarction.

- Administer epinephrine, 1 mg IV push every 3 to 5 minutes. Additional pharmacological support includes atropine, 1 mg IV, if bradycardia is present.
- Continue the ABCD of the secondary survey while identifying underlying causes and initiating related intervention.

Asystole

The absence of electrical activity in the heart continues to carry a grim prognosis. The rescuer must focus aggressively on the differential diagnosis of the secondary survey.

Critical Actions

- Perform cardiopulmonary resuscitation, intubation, IV access, and confirmation of asystole in more than one monitoring lead. An additional lead confirms or rules out the possibility of a fine VF.
- Ensure adequate ventilation.
- Consider possible causes, including hypoxia, hyperkalemia or hypokalemia, preexisting acidosis, drug overdose, or hypothermia.
- Consider transcutaneous pacing. It may be effective if it is early and in conjunction with medications.
- Administer medications: epinephrine, 1 mg IV push every 3 to 5 minutes, and atropine 1 mg IV every 3 to 5 minutes up to a total dose of 0.03 to 0.04 mg/kg.
- Consider termination of efforts.

Symptomatic Bradycardia

This category encompasses two types: the classic bradycardia, i.e., a heart rate of less than 60 that causes symptoms, or any heart rhythm that is slow enough to cause hemodynamic compromise. The cause of the bradycardia should be considered. For example, hypotension associated with bradycardia may be caused by dysfunction of the myocardium or hypovolemia rather than by a conduction system or autonomic nervous system disturbance.

Critical Actions

- Assess the ABC of the primary survey. Secure the airway, administer oxygen, start an IV line, and assess vital signs. The use of a pulse oximeter is encouraged.
- Administer Atropine, 0.5 to 1 mg IV, the initial drug of choice. It may not be effective, however, in second-degree atrioventricular (AV) block type II or third-degree AV block.

- Identify the causative rhythm. Symptomatic bradycardias include sinus rhythm with a rate of less than 60, second-degree AV block types I or II, and third-degree AV block.
- Consider transcutaneous pacing for all symptomatic bradycardias. If used, analgesics or sedatives may need to be given because patients often find the pacing stimulus that is delivered with this therapy uncomfortable.
- Dopamine is acceptable for blood pressure support. Epinephrine may be administered instead if clinical symptoms are severe.
- Avoid lidocaine. Lidocaine may be lethal if the underlying bradycardia is a ventricular escape rhythm. The ventricular escape rhythm indicates the failure of higher pacemakers. In this instance, lidocaine would suppress the patient's only rhythm that is providing any cardiac output, leaving asystole.

Symptomatic Tachycardia

The treatment of this group of dysrhythmias involves the rapid assessment of the patient and identification of the dysrhythmia. Synchronized cardioversion and antiarrhythmic therapy may be needed.

Critical Actions

- Initiate the ABCD survey. Assess the patient and recognize the signs and symptoms of cardiovascular instability. Establish IV access, and prepare suction and intubation equipment.
- Recognize the unstable tachycardia from the monitor. This group of dysrhythmias includes atrial fibrillation and flutter, supraventricular tachycardia, wide-QRS tachycardia of uncertain type, and VT.
- Premedicate with sedation or anesthesia whenever possible. Cardioversion is an uncomfortable procedure. Therefore, a fully conscious patient should be sedated before electrical intervention.
- Perform synchronized cardioversion at the appropriate energy level. Supraventricular tachycardia and atrial flutter often respond to lower energy levels, so it would be feasible to initiate therapy with 50 J. Cardioversion for the other tachydysrhythmias should be initiated at 100 J, increasing to 200 J, 300 J, and 360 J for subsequent attempts.
- Reassess the patient and consider the need for follow-up monitoring and antiarrhythmic therapy.

ELECTRICAL THERAPY

The therapeutic use of electrical current has expanded over the past several years with the addition and increased use of the automatic external defibrillator. This section addresses the use of electricity in code management for the purposes of defibrillation, cardioversion, and transcutaneous (external) pacing. Defibrillation of the patient with an implantable cardioverter-defibrillator (ICD) is also discussed.

Defibrillation

The primary treatment for VF and pulseless VT is defibrillation. VF may occur as a result of coronary artery disease, myocardial infarction, electrical shock, drug overdose, near drowning, and acid-base imbalance.

Definition. *Defibrillation* is the delivery of an electrical current to the heart through the use of a defibrillator (Fig. 7–9); it is sometimes referred to as *countershock*. The current can be delivered through the chest wall by use of external paddles or adhesive electrode pads connected to cables. Smaller, internal paddles may be used to deliver current directly to the heart during cardiac surgery. Defibrillation works by completely depolarizing the heart and disrupting the impulses that are causing the dysrhythmia. Because the heart is completely depolarized, the sinoatrial node or other pacemaker can resume control of the heart's rhythm.

Procedure. Two methods exist for paddle placement for external defibrillation. Transverse, or anterior, paddle placement is used most often. In the transverse method, one paddle is placed at the second intercostal space to the right of the sternum, and the other paddle is placed at the fifth intercostal space, in the midclavicular line, to the left of the sternum (Fig. 7–10). The alternate method is anteroposterior paddle placement. When this method is used, an anterior paddle is placed at the anterior precordial area, and the posterior paddle is placed at the posterior-infrascapular area (Fig. 7–11). When the anteroposterior method is used, less energy may be needed for successful defibrillation. Some defibrillators permit "hands-off" defibrillation. Countershocks are delivered through special adhesive electrodes attached to the patient's chest rather than through paddles.

Energy is delivered to the patient through the paddles or special electrodes. The amount of energy delivered is referred to as joules, or watt seconds. Most defibrillators deliver up to 360 J.

For the shock to be effective, some type of conductive medium is placed between the paddles and the skin. In the past, gel and saline pads have been used

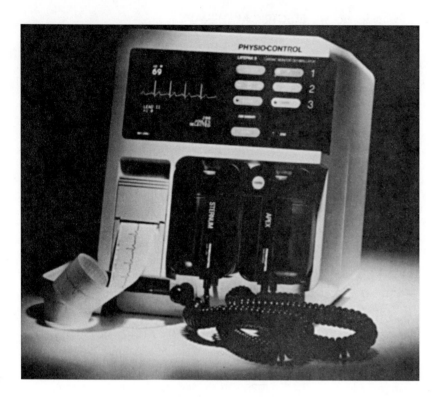

Figure 7–9. Defibrillator. (Courtesy of Physio-Control, Redmond, WA.)

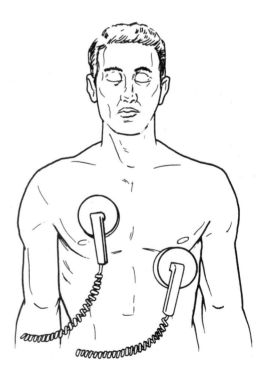

Figure 7–10. Paddle placement for defibrillation. (Redrawn from Sheehy, S. B. (1990). *Mosby's manual of emergency care* (p. 76). St. Louis: C. V. Mosby Co.)

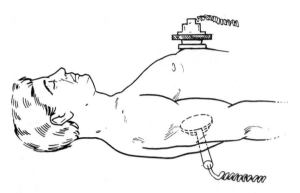

Figure 7-11. Anteroposterior paddle placement. (Redrawn from Sheehy, S. B. (1990). *Mosby's manual of emergency care* (p. 77). St. Louis: C. V. Mosby Co.)

Table 7–5. PROCEDURE FOR EXTERNAL DEFIBRILLATION

1. Apply defibrillator pads to the patient's chest (*or* apply conductive gel to paddles).
2. Turn on defibrillator.
3. Charge the defibrillator to the desired setting.
4. Position paddles on chest and apply 25 pounds of pressure.
5. Ensure that all personnel (including yourself) are clear of the patient, the bed, and any equipment that might be connected to the patient.
6. Shout ``All clear!''and look to verify.
7. Deliver countershock by depressing buttons on each paddle simultaneously.
8. After the defibrillation, observe patient's rhythm and feel for a pulse.

to conduct the electricity. If gel is used, it is important to cover the paddles completely with the gel. Commercially prepared defibrillator pads are also available and can be used for multiple shocks in order to prevent burns on the patient's skin.

The defibrillator is charged to the desired setting. The paddles are placed firmly on the patient's chest. Firm pressure is needed to facilitate skin contact and to reduce the impedance to the flow of current.

Safety is essential during the procedure to prevent injury to the patient and the personnel assisting with the procedure. The person performing the defibrillation ensures that all personnel are standing clear of the bed by shouting "all clear" and visually checking to see that no one is in contact with the patient or bed. The countershock is then delivered. The patient's rhythm is assessed after each defibrillation. After the initial triad of shocks for VF and pulseless VT, and after subsequent shocks, the pulse is assessed. It is helpful if one of the team members obtains rhythm strips during the procedure in order to document effectiveness. The procedure for defibrillation is summarized in Table 7–5.

Complications of defibrillation include burns on the skin and damage to the heart muscle. Arcing of electricity can occur if the paddles are not firmly placed on the skin, excessive conductive gel is used, or the skin is wet. Arcing has also been noted when patients have nitroglycerin patches or paste on the chest; therefore, topical nitroglycerin should be removed before defibrillation.

Cardioversion

Definition. *Cardioversion* is the delivery of a countershock that is synchronized with the patient's cardiac rhythm. The purpose of cardioversion is to disrupt an ectopic pacemaker that is causing a dysrhythmia and to allow the sinoatrial node to take control of the rhythm. During an emergency situation, cardioversion is used to treat patients with VT or supraventricular tachycardia who have a pulse but are developing symptoms related to a low cardiac output, such as hypotension, cool clammy skin, and decreased level of consciousness. Elective cardioversion is used to treat atrial flutter and fibrillation.

Cardioversion is similar to defibrillation with two major exceptions: (1) the countershock of cardioversion is *synchronized* to occur during ventricular depolarization (QRS complex) and (2) less energy is used for the countershock. The rationale for delivering the shock during the QRS complex is to prevent the shock from being delivered during repolarization (T wave), often termed the *vulnerable period*. If a shock is delivered during this vulnerable period (Fig. 7–12), VF may occur. Because the purpose of cardioversion is to disrupt the rhythm rather than completely depolarize the heart, less energy is required. Cardioversion can be performed with energy levels as low as 50 J. The

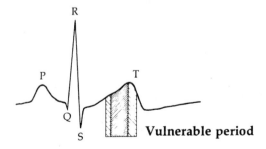

Figure 7–12. Vulnerable period during the cardiac cycle. If a countershock is delivered during this time, it may result in ventricular fibrillation. (From Crockett, P. J., Droppert, B. M., Higgins, S. E. (1991). *Defibrillation: What you should know* (3rd ed.) (p. 4). Redmond, WA: Physio-Control.

amount of energy is gradually increased until the rhythm is converted.

Procedure. The procedure for cardioversion (Table 7–6) is similar to that for defibrillation. However, the defibrillator is set in the "synchronous" mode for the cardioversion. The R waves are sensed by the machine and are noted by "spikes" or other markings on the monitor of the defibrillator. It is important to assess that all R waves are properly sensed. When it is time to deliver the shock, the buttons on the paddles must remain depressed until the shock is delivered because energy is discharged only during the QRS complex. When a patient is undergoing cardioversion nonemergently, sedation should be given before the procedure.

Automatic External Defibrillation

The principle of early defibrillation states that all basic life support personnel must be trained and permitted to operate a defibrillator if their professional activities require a response to people in cardiac arrest (AHA, 1994b).

Definition. Automatic external defibrillators are external defibrillators with rhythm analysis capabilities (Fig. 7–13). They are used by BCLS-trained personnel who have been trained in their operation. The AED may be used in an area of the hospital in which cardiac arrest may occur but personnel are not required to

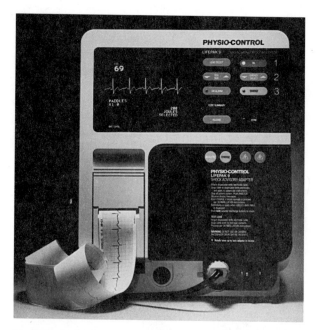

Figure 7–13. Monitor-defibrillator with automated external defibrillator. (Courtesy of Physio-Control, Redmond, WA.)

be trained in ACLS measures (e.g., general medical-surgical patient areas).

Procedure. All AEDs are attached to the patient by two adhesive pads and connecting cables, similar to the pads used for "hands-off" traditional defibrillation. These pads serve a dual purpose: recording the rhythm and delivering the countershock. The AED may be fully automated or semiautomated (also known as shock-advisory). The fully automated model requires only that the operator attach the defibrillation electrodes and turn on the device. Semiautomated devices require the operator to initiate analysis of the rhythm and discharge the defibrillator if a shock is advised. Both models deliver AHA-recommended energy levels for the treatment of VF/pulseless VT.

Special Situations

Defibrillation of the Patient with an Implantable Cardioverter-Defibrillator

Patients with ICDs are at high risk for lethal dysrhythmias. Numerous devices are available today with multiprogrammable levels of therapy. Nurses must become familiar, whenever possible, with the type of therapy the patient's device has been programmed to deliver. When caring for a patient with an ICD, some important points must be considered. By the time VF/VT is recognized on the monitor, the rhythm should also have been recognized by the ICD.

Table 7–6. PROCEDURE FOR SYNCHRONOUS CARDIOVERSION

1. Ensure that emergency equipment is readily available.
2. Explain the procedure to the patient.
3. Consider sedating the patient.
4. Turn on defibrillator to "synchronous" mode.
5. Observe the rhythm on the monitor to determine that the R wave is properly sensed and marked (usually with a spike).
6. Apply defibrillator pads to the patient's chest (or apply conductive gel to paddles).
7. Charge the defibrillator to the desired setting.
8. Position paddles on chest and apply 25 pounds of pressure.
9. Ensure that all personnel (including yourself) are clear of the patient, the bed, and any equipment that might be connected to the patient.
10. Shout "All clear" and look to verify.
11. Deliver synchronized countershock by depressing buttons on each paddle simultaneously. Keep buttons depressed until the shock has been delivered.
12. After the cardioversion, observe the patient's rhythm to determine effectiveness.

If a successful countershock by the ICD has not occurred when the rhythm is noted on the monitor, one should proceed with standard code management. If external defibrillation is unsuccessful, the placement of the paddles on the chest should be changed. Anteroposterior paddle placement may be more effective than anterior-apex placement. External defibrillation of a patient while the ICD is firing does not harm the patient or the ICD. ICDs are insulated from damage caused by conventional external defibrillation, but the unit should be checked if these episodes occur. There is no danger to personnel if the ICD discharges while personnel are touching the patient. However, the shock may be felt and has been compared to the sensation of contact with an electrical outlet.

Defibrillation of the Patient with a Permanent Pacemaker

When a patient with a permanent pacemaker requires defibrillation, placing the paddle near the pacemaker generator should be avoided. Although damage is rarely caused to the pacemaker, the generator can absorb much of the current of defibrillation from the pads or paddles and reduce the chance of success (AHA, 1994b). The pacing and sensing thresholds of the pacemaker should be assessed after external defibrillation.

Transcutaneous Cardiac Pacing

Definition. *Transcutaneous (external noninvasive) cardiac pacing* is used during emergency situations to treat symptomatic bradycardia and asystole. In this method of pacing, the heart is stimulated with externally applied cutaneous electrodes that deliver the electrical impulse. Impulse conduction occurs across the chest wall to stimulate the myocardium. Pacing should be considered for symptomatic bradycardia caused by drug overdose, electrolyte abnormalities, or acidosis. The myocardium may be normal, but the metabolic insult has disturbed the conduction system. Pacing the heart after correction of the underlying abnormality can stimulate effective myocardial contractions until the conduction system recovers (AHA, 1994b).

The transcutaneous pacemaker may be a freestanding unit with a monitor and a pacemaker. Some models incorporate a monitor, a defibrillator, and an external pacemaker into one system (Fig. 7–14).

Advantages of transcutaneous pacemakers include the following:

1. It is easy to operate.
2. It requires minimal training.

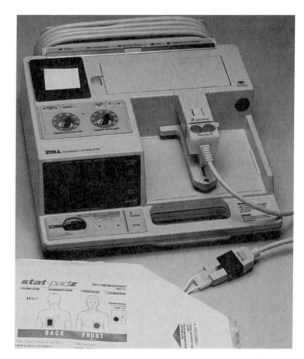

Figure 7–14. Transcutaneous pacemaker-defibrillator. (Courtesy of Zoll Medical, Burlington, MA.)

3. It can be initiated immediately in emergency situations.
4. It eliminates the risks associated with invasive pacemakers.

Procedure. The procedure (Table 7–7) for transcutaneous pacing involves the placement of large electrodes anteriorly and posteriorly on the patient (Fig. 7–15). The electrodes are connected to the external pacemaker. The pacemaker is set in either asynchronous or demand modes. (Some devices permit only demand pacing). In the asynchronous mode, the pacemaker generates a rhythm without regard to the patient's own rhythm. In the demand mode, the pacemaker fires only if the patient's heart rate falls below a preset limit determined by the operator (e.g., 50 beats/min). The electrical output is adjusted to stimulate a paced beat.

The electrical and mechanical effectiveness of pacing is assessed. The electrical activity is noted by a pacemaker "spike" that indicates that the pacemaker is initiating electrical activity. The spike is followed by a broad QRS complex (Fig. 7–16). Mechanical activity is noted by palpating a pulse during electrical activity. Additionally, the patient has signs of improved cardiac output, including increased blood pressure, improved skin color, and temperature. If the external pacemaker is effective, the patient may need to have a

Table 7–7. PROCEDURE FOR TRANSCUTANEOUS PACEMAKER

1. Obtain transcutaneous pacemaker, pacemaker electrodes, and emergency equipment.
2. If the patient is alert, explain the procedure.
3. Clip excess hair from the patient's chest. *Do not shave hair.*
4. Apply anterior electrode to the chest. Electrode is centered at the fourth intercostal space to the left of the sternum.
5. Apply the posterior electrode on the patient's back in the left subscapular region.
6. Connect electrode to pacemaker generator.
7. Set pacemaker parameters for mode, heart rate, and output according to the manufacturer's instructions.
8. Turn unit on. Choose pacing mode (if applicable).
9. Assess adequacy of pacing:
   Assess for pacemaker spike and QRS complex (capture).
   Heart rate and rhythm
   Blood pressure
   Level of consciousness
10. Observe for patient discomfort. May need to sedate patient.
11. Anticipate follow-up treatment, e.g., insertion of a temporary transvenous pacemaker.

temporary transvenous pacemaker inserted, depending on the cause of the bradycardia.

The alert patient who requires transcutaneous pacing may experience some discomfort. Because the skeletal muscles are stimulated as well as the heart muscle, the patient may experience a tingling, twitching, or thumping feeling that ranges from mildly uncomfortable to intolerable. The patient may require sedation, analgesia, or both.

Pharmacological Intervention/ Code Drugs

Medications that are administered to the patient during a code depend on several factors: the cause of the arrest, the patient's cardiac rhythm, the physician's preference, and the patient's response. The goals of treatment with code drugs are to reestablish and maintain optimal cardiac function, to correct hypoxemia and acidosis, and to suppress dangerous cardiac ectopic activity. Additionally, drugs are used to achieve a balance between myocardial oxygen supply and demand, to maintain adequate blood pressure, and to relieve congestive heart failure. Because of the rapid and profound effects these drugs can have on cardiac activity and hemodynamic function, ECG monitoring is essential, and hemodynamic monitoring should be

instituted as soon as possible after the code. If IV push drugs are given peripherally, they should be flushed with 20 to 30 ml of IV fluids to ensure central circulation. Additionally, because of the precise dosages and careful administration required with these medications, volumetric infusion pumps should be used when continuous infusions are given. IV infusion rates should be tapered slowly, with frequent monitoring of clinical effect.

The following drugs are included in ACLS guidelines (AHA, 1994b) and represent those drugs most frequently used in code management. Indications, mechanisms of action, and dosages for each drug are discussed in this section. Table 7–8 summarizes the code drugs and also presents other medications that are frequently used to treat acute myocardial infarction according to AHA guidelines and current texts.

OXYGEN

Oxygen is treated as a drug because it is essential to resuscitation and has several pharmacological con-

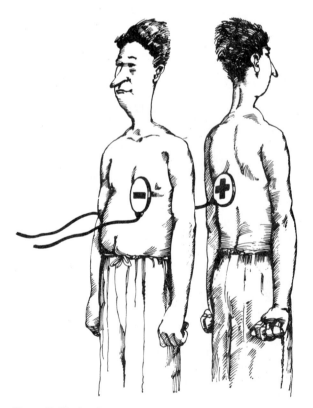

Figure 7–15. Application of electrodes for transcutaneous pacing. Electrodes are placed anteriorly and posteriorly. (From Crockett, P., & McHugh, L. G. (1988). *Noninvasive pacing: What you should know* (p. 19). Redmond, WA: Physio-Control.)

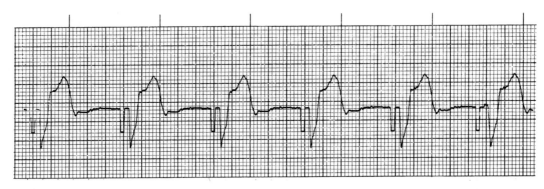

Figure 7–16. Electrical capture of transcutaneous pacemaker. Note the pacemaker spikes followed by a wide QRS complex and a tall T wave.

siderations. Oxygen is used to treat hypoxemia, which exists in any arrest situation as a result of lack of adequate gas exchange, or inadequate cardiac output, or both. Artificial ventilation without supplemental oxygen does not correct hypoxemia.

Oxygen is used to improve tissue oxygenation. Additionally, the success of other medications and interventions, such as defibrillation, depend on adequate oxygenation and normal acid-base status.

Oxygen can be delivered via mouth to mask, BVD with mask, BVD to ETT, or other airway adjuncts. During an arrest, 100% oxygen is administered.

EPINEPHRINE (ADRENALIN)

Epinephrine is a potent vasoconstrictor. Because of its alpha-adrenergic and beta-adrenergic effects (Table 7–9), epinephrine increases systemic vascular resistance and arterial blood pressure as well as heart rate, contractility, and automaticity of cardiac pacemaker cells. Because of peripheral vasoconstriction, blood is shunted to the heart and brain. Epinephrine also increases myocardial oxygen requirements.

Epinephrine is indicated for the restoration of cardiac electrical activity in an arrest. In addition, epinephrine increases automaticity and the force of contraction, an effect that makes the heart more susceptible to successful defibrillation. Epinephrine is used to treat VF or pulseless VT that is unresponsive to initial defibrillation, asystole, and pulseless electrical activity.

During a code, epinephrine may be given by the IV route or through an ETT. The IV dosage is 1.0 mg (10 ml of a 1:10,000 solution) and is repeated every 3 to 5 minutes as needed. When given through the ETT, 2 to 2.5 times the IV dose of epinephrine should be diluted in 10 ml of normal saline or sterile water. (Either diluent should be preservative free in order to prevent injury to the lungs.) A follow-up dose of up to 5 mg is acceptable.

Occasionally, epinephrine is administered by continuous infusion in order to increase heart rate or blood pressure. Dilution is 1 mg in 250 ml or 500 ml of 5% dextrose in water or normal saline. The infusion is started at 1 μg/min and is titrated according to the patient's response in a range of 2 to 10 μg/min. In a non–cardiac arrest situation, because epinephrine increases myocardial oxygen requirements, the nurse must monitor the patient closely for signs of myocardial ischemia.

ATROPINE

Atropine is used to increase the heart rate by decreasing the vagal tone. It is indicated for patients with symptomatic bradycardia. In an arrest, atropine may be used for asystole because it may initiate electrical activity or restore conduction through the AV node.

For symptomatic bradycardia, atropine is given in 0.5-mg doses IV and repeated every 5 minutes as needed (for a total of 0.03 to 0.04 mg/kg) to maintain a heart rate greater than 60 beats per minute, or until adequate tissue perfusion is achieved (as indicated by blood pressure, level of consciousness, and so forth). External pacing should be considered to maintain an adequate heart rate after the initial atropine dose in patients with myocardial ischemia in order to minimize the increased myocardial oxygen consumption caused by atropine. Doses lower than 0.5 mg can cause a paradoxical bradycardia and may precipitate VF.

In asystole, a 1-mg dose is given and repeated every 3 to 5 minutes, if necessary, up to a maximum of 0.03 to 0.04 mg/kg. If necessary, atropine may be given via an ETT. The dose for ETT administration is 1 to 2 mg diluted in 10 ml of normal saline or sterile water (without preservatives).

Text continued on page 192

Table 7-8. DRUGS FREQUENTLY USED IN CODE MANAGEMENT AND ACUTE MYOCARDIAL INFARCTION

Drug	Indication	Mechanism of Action	Dosage/Route	Side Effects	Nursing Implications
Adenosine (Adenocard)	Initial drug of choice for supraventricular dysrhythmias	Slows conduction in AV node and interrupts AV nodal reentry circuits	6 mg rapid IV bolus over 1–3 sec, followed by 20-ml rapid flush. If no response in 1–2 min, give 12-mg repeat dose and flush	Transient flushing, dyspnea, and chest pain; may cause asystole up to 15 sec	Half life < 5 seconds; higher dose needed with theophylline, lower dose with dipyridamole or cardiac transplantation
Amrinone (Inocor)	Severe congestive heart failure uncorrected by other drugs	Increases contractility, decreases preload and peripheral resistance	Loading dose of 0.75 mg/kg IV push over 2–15 min, followed by continuous infusion at 2–15 µg/kg/min, titrated to effect	Thrombocytopenia (2–3%)	Mix only in saline, monitor for myocardial ischemia
Atropine	Symptomatic bradycardia, asystole, bradycardic pulseless electrical activity	Increases SA node automaticity and AV node conduction activity	*Bradycardia:* 0.5–1 mg IV push *Asystole:* 1 mg IV push or 1–2 mg in 10 ml via ET; may repeat every 5 min up to 0.03–0.04 mg/kg	Tachycardia, increased myocardial oxygen consumption and ischemia	Consider external pacing if repeated doses needed; 3 mg is a fully vagolytic dose
Beta-blockers propranolol, metoprolol, atenolol, esmolol	Recurrent ventricular tachycardia or ventricular fibrillation, supraventricular tachycardia unresponsive to other therapies, hypertension	Reduces heart rate, blood pressure, contractility, and myocardial oxygen consumption; may control ventricular dysrhythmias	*Propranolol:* 1–3 mg IV push over 2–5 min; may be repeated after 2 min, not to exceed a total of 1 mg/kg *Metoprolol:* 5 mg IV push over 2–5 min, every 5 min not to exceed a total of 15 mg *Atenolol:* 5 mg IV over 5 min, repeat in 10 min *Esmolol:* dilute to 10 mg/ml; infuse 250–500 µg/kg for 1 min, followed by a continuous infusion of 25–50 µg for 4 min, then titrated up to 300 µg/kg/min	Hypotension, myocardial depression, bronchospasm (propranolol only)	Esmolol has rapid onset, short half-life for short-term use only; calcium channel blockers potentiate effect

Drug	Indications	Action	Dose	Side effects	Nursing considerations
Bretylium (Bretylol)	Ventricular fibrillation or pulseless ventricular tachycardia unresponsive to defibrillation and lidocaine, ventricular tachycardia with a pulse uncontrolled by lidocaine and procainamide	Raises fibrillation threshold, suppresses ventricular dysrhythmias	Ventricular fibrillation: initially, 5 mg/kg IV push; increase to 10 mg/kg and repeat every 5–30 min, up to a total of 35 mg/kg; may follow with a continuous infusion at 2 mg/min	Postural hypotension, nausea, vomiting	Ensure supine position and IV fluids available; dilution, 1 g/500 ml = 2 mg/ml
Calcium chloride	Acute hyperkalemia, hypocalcemia, calcium channel blocker toxicity	Increases myocardial contractility	8–16 mg/kg of 10% solution slow IV push; 10 ml of 10% solution = 100 mg/ml; repeat as needed.		Rapid administration can slow heart rate
Digitalis (Digoxin)	Atrial fibrillation or flutter with rapid ventricular response, supraventricular tachycardia	Depresses conduction through AV node	10–15 µg/kg IV push loading dose	Dysrhythmias, changes in mental status, anorexia, nausea, vomiting	Monitor drug levels; ensure normal potassium levels; onset of action, 5–30 min; peak, 1-1/2–3 hours
Diltiazem (Cardizem)	Reentrant supraventricular tachycardias, atrial fibrillation and flutter with rapid ventricular response	Calcium channel blocker, slows conduction and prolongs refractoriness in the AV node	0.25 mg/kg (approx. 20 mg) IV over 2 min for rapid atrial fibrillation/flutter, follow with maintenance infusion at 5–15 mg/h titrated to heart rate; if initial dose not effective within 15 min, follow with a 0.35 mg/kg dose	Myocardial depression	Beta-blockers have synergistic effects; use with caution with left ventricular failure
Dobutamine (Dobutrex)	Low cardiac output, pulmonary congestion	Alpha, beta$_1$, beta$_2$ agonist, increases contractility and cardiac output without increasing myocardial oxygen consumption, causes mild vasodilation	Continuous IV infusion at 2–20 µg/kg/min	Tachycardia, dysrhythmias, myocardial ischemia at high doses	Dilution; 500–1000 mg in 250 ml 5% D/W = 2000–4000 µg/ml; use lowest effective dose; avoid > 10% increase in heart rate
Dopamine (Intropin)	Hypotension not related to hypovolemia	Low doses (1–2 µg/kg/min): renal, mesenteric, and cerebral vasodilation; urine output increases Moderate doses (2–10 µg/kg/min): increases contractility and cardiac output High doses (>10 µg/kg/min): vasoconstriction and increased systemic vascular resistance	Continuous IV infusion, 2–5 µg/kg/min initially and titrated as needed	Tachycardia, increased dysrhythmias	Extravasation may cause necrosis and sloughing; dilution, 400–800 mg in 250 ml 5% D/W = 1600–3200 µg/ml

Table continued on following page

189

Table 7–8. DRUGS FREQUENTLY USED IN CODE MANAGEMENT AND ACUTE MYOCARDIAL INFARCTION *(Continued)*

Drug	Indication	Mechanism of Action	Dosage/Route	Side Effects	Nursing Implications
Epinephrine (Adrenalin)	Ventricular fibrillation, pulseless ventricular tachycardia, pulseless electrical activity, asystole	Increases contractility, automaticity, systemic vascular resistance, and arterial blood pressure; vasoconstriction improves coronary and cerebral perfusion	1.0 mg IV push or 2–2.5 mg in 10 ml via ETT; may repeat every 3–5 mg at a dose, up to 5 mg maximum		Occasionally used as a continuous infusion for hypotension; dilution, 1 mg/250–500 ml 5% D/W; start at 1 µg/min and titrate as needed (range 2–10 µg/kg/min)
Furosemide (Lasix)	Pulmonary congestion from left ventricular dysfunction	Loop diuretic; inhibits sodium reabsorption in the nephron, causing diuresis; decreases venous return and central venous pressure (preload)	20–40 mg (0.5–1.0 mg/kg) IV push over at least 1–2 min, up to a total of 2 mg/kg	Hypokalemia, hypovolemia	Excessively rapid administration can cause ototoxicity; monitor all electrolytes and fluid status
Isoproterenol (Isuprel)	Symptomatic bradycardia in cardiac transplantation patients, symptomatic bradycardia when other drugs have failed and external pacing is not available	Beta agonist, increases contractility and heart rate, also greatly increases myocardial oxygen demand	Continuous IV infusion at 2 µg/min, titrated to maintain heart rate of 60 beats per minute (range 2–10 µg/min)	Myocardial ischemia, ventricular dysrhythmias	Monitor for myocardial ischemia; dilution, 1 mg in 250 ml 5% D/W = 4 µg/ml
Lidocaine (Xylocaine)	Ventricular fibrillation, ventricular tachycardia, PVCs	Suppresses ventricular dysrhythmias, raises fibrillation threshold	*Ventricular fibrillation:* 1–1.5 mg/kg IV push, followed by 0.5 mg/kg every 3–5 min if needed to total dose of 3 mg/kg; may be given by ETT; follow with continuous intravenous infusion at 2–4 mg/min	Neurologic toxicity if drug level excessive	Lower dose if impaired hepatic blood flow; dilution, 1 g in 250 ml or 2 g/500 ml = 4 mg/ml
Magnesium	Torsades de pointes, hypomagnesemia in acute myocardial infarction	Essential for enzyme reactions and sodium-potassium pump, reduces postinfarction dysrhythmias	*Torsades de pointes:* up to 5–10 g IV *Acute ventricular tachycardia:* 1–2 g in 10 ml over 1–2 min *Hypomagnesemia and MI:* 0.5–1 g/h IV infusion	Flushing, bradycardia, hypotension	Monitor serum levels
Morphine	Myocardial infarction, pulmonary edema	Analgesic effects, vasodilates and decreases systemic vascular resistance, which relieves pulmonary congestion and decreases myocardial oxygen consumption	1–3 mg slow IV push (over 1–5 minutes), repeat as needed	Respiratory depression, hypotension	Monitor vital signs

Drug	Indications	Action	Dosage	Adverse Effects	Nursing Considerations
Nitroglycerin (Nitrol, Tridil)	Unstable angina, congestive heart failure	Relaxes vascular smooth muscle, decreases preload, increases myocardial oxygen supply by coronary artery vasodilation	Continuous IV infusion at 5–20 µg/min; titrated up by 5–10 µg every 5–10 min to desired effect. An IV bolus dose of 12.5–25 µg may be given prior to infusion. Usual dose is 50–200 µg/min, although higher doses may be required.	Headache, hypotension	Use IV tubing specially made for nitroglycerin; dilution, 50–100 mg/250 ml 5% D/W = 200–400 µg/ml
Norepinephrine (Levophed)	Hypotension uncorrected by other drugs	Alpha, beta, agonist, causes arterial and venous vasoconstriction, some increase in myocardial contractility	Continuous IV infusion at 0.5–1 µg/min, titrated upward as needed to maximum of 12 µg/min	Myocardial ischemia	Administer through central line, if possible; extravasation may cause necrosis and sloughing
Oxygen	Cardiopulmonary arrest, chest pain, hypoxemia	Increases arterial oxygen content and tissue oxygenation	100% in a code via bag-valve device with mask		
Procainamide (Pronestyl)	PVCs, ventricular tachycardia uncontrolled by lidocaine, occasionally supraventricular dysrhythmias	Reduces automaticity of ectopic pacemakers, slows intraventricular conduction	Administer 20–30 mg/min until dysrhythmia is suppressed, hypotension occurs, or the QRS widens by > 50% of original width, or 17 mg/kg has been administered, followed by a continuous infusion at 1–4 mg/min or 17 mg/kg IV over 1 h, followed by continuous infusion at 2.8 mg/kg	Hypotension, heart blocks	Do not exceed recommended infusion rate; dilution, 1 g/250 ml = 4 mg/ml; decrease dose with cardiac or renal dysfunction
Sodium bicarbonate	Metabolic acidosis in cardiopulmonary arrest uncorrected by defibrillation, to correct CPR technique, oxygenation, and other drugs	Counteracts metabolic acidosis by binding with hydrogen ions to produce water and carbon dioxide	1 mEq/kg IV push initially, may repeat 0.5 mEq/kg every 10 min as needed; administration should be dictated by ABG results		Ensure adequate CPR, oxygenation, and ventilation
Sodium nitroprusside (Nipride)	Hypertensive crisis, severe heart failure	Peripheral vasodilator, decreases preload and peripheral arterial resistance	Begin with 0.5 µg/kg/min continuous IV infusion, titrate upward to effect (range, 0.5–8 µg/kg/min)	Hypotension	Protect solution from light; dilution, 50–100 mg/250 ml 5% D/W or NS = 200–400 µg/ml
Verapamil	Supraventricular tachycardia unresponsive to adenosine that does not require cardioversion	Calcium channel blocker, decreases myocardial contractility, slows AV nodal conduction, vasodilates vascular smooth muscle	Initially, 2.5–5 mg IV push over 1–2 min; repeat dose at 5–10 mg if needed in 15 to 30 min or 5 mg every 15 min, to a maximum dose of 30 mg	Hypotension, myocardial depression	Contraindicated in left ventricular failure; beta-blockers have synergistic effect; use with caution in WPW syndrome, atrial fibrillation, and flutter

AV = atrioventricular; PVC = premature ventricular contraction; SA = sinoatrial; ETT = endotracheal tube; WPW = Wolff-Parkinson-White; ABG = arterial blood gas; 5% D/W = 5% dextrose in water; NS = normal saline; MI = myocardial infarction, µg = micrograms.

Table 7–9. EFFECTS OF ADRENERGIC RECEPTOR STIMULATION

Alpha
Vasoconstriction
Increased contractility

Beta₁
Increased heart rate
Increased contractility

Beta₂
Vasodilation
Relaxation of bronchial, uterine, and gastrointestinal smooth muscle

Dopaminergic
Vasodilation of renal, mesenteric, and cerebral vessels

LIDOCAINE (XYLOCAINE)

Lidocaine is an antiarrhythmic drug that suppresses ventricular ectopic activity. It depresses the ventricular conduction system and reduces automaticity. Lidocaine is the antiarrhythmic drug of choice for ventricular ectopy (premature ventricular contractions), VT, and VF.

During a code, a bolus dose of 1 to 1.5 mg/kg of lidocaine is administered by IV push. Additional boluses of 0.5 mg/kg may be administered every 3 to 5 minutes, as needed, until a total dose of 3 mg/kg has been given. If IV access is not available, lidocaine may be given at 2 to 2.5 times the IV dose through the ETT.

If lidocaine is successful in treating the cardiac dysrhythmia, a continuous infusion should be started at 30 to 50 µg/kg/min (2 to 4 mg/min). One gram of lidocaine is mixed in 250 ml of 5% dextrose in water, or 2 g can be mixed in 500 ml. Both solutions deliver 4 mg/ml, the standard dilution.

In a nonarrest situation, an initial bolus of 1.0 to 1.5 mg/kg of lidocaine is administered. It is followed by a continuous lidocaine infusion at 2 to 4 mg/min, with a second bolus of 0.5 mg/kg given after 10 minutes.

Dosages of lidocaine should be decreased in patients with impaired hepatic blood flow (as occurs in congestive heart failure, acute myocardial infarction, shock) and in elderly patients. Blood levels should be monitored, and the patient should be assessed for central nervous system disturbances that may indicate lidocaine toxicity. Common side effects of lidocaine include lethargy, confusion, tinnitus, and paresthesias.

PROCAINAMIDE (PRONESTYL)

Procainamide is an antiarrhythmic drug that reduces the automaticity of ectopic pacemakers and slows intraventricular conduction. It is used to treat ventricular ectopy and VT that is uncontrolled by lidocaine. It may also be used to treat supraventricular dysrhythmias. Procainamide is not used initially in VF because of the length of time needed to achieve adequate blood levels; however, it may be used for recurrent VF.

Procainamide is given IV in 100-mg doses (diluted in 10 ml of sterile water for injection) at a rate of 20 to 30 mg/min until the dysrhythmia is controlled, the patient becomes hypotensive, the QRS widens by 50% of its original width, or a total of 17 mg/kg has been given. If procainamide successfully controls the dysrhythmia, a continuous infusion is given at a rate of 1 to 4 mg/min for maintenance. An alternative dosing strategy is 17 mg/kg infused over 1 hour, followed by a continuous infusion of 2.8 mg/kg/h. The infusion is prepared by mixing 1 g of procainamide in 250 ml of fluid, yielding 4 mg/ml. As with lidocaine, the drug's level should be monitored. It should be administered in reduced dosages to patients with left ventricular dysfunction or renal failure.

Hypotension may occur after rapid injection of procainamide. Procainamide may also cause widening of the QRS interval and prolongation of PR or QT intervals, resulting in AV conduction disturbances, cardiac arrest, or both. It also can induce or worsen some malignant ventricular arrhythmias, particularly if the patient is hypokalemic or hypomagnesemic (AHA, 1994b).

BRETYLIUM TOSYLATE (BRETYLOL)

Bretylium is a second-line antiarrhythmic drug that is used to treat ventricular dysrhythmias that are unresponsive to other treatments (e.g., defibrillation, lidocaine, and procainamide). In a code, it is used after repeated shocks, epinephrine, and lidocaine fail to convert VF, or if the fibrillation is recurrent. Bretylium is also considered if lidocaine and procainamide have not been successful in controlling recurrent VT.

With initial administration, bretylium causes a transient hypertension and tachycardia. After this initial sympathetic-like response, adrenergic (sympathetic) blockade occurs, resulting in significant hypotension.

In VF, a bolus dose of 5 mg/kg of undiluted bretylium is given rapidly by the IV route. After bretylium administration, defibrillation is again attempted. The dose may be increased to 10 mg/kg and repeated after 5 minutes if VF persists. Bretylium can be repeated twice further in 10-mg/kg doses every 5 to 30 minutes for a maximum total dose of 35 mg/kg.

In recurrent VT that is unresponsive to other treatment, 500 mg of bretylium is diluted in 50 ml of

5% dextrose in water or normal saline, and 5 to 10 mg/kg is injected over 8 to 10 minutes. A second dose of 5 to 10 mg/kg can be given 10 to 30 minutes later; this dose may be repeated every 6 to 8 hours if necessary. Alternatively, bretylium may be administered as a continuous infusion at 2 mg/min. One gram of bretylium is mixed in 250 to 500 ml of solution when a continuous drip is needed; this solution delivers 2 to 4 mg/ml. Whereas the onset of action of bretylium is a few minutes in the treatment of VF, 20 minutes or more may be required for it to be effective in VT.

Postural hypotension is very common with bretylium administration; the patient should be in a supine position before administration, and adequate IV fluids must be are available. Nausea and vomiting may occur in the awake patient. Bretylium may worsen dysrhythmias caused by digitalis toxicity.

ADENOSINE (ADENOCARD)

Adenosine is the initial drug of choice for the diagnosis and treatment of supraventricular dysrhythmias. Adenosine slows conduction through the AV node and interrupts AV-node reentrant electrical conduction, which is the cause of most supraventricular dysrhythmias. It is effective in restoring normal sinus rhythm in patients with paroxysmal supraventricular tachycardia, including that caused by Wolff-Parkinson-White syndrome. Adenosine does not convert supraventricular rhythms that do not involve the sinoatrial or AV node, such as atrial fibrillation, atrial flutter, atrial tachycardia, and VT. However, adenosine may produce a brief AV node block, thereby assisting with the diagnosis of these rhythms.

Adenosine has a half-life of less than 5 seconds; therefore, it must be administered extremely rapidly. The initial dose is 6 mg IV push over 1 to 3 seconds, followed by a 20-ml rapid saline flush. A period of asystole lasting as long as 15 seconds may be seen after adenosine administration; this phenomenon reflects the suppression of AV node conduction. A second dose of 12 mg may be given 1 to 2 minutes later if the first dose is ineffective in converting the rhythm.

Patients receiving theophylline require higher doses of adenosine. Cardiac transplantation patients and those receiving dipyridamole are more sensitive to adenosine and need lower drug doses (AHA, 1994b). Common side effects include transient flushing, dyspnea, and chest pain.

VERAPAMIL (CALAN, ISOPTIN)

Verapamil is a calcium channel blocker that causes decreased heart rate. Unfortunately, it also causes vasodilation and decreased cardiac contractility. Verapamil slows conduction through the AV node, making it effective in the treatment of most supraventricular arrhythmias. Verapamil is useful in stable supraventricular tachycardia that does not require cardioversion.

Verapamil is ineffective in converting paroxysmal supraventricular tachycardia caused by Wolff-Parkinson-White syndrome. Verapamil may actually increase the ventricular rate in Wolff-Parkinson-White syndrome and may cause VF (AHA, 1994b). However, verapamil is useful in slowing rapid ventricular rates with atrial fibrillation or atrial flutter. Verapamil is not effective, and should not be used, in the treatment of VT. Severe hypotension, VF, or both, may result.

The initial dose of verapamil is 2.5 to 5.0 mg IV bolus given over 2 minutes. In middle-aged or older patients, verapamil should be given more slowly, at least over 3 minutes (AHA, 1994b). Maximal therapeutic response occurs within 3 to 5 minutes after injection. A repeat dose of 5 to 10 mg may be repeated 15 to 30 minutes later if needed, up to a maximum dose of 30 mg.

Because verapamil is also a vasodilator, arterial blood pressure should be monitored closely during and after administration. Verapamil is contraindicated in patients with preexisting severe heart failure because hemodynamic compromise may result. Combined use of beta-blockers and calcium channel blockers may increase myocardial depression as a result of the synergistic effects of these agents.

DILTIAZEM (CARDIZEM)

Diltiazem is a calcium channel blocker that is effective in slowing heart rate but has less effect on cardiac contractility than verapamil. Diltiazem may be as effective as verapamil in treating supraventricular tachycardias, particularly rapid atrial fibrillation or flutter (AHA, 1994b).

The initial dose for supraventricular tachycardias is 0.25 mg/kg (20 mg) by IV bolus over 2 minutes. This regimen converts the rhythm of more than 90% of patients with supraventricular tachycardia. A second dose of 0.35 mg/kg may be given 15 minutes after the initial dose, if needed. If treating atrial fibrillation or flutter, the bolus dose is followed by a continuous infusion of 5 to 15 mg/h. Continuous infusions at rates greater than 15 mg/h or for longer than 24 hours are not recommended (AHA, 1994b).

MAGNESIUM

Magnesium is essential for many enzyme reactions and for the function of the sodium-potassium pump. It also acts as a calcium channel blocker and slows neuromuscular transmission. Hypomagnesemia is associated with a high frequency of cardiac dysrhythmias, including refractory VF. Transient hypomagnesemia is seen with acute myocardial infarction (AHA, 1994b). Magnesium supplementation may decrease the number of postinfarction ventricular dysrhythmias. Magnesium is also the treatment of choice for torsades de pointes.

For torsades de pointes, doses of up to 5 to 10 g may be given intravenously. During VT, 1 to 2 g of magnesium sulfate is diluted in 10 ml of 5% dextrose and given via IV bolus over 1 to 2 minutes. In VF, it can be given more rapidly. A continuous infusion of magnesium at a rate of 0.5 to 1 g/h may be considered for the acute myocardial infarction patient with known magnesium deficiency.

The side effects of rapid magnesium administration include hypotension, asystole, flushing, and sweating. Serum magnesium levels should be monitored in order to avoid hypermagnesemia.

SODIUM BICARBONATE

A patient who has experienced an arrest quickly becomes acidotic. The acidosis results from two sources: (1) retention of carbon dioxide from inadequate ventilation and (2) build-up of acids from anaerobic metabolism induced by hypoxia. Effective ventilation with supplemental oxygen and rapid restoration of tissue perfusion (by CPR and spontaneous circulation) are the best mechanisms to correct these causes of acidosis.

Sodium bicarbonate is indicated in the treatment of metabolic acidosis *only* after interventions such as defibrillation, intubation and hyperventilation with 100% oxygen, and administration of pharmacological agents have been instituted. Sodium bicarbonate buffers the increased numbers of hydrogen ions present in metabolic acidosis. Administration and dosing of sodium bicarbonate should be based on arterial blood gas results.

If indicated, the initial dosage of sodium bicarbonate is 1 mEq/kg by IV push. Subsequent doses of half this amount may be repeated every 10 minutes, as determined by arterial blood gas results. Sodium bicarbonate should not be mixed or infused with any other drug, because it may precipitate or cause deactivation of other drugs.

DOPAMINE (INTROPIN)

The primary use of dopamine during a code is vasoconstriction; however, the drug's effects are dose related. For instance, at low doses of 1 to 2 μg/kg/ min, vasodilation of renal, mesenteric, and cerebral arteries occurs through stimulation of dopaminergic receptors (see Table 7–9). This effect increases urine output without affecting the blood pressure or heart rate. At rates of 2 to 10 μg/kg/min, myocardial contractility increases from beta-adrenergic stimulation, and cardiac output increases. At rates greater than 10 μg/kg/min, systemic vascular resistance markedly increases as a result of generalized vasoconstriction produced from alpha-adrenergic stimulation, which predominates in this dosage range. At doses greater than 20 μg/kg/min, marked vasoconstriction and increases in myocardial contractility occur. Myocardial workload is increased without an increase in coronary blood supply, a situation that may cause myocardial ischemia.

Dopamine is indicated in code situations for hypotension that is symptomatic (e.g., changes in mental status or oliguria) and not caused by hypovolemia. Dopamine is administered by continuous IV infusion starting at 2 to 5 μg/kg/min, and the dose is titrated upward. A dilution of 400 to 800 mg of dopamine in 250 to 500 ml of fluid delivers 1600 to 3200 μg/ml. Table 7–10 demonstrates the steps in the calculation of an IV infusion in micrograms per kilogram per minute. The lowest dose necessary for blood pressure control should be used in order to minimize side effects and ensure adequate perfusion of vital organs. Vasodilators (e.g., nitroprusside) may be used in conjunction with dopamine to lower vascular resistance while improving cardiac output.

In addition to causing myocardial ischemia, dopamine may also cause cardiac dysrhythmias, such as tachycardia and premature ventricular contractions. Necrosis and sloughing of tissue may occur if the drug infiltrates; therefore, it should be infused into a central line if possible. Phentolamine, 5 to 10 mg in 10 to 15 ml of normal saline, can be injected into the infiltrated area to prevent necrosis.

CALCIUM CHLORIDE

Calcium increases the force of myocardial contraction. The only use of calcium chloride in a code is the treatment of underlying hypocalcemia, hyperkalemia, or calcium channel blocker toxicity that may be a cause of the arrest. Unless these conditions are present, calcium chloride should not be used in resuscitation efforts.

For hyperkalemia and calcium channel overdose in a code, 8 to 16 mg/kg of a 10% solution is administered via IV push. (A 10-ml prefilled syringe of 10% calcium chloride yields 100 mg/ml.) This dose may be repeated if necessary. Calcium must be administered slowly in order to prevent a decrease in the heart rate

Table 7–10. DRUG CALCULATION CASE

A 55-year old man has been successfully defibrillated. He remains hypotensive with a blood pressure of 78/40 mm Hg despite two fluid challenges (each with 250 ml of normal saline). The decision is made to initiate a dopamine infusion at 5 µg/kg/min. The patient weighs 165 pounds. Your crash cart contains premixed dopamine with 800 mg in 250 ml of 5% dextrose in water.

Step 1. Determine the patient's weight in kilograms. 2.2 lbs/kg

$$\frac{165}{2.2} = 75\,kg$$

Step 2. Determine the concentration of solution.

$$\frac{Total\ Amount\ of\ the\ Drug}{Total\ Amount\ of\ the\ Solution}$$

    a. Convert mg to µg to determine total amount of drug in solution

        mg × 1000 = µg

        800 mg × 1000 = 800,000 µg

    b. Divide this number by the total number of ml in the IV bag

$$\frac{800,000}{250} = 3200$$

    c. The solution contains 3200 µg dopamine per ml

Step 3. Determine the number of milliliters per hour that must be delivered in order for 5 µg/kg/min to be provided.

$$\frac{Desired\ Dose \times 60\ (Minutes\ in\ 1\ Hour) \times Body\ Weight\ in\ kg}{Concentration/ml\ of\ Drug}$$

$$\frac{5 \times 60 \times 75}{3200\ µg/ml} = \frac{22,500}{3200} = 7.03\ or\ 7\ ml/h$$

(when the heart is beating). Ventricular irritability and coronary or cerebral vasospasm may also occur after administration.

Calcium gluceptate and calcium gluconate may also be used in doses of 5 to 7 ml and 5 to 8 ml, respectively. Calcium chloride is preferred over calcium gluceptate and calcium gluconate because higher plasma levels are achieved.

MORPHINE

Morphine is an analgesic used in the treatment of ischemic chest pain. It is also used in pulmonary edema because it increases venous capacitance and decreases systemic vascular resistance. These effects result in venous pooling and decreased blood return to the heart, thereby reducing pulmonary congestion and myocardial oxygen demand.

Morphine is given in small increments of 1 to 3 mg by IV push over 1 to 5 minutes; this dosage is repeated until symptomatic relief is obtained. Respiratory depression, hypotension, or both, may result from the use of morphine, but these effects are less likely to occur with smaller, frequent doses.

Special Problems During a Code

In addition to electrical and pharmacological interventions carried out in a code, immediate treatment of the underlying cause of the arrest may be necessary. Tension pneumothorax and cardiac tamponade are two such problems that require rapid invasive therapeutic techniques.

TENSION PNEUMOTHORAX

A tension pneumothorax occurs when air enters the pleural space but cannot escape (Fig. 7–17). Pressure increases in the pleural space, causing the lung to collapse. Tension pneumothorax is a life-threatening emergency. It may be caused by barotrauma from mechanical ventilation, blunt or penetrating trauma, or invasive procedures that inadvertently cause air to enter the pleural space. Symptoms of a tension pneumothorax include dyspnea, chest pain, tachypnea, tachycardia, and jugular venous distension. On assessment, breath sounds on the affected side are diminished, and the trachea may be shifted to the opposite side. If left

TENSION PNEUMOTHORAX

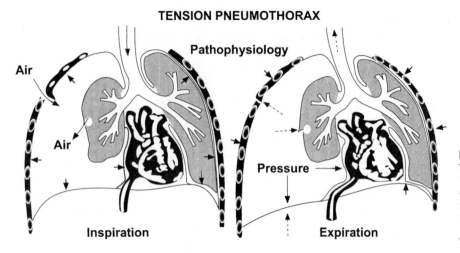

Figure 7–17. Tension pneumothorax. (From Alspach, J. G. (Ed.) (1992). *AACN instructor's resource manual for the AACN core curriculum for critical care nursing* (Transparency 168). Philadelphia: W. B. Saunders Co.)

untreated, the tension pneumothorax may progress and cause cardiovascular collapse and cardiac arrest. Because little time exists for radiographic confirmation, a needle may be inserted into the second or third anterior intercostal space on the affected side for relief of the tension pneumothorax. If air is under pressure in the pleural space, it escapes through the needle, making a hissing noise. As soon as possible after needle placement, a chest tube must be inserted and placed for suctioning in order to restore negative pressure in the chest and reexpand the lung.

PERICARDIAL TAMPONADE

Pericardial tamponade is the accumulation of fluid in the pericardial sac. The fluid causes a decrease in ventricular filling and results in decreased cardiac output. Pulseless electrical activity or cardiac arrest may follow. Tamponade can be caused by such events as trauma, pericarditis, CPR, or invasive procedures. The patient with cardiac tamponade has an increased central venous pressure, hypotension with narrowing of the arterial pulse pressure, and paradoxical pulse. Paradoxical pulse is the exaggerated fluctuation of arterial pressure during the respiratory cycle. It is defined as a peak systolic blood pressure drop of greater than 10 mm Hg during normal inspiration. Further assessment may reveal distant or muffled heart tones. Pericardiocentesis, or needle aspiration of pericardial fluid, is performed to alleviate the pressure around the heart. Additionally, rapid administration of IV fluids (to increase preload and stroke volume) and drugs such as epinephrine or isoproterenol may be used in order to temporarily increase stroke volume and cardiac output.

Documentation of Code Events

A detailed chronological record of all interventions must be maintained during a code. This task is sometimes forgotten; therefore, one of the first actions of the nurse team leader or nursing supervisor is to ensure that someone is assigned to record information throughout the code.

Documentation should include the time the code is called, the time CPR is started, any actions that are taken, and the patient's response (e.g., pulse, blood pressure, cardiac rhythm). Intubation and defibrillation (and the energy used) must be documented with the patient's response. The time and sites of IV initiations, the types and amounts of fluids administered, and the medications given to the patient are all accurately recorded. Many hospitals have standardized code records (Fig. 7–18) that list actions and medications and include spaces for the time of interventions and any comments. It is best if information can be recorded directly on the code record during the code to ensure that all information is obtained. Code records become part of the patient's permanent record.

Care of the Patient After Resuscitation

The survivor of a cardiac or respiratory arrest requires intensive monitoring and care. If the patient is not already in a critical care unit, he or she is transferred to one as soon as possible. Postresuscitation care includes airway and blood pressure maintenance, oxygenation, and control of dysrhythmias. Underlying abnormalities that may have caused the arrest, such as hypokalemia and myocardial ischemia, are corrected.

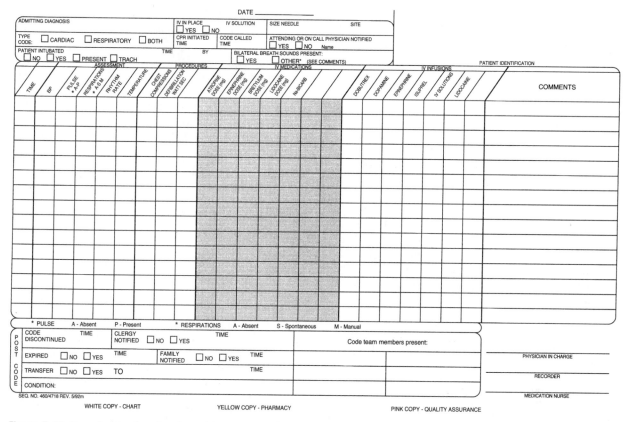

Figure 7–18. Sample of a flowsheet used for documenting activities during a cardiac arrest. (Reproduced with permission of Orlando Regional Healthcare System, Orlando, FL.)

Oxygen is given at a concentration of 100%. It is adjusted according to blood gas and pulse oximeter values. Dopamine or other pharmacological intervention may be needed for the maintenance of systolic blood pressure at or greater than 90 mm Hg. Blood pressure and heart rate should be recorded every 15 minutes during continuous infusion of vasoactive medications. If antiarrhythmic drugs were used successfully during the code, boluses may be repeated in order to achieve adequate blood levels, or continuous infusions may be administered for 24 hours. Other drugs may be given in order to improve cardiac output and myocardial oxygen supply. Arterial lines and pulmonary artery catheters are frequently inserted after a code in order to facilitate hemodynamic assessment and patient treatment.

Cerebral resuscitation is a term used for the interventions that are carried out to optimize cerebral recovery after an arrest. When a patient suffers a cardiac arrest, blood flow to the brain is interrupted, causing a lack of oxygen and glucose. Even with correct CPR, blood flow may not be sufficient. Hypoxemia and a lack of an energy source result, leading to ischemia,

lactic acid accumulation, and leaky cell membranes. Cerebral edema may occur, causing further damage and impedance to cerebral blood flow. Research is being conducted to determine which interventions and pharmacological agents improve cerebral recovery because brain injury often results from cardiac or respiratory arrest (AHA, 1994b).

The overall goals of cerebral resuscitation are promotion of cerebral perfusion and oxygenation. Adequate cerebral perfusion is accomplished through maintenance of blood pressure and prevention or reduction of increased intracranial pressure. Mean arterial pressure should be maintained between 60 and 150 mm Hg through the use of plasma volume expanders, vasopressors, or both.

The patient's ventilatory status is supported in order to promote improved tissue oxygenation and normal acid base status. This measure facilitates normal cellular cerebral function and repair. In addition to promoting tissue oxygenation, hyperventilation and the resultant decreased arterial pressure of carbon dioxide also causes cerebral vasoconstriction and may help to reduce intracranial pressure.

Other nursing measures in cerebral resuscitation include maintenance of normal body temperature, monitoring for glucose and electrolyte abnormalities, and thorough neurological assessments. Cooling blankets, antipyretic drugs, or both, should be used to maintain normothermia. Glucose and electrolyte monitoring is essential because disturbances can alter cerebral functioning. Neurological assessment should include the patient's level of consciousness, orientation, motor function, pupillary response, and respiratory patterns.

Emotional support is an important aspect of care after an arrest. Fear of death or a recurrence of the arrest is common. Some patients have out-of-body experiences during the code (Martens, 1994). Although this phenomenon is poorly understood, it may have a significant impact on the patient. Survivors often feel the need to discuss their experience in depth, and they should be listened to objectively and provided with psychological support.

Psychosocial/Legal/Ethical Implications

PSYCHOSOCIAL CONCERNS

In addition to the patient, many other people are affected when a code occurs. Family members, roommates and other patients, and staff members are all affected by the emergency.

If the family is with the patient when the arrest occurs, they should be tactfully removed from the scene as quickly as possible. A staff member, chaplain, volunteer, or friend should remain with the family during this time and keep them informed of the patient's progress. Honesty is crucial, and it is important that they know that their family member is receiving the best possible care. Debate exists over whether the family member should be allowed to stay in the patient's room during a code. Advocates believe that it helps the family members cope with the patient's critical status and possible death (Back and Rooke, 1994). Decisions should be made on an individual basis after assessment of family coping and preferences. If the family is not present, the next of kin should be called as soon as possible and informed of the patient's critical status.

If the patient is successfully resuscitated, the family should be allowed to see the patient as soon as is feasible. If the patient does not survive, the family should be encouraged to see the patient; this measure may facilitate the grief process.

All efforts should be made to remove a roommate or alert patients from the scene. If this is not feasible,

the curtains should be drawn. These patients may experience fear and usually want to talk about the experience. As do the survivor and family members, these patients require emotional support. Patient privacy must also be protected; it suffices to tell curious patients that an emergency is in progress. Also, it is easy to overlook other patients and their needs during a code. If staff members are not performing a specific role in the code, they should clear the area and tend to other patients.

Staff members are also affected by a code. In addition to the grief that may be felt over the loss of a patient, guilt, anger, and anxiety may also be felt. It is helpful for the staff involved in a code to be "debriefed," not only to evaluate how well the code went but also to discuss feelings about the events (Spitzer and Burke, 1993). Here, too, emotional support is needed.

LEGAL AND ETHICAL CONCERNS

In the absence of a written order from a physician to withhold resuscitative measures, CPR and a code must be initiated when a patient arrests. The physician generally makes the decision as to whether or not a patient is resuscitated. Likewise, it is the physician who makes the decision to terminate resuscitation efforts in progress. Decisions about resuscitation status often create ethical dilemmas for the nurse, patient, and family (see Chapter 3).

In situations of terminal or prolonged catastrophic illness, the patient may wish not to be resuscitated. A competent patient is legally and ethically allowed to make this choice. If the patient is comatose or otherwise unable to make end-of-life decisions (e.g., from irreversible brain damage), the health care team seeks to determine whether the patient would have wanted to be resuscitated in the present situation. Previously expressed wishes may exist in written form through advanced directives. The patient may have written a living will or may have assigned a health care surrogate to make decisions for him. In addition to discussing what their wishes are, the family may be able to express what they believe the patient would have wanted. The patient and/or family members need to voice their wishes to the physician and discuss these issues. Often, it is the nurse who must approach a physician regarding a "do not resuscitate" order and must encourage open communication with the patient and family. It is best if discussions regarding code status occur as soon as it is evident that a cardiac or respiratory arrest is possible, so that the decision can be made well before a code occurs. The patient and the patient's family should understand and agree with the decision, whether it be to withhold CPR or to do

RESEARCH APPLICATION

Article Reference

Rogove, H. J., Safar, P., Sutton-Tyrell, K., Abramson, N. S., & the Brain Resuscitation Clinical Trial I and II Study Groups. (1995). Old age does not negate good cerebral outcome after CPR: Analyses from the brain resuscitation clinical trials. *Critical Care Medicine, 23*, 18-25.

Study Overview

This study performed analyses on data from 774 patients who participated in the Brain Resuscitation Clinical Trials (BRCT) I or II. The BRCT I and II were multisite studies: data were collected in eight countries for BRCT I and in nine countries for BRCT II. The main purpose of these clinical trials was to evaluate different cerebral resuscitation methods. Patients without prior neurological problems who had no purposeful response to pain after successful resuscitation from cardiac arrest were eligible for entry in the study. Subjects were followed up regarding physical and neurological function for up to 1 year.

Eighty-one percent of the subjects died within the first 6 months after arrest. The mortality increased by age: 68% for subjects younger than 45 years of age; 94% for subjects older than 80 years of age. Significant independent predictors of mortality in all groups included history of diabetes mellitus, history of congestive heart failure, in-hospital arrests, time from arrest until initiation of resuscitation (CPR) of greater than 5 minutes, noncardiac cause of arrest, and CPR time of greater than 20 minutes.

Neurological outcome was also evaluated: 27% of subjects recovered "good" neurological function, which was defined as rendering the subject capable of independent functioning outside of an institutional setting. No difference in neurological outcomes were found between the different age groups. Also, the time to cerebral recovery after the arrest did not vary by age. Predictors of poor neurological outcome included history of diabetes, noncardiac cause of arrest, arrest time of greater than 5 minutes, and initial electrocardiographic readings during arrest of other than VT or fibrillation. Of the subjects surviving at 6 months, 86% had a "good" neurological outcome.

Critique

The strengths of this study include its prospective nature, the large sample size obtained from multiple settings, and the diligence of the investigators in following up on postarrest outcomes. The researchers spoke directly with the health care providers involved in resuscitation in order to verify the accuracy of arrest time. Similarly, they spoke to family members and close friends of the subjects to determine the subjects' prearrest neurological status. All investigators used the same resuscitation methods to allow valid comparisons across data collection sites.

Nursing Implications

This study scientifically confirms a widely held belief among health care providers that chances of survival are poor in arrest patients with preexisting diabetes mellitus or congestive heart failure, prolonged time before initiation of resuscitation, or prolonged resuscitation time. This information is helpful in clinical and ethical decision making regarding patient prognosis and code status. However, the most striking finding is that neurological outcome after resuscitation does not vary by age. Therefore, a commonly held belief that level of functioning is worse in the older resuscitated patient must be questioned.

everything possible to sustain life. Discussions and orders related to treatment in the event of an arrest should be clearly documented in the medical record according to hospital policy.

Summary

Positive patient outcomes depend on the health care team members' ability to rapidly recognize problems and intervene effectively. When a patient suffers a cardiac or respiratory arrest, or both, in the hospital, basic and advanced life support measures must be initiated immediately. How the code team functions and how interventions are carried out affect the patient's potential for recovery. Thus, code management is an important topic for anyone involved in the care of patients, especially those in critical care areas.

CRITICAL THINKING QUESTIONS

1. Discuss nursing strategies to be implemented during and after a code in order to provide psychosocial support to family members of patients suffering a cardiopulmonary arrest.
2. A surgical patient on a general nursing unit has just been successfully resuscitated after a respiratory arrest. He is intubated and is being manually ventilated with a BVD. Identify the current nursing priorities and their rationales.
3. You are the second nurse to respond to a code. The first nurse is administering CPR. Describe your first actions and their rationales.
4. Your patient has a permanent pacemaker generator. How would care and treatment of this patient differ in a code situation?
5. Some hospitals are now considering allowing family members to be present during a code.
   a. How might the presence of family members affect the management of the code?
   b. What factors should you consider before permitting family members to be present?

REFERENCES

American Heart Association (1994a). *Basic life support for healthcare providers.* Dallas: Author.

American Heart Association (1994b). *Textbook of advanced cardiac life support.* Dallas: Author.
Back, D., & Rooke, V. (1994). The presence of relatives in the resuscitation room. *Nursing Times, 90*(30), 34–35.
Crockett, P., & McHugh, L. G. (1988). *Noninvasive pacing: What you should know.* Redmond, WA: Physio-Control.
Crockett, P. J., Droppert, B. M., & Higgins, S. E. (1991). *Defibrillation: What you should know* [3rd ed.]. Redmond, WA: Physio-Control.
Kersten, L. D. (1989). *Comprehensive respiratory nursing.* Philadelphia: W. B. Saunders Co.
Martens, P. R. (1994). Near-death-experiences in out-of-hospital cardiac arrest survivors: Meaningful phenomena or just fantasy of death? *Resuscitation, 27*(2), 171–175.
Spitzer, W. J., & Burke, L. (1993). A critical-incident stress debriefing program for hospital-based health care personnel. *Health and Social Work 18*(2), 149–156.

RECOMMENDED READINGS

Angelini, K. M., & Boecklen, S. (1994). Take it to heart: how to operate an automated external defibrillator. *Nursing, 24*(3), 50–53.
Appel-Hardin, S., & Dente-Cassidy, A. M. (1991). How to use a noninvasive temporary pacemaker. *Nursing, 21*(5), 58–64.
Beeler, L. (1993). Noninvasive temporary cardiac pacing in the emergency department: A review and update. *Journal of Emergency Nursing, 19*(3), 202–205.
Campbell, C. D., & Newsome, J. A. (1990). Detecting life-threatening arrhythmias. *Nursing, 20*(12), 34–39.
Corcoran, J. R. (1994). The new ACLS tachycardia algorithm: Flexible guidelines for an old problem. *Journal of Emergency Nursing, 20*(2), 93–104.
Handerhan, B. (1993). Managing pericardial tamponade. *Nursing, 23*(4), 77–81.
Herrmann, D. J., & Raehl, C. L. (1993). Optimizing resuscitation outcomes with pharmacologic therapy. *Critical Care Nursing Clinics of North America, 5*(2), 247–259.
Mancini, M. E. (Ed.) (1996). Cardiac resuscitation issues. *Journal of Cardiovascular Nursing, 11*(2).
Michal, D. M. (1993). Automated external defibrillators: Prehospital use in advanced cardiac life support. *Journal of Emergency Nursing, 19*(2), 96–101.
Mitchell, L. (1995). Cardiac arrest during pregnancy: Maternal fetal physiology and advanced cardiac life support for the obstetric patient. *Critical Care Nurse, 15*(1), 56–60.
O'Neil, M. (1994). Administering code drugs confidently. *Nursing, 24*(7), 30.
Porterfield, L. M., & Porterfield, J. G. (1995). Third-generation pacemaker-cardioverter-defibrillator: A case study. *Critical Care Nurse, 15*(1), 43–45.
Repasky, T. M. (1994). Tension pneumothorax. *American Journal of Nursing, 94*(9), 47.
Saver, C. L. (1994). Decoding the ACLS algorithms: Advanced cardiac life support. *American Journal of Nursing, 94*(1), 26–36.

PART

3

Nursing Care During Critical Illness

CHAPTER

8

Shock

Mary G. McKinley, M.S.N., R.N., CCRN
Catherine F. Robinson, M.S., R.N., CCRN, CEN
Mary Lou Sole, Ph.D., R.N., CCRN

OBJECTIVES

- Describe the pathophysiology of shock.
- Differentiate the four classifications of shock.
- Discuss the progression of shock through the four stages.
- Identify clinical manifestations that may be seen in patients in shock.

- Discuss the nursing assessment of patients in shock.
- Discuss nursing diagnoses, treatment modalities, and potential outcomes for patients experiencing shock.
- Develop a plan of care for a patient in shock.

Introduction

Shock is a clinical syndrome characterized by inadequate tissue perfusion that results in impaired cellular metabolism. This syndrome is a severe, life-threatening complication that results from many patient conditions. The nurse's understanding of the pathophysiology of shock and the recognition of its clinical manifestations are essential for the prevention of shock and for the initiation of therapeutic interventions early in the course of shock.

The effects of shock are not isolated to one organ system; instead, all body systems are affected. Shock is best described by its symptomatology, the complex clinical picture that results from the underlying cause of the shock state, and the compensatory mechanisms initiated by the body in an attempt to restore homeostasis.

Although the causes of shock differ, the endpoints of poor nutritional blood flow and impaired cellular metabolism are common to all cases. Patient responses to the shock syndrome and its treatment vary, pre-senting a challenge to the patient and the nurse. Nursing care of patients in shock requires critical thinking based on knowledge, skills, and the application of research.

The purpose of this chapter is to introduce the nurse to the complex syndrome of shock and its management. The etiology, pathophysiology, and clinical manifestations of shock are reviewed. Nursing assessment and diagnoses are reviewed in order to provide a plan of care. The complex treatment of the patient in shock is also discussed, including fluids, pharmacological therapy, mechanical modalities, and supportive nursing care. An overview of patient outcomes and complications and a comprehensive nursing care plan complete the chapter.

Review of Anatomy and Physiology

The cardiovascular system continually provides cells with the oxygen and the nutrients necessary for

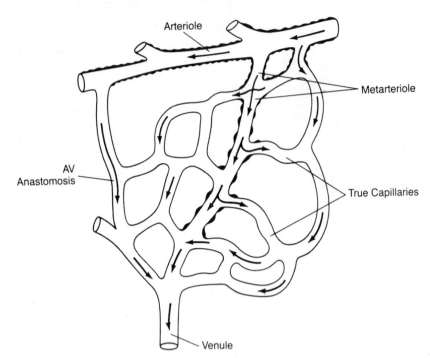

Figure 8–1. Microcirculation. AV = atrioventricular. (Redrawn from Perry, A. G., & Potter, P. A. (1983). *Shock: Comprehensive nursing management.* St. Louis: C. V. Mosby Co.)

survival and rids the body of the waste products of metabolism. It is a closed, interdependent system composed of the heart, blood, and vascular bed. Arteries, arterioles, capillaries, venules, and veins make up the vascular bed. The microcirculation, the portion of the vascular bed between the arterioles and the venules, is the most significant portion of the circulatory system for cell survival (Fig. 8–1). Its functions are the delivery of nutrients to cells, the removal of wastes from cells, and the regulation of blood volume. Additionally, the vessels of the microcirculation constrict or dilate in order to selectively regulate blood flow to cells in need of oxygen and nutrients.

The structure of the microcirculation differs according to the function of the tissues and organs it supplies; however, all of the vascular beds have common structural characteristics (see Fig. 8–1). As oxygenated blood leaves the left side of the heart and enters the aorta, it flows through progressively smaller arteries until it flows into an arteriole. Arterioles are lined with smooth muscle, which allows these small vessels to change diameter, and as a result, direct and adjust blood flow to the capillaries. From the arteriole, blood then enters a metarteriole, a smaller vessel that branches from the arteriole at right angles. Metarterioles are partially lined with smooth muscle, which allows them to also adjust diameter size and regulate blood flow into capillaries.

Blood next enters the capillary network by passing through a muscular precapillary sphincter. Capillar-

ies are narrow, thin-walled vascular networks that branch off the metarterioles. This network configuration increases the surface area to allow for greater fluid and nutrient exchange. It also decreases the velocity of the blood flow in order to prolong transport time through the capillaries. Capillaries have no contractile ability and are not responsive to vasoactive chemicals, electrical or mechanical stimulation, or pressure across their walls. The precapillary sphincter is the only means of regulating blood flow into a capillary. When the precapillary sphincter constricts, blood flow is diverted away from a capillary bed and directed to one that supplies tissues in need of oxygen and nutrients. The capillary bed lies close to the cells of the body, a position that facilitates the delivery of oxygen and nutrients to the cells.

Once nutrients are exchanged for cellular waste products in the capillaries, blood enters a venule. These small muscular vessels are able to dilate and constrict, offering postcapillary resistance for the regulation of blood flow through capillaries. Blood then flows from the venule and enters the larger veins of the venous system.

Another component of the microcirculation is the arteriovenous anastomoses that connect arterioles directly to venules. These muscular vessels are able to shunt blood away from the capillary circulation, sending it directly to tissues in need of oxygen and nutrients.

The flow of blood is facilitated by changing pressures within the vessels as blood moves from an area of high pressure within the arteries and passes to the venous system, which has lower pressures. Blood flow is opposed, however, by the force of resistance. As resistance increases, blood flow decreases. Resistance is determined by three factors: (1) vessel length, (2) blood viscosity, and (3) vessel diameter (Emerson, 1995). Increased resistance occurs with increased vessel length, increased blood viscosity, and decreased blood vessel diameter.

Vessel diameter is the most important determinant of resistance. As the pressure of blood within the vessel decreases, the diameter of the vessel decreases, resulting in decreased blood flow. The critical closing pressure and the resultant cessation of blood flow occurs when blood pressure decreases to a point at which it is no longer able to keep the vessel open.

Shock begins when the cardiovascular system fails to function properly because of an alteration in at least one of the four essential circulatory components: blood volume, myocardial contractility, blood flow, and vascular resistance. Under healthy circumstances, these components function together to maintain circulatory homeostasis. When one of these components fails, the others compensate. However, as compensatory mechanisms fail, or if more than one of the circulatory components are affected, a state of shock ensues. Shock is not a single clinical entity but a life-threatening response to alterations in circulation, resulting in impaired tissue oxygenation and cellular metabolism.

Pathophysiology

CLASSIFICATIONS OF SHOCK

Various diverse events can initiate the shock syndrome. These events are classified according to the affected circulatory component (Table 8–1) (Bongard, 1994; O'Rourke and McCall, 1994; Parrillo, 1994; Summers, 1995; Tierney, 1995; Trunkey et al., 1992).

Hypovolemic Shock

Hypovolemic shock occurs when the circulating blood volume is inadequate to fill the vascular net-

Table 8–1. CLASSIFICATION OF SHOCK

Altered Circulatory Component	Type of Shock
Blood volume	Hypovolemic shock
Myocardial contractility	Cardiogenic shock
Blood flow	Obstructive shock
Vascular resistance	Distributive shock

Table 8–2. CAUSES OF HYPOVOLEMIC SHOCK

External Losses	Internal Losses
Blood	Third-space sequestration
Plasma	Fluid loss into intestinal lumen
Body fluid	Internal hemorrhage

work. Intravascular volume deficits may be caused by either external or internal losses (Table 8–2) (Rice, 1991a). In either case, the blood volume is depleted and is unavailable for the transport of oxygen and nutrients to tissues.

External volume deficits include loss of blood, plasma, or body fluids. The most common cause of hypovolemic shock is hemorrhage (Rice, 1991a). External loss of blood may occur after traumatic injury, surgery, or delivery of a baby, or with coagulation alterations (e.g., hemophilia, thrombocytopenia, disseminated intravascular coagulation, and anticoagulant medications). Hypovolemic shock resulting from hemorrhage is classified according to the volume of blood lost and the resultant effects on level of consciousness, vital signs, capillary refill, and urine output (Table 8–3).

External plasma losses may be seen in patients with exudative lesions or burn injuries. Excessive external loss of fluid may occur through the gastrointestinal tract (e.g., via suctioning, vomiting, diarrhea, reduction in oral fluid intake, fistulas), the genitourinary tract (e.g., as a result of excessive diuresis, diabetes mellitus with polyuria, diabetes insipidus, diuretic therapy, Addison's disease), or the skin (e.g., as a result of diaphoresis without fluid and electrolyte replacement).

Internal volume deficits caused by third-space sequestration, fluid leakage into the intestinal lumen, and/or internal hemorrhage may also result in hypovolemic shock. Third-space sequestration is seen in patients with ascites, peritonitis, and edema. Intestinal obstruction causes fluid to leak from the intestinal capillaries into the lumen of the intestine. Internal hemorrhage may be seen in patients with a ruptured spleen or liver, hemothorax, hemorrhagic pancreatitis, fractures of the femur or pelvis, and lacerations of the great vessels.

The severity of hypovolemic shock depends on the volume lost, the rate of volume loss, the patient's age, and the presence of other preexisting conditions (Bongard, 1994). Hypovolemic shock results in a reduction of intravascular volume and a decrease in venous return to the right side of the heart. Ventricular filling pressures are reduced, resulting in a decrease in stroke volume and cardiac output. As the cardiac output decreases, the blood pressure decreases and the

Table 8–3. CLASSIFICATION OF HYPOVOLEMIC SHOCK AND ESTIMATED FLUID AND BLOOD REQUIREMENTS*

	Class I	Class II	Class III	Class IV
Blood loss (ml)	≤750	750–1500	1500–2000	≥2000
Blood loss (% blood volume)	≤15%	15–30%	30–40%	≥40%
Pulse rate	<100	>100	>120	≥140
Blood pressure	Normal	Normal	Decreased	Decreased
Pulse pressure (mm Hg)	Normal or increased	Decreased	Decreased	Decreased
Capillary refill test	Normal	Delayed	Delayed	Delayed
Respiratory rate	14–20	20–30	30–40	>35
Urine output (ml/h)	≥30	20–30	5–15	Negligible
Mental status	Slightly anxious	Mildly anxious	Anxious and confused	Confused, lethargic
Fluid replacement (3:1 rule)	Crystalloid	Crystalloid	Crystalloid + blood	Crystalloid + blood

*For a 70-kg male.
Adapted from American College of Surgeons. (1993). *Advanced trauma life support for physicians*. Chicago: Author.

tissue perfusion decreases. The end result is impaired cellular metabolism as a result of the decrease in nutritional blood flow through capillaries that supply the cells with oxygen and nutrients.

Cardiogenic Shock

Cardiogenic shock is caused when the heart fails to act as an effective pump. A decrease in myocardial contractility results in a decrease in cardiac output and an impairment in tissue perfusion. Cardiogenic shock is one of the most difficult types of shock to treat and carries a mortality of 75 to 85% (Tierney, 1995).

Most causes of cardiogenic shock occur when diseased coronary arteries are not capable of meeting the oxygen demand of the working myocardial cells, such as occurs in acute myocardial infarction. A correlation exists between the amount of myocardial damage and the likelihood of cardiogenic shock. If 40% or more of the left ventricle is damaged, the likelihood that cardiogenic shock may develop increases (Suhl, 1993).

Other causes of cardiogenic shock include conditions that result in ineffective myocardial cell function. These conditions include dysrhythmias, cardiomyopathy, myocarditis, metabolic derangement, valvular disease, structural disorders, and vitamin deficiencies.

The pathophysiology of cardiogenic shock can be understood by review of cardiac dynamics. Contractile force is responsible for the amount of blood ejected from the heart each minute, termed the *stroke volume*. Ventricular filling pressure is the pressure in the ventricles as they fill. When contractile force is reduced, damage to the myocardium occurs, and stroke volume and ventricular filling pressure are affected. Stroke volume is decreased because the heart is unable to pump effectively and eject adequate amounts of blood. Ventricular filling pressures begin to increase as the stroke volume decreases. This increase occurs because blood remains in the cardiac chambers and increases pressure in the ventricles. As these two mechanisms occur, the cardiac output decreases and causes hypotension. This hypotension brings about a reflex compensatory peripheral vasoconstriction, resulting in an increase in the afterload, or the resistance against which the heart must pump. At the same time, backup of blood into the pulmonary circulation causes a decrease in the perfusion of oxygen across alveolar membranes, thereby reducing the oxygen tension in the blood.

The already failing heart is now in a crisis situation (Fig. 8–2). An increased demand is placed on the myocardium as it attempts to increase perfusion to the cells. The heart rate increases as a compensatory mechanism, a phenomenon that increases the oxygen demand on an overworked myocardium, thereby compounding the problem. In patients with cardiogenic shock secondary to acute myocardial infarction, the increased demand may increase infarction size.

Obstructive Shock

Obstructive shock occurs when the heart or great vessels (i.e., aorta, vena cava, pulmonary arteries) are compressed, causing a mechanical obstruction to central blood flow (Bongard, 1994; O'Rourke and McCall, 1994; Parrillo, 1994; Tierney, 1995; Trunkey, et al., 1992). Causes of obstructive shock are noted in Table 8–4.

Compression of the heart or great vessels either impedes venous return to the right side of the heart or prevents effective pumping action of the heart. This

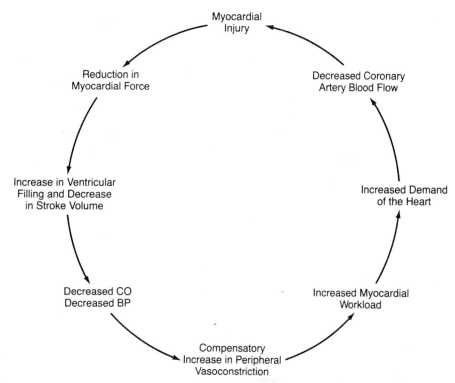

Figure 8–2. Cycle of cardiogenic shock. CO = cardiac output; BP = blood pressure.

results in a decrease in cardiac output, a decrease in blood pressure, and a reduction in tissue perfusion.

Distributive Shock

Distributive shock describes several different types of shock that have in common widespread vasodilatation and a decrease in peripheral vascular resistance. Vasodilatation increases the vascular capacity; however, the blood volume is unchanged, resulting in a relative hypovolemia. Neurogenic, anaphylactic, and septic shock are forms of distributive shock.

Table 8–4. CAUSES OF OBSTRUCTIVE SHOCK

Pericardial tamponade
Aortic dissection
Positive end-expiratory pressure
Atrial myxoma
Prosthetic valve thrombus
Pulmonary embolus
Tension pneumothorax
Abdominal distention
Aortic stenosis
Mitral stenosis

Neurogenic Shock

Neurogenic shock occurs when a disturbance in the nervous system affects the vasomotor center in the medulla. In healthy individuals, the vasomotor center in the medulla initiates sympathetic stimulation of nerve fibers that travel down the spinal cord and out to the periphery. There, they innervate the smooth muscles of the blood vessels to cause vasoconstriction. In neurogenic shock, disturbances that interrupt sympathetic nerve impulses result in vasodilatation. Consequently, a decrease in systemic vascular resistance, venous return, preload, and cardiac output occurs.

Causes of neurogenic shock include injury or disease of the upper spinal cord, spinal anesthesia, nervous system damage, ganglionic and adrenergic blocking agents, and vasomotor depression (Bongard, 1994; O'Rourke and McCall, 1994; Rice, 1991a; Summers, 1995; Trunkey, et al., 1992). Patients who have a cervical spinal cord injury may experience a permanent or temporary interruption in sympathetic nerve stimulation. Spinal anesthesia may extend up the spinal cord and block sympathetic nerve impulses from the vasomotor center. Vasomotor depression may be seen with deep general anesthesia, injury to the medulla, administration of drugs, severe pain, and hypoglycemia.

Table 8–5. CLASSIFICATIONS OF ANTIGENS

Route	Substance
Injection	
Drugs	Antibiotics, analgesics, anesthetics, vaccine, hormones
Contrast media	Iodine based radiologic dye
Blood transfusions	Sensitivity to antigens in donor blood
Ingestion	Antibiotics, milk, egg, egg whites, oranges, mangos, bananas, beans, soybeans, sesame and sunflower seeds, seafood, shellfish
Bites/stings	Venomous snakes, wasps, bees, hornets, yellow jackets

Anaphylactic Shock

A severe allergic reaction can precipitate a second form of distributive shock, known as anaphylactic shock. Antigens, which are foreign substances to which the individual is sensitive, initiate an antigen-antibody response. Table 8–5 lists some common antigens grouped by the route in which they enter the body.

Once an antigen enters the body, antibodies are produced that attach to mast cells and basophils. The greatest concentrations of mast cells are found in the lungs, around blood vessels, in connective tissue, and in the uterus. Mast cells are also found to a lesser extent in the kidneys, heart, skin, liver, and spleen and in the omentum of the gastrointestinal tract. Basophils circulate in the blood. Both mast cells and basophils contain histamine and histamine-like substances, which are potent vasodilators.

The initial exposure to the antigen may not cause any harmful effects. However, subsequent exposures to the antigen cause the anaphylactic reaction. The antigen-antibody reaction causes cellular breakdown and the release of powerful vasoactive substances from the cells. These substances cause vasodilatation, increased capillary permeability, and smooth muscle contraction. The combined effects are a decrease in blood pressure, a relative hypovolemia caused by the vasodilatation and fluid shifts, and symptoms of anaphylaxis that primarily affect the skin, respiratory, and gastrointestinal systems.

Septic Shock

A third type of distributive shock, septic shock, is caused by a systemic inflammatory response syndrome, usually from an infectious process. Systemic inflammatory response syndrome is the initial stage of progressive deterioration, which leads to multiple organ dysfunction syndrome (American College of Chest Physicians/Society of Critical Care Medicine [ACCP/SCCM] Consensus Conference Committee, 1992). Terms commonly used in discussions of septic shock are presented in Table 8–6. Severe sepsis and septic shock are the most common causes of death in intensive care units in the United States, where the mortality rate is between 40 and 80% (Tierney, 1995).

Nosocomial infections are a major cause of sepsis in critically ill patients. Factors that increase the risk of developing nosocomial infections include underlying chronic disease, alteration in host defenses, long hospital stays, use of invasive catheters and devices, trauma, and surgical wounds (Hazinski et al., 1993). Additionally, the increased use of more potent and broader-spectrum antibiotics, immunosuppressive agents, and invasive technology for the treatment of inflammatory, infectious, and neoplastic diseases has contributed to the increased incidence of infection and sepsis (ACCP/SCCM Consensus Conference Committee, 1992).

Infection with gram-negative bacteria is a common cause of nosocomial infections in adults (Hazinski et al., 1993). Common sites of infection include the pulmonary system, urinary tract, gastrointestinal system, and wounds. Predisposing risk factors are summarized in Table 8–7.

Table 8–6. DEFINITIONS RELEVANT TO SEPTIC SHOCK

Infection—inflammatory response to microorganisms.
Bacteremia—presence of bacteria in the blood.
Systemic inflammatory response syndrome (SIRS)—systemic response to a clinical insult, e.g., infection, pancreatitis, ischemia, trauma, and hemorrhagic shock. Symptoms include fever or hypothermia, tachycardia, tachypnea, leukocytosis, and leukopenia.
Sepsis—systemic response to infection manifested by two or more of the symptoms noted with SIRS.
Severe sepsis—sepsis associated with organ dysfunction, hypoperfusion, or hypotension. Alterations may include lactic acidosis, oliguria, or changes in mental status.
Septic shock—sepsis associated with hypotension despite adequate fluid resuscitation, along with perfusion abnormalities. Patients receiving inotropes or vasopressors may not exhibit hypotension.
Hypotension—a systolic blood pressure of <90 mm Hg or a reduction of >40 mm Hg from normal baseline.
Multiple organ dysfunction syndrome—altered organ function in acutely ill patients.

Adapted from American College of Chest Physicians/Society of Critical Care Medicine Consensus Conference Committee (1992). Definitions for sepsis and organ failure and guidelines for the use of innovative therapies in sepsis. *Chest*, 101:1644–1655.

Table 8–7. PREDISPOSING RISK FACTORS FOR SEPTIC SHOCK

Compromised Immunity	Invasive Procedures

Chronic debilitating diseases
  Neoplastic disease, leukemia, cirrhosis, diabetes mellitus, cardiovascular disease, pulmonary disease, renal failure, lupus, alcoholism, human immunodeficiency virus infection
	Surgical procedures
	
	Invasive diagnostics
	  Urologic procedures
	  Bronchoscopies
	
	Obstetrical-gynecological procedures
	  Septic abortions, cesarean sections
	  Hysterectomy for pelvic inflammatory disease

Anemia, malnutrition	

Skin alterations
  Burns, ulcerations
	Invasive lines/tubes
	  Indwelling catheters
	  Pulmonary artery catheters

Drug therapy
  Antibiotics, immunosuppressives
  Cytotoxics, corticosteroids
	Central venous lines
	  Endotracheal tube/ tracheostomy

Extremes of age <1 years >65 years	

The cascade of infection that leads to septic shock and multiple organ dysfunction syndrome, clinical signs, and treatment is shown in Figure 8–3. In septic shock, the invading bacteria multiply faster than the body can kill them. As bacteria are destroyed, endotoxins are released into the bloodstream, damaging tissues and altering cellular metabolism. The cells are unable to use the oxygen and other nutrients, resulting in cellular hypoxia and decreased energy production. In addition, endotoxins cause the release of histamine and other cellular mediators (e.g., prostaglandin, leukotriene, thromboxane, protacycleine, and bradykinin), which are vasoactive substances that cause increased capillary permeability (Hazinski et al., 1993; Summers, 1995). As a result, a decrease in systemic vascular resistance, hypotension, and venous pooling occurs, which reduces venous return. The cardiac output may be normal to high because of a compensatory tachycardia response and the fact that the heart does not have to pump as hard against the low systemic vascular resistance.

Toxic shock syndrome is caused by a gram-positive bacteria, *Staphylococcus aureus*. The bacteria release a potent toxin that exerts its effects within hours. It has been associated with the use of tampons in menstruating women; however, toxic shock syndrome is also seen in patients with surgical wounds, deep and superficial abscesses, infected burns, abrasions, insect bites, herpes zoster, cellulitis, septic abortion, and osteomyelitis; after vaginal and cesarean delivery; and in some newborns in whom the bacteria are transmitted from the mother.

Distributive shock results in a relative hypovolemia. Blood volume remains normal, but because of massive vasodilatation and decreased peripheral vascular resistance, the blood is abnormally distributed in this enlarged vascular space. The result is a decrease in venous return to the right side of the heart and a reduction in ventricular filling pressures. Anaphylactic shock and septic shock are also complicated by an increase in capillary permeability, which decreases intravascular volume, further compromising venous return. Eventually, in all forms of distributive shock, stroke volume, cardiac output, and blood pressure decrease resulting in decreased tissue perfusion. The end result is impaired cellular metabolism that results from decrease in nutritional blood flow through capillaries that supply the cells with oxygen and nutrients.

STAGES OF SHOCK

While the response to shock is highly individualized, the clinical picture presents in stages that progress at unpredictable rates (Rice, 1991b; O'Rourke and McCall, 1994; Summers, 1995). These stages of shock result, regardless of the type of shock experienced (Table 8–8).

Stage I: The Initial Stage

During the initial stage of shock, cardiac output is reduced. Increased sympathetic stimulation occurs in an attempt to maintain tissue perfusion. At this stage, shock may be reversed by infusion of blood, fluids, and/or pharmacological therapy (O'Rourke and McCall, 1994).

Stage II: Early or Compensatory Stage

As shock progresses, the sustained reduction in cardiac output initiates a set of neural, endocrine, and chemical compensatory mechanisms in an attempt to maintain blood flow to vital organs and restore homeostasis (Rice, 1991b). During this stage, symptoms become more apparent. At this stage, shock may still be reversed if appropriate interventions are initiated (O'Rourke and McCall, 1994). Figure 8–4 shows the physiologic responses that occur during this stage.

Neural Compensation. Baroreceptors (which are sensitive to pressure changes) and chemoreceptors (which are sensitive to chemical changes) located in the carotid sinus and aortic arch detect the reduction in arterial blood pressure. Impulses are relayed to the vasomotor center in the medulla oblongata, stimulating

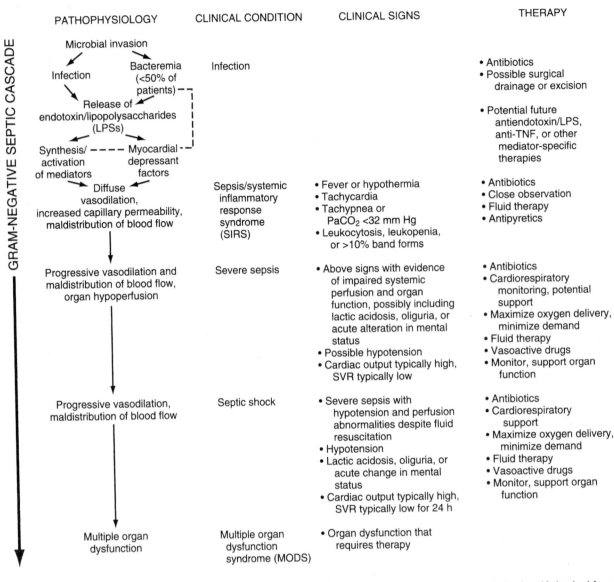

Figure 8–3. Progression of septic shock. SVR = systemic vascular resistance; TNF = tumor necrosis factor. (Adapted from Hazinski, M., Iberti, T., MacIntyre, N., Parker, M., Tribett, D., Prion, S., & Chmel, H. (1993). Epidemiology, pathophysiology and clinical presentation of gram-negative sepsis. *American Journal of Critical Care, 2*(3), 224–235.)

the sympathetic branch of the autonomic nervous system to release epinephrine and norepinephrine from the adrenal medulla. In response to these catecholamines, the heart increases the rate and the force of contractions in order to improve cardiac output and supply the heart muscle with more oxygen. Vasoconstriction occurs. Arterial vasoconstriction improves blood pressure, whereas venous vasoconstriction augments venous return to the heart, thereby increasing

cardiac output. Blood is shunted from the kidneys, gastrointestinal tract, and skin to the heart and brain. Bronchial smooth muscles are relaxed, and respiratory rate and depth are increased, thus improving oxygenation and gas exchange. Additional catecholamine effects are an increase in blood glucose level as the liver is stimulated to convert glycogen to glucose; dilation of pupils; and cool, moist skin that is caused by peripheral vasoconstriction and increased sweat gland activ-

Table 8–8. STAGES OF SHOCK

Stage of Shock	Physiological Event
Initial stage	Decrease in baseline mean arterial pressure (MAP) of 5–10 mm Hg Increased sympathetic stimulation Mild vasoconstriction Increase in heart rate
Compensatory stage	Decrease in MAP of 10–15 mm Hg from the client's baseline value Continued sympathetic stimulation Moderate vasoconstriction Increased heart rate Decreased pulse pressure Chemical compensation Renin, aldosterone, and antidiuretic hormone secretion Increased vasoconstriction Decreased urinary output Stimulation of the thirst reflex Some anaerobic metabolism in nonvital organs Mild acidosis Mild hyperkalemia
Progressive stage	Decrease in MAP of >20 mm Hg from the client's baseline value Anoxia of nonvital organs Hypoxia of vital organs Overall metabolism is anaerobic Moderate acidosis Moderate hyperkalemia Tissue ischemia
Refractory stage	Severe tissue hypoxia with ischemia and necrosis Release of myocardial depressant factor from pancreas Build-up of toxic metabolites

Adapted from Ignatavicius, D. D., Workman, M. L., & Mishler, M. A. (1995). *Medical-surgical nursing: A nursing process approach* (2nd ed.) (p. 970). Philadelphia: W.B. Saunders Co.

ity. Stimulation of the sympathetic nervous system attempts to combat shock by vasoconstriction, increased cardiac output, improved blood pressure, and increased perfusion to the heart and brain.

Endocrine Compensation. In response to the reduction in blood pressure, messages are also relayed to the hypothalamus, which stimulates the anterior and posterior pituitary gland. The anterior pituitary gland releases adrenocorticotropic hormone, which acts on the adrenal cortex to release glucocorticoids and min-eralocorticoids (aldosterone). Glucocorticoids increase the blood glucose level by increasing the conversion of glycogen to glucose (glycogenolysis). Mineralocorticoids act on renal tubules to reabsorb sodium and chloride, causing water to be reabsorbed, thus conserving intravascular volume and improving blood pressure. Aldosterone is also released in response to a reduction of pressure in the renal arterioles that supply the glomeruli of the kidneys and/or by a decrease in sodium levels as sensed by the kidney's juxtaglomerular apparatus. In response to decreased renal perfusion, the juxtaglomerular apparatus releases renin. Renin circulates in the blood and reacts with angiotensinogen to produce angiotensin I. Angiotensin I circulates through the lungs, where it forms angiotensin II, a potent arterial and venous vasoconstrictor that increases blood pressure and improves venous return to the heart. Angiotensin II also activates the adrenal cortex to release aldosterone. Stimulation of the posterior pituitary gland releases antidiuretic hormone, which is secreted in response to the increased osmolarity of the blood that occurs in shock. The overall effects of endocrine compensation result in an attempt to combat shock by providing the body with glucose for energy and by increasing the intravascular blood volume.

Chemical Compensation. As cardiac output decreases, pulmonary blood flow is reduced, resulting in ventilation-perfusion imbalances. The alveoli may be adequately ventilated with oxygen, but the perfusion of blood through the alveolar capillary bed is decreased. Chemoreceptors located in the aorta and carotid arteries are stimulated in response to this low oxygen tension in the blood. Consequently, the rate and depth of respirations increase. As the patient hyperventilates, carbon dioxide is excreted, and respiratory alkalosis occurs. A reduction in carbon dioxide levels and the alkalotic state cause vasoconstriction of cerebral blood vessels. This vasoconstriction, coupled with the reduced oxygen tension, leads to cerebral hypoxia and ischemia. The overall effects of chemical compensation result in an attempt to combat shock by increasing oxygen supply; however, in doing so they cause negative effects on cerebral perfusion.

Stage III: Intermediate or Progressive Shock

If the cause of shock is not corrected, or if compensatory mechanisms continue without reversing the shock, further patient deterioration occurs. Whereas during the compensatory stage, the systemic and microcirculation worked together with vasoconstriction to increase venous return, they now begin to function independently and in opposition (Rice, 1991b).

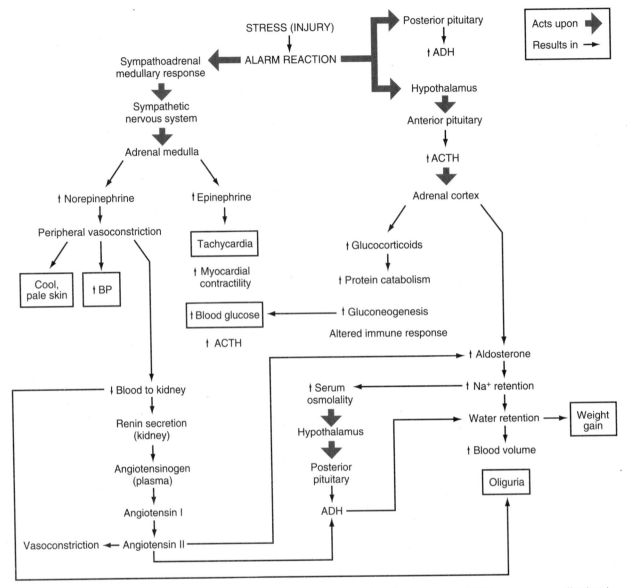

Figure 8–4. Physiologic responses to stressors in shock. ADH = antidiuretic hormone; ACTH = adrenocorticotropic hormone. (Adapted from Polaski, A. L., & Tatro, S. E. (1996). *Luckmann's core principles and practice of medical-surgical nursing*. Philadelphia: W. B. Saunders Co.)

The systemic circulation continues to vasoconstrict. Although this effect shunts blood to vital organs, the decrease in cutaneous blood flow leads to ischemia in peripheral extremities, weak or absent pulses, and altered body defenses. Prolonged vasoconstriction results in decreased capillary blood flow and eventually results in cellular hypoxia. The cells convert to anaerobic metabolism, which leads to a local metabolic acidosis.

The microcirculation exerts the opposite effect and dilates in order to obtain the blood supply for local tissue needs. Whereas the arterioles remain constricted in an attempt to keep vital organs perfused, the precapillary sphincters relax, allowing blood to flow into the capillary bed. Meanwhile, postcapillary sphincters remain constricted. As a result, blood flows freely into the capillary bed but accumulates in the capillaries as blood flow from the capillary bed is impeded. Capillary hydrostatic pressure increases, and fluid is pushed from the capillaries into the interstitial space, causing edema. Fluid shifting from the intravascular space is further aggravated as histamine release increases capillary permeability, and the loss of proteins through enlarged capillary pores lowers colloidal osmotic pressure. As intravascular blood volume decreases, the blood becomes more viscous, and blood flow is slowed. This situation causes capillary sludging as red blood cells, platelets, and proteins clump together. Blood flow is further impaired and later contributes to coagulation alterations. The loss of intravascular volume and capillary pooling further reduce the venous return to the heart and cardiac output. Coronary perfusion is impaired, and ischemia results when the systolic pressure is less than 60 mm Hg. Cardiac contractility, cardiac output, and blood pressure decrease. The vicious cycle of shock begins as the body attempts to compensate with further vasoconstriction. At this point, the patient presents with classic shock signs and symptoms that affect all body systems (see Assessment). This phase of shock responds poorly to fluid replacement alone and requires aggressive medical and nursing management if it is to be reversed (O'Rourke and McCall, 1994).

Stage IV: Refractory or Irreversible Shock

Prolonged inadequate tissue perfusion that is unresponsive to therapy ultimately contributes to multiple organ failure and death. A large volume of the blood remains pooled in the capillary bed, and the arterial blood pressure is too low to support perfusion of the vital organs. Poor renal function, respiratory failure, and impaired cellular function aggravate the existing state of acidosis, which in turn contributes to further fluid shifts, loss of vasomotor tone, and relative hypovolemia. Coronary artery perfusion and oxygen delivery to the heart muscle are reduced, causing myocardial ischemia and dysrhythmias. Myocardial depressant factor is released. These alterations in the cardiovascular system and continued acidosis cause a reduction in heart rate, an impaired contractility, and a further decrease in cardiac output. Acidosis, decreased intravascular fluid volume, and sluggish blood flow through the capillaries leads to clumping of platelets and red blood cells. These aggregates form fibrin clots that occlude small vessels and further impede blood flow. This cycle depletes clotting factors and may result in disseminated intravascular coagulation. Cerebral ischemia occurs as a result of the reduction in cerebral blood flow. Consequently, the sympathetic nervous system is stimulated, an effect that aggravates the existing vasoconstriction, thereby increasing afterload and decreasing cardiac output. Prolonged cerebral ischemia eventually causes the loss of sympathetic nervous system response, and vasodilatation and bradycardia result. The patient's decreasing blood pressure and heart rate cause a lethal decrease in tissue perfusion, multisystem organ failure, and ultimately brain death and cardiopulmonary arrest.

Assessment

Shock is a common threat to all patients. Shock is not selective in its effects—all tissues and cells suffer as a result of the decreased tissue perfusion. Assessment of the patient at risk can make the difference between life and death. An understanding of how cells and organ systems are affected facilitates assessment. Assessment focuses on three areas: history, clinical picture, and laboratory diagnosis. The logical approach for assessment is to examine the history of the patient and then look at the systems most sensitive to a lack of oxygen and nutrients.

HISTORY AND PREVENTION

An accurate and detailed history is essential for guiding medical and nursing interventions. An assessment of patients with a high likelihood of developing shock, and information about the causative event must be obtained. Identification of high-risk patients increases the likelihood that preventive steps can be taken.

Hypovolemic Shock

Hypovolemic shock can be prevented by assessment of fluid balance, hemodynamic values, and vital signs. Recognizing the need for fluid administration in those experiencing rapid or large volume losses is essential (Rice, 1991d). Fluid losses occur in frank or subtle ways. Assessment includes weighing dressings; considering insensible losses, such as perspiration; and measuring drainage, such as from chest or nasogastric tubes. Abdominal girth is measured periodically in patients in whom hidden bleeding may be suspected or in those with ascites. Daily weights should be obtained by use of the same scale with the patient wearing the same clothing at approximately the same time each day.

Cardiogenic Shock

Prevention of cardiogenic shock is aimed at decreasing the myocardial oxygen demand and increasing oxygen supply to the damaged tissue (Rice, 1991d). Aggressive therapy, such as thrombolytic agents, beta blockers, and percutaneous transluminal coronary angioplasty, may help to reduce the size of the infarction. Pain relief and rest are significant aids in reducing the workload of the heart and therefore infarct size. Oxygen administration increases the supply to the ischemic muscle and may help save myocardial tissue.

Obstructive Shock

Obstructive shock can be prevented by aggressive interventions to relieve the source of the compression or obstruction. Pericardiocentesis, or the removal of fluid in the pericardial sac, is performed for the treatment of cardiac tamponade. Surgical repair of aortic dissection eliminates the occlusion to the lumen of the aorta. A needle thoracentesis relieves the accumulated intrathoracic pressure associated with a tension pneumothorax that results from blunt or penetrating chest injuries. Early surgical reduction of long bone fractures, measures to enhance circulation in immobile patients (e.g., use of antiembolism hose, range-of-motion exercises), and prophylactic anticoagulant therapy reduce the risk for pulmonary emboli.

Distributive Shock

Immobilization of spinal injuries may assist in preventing severe neurogenic shock. Such measures include the use of traction devices, such as skull tongs or a halo brace (to maintain alignment) or surgical intervention to stabilize the injury. Frequent assessment of patients receiving spinal anesthesia can prevent the occurrence of neurogenic shock. These patients may be positioned with the head of the bed at a 20° elevation in order to prevent the upward progression of the agent up the cord.

The nurse can prevent anaphylactic shock by collecting detailed information about allergies and drug reactions. The nurse inquires about reactions to drugs with similar structures. For example, if patients are allergic to penicillin, they are likely to have a reaction to ampicillin (Principen), carbenicillin (Geopen), or nafcillin sodium (Nafcil). Response to intravenous (IV) administration of medications, particularly antibiotics, is monitored. Injecting small amounts of a drug before the entire dosage is given is recommended in order to assist in detecting a possible reaction. Care is taken during the transfusion of blood or blood products, which can result in allergic reactions. The patient receiving any of these products is observed closely for any signs of an allergic reaction (see Table 8–14).

Prevention of septic shock is promoted through proper hand washing and use of aseptic technique. The critical care patient is debilitated and has many potential portals of entry for bacterial invasion. Meticulous technique is required during procedures (i.e., suctioning, dressings, and wound care) and when handling catheters or tubes. Frequent assessment of temperature

and laboratory results (e.g., white cell and differential counts) are important for the identification of response to infection.

CLINICAL PICTURE

Multiple body systems are affected by the shock syndrome. Effects are summarized.

Central Nervous System

The central nervous system is the most sensitive to changes in the supply of oxygen and nutrients. Thus, it is the first system affected by changes in cellular perfusion. Initial responses of the central nervous system to shock include agitation, anxiety, nervousness, and restlessness. As the shock state progresses, the patient becomes drowsy, confused, and lethargic because of the decreased blood flow to the brain. In stage III of shock, the patient becomes unresponsive.

Cardiovascular System

Blood Pressure. A major focus of assessment is blood pressure. It is important for the nurse to know the patient's baseline blood pressure. The initial blood pressure is usually normal to hypertensive because of the compensatory effects of the sympathetic nervous system. As the shock state progresses, the systolic blood pressure drops, whereas the diastolic pressure remains normal, resulting in a narrowed pulse pressure. Recommendations vary, but a drop in systolic blood pressure to less than 80 mm Hg is considered hypotensive. For hypertensive patients, a decrease in systolic pressure to less than 100 mm Hg from their usual pressure may be considered severely hypotensive.

A point to consider is that cuff pressures may be very inaccurate. One of the chief compensatory mechanisms occurring early in the shock state is vasoconstriction, which can lead to inaccuracies in blood pressure measurement. If a blood pressure is not heard via auscultation, the pressure is assessed by palpation or ultrasound (Doppler) devices. Intra-arterial lines may also be used for assessing blood pressure.

Palpable pulses can give an approximation of the blood pressure. If the brachial pulse is readily palpable, the approximate systolic pressure is 80 mm Hg. Corresponding blood pressure for the femoral and carotid pulses are 70 and 60 mm Hg, respectively (McQuillan and Wiles, 1994).

Another assessment of the blood pressure is the tilt test or orthostatic vital sign assessment. The patient is taken from a lying to a sitting position very quickly, and blood pressure and pulse before and after positioning are compared. A 10 mm Hg decrease in systolic pressure is correlated with a mild degree of shock. A decrease of 25 to 50 mm Hg approximates a moderate degree of shock, and a decrease of 50 mm Hg or greater indicates a severe state of shock. An increase in the pulse rate of 10 to 20 beats per minute is also considered to be a positive tilt or orthostatic sign.

Pulsus paradoxus is assessed in patients with suspected obstructive shock caused by cardiac tamponade. Pulsus paradoxus is a decrease in systolic blood pressure of more than 10 mm Hg during inspiration.

Pulse. The rate, quality, and character of major pulses are evaluated: carotid, radial, femoral, dorsalis pedis, and posterior tibial. In shock states, the pulse is generally weak and thready (Summers, 1995; Rice, 1991d). The pulse is increased, usually greater than 100 beats per minute, in a compensatory response to the decreased cardiac output and demand of the cells for increased oxygen. In later stages of shock, the pulse slows. The decrease in pulse rate may be related to myocardial depressant factor, which is released in severe cases of metabolic acidosis (Suhl, 1993).

Heart Sounds. Cardiac auscultation reveals abnormal heart sounds if the patient is in cardiogenic shock. A third heart sound (S_3) indicates filling of a flabby ventricle, which occurs with myocardial muscle damage. A fourth heart sound (S_4) reflects a noncompliant ventricle. Murmurs may be present in the patient with valvular diseases. Pulsus paradoxus may be present in the patient with obstructive shock related to cardiac tamponade.

Neck Veins. Assessment of the neck veins provides information regarding the volume and pressure in the right side of the heart. It is an indirect method of evaluating the central venous pressure. Neck veins are distended in patients with obstructive or cardiogenic shock and are nondistended in hypovolemic shock.

Capillary Refill. Capillary refill assesses the ability of the cardiovascular system to maintain perfusion to the periphery. The normal response to pressure on the nail beds is blanching; the color returns to a normal pink hue 1 to 2 seconds after the pressure is released. A delay in the return of color indicates peripheral vasoconstriction. Capillary refill provides a quick assessment of the patient's overall cardiovascular status, but this assessment is not reliable in a patient who is hypothermic or has peripheral circulatory problems.

Central Venous Pressure. Central venous catheters may be inserted in order to aid in the differential diagnosis of shock, to administer and monitor therapies, and to provide an evaluation of the preload of the heart. Normally, the central venous pressure is 0 to 8 mm Hg. When blood volume decreases, such as in hypovolemic shock, the central venous pressure

decreases. In cardiogenic shock, the central venous pressure may be increased owing to the poor myocardial contractility and high filling pressure in the ventricles.

Pulmonary Artery Pressures. A pulmonary artery catheter is one of the most useful tools for diagnosing and treating the patient in shock. The flow-directed, balloon-tipped catheter can give information regarding fluid balance, pumping ability of the heart, and effects of vasoactive agents. Table 8–9 lists normal values and alterations seen in the various types of shock.

Preload, which is measured by the mean right atrial pressure for the right ventricle and by the pulmonary capillary wedge pressure for the left ventricle, is used for assessing fluid balance. Systemic vascular resistance, which is a calculated value, offers information on the afterload or workload of the left ventricle. Pulmonary vascular resistance measures right ventricular workload or afterload. Cardiac output and cardiac index give information regarding contractility and how the heart is handling the cell's demands for nutrients.

A fiberoptic pulmonary artery catheter, which measures mixed venous oxygen saturation, is used to evaluate whether or not oxygen supply is meeting the demands of the tissues. Mixed venous oxygen saturation is useful in identifying the type of shock and in evaluating the effectiveness of treatments.

Respiratory System

Respirations in the early stage of shock are rapid and deep. The respiratory center responds to the shock state and metabolic acidosis with an increase in respiratory rate in order to eliminate carbon dioxide. Direct stimulation of the medulla by the chemoreceptors is responsible for the alteration of the respiratory pattern. As the shock state progresses, metabolic wastes build up and cause generalized muscle weakness. The respiratory muscles are affected, leading to shallow breathing with poor air exchange.

Pulse oximetry is frequently used to measure arterial oxygen saturation. A probe is placed on a finger, toe, or earlobe, and a fiberoptic sensor evaluates the saturation of the red blood cell with oxygen. Pulse oximetry should be used with caution in patients in shock because the peripheral circulation is decreased in these patients, which may result in inaccurate readings. Arterial blood gas analysis may be required for the assessment of oxygenation.

Renal System

A urine output of less than 30 ml/h is considered a sign of shock. In shock, the urine output decreases

Table 8–9. HEMODYNAMIC ALTERATIONS IN SHOCK STATES

Parameter/ Normal Range	Cardiogenic	Hypovolemic	Obstructive	Distributive	
				Septic	Anaphylactic Neurogenic
Cardiac output, 4–8 L/min	Low	Low	Low	High then low	Low
Cardiac index, 2.8–4.2 L/min/m²	Low	Low	Low	High then low	Low
Right atrial pressure, 0–8 mm Hg	High	Low	High	Low then high	Low
Pulmonary artery diastolic pressure, 4–12 mm Hg	High	Low	High	Low then high	Low
Pulmonary capillary wedge pressure, 1–10 mm Hg	High	Low	High	Low then high	Low
Systemic vascular resistance, 900–1400 dynes/sec/cm⁻⁵	High	High	Low	Low	Low
Mixed venous oxygen saturation, 60–80%	Low	Low	High	High then low	Low

because of reduced renal perfusion. The kidneys compensate by reducing excreted fluids and concentrating urine. In addition, a hormonal response aids the body in shock. Aldosterone promotes the retention of sodium and the reabsorption of water. Renal failure can result if shock is not treated.

Skin and Mucous Membranes

Skin color, temperature, texture, turgor, and moisture level are evaluated. Characteristic skin changes occur, depending on the type of shock involved. In septic shock, the skin is often moist, flushed, and warm. In hypovolemic or cardiogenic shock, the skin is pale, cool, and moist. The mucous membranes are dry and pale in shock as a result of the decreased perfusion. In toxic shock syndrome, the patient displays a red macular rash, desquamation of the skin, and, occasionally, bright red mucous membranes (Broscious, 1991). Cyanosis may be present; however, it is a late and unreliable sign. The patient may exhibit *central* cyanosis, seen in the mucous membranes of the mouth and nose, or *peripheral* cyanosis, evident in the nails and earlobes.

Musculoskeletal System

The patient in shock suffers from fatigue in all muscle systems. Generalized weakness and fatigue are major complaints. Alterations in perfusion to the gas-

trointestinal musculature result in a slowing of intestinal activity and cause symptoms of decreased bowel sounds, distention, nausea, and constipation. Prolonged decrease in perfusion can lead to paralytic ileus and ulceration. Patients with toxic shock exhibit neuromuscular symptoms, such as arthralgia, general aching, malaise, abdominal discomfort, and neck stiffness (Broscious, 1991).

DIAGNOSTIC TESTS

Additional tests may assist in the differential diagnosis of the patient in shock. These include laboratory tests and a variety of other tests.

Laboratory Studies

Various laboratory tests aid in the diagnosis of shock. (Tables 8–10 and 8–11). By the time many of the laboratory test results are altered, patient is in the later stages of shock. The clinical picture is more useful for early diagnosis and immediate treatment.

Other Diagnostic Tests

Additional diagnostic tests and assessment parameters include urine studies, chest x-ray studies, echocardiography, peritoneal lavage, and computed tomography (CT).

Table 8–10. LABORATORY VALUES COMMON IN SHOCK

Test	Normal Value	In Shock
Blood glucose	70–100 mg/dl	Early: increased Late: decreased
Blood urea nitrogen	5–20 mg/dl	Increased
Creatinine	0.6–1.2 mg/dl	Increased
Sodium	136–142 mEq/L	Increased
Chloride	95–103 mEq/L	Decreased
Carbon dioxide	21–28 mEq/L	Early: increased Late: decreased
Arterial blood gases		
pH	7.35–7.45	Early: increased Late: decreased
$PaCO_2$	35–45 mm Hg	Early: decreased Late: increased
PaO_2	80–100 mm Hg	Decreased
HCO_3	22–26 mEq/L	Late: decreased

$PaCO_2$ = partial pressure of arterial carbon dioxide; PaO_2 = partial pressure of arterial oxygen; HCO_3 = bicarbonate.

Urine studies may be ordered for the examination of renal status. The urine specific gravity and osmolarity may be high as a result of decreased urine production, resulting from impaired renal perfusion, as well as increased release of antidiuretic hormone and aldosterone.

Chest x-ray studies are helpful for assessing respiratory status. They can be used to identify pulmonary edema in the patient in cardiogenic shock. Pulmonary edema can further compromise the patient's cellular oxygenation. In obstructive shock, a chest film may help to identify a tension pneumothorax or cardiac tamponade. Chest x-ray studies are also helpful in the early recognition of acute respiratory distress syndrome, which is a common complication of the shock syndrome. In the patient admitted with chest injuries, an x-ray study assists in the diagnosis of a pneumothorax or a hemothorax.

An echocardiogram is useful in the diagnosis of cardiac tamponade. It shows a collection of fluid in the pericardial sac.

A diagnostic peritoneal lavage may be performed for the assessment of abdominal bleeding. Diagnostic peritoneal lavage is indicated in cases of severe trauma and is performed in the emergency department. Abdominal girth is also assessed. An increase in the girth may be an indicator of abdominal bleeding or fluid loss into the abdomen.

Computed tomography is useful in assisting with the differential diagnosis of shock. CT can pinpoint sources of bleeding, which can cause hypovolemic shock, or abcess formation, which can cause septic shock. A CT can also show spinal injuries that can precipitate spinal shock.

Nursing Diagnosis

Alteration in tissue perfusion (cellular) is related to decreased blood volume, myocardial contractility,

Table 8–11. LABORATORY TESTS FOR DIFFERENTIAL DIAGNOSIS OF SHOCK

Test	Normal Value	In Shock
Blood culture	No growth	Positive in septic shock
Hemoglobin	14–18 g/dl (men) 12–16 g/dl (women)	Decreased in hypovolemic shock caused by hemorrhage
Hematocrit	42–52% (men) 35–47% (women)	Decreased in hypovolemic shock caused by hemorrhage
Red blood cells	4.5–6.2 million/µl (men) 4.0–5.5 million/µl (women)	Decreased in hypovolemic shock caused by hemorrhage
Cardiac enzymes		
CK	20–170 U/L (men) 10–135 U/L (women)	All enzymes may be increased in cardiogenic shock as a result of decreased coronary artery perfusion and myocardial injury
CK-MB	0–7 µg/dl 0–6% of total CK	
LDH	150–450 µg/dl	
LDH$_1$	22–36%	
LDH$_2$	35–46%	

CK = creatine kinase; LDH = lactate dehydrogenase.

vascular resistance, obstruction, or a combination of these.

Medical Interventions

Treatment of the patient in shock consists of treating the cause of the shock. Care is directed toward correcting and/or reversing the altered circulatory component, (e.g., blood volume, cardiac contractility, obstruction, and vascular resistance) and treating clinical symptoms. Care includes a combination of fluid, pharmacological, and mechanical therapies in order to maintain tissue perfusion. Oxygen consumption decreases in shock as oxygen delivery decreases, a phenomenon that has been associated with poor prognosis. Current medical management of shock includes interventions to increase oxygen delivery. These interventions include increasing cardiac output and index, increasing hemoglobin value, and increasing arterial oxygen saturation (Barone and Snyder, 1991).

Hypovolemic Shock

Treatment for hypovolemic shock includes locating and controlling the source of fluid loss while restoring circulatory blood volume. A combination of crystalloids, colloids, plasma expanders, and blood and/or blood products may be used, depending on whether the hypovolemic state is caused by hemorrhage, plasma losses, or dehydration.

Cardiogenic Shock

Treatment for cardiogenic shock focuses on protecting the ischemic myocardium. A combination of pharmacologic agents, mechanical assist devices, and surgery may be used for reestablishing circulation to the myocardium, increasing cardiac output, decreasing afterload, and increasing oxygenation to the myocardium.

Obstructive Shock

Treatment for obstructive shock includes interventions for relieving the obstruction and restoring blood flow. Definitive treatment varies for each of the causes of obstructive shock.

Distributive Shock

The primary treatment for distributive shock is the restoration of vascular tone. Vasopressor therapy and measures for correcting the cause of the vascular alteration are directed toward reversing the relative hypovolemia caused by vasodilation.

The cause of shock in patients with spinal cord injury must be determined so that the appropriate intervention can be chosen. Vasopressor therapy is indicated for neurogenic shock resulting from spinal cord injury. However, these patients frequently have multiple injuries and altered host defenses with portals of entry for microorganisms that are related to injuries and to therapeutic measures, such as central lines and Foley catheters. Therefore, shock caused by hypovolemia or sepsis must be ruled out.

Interventions for anaphylactic shock include prevention of the further introduction of the antigen and reversal of the allergic reaction. Medications are administered in order to restore vascular tone, neutralize the effects of histamine, promote bronchial dilation, and stabilize capillary walls.

In septic shock, cultures from potential sites of infection (e.g., urine, blood, sputum, and wounds) are obtained in order to locate the source. Sensitivity studies are performed in order to determine the antibiotic therapy that will eradicate the causative organism.

FLUID THERAPY

Regardless of the cause, shock produces profound alterations in fluid balance that affect tissue perfusion. Therefore, patients experiencing absolute hypovolemia (hypovolemic shock) or relative hypovolemia (distributive shock) require the administration of IV fluids for the restoration of intravascular volume, the maintenance of oxygen-carrying capacity, and the establishment of the hemodynamic stability necessary for optimal tissue perfusion. The choice of fluid and the volume and rate of infusion depend on the type of fluid lost, the patient's concurrent medical problems, and the fluid's availability.

Benefits of parenteral fluid administration include increased intravascular volume, increased venous return to the right side of the heart, optimal stretching of the ventricle, improved myocardial contractility, and increased cardiac output. The end result is enhanced tissue perfusion. However, these effects may be dangerous to the patient in cardiogenic shock because large volumes of fluid overwork an already failing heart. Instead, cardiogenic shock is managed primarily with medications that reduce both preload and afterload.

Patients in severe shock may require immediate rapid volume replacement, although recent research calls into question the value of immediate versus delayed fluid administration in selected populations experiencing hemorrhagic shock with hypotension (Bickell et al., 1994). The IV flow rate can be increased by infusion of fluids under pressure by use of a blood pump, large-bore infusion tubing, or rapid-infusion devices. Infusion pumps can be used for the accurate administration of large volumes at fast rates. Consideration should be given to infusing fluids through a warmer when rapid, massive parenteral infusions are administered.

Intravenous Access

Intravenous access is needed for the administration of fluids and medications. The patient in shock requires a minimum of two IV catheters: one in a peripheral vein and one in a central vein. Peripheral access via a large-gauge catheter (No. 14 or 16) provides a route for immediate, rapid administration of fluids and medications. Establishing IV routes in a patient in shock is challenging because peripheral vasoconstriction and venous collapse make access difficult. Initially, it is usually necessary to use the large peripheral veins in the antecubital fossa (i.e., the basilic, cephalic, or accessory cephalic). In extreme emergencies, the physician may need to perform a venous cut-down.

A central venous access is established for large-volume replacement and can be used for monitoring central venous pressure or for placing a pulmonary artery catheter in order to guide fluid replacement. Central venous catheters are commonly inserted into the subclavian, internal jugular, or femoral veins. Multilumen catheters, which provide multiple access ports, are often used in order to allow the concurrent administration of fluid, medication, and blood products.

Fluid Challenge

Once IV access is established, a fluid challenge may be performed for the assessment of the patient's hemodynamic response to the rapid administration of fluid. Various methods for administering a fluid challenge exist. Typically, the physician orders a rapid infusion of 250 to 500 ml of normal saline, followed by repeated boluses, based on blood pressure or central venous pressure response (Suhl, 1993). Nursing responsibilities include obtaining the baseline hemodynamic measurements, administering the fluid challenge, and assessing the patient's response.

Types of Fluids

The choice of fluid or fluids depends on the cause of the volume deficit, the patient's clinical status, and the physician's preference. Although the nurse is not responsible for selecting the infusion or transfusion,

---

Table 8–12. DESIRABLE OUTCOMES FOR THE PATIENT IN SHOCK

1. Alert and responsive (in the absence of head injury)
2. Warm, dry, normal-colored skin with good turgor
3. Pink, moist mucous membranes
4. Capillary refill <2 sec
5. Nondistended, not collapsed jugular veins
6. Blood pressure ± 20 mm Hg as compared with preshock
7. Mean arterial pressure, 80 mm Hg
8. Heart rate, 60–100 beats per minute, strong and regular
9. Respirations, 10–20 breaths per minute, regular and unlabored
10. Balanced intake and output
11. Stable weight
12. Urinary output, 30–60 ml/h, specific gravity, 1.010–1.025

---

an understanding of the rationale for the prescribed fluid as well as the expected effects is needed for the assessment of patient outcomes. The nurse needs to carefully monitor the patient's response to fluid therapy. A return to normal of the laboratory and hemodynamic values, as well as the patient outcomes described in Table 8–12, are the goals of fluid therapy.

Crystalloids, colloids, blood, and blood products are used alone or in combination in order to restore intravascular volume. Initially, crystalloids and/or colloids are infused until diagnostics, typing, and cross-matching are completed as a guide to further treatment.

Crystalloids. Crystalloids are inexpensive and readily available solutions. Lactated Ringer's solution and 0.9% normal saline are isotonic electrolyte solutions that are used initially in order to expand intravascular volume. These solutions move freely from the intravascular space into the tissues; therefore, 3 ml of crystalloid solution is used to replace each 1 ml of blood loss (Advanced Trauma Life Support for Physicians, 1993). Lactated Ringer's solution closely resembles plasma, rarely causes side effects, and may be the only fluid replacement required if the blood loss is less than 1500 ml (Advanced Trauma Life Support for Physicians, 1993). Although 0.9% normal saline is an isotonic solution, its side effects include hypernatremia, hypokalemia, and metabolic acidosis. Solutions of 5% dextrose in water and 0.45% normal saline solutions are hypotonic and should be used only temporarily because they rapidly leave the intravascular space, causing interstitial and intracellular edema.

If large volumes of crystalloids are the only parenteral fluids infused, the patient is at risk for developing hemodilution of red blood cells and plasma proteins. Hemodilution of red blood cells impairs delivery of oxygen to the cells if the hematocrit value is decreased to such an extent that the cardiac output cannot increase enough to compensate. Hemodilution of plasma proteins decreases the colloidal osmotic pressure, a phenomenon that places the patient at risk for pulmonary edema.

Colloids. Colloids contain proteins that increase osmotic pressure. Osmotic pressure holds and attracts fluid into blood vessels, thereby expanding plasma volume. Because colloids remain in the intravascular space longer than crystalloids, smaller volumes of colloids are given.

Albumin and Plasmanate are naturally occurring colloid solutions that are given when the volume loss is caused by a loss of plasma rather than blood, such as occurs in burns, peritonitis, and bowel obstruction. Typing and cross-matching of albumin and Plasmanate are not required. Pulmonary edema may occur as a complication of colloid administration because of increased pulmonary capillary permeability seen in some stages of shock, or because of increased capillary hydrostatic pressure in the pulmonary vasculature created by rapid plasma expansion.

Dextran is a synthetic colloid used as a plasma expander. Dextran solutions contain glucose polymers that draw water into the vascular space. Low-molecular-weight dextran (dextran 40, Rheomacrodex) has a duration of 12 hours. Its use is contraindicated in hemorrhagic shock because it causes a decrease in platelet adhesiveness and consequently increases bleeding from wounds. High-molecular-weight dextran (dextran 70, Macrodex) is effective for 24 hours, but it increases platelet aggregation and interferes with blood typing and cross-matching; therefore, these assessments should be performed before dextran 70 is infused. No more than 1 L of dextran should be given in a 24-hour period. Additional complications associated with this plasma expander include allergic reactions and renal damage.

Hetastarch (Hespan) is a synthetic colloid that acts as a plasma expander but carries less risk for the development of pulmonary edema. Compared with dextran, hetastarch has no apparent effect on renal function and is less likely to cause allergic reactions. Side effects of hetastarch include altered prothrombin time and partial thromboplastin time and the potential for circulatory overload. No more than 1 L should be given in a 24-hour period.

Blood and Blood Products. Whole blood, packed red blood cells, washed red blood cells, fresh frozen plasma, and platelets are given for the treatment of major blood loss. Typing and cross-matching are performed for these products in order to identify the patient's blood type (A, B, AB, O), to determine the presence of the Rh factor, and to ensure compatibility with the donor blood in order to prevent transfusion reactions. In extreme emergencies, the patient may be transfused with O negative blood, which is considered to be the universal donor.

Transfusions require an IV access with at least a 20-gauge, and preferably an 18-gauge or larger, catheter (a 22- or 23-gauge needle or catheter may be used in neonates, children, or adults with small veins). The use of a Y-set allows the concurrent administration of blood with a 0.9% normal saline solution; it also permits the transfusion to be stopped and the vein kept open. Additionally, 50 to 100 ml of 0.9% normal saline solution may be injected directly into the unit of blood in order to decrease the viscosity and facilitate a more rapid infusion rate. Solutions other than 0.9% normal saline should not be infused into blood because they cause red blood cells to clump, swell, and burst. In addition, IV medications should never be infused in the same port with blood. Transfusions are administered with a blood filter, which traps debris and tiny clots found in blood. Hospital protocols are followed for obtaining baseline vital signs before the transfusion, and vital signs and assessments are repeated during the transfusion. Before any transfusion is begun, hospital policy is followed to ensure accurate administration (Table 8–13). Frequent assessment of the patient receiving a blood transfusion is necessary in order to identify adverse reactions (Table 8–14) (Dressler, 1993; Kotter and Osguthorpe, 1995). In the event of a reaction, the transfusion is stopped, the transfusion tubing is disconnected from the IV access site, and the vein is kept open with an IV of 0.9% normal saline solution. The patient is assessed, and the physician and the laboratory are notified. All transfusion equipment (bag, tubing, solutions) and any blood or urine specimens obtained are sent to the laboratory

---

Table 8–13. PROCEDURE FOR CHECKING BLOOD TRANSFUSIONS

Usually the blood product must be double checked (generally by two nurses) for the following:

1. The blood product matches the order on the patient's chart.
2. The name and the donor unit identification number on the transfusion form matches that on the patient's wristband/blood bracelet (if the patient can respond, ask the patient his or her name).
3. The ABO group, Rh type, and donor unit identification number on the transfusion form matches those on the donor unit with its compatibility tag and blood bag label.
4. The expiration date on the blood bag has not passed.
5. The blood product has no clots, bubbling, or purplish tinge, which indicates bacterial contamination.

Table 8–14. ADVERSE REACTIONS TO BLOOD TRANSFUSIONS

Type	Signs and Symptoms
Circulatory overload	Pulmonary edema, dyspnea, crackles, hypertension, dysrhythmias, dry cough, cyanosis, distended neck veins, tightness in chest
Hemolysis	Fever, chills, shock, disseminated intravascular coagulation, chest pain, dyspnea, low back pain, headache, pain at intravenous access and along vein, headache, nausea, vomiting
Allergy	Urticaria, flushing, pruritis, wheezing, laryngeal edema, anaphylaxis
Febrile hypothermia	Fever, chills, headache, flushing chills, low body temperature, ventricular dysrhythmias, possible cardiac arrest
Hyperkalemia	Peaked T waves, bradycardia, cardiac arrest, muscular weakness, flaccid paralysis, paresthesia, nausea, diarrhea
Hypocalcemia (citrate intoxication)	Tingling in fingers, tetany, muscle cramps, carpopedal spasms, hyperactive reflexes, convulsions, laryngeal spasms, respiratory arrest
Air emboli	Acute dyspnea, chest pain, shock, respiratory/cardiac arrest
Bacteria	Fever, hypotension, chills, shock

according to hospital policy. The events of the reaction, the interventions used, and the patient's response to treatment are documented.

Blood and blood products are given until the hematocrit value returns to 30% or higher (Suhl, 1993). The transfusion administration time varies with the particular blood product used and the individual patient circumstances. Documentation of the transfusion includes the blood product administered, the baseline vital signs, the time the transfusion was started and completed, the volume of blood and fluid administered, the results of assessment of the patient during the transfusion, and any nursing actions taken.

Whole blood is indicated for the treatment of both rapid-bleeding and slow-bleeding conditions. It restores blood volume and oxygen-carrying capacity; however, side effects include volume overload. Acidosis, hyperkalemia, and coagulation problems are associated with transfusions of banked blood more than 24 hours old. Typing and cross-matching of whole blood are required.

Packed red blood cells increase the blood volume and oxygen-carrying capacity without causing the problems of volume overload associated with the ad-

ministration of whole blood. One unit of packed red blood cells increases the hematocrit value by about 3% and the hemoglobin value by 1 g/dl (Orsi, 1993). Typing and cross-matching of packed red blood cells are required. Because red blood cells tend to aggregate because of the fibrinogen coating, washed red blood cells may be given in order to decrease capillary sludging.

Fresh frozen plasma is administered in order to replace all clotting factors except platelets. When massive transfusions are infused, fresh frozen plasma is given rapidly in order to restore coagulation factors. One unit of fresh frozen plasma is given for every 4 to 5 units of blood transfused. Typing and cross-matching of fresh frozen plasma are required.

Platelets are given rapidly in order to help control bleeding caused by low platelet counts (usually < 50,000). Typing of platelets, but not cross-matching, is required.

PHARMACOLOGICAL THERAPY

Pharmacological management of shock is based on the manipulation of four variables: contractility, preload, afterload, and heart rate (Burns, 1990). No drugs magically restore cellular nutrition, but agents are available that assist in the manipulation of the four circulatory variables, thereby making nutrients available to the cells. A list of commonly used medications is found in Table 8–15 (see Chapter 7). Hemodynamic monitoring is commonly used to assess the effectiveness of medications.

Drugs That Affect Contractility

Positive inotropic agents, which increase the contractile force of the heart, are used in the management of cardiogenic and distributive shock (Rice, 1991c). As contractility increases, two things occur: (1) ventricular emptying increases, and filling pressures of the heart decrease, and (2) improved stroke volume increases cardiac output, which in turn increases blood pressure. The increase in blood pressure improves tissue perfusion.

Positive inotropic agents increase myocardial oxygen demand, which increases the workload of the heart. Therefore, the agents must be used cautiously in patients with ischemic heart disease and in those with cardiogenic shock.

Negative inotropic agents, such as propranolol and metoprolol, are not used to treat shock but are discussed here because of the widespread use of these agents in the treatment of angina, hypertension, and dysrhythmias and their effect on the patient in shock. Negative inotropes work primarily by blocking the

---

Table 8–15. PHARMACOLOGICAL MANAGEMENT OF SHOCK

Commonly used positive inotropic agents
  Dopamine (in mid-range doses: 5–10μg/kg/min)
  Dobutamine
  Amrinone
  Norepinephrine
  Epinephrine
  Isoproterenol
  Digoxin

Commonly used drugs to reduce preload
  Diuretics—furosemide
  Nitroprusside
  Nitrates
  Morphine sulfate

Commonly used agents to increase afterload
  Dopamine (in high doses: 10–20 μg/kg/min)
  Norepinephrine
  Phenylephrine
  Metaraminol

Commonly used agents to decrease afterload
  Amrinone
  Nitroprusside
  Hydralazine
  Captopril
  Nifedipine

Commonly used positive chronotropic agents
  Atropine
  Isoproterenol

Commonly used negative chronotropic agents
  Verapamil
  Propranolol
  Adenosine
  Digitalis

Commonly used antiarrhythmic agents
  Lidocaine
  Procainamide
  Bretylium

---

effects of the beta branch of the sympathetic nervous system, causing a decrease in cardiac output. The nurse must know the effects of these medications because a patient who is taking them has an altered ability to respond to the stress of shock and may not exhibit typical signs and symptoms.

Drugs That Affect Preload

Treatment aimed at increasing preload is instituted for the treatment of hypovolemic and distributive shock. The primary treatment to increase preload is the administration of fluids. Vasopressors, such as epinephrine and norepinephrine, are also used to increase preload. These drugs cause vasoconstriction and increase the venous return to the heart. Vasopressors are used in the treatment of distributive shock. These drugs should be used with caution in patients with hypovolemic shock; such patients need volume replacement.

In patients in cardiogenic shock, drugs are administered in order to reduce preload. Drugs such as nitroprusside are given in order to reduce the venous return to the heart. A serious side effect of these drugs is that they may reduce the preload to such an extent that the patient has an extreme loss of volume, thereby increasing hypoperfusion to the cells; the results may be seriously detrimental to the patient.

Drugs That Affect Afterload

Afterload is the force the heart must overcome in order to pump effectively. Afterload is low in distributive shock. In this situation, drugs such as epinephrine are used to increase vascular tone, improve venous return, and consequently increase cardiac output. As with other agents, a negative side to drugs that increase afterload exists. Although the individual needs an increase in vascular resistance, this increase can put too much workload on the heart, causing an increase in the myocardial oxygen demand. Accurate measurement of systemic vascular resistance and pulmonary vascular resistance via a pulmonary artery catheter assists in assessment.

In cardiogenic shock, drugs are given in order to reduce afterload. Increased afterload can cause an already ischemic heart to suffer more insult. Nitroprusside is a commonly used afterload-reducing agent.

Drugs That Alter Heart Rate

Heart rate is the fourth variable that can be altered in the treatment of shock. Extremes in heart rate and dysrhythmias result in decreased cardiac output, which can be deleterious to the patient in shock. Chronotropic drugs and antiarrhythmic drugs are given as indicated.

OTHER PHARMACOLOGIC THERAPY

Some additional drugs are useful in the treatment of the patient in shock. Oxygen is administered in order to elevate the arterial oxygen tension and to increase the arterial oxygen content of the blood, thereby improving tissue oxygenation (Cummins, 1994). Oxygen is administered by methods ranging from nasal cannulation to mechanical ventilation, depending on the patient's condition.

Antibiotics are used in the treatment of septic shock. The antibiotic ordered is determined by culture and sensitivity tests. If the source of infection cannot be identified, broad-spectrum therapy is instituted in order to eradicate organisms commonly encountered (Bongard, 1994).

Steroids have had a controversial place in the treatment of shock, and current evidence provides no support for the use of corticosteroids in the treatment of shock (O'Rourke and McCall, 1994). The only indication for their use is shock associated with acute adrenal insufficiency (Tierney, 1995; Bongard, 1994).

Sodium bicarbonate is sometimes given for the treatment of metabolic acidosis associated with the lactic acid production that occurs in shock. Sodium bicarbonate combines with hydrogen ions to form water and carbon dioxide in order to buffer metabolic acidosis. Sodium bicarbonate is administered cautiously because the carbon dioxide produced crosses rapidly into the cells and may cause a paradoxical worsening of intracellular hypercarbia and acidosis (Cummins, 1994). Other methods for treating acidosis, such as increasing the ventilatory rate, are used before sodium bicarbonate is given. Arterial blood gas analysis is used to guide treatment.

Pharmacological treatment of shock includes a wide range of agents. The major drugs, actions, dosages, side effects, and nursing implications are found on Table 8–16.

MECHANICAL MANAGEMENT OF SHOCK

The management of shock includes the use of mechanical devices that aid in the restoration of perfusion to the cells. The mechanical devices are the intra-aortic balloon pump (IABP), the ventricular assist device (VAD), and the pneumatic antishock garment (PASG).

Intra-aortic Balloon Pump

A common method for mechanically assisting the heart is the use of counterpulsation via the IABP (Suhl, 1993; O'Rourke and McCall, 1994). This device is most often used in the treatment of cardiogenic shock. It is more effective if it is inserted early in the course of treatment.

The IABP is a dual-chambered balloon that is inserted into the descending thoracic aorta via the femoral artery (O'Rourke and McCall, 1994). The tip of the balloon is positioned just distal to the left subclavian artery (Fig. 8–5). The IABP may be inserted by use of fluoroscopy at the patient's bedside, and placement is verified via chest x-ray study.

The IABP assists the patient in shock in several ways: it improves the coronary artery perfusion, it reduces afterload, and it improves perfusion to vital organs. The balloon is inflated mechanically with either carbon dioxide or helium. Inflation and deflation are automatically timed with the cardiac cycle. The IABP inflates during diastole and deflates before systole. The inflation cycle displaces an amount of blood and forces it backward and forward simultaneously. The backward flow increases perfusion to the coronary arteries, and the forward flow increases perfusion to vital organs (Lynn-McHale and McGrory, 1993).

The balloon pump also assists the heart during systole. The balloon deflates just before contraction. This sudden deflation reduces the pressure in the aorta. The workload of the heart is decreased, resulting in reduced myocardial oxygen demand (Lynn-McHale and McGrory, 1993).

Despite its usefulness, the IABP has its limitations. Its use requires a high degree of nursing skill because of the complexity of the equipment and need for frequent monitoring. Limb ischemia and embolic phenomena are potential complications that must be assessed. Other complications include dissection of the aorta, infection, ineffective pumping, leakage of gas, and technical problems. Use of the IABP is contraindicated in patients with aortic insufficiency and thoracic and abdominal aneurysms (Lynn-McHale and McGrory, 1993).

The IABP is used concurrently with definitive measures, such as drugs. Long-term use can result in patients' becoming pump dependent. Weaning is performed by gradually decreasing the pump to cardiac cycle ratio from 1:1, in which the IABP supports every heartbeat, to 1:3 or 1:4, in which the IABP supports every third or fourth beat.

Ventricular Assist Device

Ventricular assist devices are inserted in order to assume cardiac pumping function. They are used to temporarily support a failing ventricle that has not responded to IABP and pharmacological therapy (Ley, 1993). Ventricular assist devices are used to treat cardiogenic shock by allowing the ventricle to recover. They can be used to support the left ventricle, the right ventricle, or both ventricles.

Ventricular assist devices vary in design and technology. In general, they consist of an external pump, which diverts blood from the failing ventricle or ventricles and pumps it back into the aorta (left ventricular assist device [LVAD]), the pulmonary artery (right ventricular assist device [RVAD]), or both great vessels [Bi-VAD] (Ley, 1993). The use of ventricular assist devices requires extensive training and advanced nursing care. These devices are not typically available in community hospitals.

Pneumatic Antishock Garment

The pneumatic antishock garment is another device that may be used for circulatory assistance in

Table 8–16. DRUGS COMMONLY USED IN SHOCK

Drug	Action	Use	Dosage/Route	Standard Mix	Side Effects	Nursing Implications
Dopamine	Renal vasodilator	Increases renal perfusion	1–2 µg/kg/min IV drip	400 mg/250 ml 5% D/W	Increased heart rate, increased dysrhythmias, increased myocardial oxygen consumption, nausea/vomiting	Do not administer with alkaline solutions. Monitor for myocardial ischemia. Monitor BP at least every 15 min. If IV infiltrates, may cause extravasation. Administer via volumetric pump. Should be tapered gradually. Administer via central catheter if possible. Low BP associated with hypovolemia should be treated with aggressive fluid resuscitation prior to drug administration.
	Positive inotropic	Increases myocardial contractility	2–10 µg/kg/min IV drip			
	Vasopressor	Increases BP when not caused by hypovolemia	10–20 µg/kg/min IV drip			
Dobutamine	Positive inotropic	Increases BP in low cardiac output states	2–20 µg/kg/min IV drip	500–1000 mg/250 ml 5% D/W or NS	Increased heart rate, increased dysrhythmias, increased myocardial oxygen consumption, headache, tremors, nausea	Monitor for myocardial ischemia. Monitor BP at least every 15 min. Administer via volumetric pump. Should be tapered gradually. Administer via central catheter, if possible.
Norepinephrine	Vasopressor, some positive inotropic effects	Increases BP; refractory to other drugs	2–12 µg/min IV drip	4 mg/250–1000 ml 5% D/W or NS	Increased myocardial oxygen consumption, increased dysrhythmias, severe vasoconstriction	Monitor for myocardial ischemia. Monitor BP at least every 15 min. Administer via volumetric pump. Should be tapered gradually. Administer via central catheter, if possible. If IV infiltrates, may cause extravasation.
Nitroglycerin	Venodilator	Reduces preload, pump failure	Start at 5 µg/min and titrate to effect; 50–200 µg/min is range for most patients. An IV bolus dose of 12.5–25 µg may be given prior to infusion	50–100 mg/250 ml 5% D/W	Headache, hypotension, bradycardia	Monitor BP at least every 15 min. Administer via volumetric pump. Should be tapered gradually. Administer via central catheter, if possible.
Nitroprusside	Vasodilator	Reduces preload and afterload	0.5–10 µg/kg/min IV drip	50 mg/250 ml 5% D/W or NS	Myocardial ischemia, hypotension, nausea	Monitor for myocardial ischemia. May cause thiocyanate intoxication in large dosages or prolonged administration. Monitor BP at least every 15 min. Administer via volumetric pump. Should be tapered gradually. Administer via central catheter, if possible.

BP = blood pressure; 5% D/W = 5% dextrose in water; NS = normal saline.

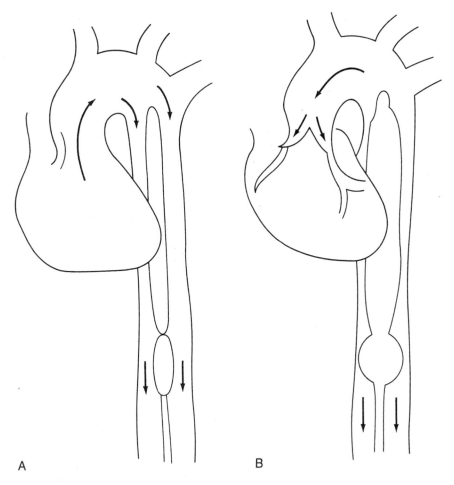

Figure 8–5. Intra-aortic balloon pump. The balloon is deflated during systole *(A)* and inflated during diastole *(B)*.

A

B

shock (Fig. 8–6). Other names for the PASG include military antishock trousers, external counter pressure devices, and G suits. The PASG raises the mean arterial pressure by increasing the peripheral vascular resistance in the lower portion of the body. The PASG also provides a splinting action and decreases blood flow to torn vessels under the garment (Hankins and Freeman, 1996). Thus, it is particularly useful in the treatment of hypovolemic shock associated with traumatic injury. The device is used only as a temporary measure until definitive treatment is given because it can compromise blood flow to the lower half of the body. Although the PASG is still used, a recent study recommends that the device no longer be routinely used for the treatment of shock (Chang et al., 1995).

An absolute contraindication for using the PASG is pulmonary edema. Relative contraindications include pregnancy, the presence of impaled objects, evisceration of the abdomen, and thoracic and diaphragmatic injury (Hankins and Freeman, 1996).

The PASG consists of an inflatable bladder that maintains a high internal pressure when it is inflated. Most models have three compartments that can be inflated individually in order to compress the lower extremities and the abdomen. The suit is inflated with a foot pump and has pop-off valves that assist in regulating the internal pressure.

The PASG is usually instituted in emergency situations in the field or the emergency department and may be removed before the patient's admission to the critical care unit. However, it is important for the nurse to be aware that the garment has been used. The nurse closely monitors the vascular status of the lower extremities and assesses for the reappearance of shock symptoms.

If the patient is admitted to the critical care unit with a PASG in place, the nurse monitors the circulatory status of the patient and assists with the removal of the device when the patient stabilizes. The PASG is removed by a gradual reduction in the pressure in the compartments. The abdominal section is deflated first in order to allow the gradual redistribution of blood

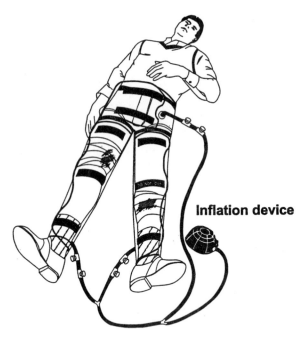

Inflation device

Figure 8–6. Pneumatic antishock garment with abdominal and leg compartments and foot pump.

volume and to avoid the trapping of large volumes of blood in the lower extremities. The vital signs of the patient are closely monitored. Removal of the PASG from a patient who is not fully stabilized may cause a sudden relapse.

Nursing Interventions

The nurse provides care to support tissue perfusion of the patient in shock until definitive care is underway. Supportive care is aimed at maintenance of organ function (see Nursing Care Plan).

MAINTENANCE OF A PATENT AIRWAY

Airway maintenance is the top priority. The airway is maintained by proper head position, use of oral or nasopharyngeal airways, or intubation, depending on the patient's condition (see Chapter 6). Supplemental oxygen is provided. Secretion removal is facilitated by suctioning and possibly chest physiotherapy.

PATIENT POSITIONING

Proper positioning can assist in improving venous return. Traditionally, the patient in shock has been placed in the Trendelenburg position (head down and feet up). This position was thought to increase the venous return to the heart and to increase the cardiac

output. However, the Trendelenburg position can actually worsen the shock state. By raising the legs, diaphragmatic movement is restricted, which may impair ventilation. A reflex inhibition of the baroreceptors may occur by the dramatic increase in venous return caused by the elevation of the legs. This pseudoincrease in blood volume fools the baroreceptors that blood volume is adequate, which causes the blood pressure to decrease even more.

The best position for the patient in shock is one that elevates the lower extremities slightly. This elevation increases venous return without compromising the ventilatory status.

MAINTENANCE OF BODY TEMPERATURE

Care is directed toward maintaining normal body temperature. The patient's temperature is checked frequently, and he or she is covered with light blankets. Patients need to be kept warm and comfortable and yet not be overly warmed: excessive warmth increases the metabolic needs and places a larger demand on an already stressed cardiovascular system. The nurse observes for hypothermia when fluids are infused rapidly and considers warming the fluids before their administration.

MAINTENANCE OF SKIN INTEGRITY

Nursing actions for the maintenance of skin integrity—the first line of defense—are important. Decreased peripheral perfusion seen in shock can precipitate injury to this important defense mechanism. Meticulous skin care is required in order to ensure that no breaks occur in the patient's skin. The patient is turned at frequent intervals, and lotion is applied. Pressure-relieving devices, such as foam egg crates, air mattresses, and therapeutic beds, may be warranted, depending on the condition of the patient and his or her risk for skin breakdown.

PSYCHOLOGICAL SUPPORT

A section on supportive care would be remiss if it did not address the area of psychological support. Nursing interventions focus on identifying the impact of the illness on the patient and the family. Nursing interventions include providing information, such as specifics about the patient's status, the necessity for procedures, explanations of tests and test results, and an understanding of routines within the unit. Information is essential for the psychological well-being of the patient and the family and may help to give them a sense of understanding and control of the situation. Additional supportive actions include providing time, space, and privacy for family discussions and allowing ventilation, encouragement, and acceptance.

NURSING CARE PLAN FOR THE PATIENT WITH HYPOVOLEMIC SHOCK		
Nursing Diagnosis	Patient Outcomes	Nursing Interventions
Altered tissue perfusion related to decreased blood volume.	Tissue perfusion will be optimized as evidenced by: Balanced fluid intake and output. Controlled bleeding or fluid loss. Normal serum and urine laboratory values and arterial blood gas results. Normal vital signs. Normal mentation and cognition for patient. Normal elimination pattern. Normal mobility for patient. Managed pain. Absence of complication (ARDS, e.g., acute respiratory distress syndrome, renal and hepatic failure, disseminated intravascular coagulation, multiple organ dysfunction).	Assess vital signs, skin color and temperature, capillary refill, level of consciousness/ neurological status. Assess hemodynamic values if pulmonary artery catheter is inserted. Assess cardiac rhythm. Assess fluid balance and intake and output every hour. Obtain daily weights. Assess amount and type of drainage (e.g., chest tube, nasogastric, dressings). Perform abdominal girth measurements. Assess bowel sounds. Assess serial serum and urine values. Assess pain levels. Establish or maintain patent airway. Administer oxygen. Apply pressure, use pneumatic antishock device, or surgical intervention for the control of bleeding. Establish intravenous access, use large-gauge catheters (No. 14 or 16), peripherally, obtain central venous access, if possible. Obtain type and cross-match for blood replacement. Administer fluids as ordered (e.g., crystalloids, colloids, blood, plasma expanders); consider warming fluids before infusing. Insert urinary catheter. Administer vasoactive agents as prescribed. Administer analgesics and implement comfort measures; evaluate patient's response. Administer antibiotics and/or tetanus prophylactically as indicated. Position in modified Trendelenburg's position. Provide wound care as indicated. Collaborate with dietitian about patient's nutritional needs. Provide psychological support for patient, family, and others. Evaluate patient's response to fluid challengers and fluid and blood product administration via changes in vital signs, level of consciousness, urinary output, hemodynamic values, and serum and urine laboratory values. Evaluate wound healing. Assess patient for the development of complications.

Patient Outcomes

The expected outcome is that the patient will have improved tissue perfusion (see Table 8–12). Specific patient outcomes include alertness and orientation, normotension, warmth, dry skin, adequate urine output, hemodynamic and laboratory values within normal limits, absence of infection, and intact skin. The patient should be relaxed and should be resting quietly.

Complications

Complications of shock are related to the metabolic and tissue changes that result. If the normal compensatory mechanisms are not supported by effective therapeutic interventions, the pathological consequences perpetuate a vicious cycle of shock. The cycle is initiated by ischemia to the cells. Ischemia results in anaerobic metabolism, which leads to an accumulation of lactic acid and metabolic acidosis. This acidosis leads to irreversible changes in the cells. Many of these complications are discussed in greater depth in other chapters in this text.

CENTRAL NERVOUS SYSTEM

The brain suffers as a result of anaerobic metabolism. As lactate levels begin to increase and glucose consumption decreases, the availability of energy for cells in the central nervous system declines. The cells begin to retain sodium and water, and cerebral edema ensues. This phenomenon initiates a vicious cycle in which further compromise of the tissues occurs. Neurological deficits are the end result of severe and prolonged episodes of shock.

CARDIOVASCULAR SYSTEM

The major mechanisms for failure of the heart in shock include (1) a decrease in cardiac output, (2) a decrease in coronary blood flow, and (3) a marked decrease in myocardial contractility. The factors that contribute to these processes in shock are the decreased oxygen availability and the production of myocardial depressant factors (Suhl, 1993). The end result is heart failure.

Alterations in the clotting system are a common complication of shock. The most common occurrence is disseminated intravascular coagulation. This results in coagulation in the microcirculation and a paradoxical hemorrhage. In general, disseminated intravascular coagulation is a late occurrence in the shock syndrome.

The white blood cells are also affected by the shock syndrome. Leukopenia is a common occurrence that predisposes the patient to infections.

RESPIRATORY SYSTEM

The major respiratory complication is acute respiratory distress syndrome (Suhl, 1993). Acute respiratory distress syndrome occurs secondary to a reduced pulmonary blood flow and an increased pulmonary vascular resistance. Pulmonary capillary permeability increases, resulting in noncardiogenic pulmonary edema. Surfactant production is decreased resulting in decreased pulmonary compliance and hypoxemia that is refractory to oxygen therapy.

RENAL SYSTEM

Acute renal failure is a common complication of shock. Decreased renal perfusion leads to acute tubular necrosis.

HEPATIC SYSTEM

Decreased perfusion to the hepatic cells results in a decreased ability to produce energy, serum proteins, and clotting factors and in a decreased ability to detoxify circulating toxins (Suhl, 1993). Consequences include coagulopathy, poor wound healing, and inability to detoxify drugs.

GASTROINTESTINAL SYSTEM

Ischemia to the intestines causes two distinct problems. Reduction in blood supply affects the protective mechanism of the gastrointestinal tract, which leads to mucosal damage and ulceration of the intestines. Ischemia also increases the likelihood of bacteria and toxins' crossing the intestinal barrier and entering the circulation, leading to sepsis (Suhl, 1993).

MULTIPLE ORGAN DYSFUNCTION SYNDROME

Multiple organ dysfunction syndrome is a complication of shock or severe injury. It is a process of progressive physiological failure of several interdependent organ systems. Multiple organ dysfunction syndrome may develop through a primary insult, such as a direct injury to an organ system, or as a consequence of the systemic inflammatory response syndrome (ACCP/SCCM Conference Committee, 1992). Sepsis is a contributing factor to the development of multiple organ dysfunction syndrome.

Summary

The risk for shock is a common threat for all patients. Its causes are many, its treatment varied and complex. Prevention is the primary goal; it is accomplished through the identification of high-risk patient conditions and early interventions. Successful management relies on accurate nursing assessments, data analysis, implementation of definitive interventions, and evaluation of patient response to treatment. Shock is a crisis for the patient, family, nurse, and health care team. A collaborative approach of clinical expertise combined with caring assists the patient in reaching a positive outcome from shock.

RESEARCH APPLICATION

Article Reference

Bickell, W., Wall, M., Pepe, P., Martin, R., Ginger, V., Allen, M., et al. (1994). Immediate versus delayed fluid resuscitation for hypotensive patients with penetrating torso injuries. *New England Journal of Medicine, 331*(17), 1105–1109.

Review of Study Methods and Findings

The purpose of this prospective study was to determine the effects of delaying fluid resuscitation until the time of operative intervention in hypotensive patients with injuries to the torso. It was hypothesized that survival of hypotensive patients with penetrating injuries to the torso would be improved if fluid resuscitation was restricted until the time of operative intervention.

Subjects ($n=598$) had sustained gunshot or stab wounds to the torso and had a systolic blood pressure of less than 90 mm Hg at the time of initial assessment by paramedics. Patients injured on even-numbered days were assigned to the immediate fluid resuscitation group. Those injured on odd-numbered days were assigned to the delayed fluid resuscitation group. Other treatment protocols were identical for the groups, and demographic and clinical characteristics were well matched for the two groups.

Subjects in the immediate resuscitation group ($n=309$) were treated with intravascular fluid administration before surgical intervention in both prehospital and trauma center settings. The delayed resuscitation group ($n=289$) had intravascular access established but did not receive fluid resuscitation until surgery. Surgical procedures included thoracotomy, laparotomy, and neck and/or groin exploration.

After the patient arrived in the operating room, intravenous crystalloids and packed red blood cells were given as needed, regardless of the study group assignment, to maintain a systolic blood pressure of 100 mm Hg, a hematocrit value of greater than or equal to 25%, and a urinary output of greater than or equal to 50 ml/h.

During the prehospital phase, the immediate resuscitation group received an average of 870 ml of isotonic solution, compared with 92 ml in the delayed resuscitation group. Volumes administered in the trauma center were 1608 ml and 283 ml, respectively. Seventy patients (12%) died before reaching the operating room. Surgery was performed on 528 subjects: 87% from the immediate resuscitation group and 90% from the delayed resuscitation group. The overall survival rate (70%) was significantly greater ($P = .04$) in the delayed resuscitation group than in the immediate resuscitation group (62%). Based on these findings, the authors concluded that their hypothesis was supported.

Critique

The authors clarified that the value of fluid resuscitation was not being debated, but rather the volume, timing, and extent of that resuscitation for certain patient populations. The strengths of the study were that it was prospective and randomized, the sample size was adequate for the investigation, the experimental groups were well matched, the protocols were well defined and followed, and the time intervals between injury and operative intervention were short. The weaknesses of the study were that the mortality rate was high (34%), but the factors contributing to mortality were not clarified. For example, was mortality related to the particular organ injured, the fact that injuries were multiple, the severity of injury or injuries, the presence of coagulation disorders, the development of complications, or even the delay in fluid resuscitation itself?

Implications of the Study for Nursing Practice

These results challenge the traditional approach of sustaining tissue perfusion and vital organ function through aggressive and universal preoperative intravenous fluid for the treatment of trauma patients with hypotension due to hemorrhage. The ethical and legal implications of delaying fluid in a hypotensive bleeding patient need to be examined. Further controlled investigations need to be conducted before the practice of withholding fluid resuscitation in patients with extensive bleeding becomes common practice, particularly for the treatment of all age groups or for the treatment of hypotension due to blunt injury or in settings where time from injury to surgery may be prolonged.

CRITICAL THINKING QUESTIONS

1. Several people are admitted to the critical care unit, including (1) a 79-year-old man with a small inferior infarct and no prior cardiac history, (2) a 47-year-old man who is admitted after surgery for an open reduction and fixation of a fractured femur, (3) a 17-year-old male with cervical spine injury after a diving accident, and (4) a 23-year-old woman with sternal bruising and occasional premature ventricular contractions after a motor vehicle accident.

    Discuss what additional assessment information is needed in order to determine which of these patients have the potential to develop shock.

2. Explain the pathophysiology of the *EARLY* clinical manifestations of shock.

3. A patient has been admitted from the emergency department after a motorcycle accident in which he sustained blunt abdominal trauma. IV access had been established in the internal jugular and left antecubital veins, and lactated Ringer's solution is being infused. The results of initial CT of the abdomen were negative. On admission to the critical care unit, you review the hematologic profile for the following results:
    a. Hemoglobin, 9.1 g/dl
    b. Hematocrit, 31.1%
    c. Platelets, 274,000/mm^3
    d. Red blood cells, 2.9 million/µL
    e. White blood cells, 9,800/mm^3
    f. Prothrombin time, 15 seconds
    g. Activated partial thromboplastin time, 47 seconds

    Explain the rationale for the alterations in these values.

4. Describe factors in the critically ill patient that increase susceptibility to the development of systemic inflammatory response, bacteremia, and sepsis, and describe how these can be prevented.

5. Discuss priorities for care of the patient in shock in order to achieve desirable outcomes.

REFERENCES

American College of Surgeons. (1993). *Advanced trauma life support for physicians.* Chicago: Author.

Alspach, J. (1991). *AACN core curriculum for critical-care nursing* (4th ed.). Philadelphia: W. B. Saunders Co.

Barone, E., & Snyder, A. B. (1991). Treatment strategies in shock: Use of oxygen transport measurements. *Heart and Lung, 20*(1), 81–85.

Bickell, W., Wall, M., Pepe, P., Martin, R., Ginger, V., Allen, M., et al. (1994). Immediate versus delayed fluid resuscitation for hypotensive patients with penetrating torso injuries. *New England Journal of Medicine, 331*(17), 1105–1109.

Bongard, F. (1994). Shock and resuscitation. In F. Bongard, & D. Sue (Eds.), *Critical care diagnosis and treatment* (pp. 14–36). Norwalk, CT: Appleton & Lange.

Broscious, S. (1991). Toxic shock syndrome and its potential complications. *Critical Care Nurse, 11*(4), 28–35.

Burns, K. (1990). Vasoactive drug therapy in shock. *Critical Care Nursing Clinics of North America, 2*(2), 167–178.

Chang, F., Harrison, P., Beech, R., & Helmer, S. (1995). PASG: Does it help in the management of traumatic shock? *Journal of Trauma, Injury, Infection, and Critical Care, 39*(3), 453–456.

American College of Chest Physicians/Society of Critical Care Medicine Consensus Conference Committee (1992). Definitions for sepsis and organ failure and guidelines for the use of innovative therapies in sepsis. *Critical Care Medicine, 20*(6), 864–874.

Cummins, R. (Ed.). (1994). *Textbook for advanced cardiac life support.* Dallas: American Heart Association.

Dressler, D. (1993). Hematologic physiology. In J. Clochesy, C. Breu, S. Cardin, E. Rudy, & A. Whittacker (Eds.), *Critical care nursing,* (pp. 1047–1071). Philadelphia: W. B. Saunders Co.

Emerson, R. (1995). Alterations in blood flow. In L. Copstead (Ed.), *Perspectives on pathophysiology.* (pp. 301–324). Philadelphia: W. B. Saunders Co.

Hankins, D., & Freeman, S. (1996). Prehospital devices. In J. Tintinalli, E. Ruiz, & R. Krome (Eds.), *Emergency medicine: A comprehensive study guide* (4th ed.) (pp. 4–7). New York: McGraw Hill.

Hazinski, M., Iberti, T., MacIntyre, N., Parker, M., Tribett, D., Prion, S., et al. (1993). Epidemiology, pathophysiology and clinical presentation of gram-negative sepsis. *American Journal of Critical Care, 2*(3), 224–235.

Ignatavicius, D. D., Workman, M. L., & Mishler, M. A. (Eds). (1995). *Medical-surgical nursing: A nursing process approach* (pp. 965–983). Philadelphia: W. B. Saunders Co.

Kotter, M., & Osguthorpe, S. (1995). Alterations in oxygen transport. In L. Copstead (Ed.), *Perspectives on pathophysiology* (pp. 250–285). Philadelphia: W. B. Saunders Co.

Ley, S. J. (1993). Myocardial depression after surgery: Pharmacologic and mechanical support. *AACN Clinical Issues in Critical Care Nursing, 4*(2), 293–308.

Lynn-McHale, D., & McGrory, J. (1993). Intraaortic balloon pump management. In R. Boggs, & M. Wooldridge-King (Eds.), *AACN procedure manual for critical care* (3rd ed.) (pp. 409–433). Philadelphia: W. B. Saunders Co.

McQuillan, K., & Wiles, C. (1994). Initial management of traumatic shock. In V. Cardona, P. Hurn, P. Mason, A. Scanlon-Schlipp, & S. Veise-Berry (Eds.), *Trauma nursing from resuscitation through rehabilitation* (pp. 151–178). Philadelphia: W. B. Saunders Co.

O'Rourke, R., & McCall, D. (1994). Hypotension and cardiogenic shock. In J. Stein (Ed.). *Internal medicine* (4th ed.) (pp. 131–143). St. Louis: C. V. Mosby Co.

Orsi, A. (1993). Hematologic management. In R. Boggs, & M. Wooldridge-King (Eds.), *AACN procedure manual for critical care* (pp. 691–717). Philadelphia: W. B. Saunders Co.

Parrillo, J. (1994). Shock. In K. Isselbacher, E. Braunwald, J. Wilson, J. Martin, A. Fauci, & D. Kasper (Eds.), *Principles of internal medicine* (pp. 187–193). New York: McGraw-Hill.

Perry, A., & Potter, P. (1983). *Shock: Comprehensive nursing management.* St. Louis: C. V. Mosby Co.

Polaski, A. L., & Tatro, S. E. (1996). *Luckman's core principles and practice of medical-surgical nursing* (pp. 1539–1562). Philadelphia: W. B. Saunders Co.

Rice, V. (1991a). Shock: A clinical syndrome: An update (part I). An overview of shock. *Critical Care Nurse, 11*(4), 20–27.

Rice, V. (1991b). Shock: A clinical syndrome: An update (part II). The stages of shock. *Critical Care Nurse, 11*(5), 74–82.

Rice, V. (1991c). Shock: A clinical syndrome: An update (part III). Therapeutic management. *Critical Care Nurse, 11*(6), 34–39.

Rice, V. (1991d). Shock: A clinical syndrome: An update (part IV). Nursing care of the shock patient. *Critical Care Nurse, 11*(7), 28–39.

Suhl, J. (1993). Patients with shock. In J. Clochesy, C. Breu, S. Cardin, E. Rudy, & A. Whittacker (Eds.), *Critical care nursing* (pp. 1258–1270). Philadelphia: W. B. Saunders Co.

Summers, G. (1995). Alterations in blood flow. In L. Copstead (Ed.), *Perspectives on pathophysiology* (pp. 1082–1099). Philadelphia: W. B. Saunders Co.

Tierney, L. (1995). Blood vessels and lymphatics. In L. Tierney, S. McPhee, & M. Papadakis (Eds.), *Medical diagnosis and treatment* (pp. 391–423). Norwalk, CT: Appleton & Lange.

Trunkey, D., Salber, P., & Mills, J. (1992). Shock. In C. Saunders, & M. Ho (Eds.). *Emergency diagnosis and treatment* (pp. 51–67). Norwalk, CT: Appleton & Lange.

RECOMMENDED READINGS

Brown, K. K. (1994). Septic shock: Stopping the deadly cascade. *American Journal of Nursing, 94*(9), 20–27.

Brown, K. K. (1994). Critical interventions in septic shock. *American Journal of Nursing, 94*(10), 22–26.

Goran, S. F. (1996). From counterpulsation to paralysis: A case presentation. *Critical Care Nurse, 16*(2), 54–57.

O'Neal, P. V. (1994). How to spot early signs of cardiogenic shock. *American Journal of Nursing, 94*(5), 36–41.

9

Cardiac Alterations

Marilyn L. Lamborn, Ph.D., R.N.
Marthe J. Moseley, M.S.N., R.N., CCRN

OBJECTIVES

- Contrast the pathological cause and effect mechanisms that produce acute cardiac disturbances.
- Discuss the nursing care responsibilities related to the cardiac patient.
- Compare and contrast pharmacological, operative, and electrical treatment modalities used in cardiac disease.

- Identify specific nursing interventions designed to prevent or minimize complications of cardiac patients.
- Develop a research-related care plan for the acutely ill cardiac patient.

Introduction

Care of the seriously ill patient with alterations in cardiac status includes those cardiac patients at risk whose outcome or prognosis is uncertain. The critical care nurse needs theoretical knowledge and practice-related understanding of the common cardiac diseases in order to have the sound clinical judgment necessary for making rapid and accurate decisions. The purpose of this chapter is to identify and explore some of the more common serious cardiac alterations that are likely to be encountered by the critical care nurse caring for patients with compromised cardiac status and to describe the nursing care that optimizes the patient's outcome.

Normal Structure and Function of the Heart

An essential component of effective nursing care is a comprehensive knowledge of the normal structure and function of the heart. The heart muscle is composed of cells that are connected to each other end to end as well as side to side, giving the shape and appearance of a lattice (Fig. 9–1). The myocardial fibers or myofibrils contract and expand lengthwise as well as widen and narrow in an accordion-type movement. The heart muscle is approximately the size of a person's closed fist and lies within the mediastinal space of the thoracic cavity between the lungs, directly under the lower half of the sternum, and above the diaphragm (Fig. 9–2) (Thibodeau, 1990). It is covered by the pericardium, which has an inner visceral layer and an outer parietal layer. Certain diseases can cause this covering to become inflamed and can subsequently diminish the effectiveness of the heart as a pump. A small amount of lubricating fluid exists between these layers. Some pathological conditions can increase the amount and the consistency of this fluid, and this can also affect the pumping ability of the heart (Canobbio, 1990). The heart muscle itself is composed of three layers: the outer layer, or epicardium; the middle, muscular layer, or myocardium; and the inner endothelial layer, or endocardium (Fig. 9–3) (Skov and Vaska, 1993). These layers are damaged or destroyed when a patient has a myocardial infarction (MI).

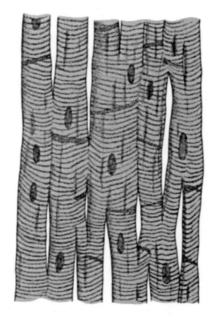

Figure 9–1. The ''syncytial,'' interconnecting nature of cardiac muscle. (From Guyton, A. C. (1986). *Textbook of medical physiology* (7th ed.). Philadelphia: W. B. Saunders Co.)

Functionally, the heart is divided into right-sided and left-sided pumps that are separated by a septum. The right side is generally considered to be a low-pressure system, whereas the left side is a high-pressure system. Each side has an atrium that receives blood and a ventricle that pumps it out. The right atrium receives deoxygenated blood from the body through the superior and inferior venae cavae. Blood travels by gravity from the atrium to the ventricles when the valves separating these chambers open. The right ventricle pumps the deoxygenated blood to the lungs through the pulmonary artery for oxygen and carbon dioxide exchange. The left atrium receives the newly oxygenated blood by way of the pulmonary veins from the lungs, and the left ventricle pumps the oxygenated blood through the aorta to the systemic circulation (Fig. 9–4) (Skov and Vaska, 1993; Vander et al., 1990).

The four cardiac valves maintain the unidirectional blood flow through the chambers of the heart. There are two types of valves: the atrioventricular (AV) valves, which separate the atria from the ventricles, and the semilunar valves, which separate the pulmonary artery from the right ventricle and the aorta from the left ventricle (Fig. 9–5). The AV valves include the tricuspid valve, which lies between the right atrium and the right ventricle, and the mitral valve, which is located between the left atrium and the

left ventricle. Each AV valve is anchored by chordae tendineae to the papillary muscles on its ventricular floor. The semilunar valves are the pulmonic valve, which lies between the right ventricle and the pulmonary artery, and the aortic valve, which is between the left ventricle and the aorta. These semilunar valves are not anchored by chordae tendineae. Instead, their closing is passive and is caused by differences in pressure between the chamber and the respective great vessel (Skov and Vaska, 1993).

HEART SOUNDS

The vibrations produced by vascular walls, flowing blood, heart muscle, and heart valves create sound waves known as heart sounds. Auscultating these sounds with a stethoscope over the heart provides valuable information about valve and cardiac functions (Fig. 9–6). Ventricular systole occurs when the pulmonic and aortic valves open to allow blood to be pumped to the lungs (right ventricle–pulmonic valve) and systemic circulation (left ventricle–aortic valve). Ventricular diastole occurs when the tricuspid and mitral valves open to allow the ventricles to fill with blood. (Skov and Vaska, 1993).

The first heart sound is known as S_1. This sound has been described as "lubb." It is caused by closure of the mitral and tricuspid valves. It is best heard at the apex (fifth intercostal space, left midclavicular line) of the heart and represents the beginning of ventricular systole.

The second heart sound is known as S_2. It has been described as "dubb" and is caused by closure of the aortic and pulmonic valves. It is best heard at the second intercostal space at the right or left sternal border and represents the beginning of ventricular diastole. The first and second heart sounds are best heard with the diaphragm of the stethoscope with the patient lying in the supine position.

A third heart sound, S_3, can be normal in a child, but it usually represents pathology in the adult. The sound may be produced at the time when the heart is already overfilled or poorly compliant. The S_3 sound can best be heard with the bell of the stethoscope at the fifth intercostal space, at the left midclavicular line. It occurs immediately after S_2. Together with S_1 and S_2, S_3 produces a sound like "lubb-dubb-a" or "ken-tuk'e." S_3 is heard in patients with congestive heart failure (CHF) or fluid overload. A fourth heart sound, S_4, is produced from atrial contraction that is more forceful than normal. Together with S_1 and S_2, S_4 produces a sound like "te-lubb-dubb" or "ten-ne'se." S_4 can be normal in the elderly, but is often heard after MI, when the atria contract more forcefully against ventricles distended with blood. In the severely failing

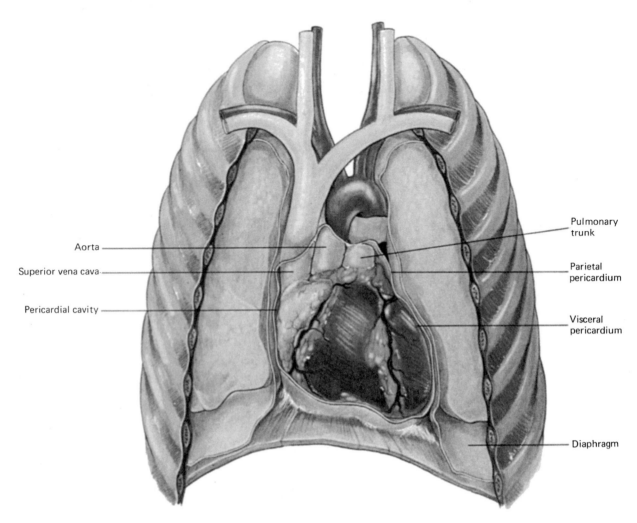

Figure 9–2. The heart lies in the mediastinum between the lungs. Its apex rests on the diaphragm. The heart and the roots of the great blood vessels are loosely enclosed by the pericardium. (From Solomon, E. P., & Phillips, G. A. (1987). *Understanding human anatomy and physiology.* Philadelphia: W. B. Saunders Co.)

heart, all four sounds (S_1, S_2, S_3, and S_4) may be heard, producing a "gallop" rhythm, so named because it sounds like the hoof beats of a galloping horse (Skov and Vaska, 1993). It can best be heard with the bell of the stethoscope at the fifth intercostal space, at the left midclavicular line.

HEART MURMUR

A heart murmur is a sound caused by a turbulence of blood flow through the valves of the heart. In children and adults, murmurs can also be heard when a septal defect is present. In adults, murmurs can be heard when a valve, usually aortic or mitral, is narrow, inflamed, stenosed, or incompetent, or when the valve leaflets fail to approximate (insufficiency). The pres-

ence of a new murmur warrants special attention, particularly in a patient with an acute MI. A papillary muscle may have ruptured, causing the valve to not approximate correctly, and can be indicative of severe damage and impending complications (e.g., CHF and pulmonary edema). A murmur is usually a rumbling, blowing, harsh, or musical sound. It is important to distinguish the sound, location, loudness, and intensity of a murmur and whether extra heart sounds are heard. This skill is developed from practice in listening to many different patients' hearts and in correlating the sounds heard with the patients' pathological conditions.

AUTONOMIC CONTROL

The autonomic nervous system exerts control over the cardiovascular system. The sympathetic ner-

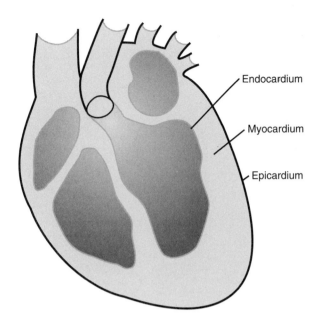

Figure 9–3. The three layers of the heart muscle.

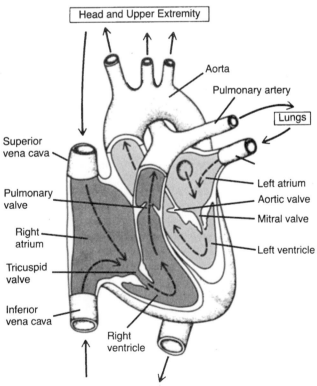

Figure 9–4. Structure of the heart and course of blood flow through the heart chambers. (From Guyton, A. C. (1986). *Textbook of medical physiology* (7th ed.). Philadelphia: W. B. Saunders Co.)

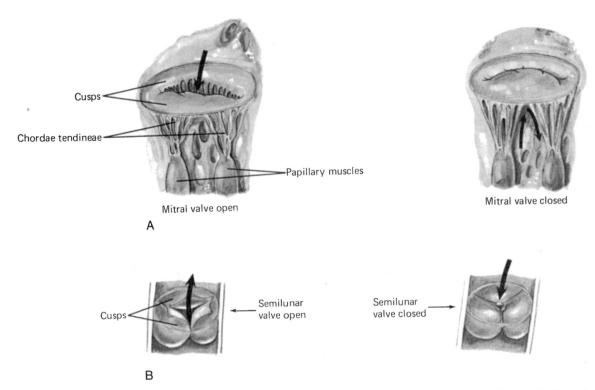

Mitral valve open

A

Mitral valve closed

Cusps

Chordae tendineae

Papillary muscles

Cusps

Semilunar valve open

Semilunar valve closed

B

Figure 9–5. How the valves of the heart work. (*A*), The mitral valve in the open and closed positions. (*B*), A semilunar valve in the open and closed positions. (From Solomon, E. P., & Phillips, G. A. (1987). *Understanding human anatomy and physiology.* Philadelphia: W. B. Saunders Co.)

vous system releases norepinephrine, which has two effects. Alpha-adrenergic effects cause arterial vasoconstriction. Beta-adrenergic effects increase sinus node discharge (positive chronotrope), increase the force of contraction (positive inotrope), and accelerate the AV conduction time (dromotrope).

The parasympathetic nervous system releases ace-

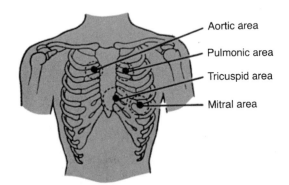

Figure 9–6. Chest areas from which each valve sound is best heard. (From Guyton, A. C. (1986). *Textbook of medical physiology* (7th ed.). Philadelphia: W. B. Saunders Co.)

Aortic area

Pulmonic area

Tricuspid area

Mitral area

tylcholine through stimulation of the vagus nerve. It causes a decrease in the sinus node discharge and slows AV conduction (Skov and Vaska, 1993; Vander et al., 1990).

In addition to this innervation, receptors help to control cardiovascular function. First are chemoreceptors, which are sensitive to changes in partial pressure of arterial oxygen, partial pressure of arterial carbon dioxide, and pH blood levels. Chemoreceptors stimulate the vasomotor center in the medulla; this center controls vasoconstriction and vasodilation. Second are baroreceptors, which are sensitive to stretch and pressure. If blood pressure increases, the baroreceptors cause the heart rate to decrease. If the blood pressure decreases, the baroreceptors stimulate an increase in heart rate (Vander et al., 1990) (Fig. 9–7).

CORONARY CIRCULATION

Because many cardiac problems arise because of an occlusion or a partial occlusion of a coronary artery, an understanding of the coronary blood supply is necessary. The blood supply to the myocardium is derived from the coronary arteries that branch off the aorta

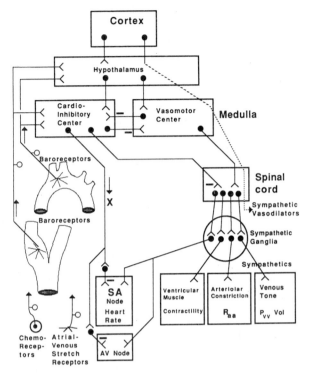

Figure 9–7. Autonomic control of circulation. AV = atrio-ventricular; SA = sinoatrial; R_{aa} = renal arterioles; P_{vv} = pulmonary venules. (Adapted from Goerke, J., & Mines, A. (1988). *Cardiovascular physiology.* New York, Raven Press.)

immediately above the aortic valve (Fig. 9–8). Two major branches exist: the right coronary artery and the left coronary artery, which splits into two branches: the left anterior descending branch and the left circumflex branch. Knowledge of the portion of the heart that receives its blood supply from a particular coronary artery allows the nurse to anticipate problems related to occlusion of that vessel (Table 9–1). The right coronary artery generally supplies the major portion of the right atrium and right ventricle, the sinoatrial and AV nodes, and the posterior portion of the left ventricle. The left anterior descending artery passes behind the pulmonary artery and provides the blood supply to the anterior two thirds of the intraventricular septum and to the anterior and lateral sections of the left ventricle. The left circumflex artery provides blood supply to the left atrium and posterior left ventricle. Variations in the branching and the exact placement of the coronary arteries are common (Skov and Vaska, 1993).

Blood flow to the coronary arteries occurs during diastole, when the aortic valve is closed and the sinuses of Valsalva are filled with blood. Myocardial

Table 9–1. CORONARY ARTERY DISTRIBUTION

Right Coronary Artery

Right atrium
Right ventricle
Sinoatrial node
Atrioventricular bundle
Posterior portion of the left ventricle

Left Anterior Descending Artery

Anterior two thirds of the intraventricular septum
Anterior left ventricle
Lateral left ventricle

Circumflex Artery

Left atrium
Posterior left ventricle

fibers are relaxed at this time, promoting blood flow through the coronary vessels. The coronary veins return blood from the coronary circulation back into the heart through the coronary sinuses to the right and left atria (Hurst and Logue, 1990).

PROPERTIES OF THE CARDIAC MUSCLE

There are five basic properties of the cardiac muscle: contractility, rhythmicity, conductivity, automaticity, and excitability.

Contractility is the ability of muscle fibers to shorten when stimulated, providing the pumping mechanism of the heart. This results in the delivery of a consistent amount of blood volume (known as stroke volume) to the pulmonic and systemic circulation with each heart beat.

Rhythmicity is the ability of the heart muscles to depolarize rhythmically.

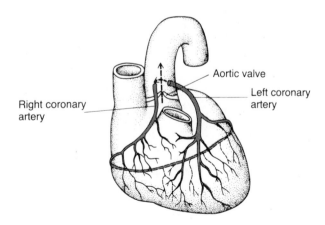

Figure 9–8. The coronary vessels. (From Guyton, A. C. (1986). *Textbook of medical physiology* (7th ed.). Philadelphia: W. B. Saunders Co.)

Conductivity is the heart cell's ability to transmit electrical impulses rapidly and efficiently to all areas of the heart.

Automaticity is the ability of the heart cell to beat spontaneously and to generate an impulse without external stimulation.

Excitability is the cell's ability to respond to electrochemical stimulation (Skov and Vaska, 1993).

CONDUCTION SYSTEM

As a consequence of the aforementioned properties of the cardiac muscle, the heart spontaneously and rhythmically initiates impulses. The cardiac impulse normally originates in the sinoatrial node, which is referred to as the natural pacemaker of the heart. These impulses travel through internodal tracts to the AV node, which is the normal route for the transmission of impulses from the atria to the ventricles.

From the AV node, the impulse spreads to the bundle of His, which divides into right and left branches. These branches terminate in a band of fibers, Purkinje fibers, which spreads impulses through the ventricles (Fig. 9–9) (Skov and Vaska, 1993).

FACTORS OF CIRCULATION

The primary function of the heart is to pump blood through the pulmonary and systemic circula-

tions. Circulation must be adequate in order to meet the fluctuating demands of the body. If the heart fails to perform, cardiac output is compromised. Cardiac output is the traditional measure of cardiac function and is equal to heart rate multiplied by the stroke volume. The average heart rate is 70 beats per minute, and the average stroke volume is 70 ml per beat. Thus, the average resting cardiac output is 4900 ml/min, or about 5 L/min.

$$70 \text{ Beats/min} \times 70 \text{ ml/Beat} = 4900 \text{ ml/min}$$
(approximately 5 L/min)

Because adequate cardiac output is dependent on body size, a more specific measure of cardiac function is the cardiac index, which is calculated by dividing the cardiac output by the body surface area obtained from a table that accounts for height and weight. The normal cardiac index is 2.8 to 4.2 L/min/m². A value of less than 1.8 reflects a hypoperfused heart (Kadota, 1993).

Stroke volume is the amount of blood ejected with each ventricular contraction, normally 60 to 100 ml. Stroke volume is determined by three variants: preload, afterload, and contractility. Preload is the amount of blood remaining in the ventricle at the end of diastole. Left-sided preload is measured by the pulmonary capillary wedge pressure (PCWP) or the left atrial pressure. Right-sided preload is measured by the right atrial pressure. The normal PCWP is approximately 6 to 12 mm Hg, and the normal right atrial pressure is zero to 8 mm Hg, but either may rise considerably in heart failure. If the failing heart is moderately distended with blood at the end of diastole (as a result of less efficient pumping by the heart), then the subsequent contraction is more forceful. This phenomenon is described as Starling's law of the heart, which states that within limits, the greater the stretch or length of the myocardial fiber (and the stretch is greater if the heart is distended with blood), the greater the force of contraction, and thus the greater the cardiac output (Skov and Vaska, 1993). Optimal contractility occurs at a PCWP of 12 to 18 mm Hg. Further stretch in cardiac muscle fibers beyond this PCWP ultimately results in poor contractile function that is analogous to the effect of overstretching a rubber band.

Afterload refers to the resistance to blood flow during ventricular ejection (Skov and Vaska, 1993). Afterload affects the rate of contraction by affecting the force-velocity relationship; that is, the less force or resistance the fiber must overcome, the more rapidly and efficiently it can contract. Therefore, a decrease in the afterload (as occurs in vasodilation) causes an increase in the cardiac output, and an increase in the afterload (as occurs in hypertension, vasoconstriction,

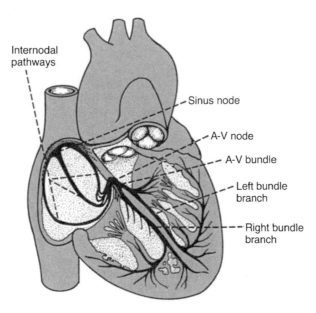

Internodal pathways

Sinus node

A-V node

A-V bundle

Left bundle branch

Right bundle branch

Figure 9–9. The SA node and the Purkinje system of the heart, showing also the AV node, the atrial internodal pathways, and the ventricular bundle branches. (From Guyton, A. C. (1986). *Textbook of medical physiology* (7th ed.). Philadelphia: W. B. Saunders Co.)

semilunar valve stenosis) decreases the cardiac output. The pulmonic and systemic circulations each have an afterload. Vascular resistance is the force that opposes blood flow within the vessels and is the measurement of afterload. It is the product of three factors: vessel radius, vessel length, and blood viscosity. Pulmonary vascular resistance is the afterload of the right side of the heart. Systemic vascular resistance is the afterload of the left side of the heart. The third factor in determining stroke volume is contractility, also known as inotropy, which was discussed earlier in this chapter (Skov and Vaska, 1993). Contractility is influenced by the balance of electrolytes within the body.

Cardiac reserve is the capacity of the heart to adjust to increased demands of the body. An example of such a demand is an increased temperature or stress, whereby cardiac output increases raising the blood pressure to meet the increasing demands of the body.

Blood pressure is the pressure exerted by the blood on the arterial wall and is a reflection of the function of the ventricles as pumps. Blood pressure is represented by systolic pressure (which is the peak pressure and occurs during contraction of the ventricles) and diastolic pressure (which is the residual pressure or the point of least pressure in the arterial system). At diastole, the myocardial muscle fibers lengthen, the heart dilates, and the ventricles fill with blood.

Coronary Artery Disease

The heart muscle requires a substantial flow of blood that can increase when physical or emotional demands on the heart increase activity. When coronary artery disease (CAD) compromises the supply of coronary blood flow, the efficiency and function of the heart muscle is jeopardized. CAD is a partial or total occlusion of the coronary arteries by atherosclerosis. The terms *CAD* and *arteriosclerotic heart disease* are used synonymously.

PATHOPHYSIOLOGY

Arteriosclerosis is a progressive, luminal narrowing that produces degeneration, hardening, or thickening of the arterial walls. Atherosclerosis is the most common form of arteriosclerosis and is characterized by lipid deposits on the intimal layer of the artery. These deposits can progress to partial or total occlusion of the lumen. Atherosclerosis is a disease that involves the aorta, its branches, and medium-sized arteries, such as those supplying blood to the brain, heart, and major internal organs (Fleury and Mur-

daugh, 1993). Atherosclerosis does not seem to involve the arterioles or the venous circulation.

The atherosclerotic lesion (atheroma, or atherosclerotic plaque) consists of an elevated mass of fatty streaks that are lipid-filled smooth muscle cells and may have secondary deposits of calcium salts and blood products. These raised fibrous plaques create changes in the arterial wall caused by chronic endothelial injury. They generally form at points where the arterial tree bifurcates. This is especially true of the carotid and iliac arteries (Fleury and Murdaugh, 1993). Coronary arteries are particularly susceptible to atherosclerosis, which is most commonly seen in individuals who also have CAD and have a history of a high-fat diet, smoking, and sedentary lifestyle.

The atheromas are derived from the lipids, cholesterol, triglycerides, and free fatty acids. An elevated level of cholesterol (>200 mg) is associated with an increased risk of CAD (Expert Panel on Detection, Evaluation, and Treatment of High Blood Cholesterol in Adults, 1993). Cholesterol and triglycerides are insoluble in plasma and must be transported by lipoproteins, which are soluble. These lipoproteins can be separated and measured. Lipoproteins are composed of lipids and proteins. High-density lipoproteins are composed mostly of protein. Serum high-density lipoprotein levels reflect the process of cholesterol removal from peripheral tissues to the liver. The lipids are removed during circulation through the liver. Because an increase in high-density lipoprotein level is thought to decrease the incidence of CAD, a higher level of high-density lipoprotein is desired in proportion to low-density lipoproteins, which carry most of the cholesterol in the plasma (approximately 60%) and deposit lipids and cholesterol in the vessels, particularly in the coronary arteries. Thus, an increase in low-density lipoprotein levels can indicate an increased risk of CAD. Very-low-density lipoproteins are largely composed of triglycerides and contain 10 to 15% of the serum cholesterol that is deposited in the coronary arteries. Increased triglyceride levels also contribute to the process of atherosclerosis, particularly in the coronary arteries (Expert Panel on Detection, Evaluation, and Treatment of High Blood Cholesterol in Adults, 1993; Fleury and Murdaugh, 1993).

During the atherosclerotic process, a thickening occurs of the intima of the coronary artery vessel wall. This thickening, along with the adherence of lipids, collagens, and elastic fibers to the wall of the damaged vessel, produces the atherosclerotic lesion. Lipids, calcium, and thrombi can be found obstructing the affected vessel, decreasing blood flow and oxygen delivery to the heart muscle and causing coronary insufficiency and ischemia that results in CAD (Fleury and Murdaugh, 1993).

ASSESSMENT

Patient Assessment

A thorough cardiovascular assessment is imperative to an understanding of the individual cardiac patient and is inherent to the planning of nursing care for that patient.

A thorough history includes subjective data regarding medical history, prior hospitalizations, allergies, and family medical history. Previous medical history of both pediatric and adult illnesses is of particular interest and includes a positive history for rheumatic fever, diabetes mellitus, hypertension, asthma, renal diseases, or cerebrovascular accident. Knowledge of prior hospitalizations is also important so that records can be obtained for review. Information regarding the patient's current medications, both prescription and over-the-counter drugs, should include information about the patient's understanding and use of these medications. It is also important to determine whether the patient has any food or drug allergies. A medical history of the patient's family can provide insight into real or potential risk factors.

A psychosocial or personal history is also important for the planning of the patient's care. This history includes possible stress events and everyday stressors. Additional information regarding activities for stress reduction is obtained. What, if any, is the individual's exercise routine, including the type, the amount, and the regularity of the activity? What is the patient's daily food pattern and intake? What is his or her sleep pattern? What are the patient's habitual patterns in using tobacco, alcohol, drugs, coffee, tea, and caffeinated sodas?

Before beginning the physical examination, the nurse determines recent and recurrent symptoms that may be related to the patient's current problems. Such information gathering should include the presence or absence of fatigue, fluid retention, dyspnea, irregular heart beat (palpitations), chest pain (including *PQRST*: *p*rovocation, *q*uality, *r*egion/*r*adiation, *s*everity, and *t*iming/*t*reatment). The physical examination itself encompasses all the body systems and is not limited to the cardiovascular system, because all of the body systems are interrelated and interdependent on one another. Although it is imperative that a total evaluation is completed regarding the physical status of the patient, a patient whose primary problems are cardiovascular most commonly exhibits alterations in circulation and oxygenation. Thus, all systems should be examined from this perspective.

The examination should be performed in an orderly, organized manner and should involve the techniques of inspection, palpation, percussion, and auscultation. A baseline assessment is provided in Table 9–2.

Table 9–2. BASELINE ASSESSMENT OF THE CARDIOVASCULAR PATIENT

Neurology	Level of consciousness, orientation to time, place, events; hallucinations, depression, withdrawal, trembling; pupils (size, equality, response); paresthesias; eye movements (nystagmus, focus, directional movement); restlessness, apprehensiveness, irritability, cooperative; hand grips; leg movement; response to tactile stimuli; location of pain, type; relieved by; patient's complaints
Skin	Color, temperature, dryness, turgor, rashes, broken areas, pressure areas, urticaria, incision site, wounds
Cardiology	BP; apical and radial pulses; pulse deficit; monitor leads on patient in correct placement; rhythm, frequency of ectopics; PR and QRS intervals; heart sounds—presence of abnormalities (e.g., rubs, gallops); neck vein distention with head of bed at what angle; edema (sacral and dependent); calf pain; varicosities; presence of pulses— bilateral carotid, radial, femoral, posterior tibial, dorsalis pedis; capillary refill in extremities; presence of invasive pressure monitoring devices; CVP; temporary pacemaker settings; medications to maintain BP or rhythm
Respiratory	Rate and quality of respirations; oxygen; accessory muscles used; cough, sputum—type, color, suctioning frequency; symmetry of chest expansion and breath sounds; describe breath sounds; current ABGs; chest tube with description of drainage, fluctuation in water seal, bubbling, suction applied; tracheostomy or endotracheal tube; ventilator used; ventilator settings; ventilator rate vs patient's own breaths; patient's spontaneous tidal volume
GI	Abdominal size and softness, bowel sounds, nausea and vomiting, bowel movement, dressing and/or drainage, NG tube with description of drainage, feeding tube—type and frequency of feedings, drains, tracheostomy tube
GU	Foley or voiding, urine color, quantity; vaginal or urethral drainage
IV	Volume of fluid, type of solution, rate; IV site condition
Wounds	Dry or drainage, type, color, amount, odor; hematoma, inflamed, drains, hemovac, dressing changes, cultures

GI = gastrointestinal; GU = genitourinary; IV = intravenous; BP = blood pressure; CVP = central venous pressure; ABG = arterial blood gas; NG = nasogastric.

Medical Assessment

Risk Factors

Coronary heart disease remains the leading cause of morbidity and mortality in the United States. Decades of research document the CAD risk factors: abnormal lipoproteins, high fat intake, hypertension, smoking, family history of CAD, diabetes mellitus, physical inactivity, obesity, sociobehavioral and environmental factors, age, and hormonal and hematological factors (Frick et al., 1987; Kannel et al., 1987; Shaten et al., 1991). Because of the current trend of health care reform that is focusing on health promotion and disease prevention, hospitals are in the unique position of offering comprehensive programs to augment cardiovascular health and quality of life for those at risk for heart disease (Lipon and Carlson, 1994). Much of the early research came from a study begun in the 1940s and 1950s, when the population of Framingham, Massachusetts, was studied for the determination of risk factors for CAD. As a result, the public has become progressively more aware and knowledgeable of the recognized risk factors.

Risk factors are divided into two areas: unmodifiable and modifiable. The unmodifiable risk factors are those that cannot be controlled. They include age greater than 45 years for men and greater than 55 years for women, gender (males have a greater incidence than females until menopause), race (African-Americans have a higher incidence), and family history of CAD, hyperlipidemia, or diabetes mellitus. The modifiable risk factors, or those that can be controlled or modified, are increased low-density lipoprotein levels, hypertension, (blood pressure > 140/90 mm Hg), smoking, obesity, sedentary lifestyle, stress/behavior, oral contraceptive use, menopause, and noncontraceptive estrogen replacement (Fleury and Murdaugh, 1993). The first three of the modifiable risk factors are considered to be the most important and most easily modified risk factors (Drown and Engler, 1994).

Diagnostic Studies. Certain diagnostic studies are fundamental for the care and treatment of patients with CAD. Following is a listing and brief description of some of the more common diagnostic studies the cardiac patient may encounter.

12-Lead Electrocardiography. This is a noninvasive test and is usually preliminary to most other testing performed. It is used as a baseline for many other tests and often as a comparison of pretest and posttest changes. This test is useful in identifying rhythm disturbances, ischemia, myocardial injury, and detection and confirmation of an infarct.

Holter Monitor. This is a noninvasive test that is used to detect suspected dysrhythmias. The patient is connected to a small portable recorder (about the size of a pocket radio) by three to five electrodes; the recorder is worn for 12 to 24 hours. The patient engages in the normal daily activities, keeps an activities log, and returns to the laboratory after the designated period of time. The recording is then analyzed.

Exercise Tolerance Test or Stress Test. This is a noninvasive test in which the patient is connected to an ongoing electrocardiography machine while exercising for 3-minute intervals (putting stress on the heart and vascular system). Physical stress causes an increase in myocardial oxygen consumption that exceeds the supply, thereby inducing ischemia. The stress test is used to document exercise-induced ischemia under a closely monitored and controlled situation (Fleury and Murdaugh, 1993). The exercising usually involves walking on a treadmill that progresses in speed and incline and/or walking up and down steps or stairs. The patient is constantly monitored, the pulse and blood pressure are checked at intervals, and the electrocardiogram (ECG) readout is analyzed at the end of the testing period. The patient usually rests in the laboratory to ensure a return to the normal state before returning to his or her room or going home.

Chest Radiography. This is a noninvasive procedure and is usually performed in the anteroposterior view. The chest x-ray study is used for detecting cardiomegaly, cardiac positioning, degree of fluid infiltrating the pulmonary space, and other structural and positional situations that may affect the physical ability of the heart to function in a normal manner.

Phonocardiogram. This is a noninvasive test involving the use of a microphone to record heart sounds that are converted to electrical activity. This procedure is used to time events of the cardiac cycle, to measure systolic time intervals, and to determine the timing and characteristics of murmurs and abnormal heart sounds. The patient may be asked to perform certain activities or may be exposed to certain medications during the recording time. The procedure takes about 30 minutes.

Echocardiogram. This is a noninvasive, acoustic imaging procedure and involves the use of ultrasound to visualize the cardiac structures and the motion and function of cardiac valves and chambers. A transducer is placed on the chest wall and sends ultrasound waves at short intervals. The reflected sound waves are termed "echoes" and are displayed on a graph for interpretation. Echocardiography is used to assess valvular function, evaluate congenital defects, measure size of cardiac chambers, evaluate cardiac disease progression, evaluate ventricular function, diagnose myocardial tumors and effusions, and, to a lesser degree, measure cardiac output.

Transesophageal Echocardiography. This test is uses a transmitter to generate high-frequency sound waves that bounce off the structures of the heart; these echoes are transformed into images of the heart's walls and valves (Hibner et al., 1993). In transesophageal echocardiography, an ultrasound probe is fitted on the end of a flexible gastroscope, which is inserted into the posterior pharynx and advanced into the esophagus. Transesophageal echocardiography shows a clear picture because the esophagus is against the back of the heart and is parallel to the aorta. Transesophageal echocardiography is indicated for pinpointing the site and the extent of a suspected aortic dissection, to rule out the heart as the source of clots in stroke patients, to visualize a valve defect, to assess prosthetic valve function, and to ensure that the left atrium is free of clots before balloon mitral valvuloplasty is performed. Patients should fast (except for medications) for 6 hours before the examination. During the procedure, vital signs, cardiac rhythm, and oxygen saturation are monitored. After the procedure, the patient is unable to eat until the gag reflex returns. A rare complication of transesophageal echocardiography is esophageal perforation with signs of sore throat, dysphagia, stiff neck, epigastric or substernal pain that worsens with breathing and movement, or pain in the back, abdomen, or shoulder.

Radioisotope Studies. These are noninvasive studies involving the use of two radioactive isotopes, thallium 201 (^{201}Tl) and technetium 99m pyrophosphate (^{99m}Tc), along with a scintillation gamma camera that follows the progression of the radioisotopes. An increase or a decrease in the uptake of a radioisotope occurs in abnormal myocardial cells. An area of increased uptake is known as a "hot spot." Technetium is used to detect hot spots that may indicate a suspected MI. An area of decreased uptake is known as a "cold spot." Thallium is used to detect cold spots that indicate decreased myocardial perfusion secondary to coronary stenosis or previous MI.

Cardiac Catheterization/Arteriography. This is an invasive procedure that can be divided into two stages. Cardiac catheterization is used to confirm and evaluate the severity of lesions of the heart muscle; to assess left ventricular function; and to measure pressures within the chambers of the heart, cardiac output, and blood gas content. The right-sided catheterization is performed by placement of a catheter in the femoral or brachial artery that is carefully advanced into the right atrium, right ventricle, and pulmonary artery. A left-sided catheterization is performed by cannulation of a femoral or brachial artery with advancement through the aorta into the left atrium and the left ventricle.

Coronary arteriography, or angiography, is performed in order to visualize coronary arteries, note the area and extent of lesions within the vessels' walls,

evaluate CAD and angina-related spasms, locate areas of infarct along with radioisotopes, and perform a percutaneous coronary angioplasty (PTCA) or intracoronary thrombolysis. The procedure entails positioning a catheter through the aorta into the proximal end of the coronary arteries. Dye is then injected into the arteries, and a radiographic picture is recorded as the dye progresses or fails to progress through the coronary circulation. In addition, dye is injected into the heart chamber, and the amount of dye ejected with the next systole is measured in order to determine the ejection fraction, that is, the fraction of the total end-diastolic volume that is ejected during systole.

Nursing care for a patient undergoing cardiac catheterization and arteriography involves the preprocedure instruction (the procedure will be performed using local anesthesia, and the patient may feel a warm or hot "flush" sensation or flutter of the catheter as it moves about) and postprocedure instruction. The postprocedure routine consists of the following:

- The patient undergoes monitoring and bed rest for 8 hours.
- The extremity used for catheter insertion is kept immobile (Hogan-Miller et al., 1995).
- The catheter insertion site is observed for bleeding or hematoma (Bogart and colleagues, 1995).
- The head of the bed is not raised greater than 30°.
- The peripheral pulses and the color and sensation of the extremities are checked.
- Fluid intake is encouraged
- Intake and output are monitored.
- If arteriography is performed, the patient is observed for an adverse reaction to the dye (Fleury and Murdaugh, 1993).

Magnetic Resonance Imaging. This is a noninvasive test used to detect aortic aneurysms and pericardiac tumors. Magnetic resonance imaging is a technique that uses magnetic resonance to create images of hydrogen, sodium, fluorine, and phosphorus. These images are created as the ions are emitted, picked up, and fed into a computer that reconstructs the image and can differentiate between healthy and ischemic tissue (Chernecky et al., 1993).

Diagnostic Measures. Diagnostic measures include serum electrolyte studies and cardiac enzymes. Because many manuals are available regarding the reading and interpretation of laboratory values, this section presents a brief overview of the more important blood studies (Chernecky et al., 1993).

Serum Electrolytes (Table 9–3)
Potassium: normal levels, 3.5 to 5.3 mEq/L

- Hypokalemia (potassium level < 3.5 mEq/L) is

Table 9–3. RELATION OF ELECTROLYTE ABNORMALITIES TO ELECTROCARDIOGRAPHIC CHANGES

Electrolyte Abnormality	Results
Hypokalemia	Increased ectopic activity
	Prominent U wave and prolonged T wave, ventricular tachycardia
Hyperkalemia	Increased block in the conduction system
Hypocalcemia	Prolonged QT interval, ventricular tachycardia
Hypercalcemia	Shortened QT interval

Adapted from Shoemaker, W. C. (1989). *Textbook of critical care* (2nd ed.). Philadelphia: W. B. Saunders Co.

probably the most common electrolyte abnormality and can be caused by vomiting, diarrhea, prolonged digitalis and diuretic therapy, prolonged nasogastric suctioning, alkalosis, and excessive steroid administration. This condition may be detected by the presence of a U wave on the ECG. A U wave follows the T wave, which may be flattened, and precedes the P wave. Untreated hypokalemia can result in premature ventricular contractions, ventricular tachycardia, ventricular fibrillation, and death.

- Hyperkalemia (potassium level > 5.3 mEq/L) is often caused by overtreatment of hypokalemia. Other causes include Addison's disease, acute renal failure, acidosis, and traumatic injuries and can be detected by the presence of tall, peaked T waves. Untreated hyperkalemia can result in a widening of the QRS until ventricular fibrillation or sudden death occurs.

Calcium: normal levels, 8.2 to 10.2 mg/dl

- Hypocalcemia (calcium level < 8.2) can occur in patients with renal failure, hypoparathyroidism, and malabsorption syndromes. Hypocalcemia can be detected by the occurrence of tetany, which begins with tingling and numbness of the mouth and the extremities and progresses to muscle spasms and seizures. Two measures for identifying a decreased serum calcium level are detection of Chvostek's sign (tapping the facial nerve below the temple anterior to the ear produces facial spasm) and Trousseau's sign (inflating the blood pressure cuff approximately 20 mm Hg > systole causes flexion and inward rotation of the hand and wrist [McCance and Huether, 1994]). The QT interval can become lengthened, and the T wave may become inverted.

- Hypercalcemia (calcium level > 10.2) can be seen in patients with hyperparathyroidism, neoplastic processes, and osteoporosis. Hypercalcemia may be detected by the presence of muscle weakness, irritability, and generalized peripheral neuropathy. The QT interval is shortened, and U waves may be present or accentuated.

Sodium: normal levels, 136 to 145 mEq/L

- Sodium concentration depends on the body's state of fluid balance as governed by release of antidiuretic hormone and by water intake. Sodium has implications for the sodium-potassium exchange in the polarization of the heart muscle (see Chapter 4) and the peripheral edema found in CHF. Generally, sodium changes that can be visualized on an ECG are incompatible with life and are therefore rarely seen.

Serum Enzymes. Enzymes are proteins that are produced by all living cells and released into the bloodstream. Injured or diseased cells increase the release of the particular enzyme into the serum. Because each cell in an organ produces a different enzyme, the identification of the particular enzyme and its elevation can suggest where in the body the damage has occurred and how extensive that damage may be. The three major cardiac enzymes are creatine kinase (CK), lactate dehydrogenase (LDH), and aspartate transaminase (AST) (Chernecky et al., 1993).

- Creatine kinase is the fastest increasing and fastest decreasing of the cardiac enzymes. Onset is 2 to 6 hours after infarction, with a peak of 5 to 12 times normal values within 18 to 36 hours. Serum levels usually return to normal within 3 to 6 days after the damage. The CK isoenzyme is second only to the LDH isoenzyme for being specific for cardiac damage. The isoenzyme of CK-MB is reported to be 100% specific (6 to 10% of the total CK value) for MI or other heart muscle damage, and it peaks in 24 hours.

- Lactate dehydrogenase is another enzyme that is released after an MI. Abnormally high levels are seen in the serum 12 hours after the MI. A peak is reached in 24 to 48 hours, and LDH level returns to normal after the CK does. LDH is present throughout the body in the heart, kidney, skeletal muscles, lung, liver, and red blood cells, and five LDH isoenzymes have been identified. LDH_1 is the isoenzyme present in the cardiac muscle and is the isoenzyme of consequence in determinations of cardiac damage. In the presence of an LDH_1-LDH_2 flip (when LDH_1 value becomes greater than LDH_2), an MI has occurred. This ratio inversion occurs 48 hours after the onset of damage.

- Aspartate transaminase is the third cardiac enzyme that increases in cases of myocardial damage. Its levels begin to increase within 6 to 8 hours of the event, peak in 24 to 48 hours, and return to normal in 72 to 96 hours. AST is present in many tissues of the body, such as the liver, skeletal muscles, renal tissue, red blood cells, brain, pancreas, and lung tissue. Because it is fairly prevalent throughout the body and has no identifiable isoenzyme that is specific to cardiac damage, the AST test tends to be not as specific and not as highly significant as the other two serum enzyme studies.

NOTE: Cardiac troponin T or cardiac troponin I has been found as a protein marker in the detection of MI (Williams and Morton, 1995) and is used in some institutions to aid in early diagnosis of MI.

NURSING DIAGNOSES

Because CAD is a very broad diagnostic area, several nursing diagnostic categories may apply. With the complications of CAD, such as angina, MI, and CHF, the diagnostic categories are more specific. Nursing diagnosis of patients with CAD include

- Acute pain related to decreased coronary artery tissue perfusion
- Anxiety/fear related to treatments and invasive procedures used for diagnostic testing
- Knowledge deficit related to understanding of anatomy and pathophysiology of the heart and its functions
- Health-seeking behaviors related to desire for information to decrease or alter ongoing disease process
- Risk for altered role performance related to possible change in physical activity secondary to illness (Fleury and Murdaugh, 1993).

INTERVENTIONS

Nursing Interventions

Nursing interventions are patient centered and encompass three areas: health assessment, patient education, and the nursing process. The format and necessity of a complete health assessment were discussed in detail earlier in this chapter. The psychosocial and family support assessment, as well as the patient's history and physical examination findings, must be used. Educating and sharing information with the patient, the family, and the support group must begin on the patient's entry into the health care system. If a patient enters the health care system through admission to a critical care unit, the patient and family members or support system may experience fear, frustration, anger, and loss of control. Informing the patient and family of the physiological events experienced by the patient, the need and method of procedures and tests and the equipment used, the medication and diet ordered, and the modification of risk factors that is needed helps alleviate some of the tension and fear that is normal in this situation. Again, communication and uncomplicated explanations are the key elements to patient and family education.

Medical Interventions

Medical interventions for the patient with CAD should also include reduction of major risk factors through patient education, related dietary management, assistance with cessation of smoking, and interpretation of diagnostic studies. Pharmacological agents, such as antilipid agents, may also be ordered (American Heart Association, 1994a):

- Bile acid binders help rid the body of cholesterol. Some commonly used agents are cholestyramine and colestipol.
- Niacin is a B vitamin called nicotinic acid. It can lower total cholesterol, low-density lipoprotein, and triglyceride levels as well as raise high-density lipoprotein cholesterol levels.
- 3-Hydroxy-3-methylglutaryl–coenzyme A (HMG-CoA) reductase inhibitors stimulate the body to process and break down cholesterol. Some commonly used agents are lovastatin, pravastatin, and simvastatin.
- Gemfibrozil is a fibric acid that is especially effective in lowering triglyceride levels.
- Probucol is another pharmacological agent used for lowering cholesterol.

Antiplatelet agents are used to inhibit platelet adhesion, to prevent problems with CAD, and to provide long-term therapy for angina, transient ischemic attacks, and valve replacement. Examples of these agents are dipyridamole (Persantine) and aspirin. If more than one antilipid agent is ordered, they should never be given together; the agents should be administered separately, and the patient should be monitored for adverse reactions (Fleury and Murdaugh, 1993).

PATIENT OUTCOMES

Expected outcomes are that the patient will

- Verbalize the absence or relief of pain.

- Experience less anxiety, related to fear of the unknown, fear of loss of control, role performance, misconceptions, or previously given misinformation.
- Describe disease process, causes, and factors contributing to symptoms and the procedures for disease or symptom control (Fleury and Murdaugh, 1993).
- Actively adhere to health behaviors determined as needing modification, include a multifaceted approach. Initially, the patient must recognize and accept personal responsibility for making lifestyle changes.

Angina

Angina is chest pain or discomfort caused by myocardial ischemia that results from an imbalance between myocardial oxygen supply and demand.

PATHOPHYSIOLOGY

Angina (from Latin, meaning "squeezing") is the chest pain associated with myocardial ischemia; it is transient, and it does not cause cell death, but it may be a precursor to cell death from MI. The neural pain receptors are stimulated by accelerated metabolism, chemical changes and imbalances, and/or local mechanical stress resulting from abnormal myocardial contractions. The oxygen circulating to the myocardial cells decreases, causing ischemia to the tissue and pain.

Myocardial oxygen requirements are dictated by myocardial contraction. The factors that influence myocardial oxygen demand include heart rate, force of cardiac contraction, and myocardial wall tension (determined by afterload, preload, and wall thickness). An increase in any of these factors increases myocardial oxygen demand. A heart at rest uses only a fraction of the oxygen that an active or stressed heart demands. Thus, patient education related to pharmacological therapy, stress reduction techniques, activity limitation, and emergency medical procedures is essential (Fleury and Murdaugh, 1993).

ASSESSMENT

Patient Assessment

Assessment of the patient with actual or suspected angina involves continual observation of the patient and monitoring of signs, symptoms, and diagnostic findings. The patient must be monitored for the type and degree of pain: chest pain or pressure; mild to severe aching of the chest, left arm, or left shoulder; sharp tingling, burning sensation in the jaw or epigastric and substernal regions; squeezing feeling in the chest; and "heartburn" lasting from 1 to 5 minutes.

The precipitating factors that can be identified as bringing on an episode of anginal pain include physical or emotional stress (including exercise), exposure to temperature extremes (particularly cold, or going suddenly from hot to cold), and ingestion of a heavy meal, particularly one rich in low-density lipoproteins and cholesterol. It is important to know what factors alleviate the anginal pain, including stopping activity or exercise and taking nitroglycerin (NTG) sublingual tablets (Fleury and Murdaugh, 1993).

Patient assessment also involves an ongoing observation and evaluation of the patient as he or she undergoes the diagnostic process as well as a complete history and physical and psychosocial examinations. Specific considerations follow.

Etiology and Precipitating Factors

- Coronary artery disease
- Coronary artery spasm
- Activity or stress
- Hypertension
- Anemia
- Dysrhythmia
- Congestive heart failure

Signs and Symptoms

- Pain is frequently retrosternal, left pectoral, or epigastric. In addition, it may radiate to the jaw, left shoulder, or left arm.
- Pain can be described as burning, squeezing, heavy, or smothering.
- Pain usually last 1 to 4 minutes.
- Classic placing of clenched fist against chest (sternum) may be seen or may be absent if the sensation is confused with indigestion.
- Pain usually begins with exertion and subsides with rest.

TYPES OF ANGINA

Different types of angina exist: unstable, variant (Prinzmetal's), or chronic exertional. Unstable, or "crescendo," angina shows a definite change in quality, severity, frequency, and duration, usually over a 3-month period. The pain may precipitate at rest and can last as long as 20 minutes. NTG tablets are not sufficient to relieve the pain. During an unstable attack, the ECG may show ST-segment depression. The patient has an increased risk for MI within 18 months of onset of the angina. Variant (Prinzmetal's) angina usually occurs at rest and without other precipitating factors because it is caused by coronary artery spasm. The

ECG shows a marked ST-segment elevation (usually seen only in an MI) during the episode. MI can occur as a result of prolonged coronary artery spasm, even when the arteries are normal. Chronic exertional angina may occur after ingestion of large meals. Digestion requires increased cardiac output, which increases myocardial oxygen demands, resulting in angina (Fleury and Murdaugh, 1993).

Diagnostic studies for angina include history and physical examination, in which patterns of pain and precipitating risk factors are sought; laboratory data, including blood studies for anemia (hemoglobin and hematocrit values), cardiac enzymes (CK, LDH, AST levels), and cholesterol and triglyceride levels; ECG studies during resting periods, precipitating events (exercise), and anginal pain episodes; exercise tolerance or stress testing; 201Tl scanning; and coronary angiography.

Complications from untreated or unstable angina include MI, CHF, dysrhythmia, and psychological depression (Fleury and Murdaugh, 1993).

NURSING DIAGNOSES/INTERVENTIONS

Nursing diagnoses and interventions for patients with angina include the following (Ulrich et al., 1994).

Pain Related to Myocardial Ischemia

- Assess for signs and symptoms of decreased myocardial tissue perfusion (chest pain, breathlessness, dysrhythmias).
- Implement measures to improve myocardial tissue perfusion, including bed rest.
- Instruct the patient to cease all activities until pain subsides.
- Record descriptions of pain and activity before the onset of pain.
- Administer NTG, up to three NTG sublingually, one every 5 minutes.
- Monitor vital signs (including apical pulse) every 4 to 6 hours, more often during pain and shortness of breath episodes.
- Assess 12-lead ECG during episodes of pain.
- Administer oxygen as ordered.
- Maintain diet (soft, low sodium, low fat, and low cholesterol); if chest pain occurs while patient is eating, encourage the eating of several small meals a day rather than three larger ones.

Anxiety Related to Knowledge Deficit Regarding Disease Process. Provide patient and family education through the following steps:

- Assess for signs and symptoms of anxiety.
- Discuss nature of angina, etiology, risk factors, and importance of modifying those risk factors.

- Discuss possible denial of critical episode by patient or family and assist in support and counseling.
- Discuss nature and characteristics of chest pain and assist in identifying precipitating factors.
- Discuss activity level: avoid isometric-type exercise, avoid heavy lifting and pushing, exercise regularly, and encourage regular home exercise program.
- Remind patient to avoid sexual activity when fatigued. If chest pain does occur during sexual intercourse, the activity is stopped, and nitrates (NTG) are administered as ordered, usually up to three NTG tablets, one every 5 minutes. If chest pain is unrelieved, recommend calling emergency medical service, and tell patient not to attempt to drive himself or herself to the emergency department.
- Discuss self-management during episodes of pain: stop the activity and rest; take nitrates as ordered, 3 NTG tablets, one every 5 minutes; if pain persists, call emergency medical service.
- Recommend following diet as ordered. Recommend avoidance of caffeine.
- Explain importance of controlling any related diseases or problems that may aggravate atherosclerosis, such as hypertension, diabetes, and hyperlipidemia.
- Explain importance of controlling weight and avoiding obesity.
- Explain role of stress in aggravating heart disease and identify individual stress-producing factors and methods of stress management, including relaxation techniques.
- Discuss medications: name, dosage (amount and times), purpose, and side effects.

Related Nursing Diagnoses

- Anxiety related to acute pain secondary to cardiac tissue ischemia
- Sleep pattern disturbances related to present status and unknown future
- Risk for constipation related to bed rest, change in lifestyle, and medications
- Activity intolerance related to fear of recurrent angina
- Risk for self-esteem disturbance related to perceived or actual role changes
- Risk for impaired home maintenance management related to angina or fear of angina
- Risk for altered family processes related to impaired ability of person to assume role responsibilities
- Risk for sexual dysfunction related to fear of angina and altered self-esteem

MEDICAL INTERVENTIONS

Medical interventions for the patient experiencing angina include the administration of nitrates, beta-adrenergic blocking agents, and calcium channel blocking agents.

Nitrates are the most common medications for angina. They are direct-acting, smooth muscle relaxants that cause vasodilation of the peripheral vascular bed (Fleury and Murdaugh, 1993). Nitrate therapy is beneficial because it decreases myocardial oxygen demand. The vasodilating effect causes relief of pain and lowering of blood pressure. Examples of nitrates are sublingual, intravenous (IV), transdermal, spray, or ointment NTG and sublingual or oral isosorbide (Isordil). Side effects of these vasodilators include headaches, flushing, tachycardia, dizziness, and orthostatic hypotension. The patient should be instructed to take NTG before engaging in activity, to replace the NTG every 3 months, and to avoid wearing NTG patches near microwave ovens (leaking waves may cause an explosion of the patch!). If an acute attack of angina occurs, the patient should take up to three tablets NTG sublingually, one every 5 minutes—if the patient experiences no relief, he or she should seek medical attention immediately.

Beta-adrenergic blocking agents may also be used to treat angina. They block adrenergic receptors, thereby decreasing heart rate, blood pressure, and cardiac contractility (Fleury and Murdaugh, 1993). Examples include nadolol, timolol maleate, propranolol, labetalol hydrochloride, and pindolol. The side effects of these agents include bradycardia, AV block, asthma attacks, depression, hypotension, memory loss, and masking of hypoglycemic attacks. The patient is taught to take these agents as prescribed, not to abruptly stop taking them, and to monitor heart rate and blood pressure at regular intervals while taking these agents.

Calcium channel blockers inhibit the flow of calcium ions access cellular membranes, an effect that causes direct increases in coronary blood flow and myocardial perfusion as well as decreases in myocardial oxygen requirements (Fleury and Murdaugh, 1993). They are used for treating tachydysrhythmias, vasospasms, CHF, and hypertension as well as for treating angina. Examples of calcium channel blockers include verapamil (Calan, Isoptin), nifedipine (Procardia), and diltiazem (Cardizem). The side effects of calcium channel blockers include dizziness, flushing, headaches, decreased heart rate, and hypotension. The patient is taught to monitor blood pressure for hypotension, especially if the agents are taken in combination with nitrates and beta-blockers.

OUTCOMES

The outcomes for the patient with angina are that the patient will

- Experience adequate myocardial tissue perfusion, as evidenced by the absence of chest discomfort.
- Not experience cardiac dysrhythmias.
- Actively participate in the health behaviors prescribed.
- Experience less anxiety related to fear of the unknown, fear of loss of control, misconceptions, or previously given misinformation.
- Describe the disease process, causes, and factors contributing to symptoms and the procedure for symptom control through rest, medication, progressive activity, diet, stress control, and control of related physiological problems (Ulrich et al., 1993).

Myocardial Infarction

An MI is ischemia with death to the myocardium that is caused by lack of blood supply from the occlusion of a coronary artery and its branches. Cardiovascular disease accounts for more than 930,000 deaths in the United States annually, with 500,000 of these deaths resulting from CAD. Of these 500,000, 489,171 are deaths from heart attack. Every 34 seconds, someone dies from heart and blood vessel diseases; two thirds of sudden deaths resulting from coronary heart disease occur out of the hospital, and most occur within 2 hours of onset of cardiovascular symptoms (American Heart Association, 1994). One in six men and one in eight women older than 45 years have had an MI or stroke. The incidence of complications in women after an MI is approaching that of men. Within 6 years after an MI, 23% of men and 31% of women have another MI, 41% of men and 34% of women experience angina, 20% of men and 20% of women are disabled with heart failure, 9% of men and 18% of women have a stroke, and 13% of men and 6% of women experience sudden death (American Heart Association, 1995).

PATHOPHYSIOLOGY

An acute MI is caused by an imbalance between myocardial oxygen supply and demand. This imbalance is the result of decreased coronary artery perfusion, which is usually the result of atherosclerosis, coronary artery vasospasm, coronary artery thrombus, dysrhythmias, or a combination of any of these factors. Atherosclerotic CAD is the most common cause of the acute MI. Reduced blood flow to an area of the myocardium causes significant and sustained oxygen deprivation to myocardial cells. Normal functioning is disrupted as ischemia and injury lead to eventual cellular death. Myocardial dysfunction occurs as more cells are involved.

Prolonged ischemia from a total decrease in blood flow is called infarction and evolves over approximately 3 hours (Riegel, 1993). It causes irreversible cellular damage and muscle death (necrosis) (Fig. 9–10). Permanent cessation of contractile function occurs in the necrotic or infarcted area of the myocardium. The infarct is surrounded by a nonfunctional zone as well as a zone of mild ischemia in potentially viable tissue. The ultimate size of the infarct depends on the fate of this ischemic zone. If the infarct is unsuccessfully treated, this margin increases as tissue death occurs. If the infarct is successfully treated, the residual necrosis can be minimized (see Fig. 9–10). Two types of MIs exist: transmural, which involves the entire thickness of the heart muscle, and nontransmural, which involves a partial thickness of inner half of the myocardial muscle thickness. The severity of the MI is determined by the success or lack of success of the treatment, as stated earlier, and the degree of collateral circulation that is present at that particular part of the heart muscle. The collateral circulation consists of the alternative routes or channels that can develop in the myocardium in response to chronic ischemia or regional hypoperfusion. Through this small, tiny network of "extra" vessels, blood flow can be improved to the threatened myocardium (Riegel, 1993).

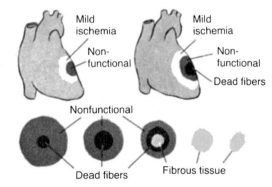

Figure 9–10. *Top:* Small and large areas of coronary ischemia. *Bottom:* Stages of recovery from myocardial infarction. (From Guyton, A. C. (1986). *Textbook of medical physiology* (7th ed.). Philadelphia: W. B. Saunders Co.)

ASSESSMENT

Patient Assessment

Patient assessment includes close observation in order to identify the classic signs and symptoms of an acute MI. Chest pain is the paramount sign and symptom. It may be severe, crushing, tight, squeezing, or simply a feeling of pressure. It can be precordial, substernal, or in the back; radiating to arms, neck or jaw; and/or unrelated to exertion and respirations. It does not cease with rest or nitrate administration and thus can be distinguished from the pain of an angina attack. Chest pain does not always occur, but when it does, it is usually associated with 70% or greater occlusion of the lumen of the involved coronary artery (Riegel, 1993). The longer the duration and the more severe the pain, the greater the likelihood that an MI is occurring.

The skin may be cool, clammy, pale, and diaphoretic; the color may be dusky or ashen; and slight hyperthermia may be present. The patient may be short of breath, dyspneic, and tachypneic; may feel faint; or may have intermittent loss of sensorium. Hypotension may be present, often accompanied by dysrhythmias, particularly ventricular ectopy, bradycardia, or tachycardia, and by heart blocks of varying degrees. The type of dysrhythmia experienced depends on the area of the MI. The patient may be anxious or restless or may exhibit certain behavioral responses, including denial, depression, and sense of impending doom. Nausea and vomiting are other common features.

Note: Approximately 20% to 60% of MIs are silent; these can occur with no presenting signs or symptoms (Riegel, 1993).

The types of MIs can be determined by the particular coronary artery involved and the blood supply to that area (Table 9–4).

Assessment of a patient experiencing an MI takes all of the above signs and symptoms into account during the history and physical examination. Risk factors for an MI (CAD, coronary spasm, and embolism) are also considered in the determination of a diagnosis. Other areas of assessment imperative for accurate diagnosis include those in the medical assessment.

Medical Assessment

Electrocardiographic Changes

- Ischemia—T-wave inversion
- Injury—ST-segment elevation
- Infarct—pathological or well-defined and deep Q wave

Cardiac Enzyme Levels (Chernecky et al., 1993)

Table 9–4. MYOCARDIAL INFARCTION (MI) BY SITE, ELECTROCARDIOGRAPHIC (ECG) CHANGES, AND COMPLICATIONS

Location of MI	Primary Site of Occlusion	Primary ECG Changes	Complications
Inferior MI	RCA (80–90%)	Leads: II, III, aVF	First- and second-degree heart block, right ventricular infarct
Inferolateral MI	LCX (10–20%) LCX	II, III, aV_5, V_6	Third-degree heart block, left CHF, cardiomyopathy, left ventricular rupture
Posterior MI	RCA or LCX	No lead truly looks at posterior surface. Look for reciprocal changes in V_1 and V_2—tall, broad R waves; ST depression and tall T waves. Posterior leads V_7, V_8, and V_9 may be recorded and evaluated.	First-, second-, and third-degree heart blocks, CHF, bradyarrhythmias
Right ventricular infarct	RCA	V_4–V_6 Right precordial leads V_1R–V_6R may be recorded and evaluated.	Increased CVP, decreased cardiac output, bradyarrhythmia, heart blocks, hypertension, cardiogenic shock
Anterior MI	LAD	V_2–V_4	Third-degree heart block, CHF, left bundle branch block
Anterior-septal MI	LAD	V_1–V_3	Second- and third-degree heart block
Anterior-lateral and lateral	LAD or LCX	V_5, V_6, aVL, I	CHF, cardiomyopathy

AV = atrioventricular; CHF = congestive heart failure; RCA = right coronary artery; LAD = left anterior descending; LCX = circumflex; RV = right ventricular.

The isoenzymes that are specific for cardiac damage are CK-MB and LDH_1 (see CAD section).

Diagnostic Studies

- Almost all patients who have had an MI eventually undergo coronary angiography so that the coronary anatomy can be visualized in order to determine if other areas of myocardium are in jeopardy. They also undergo ventriculography in order to determine the function of the myocardium (Riegel, 1993). Indications for coronary angiography and its timing after an acute MI require correction of prothrombin time, digitalis toxicity, severe hypertension, fever, severe left ventricular failure, gastrointestinal bleeding, anemia, renal failure, and electrolyte imbalances (Riegel, 1993).
- Pyrophosphate scanning is considered noninvasive and is used to determine the occurrence, extent, and prognosis of an MI. ^{99m}Tc stannous pyrophosphate is thought to combine with the calcium in damaged myocardial cells, forming a spot on the scan. Such spots appear within 12 hours of infarction. A spot that does not disappear indicates continued myocardial damage (Chernecky et al., 1993; Williams and Morton, 1995).
- Multiple-gated acquisition scanning is also noninvasive. The procedure uses radioisotope tagging of red blood cells with ^{99m}Tc, and images of cardiac volumes are collected during the cardiac cycle. The purpose of a multiple-gated acquisition scan is to collect information about the ejection fraction and left ventricular wall motion. Ejection fraction is a measurement of left ventricular systolic pump performance. The normal ejection fraction is greater than 65%; an ejection fraction less than 50% indicates the presence of ventricular dysfunction. A NTG scan is an additional feature of the multiple-gated acquisition scan. A series of images is taken for the evaluation of the effectiveness of sublingual NTG administration. (Chernecky et al., 1993).
- Myocardial perfusion imaging is a radioisotope study that uses ^{201}Tl. Ischemic areas show decreased radioactivity, or a "cold spot." This assessment is sometimes used in conjunction

with exercise tolerance testing to initiate the ischemic process. It is used to detect areas of infarct when no ECG changes or normal enzyme levels are present.

- Electrophysiological study is another diagnostic study; it is an invasive procedure that involves the introduction of an electrode catheter percutaneously from a peripheral vein or artery into the cardiac chamber or sinuses and the performance of programmed electrical stimulation of the heart. Use of electrophysiological study aids in the diagnosis of cardiac conduction defects, the evaluation of effectiveness of antidysrhythmic medications or ablation, the determination of proper choice of pacemaker; the mapping of the cardiac conduction system before ablation; and the recording of intracardiac ECGs (Chernecky et al., 1993).

NURSING DIAGNOSES/INTERVENTIONS

Nursing diagnoses and interventions for the MI patient include the following.

Pain Related to Myocardial Ischemia or Necrosis. It is essential that pain be relieved.

- Administer drug therapy as ordered and note response. Usually oxygen, NTG (IV), and morphine sulfate (IV) are given.
- Monitor blood pressure, hemodynamics, and heart sounds as pain occurs.
- Use nonpharmacological pain relief techniques and promote a relaxed, quiet, restful environment.
- Maintain bed rest during episodes of pain, and allow the patient to assume a position of comfort.
- Record the patient's description of the pain and determine aggravating factors, including breathing patterns.

Risk for Alteration in Cardiac Output Related to Loss of Myocardial Contractility

- Plan all activities to minimize oxygen demands.
- Identify, report, and assist in the correction of signs and symptoms of decreased cardiac output; tachycardia, fatigue, dyspnea, restlessness, hemodynamic changes.
- Monitor blood pressure, temperature, pulse, respiration, and apical pulse every 2 to 4 hours.
- Monitor cardiac rhythm for elevated ST segment, T-wave inversion, and/or presence of pathological Q wave.
- Administer oxygen as ordered.
- Monitor breath sounds at least every 4 to 6 hours.

- Monitor heart sounds at least every 4 to 6 hours.
- Monitor arterial blood gases (ABGs), electrolytes, cardiac enzymes.
- Monitor pulmonary artery pressure, PCWP, central venous pressure.
- 12-lead ECG.
- Intake and output every 2 to 4 hours.
- Monitor IV fluids.
- Administer medications as ordered and monitor response.
- Encourage appropriate diet—avoid ice and very cold fluids.
- Instruct patient to avoid activities that increase cardiac workload, such as the Valsalva maneuver. Provide stool softeners or laxatives.

Anxiety Related to Perceived or Actual Threat of Loss of Biological Integrity

- Use comfort measures, maintain quiet environment, and promote relaxation.
- Facilitate contact with family members and significant others who will comfort and support the patient.
- Use a calm voice and reassuring actions during care.
- Explain procedures and tests to the patient and family; orient them to critical care area.
- Administer sedative as needed to lessen anxiety.
- Explain care and procedures.
- Encourage expression of feelings.

Knowledge Deficit Regarding Disease Process

- Begin patient and family teaching as soon as the patient is stable. Refer to a formal cardiac rehabilitation program, if available.
- Review explanation of heart condition: the extent of infarct; associated complications, such as dysrhythmias, angina, CHF, pulmonary edema, cardiogenic shock, and post-MI syndrome; and the nature of disease process, such as risk factors and precipitating factors.
- Explain the importance of rest balanced with limits of exercise and activity as he or she progresses through the rehabilitation program.
- Explain the importance of controlling existing conditions that aggravate recovery, such as hyperlipidemia, diabetes, and hypertension.
- Explain the importance of weight control.
- Explain the importance of stress management.
- Explain the importance of avoiding or modifying activity after heavy meals, alcohol con-

sumption, emotional stress, and extreme temperatures.

- Explain the importance of independence and the responsibility for self-care.
- Explain the importance of modifying activity during sexual intercourse including approaching sex gradually, having intercourse when patient is well rested, practicing avoidance when patient is physically or emotionally stressed or after a heavy meal or alcohol consumption, providing a comfortable atmosphere, choosing a comfortable position, and recognizing warning signs of heart strain.
- Encourage the patient to communicate feelings and concerns with family or support group.
- Discuss the signs and symptoms of extending MI versus those of angina.
- Explain the importance of seeking emergency care if chest pain is unrelieved with rest and NTG.
- Explain the importance of diet—avoiding caffeine, high-fat, high-cholesterol, high-sodium foods.
- Explain the importance of avoiding tobacco.
- Explain the importance of resting after meals.
- Explain medications prescribed, including name, dosage (amount and time), purpose, and side effects.
- Explain why over-the-counter medications should be avoided until they are checked by a physician.
- Explain why constipation and straining should be avoided.
- Explain why a physician should be consulted before patient resumes sexual activity, travel, and driving.
- Explain why isometric-type exercises and heavy lifting and pushing should be avoided.
- Explain monitoring of daily activities and the spacing of activities throughout the day in order to avoid fatigue (Ulrich et al., 1994).

Treatment of the patient with an acute MI consists of maintaining adequate myocardial oxygenation and decreasing myocardial workload; relieving pain and anxiety; managing dysrhythmias; and observing for, and intervening promptly to, prevent or minimize complications (see Nursing Care Plan, p. 261).

COMPLICATIONS

Complications include cardiac dysrhythmias, heart failure, thromboembolism, rupture of a portion of the heart (e.g., ventricular free wall, interventricular septum, and papillary muscle), pericarditis, infarct ex-

tension or recurrence, and cardiogenic shock (see Chapter 8) (Ulrich et al., 1994).

Three complications of MI are discussed in greater detail: pericarditis, endocarditis, and Dressler's syndrome.

Pericarditis

Inflammation of the pericardium may occur as a complication of MI. The patient usually presents with precordial pain (this pain frequently radiates to the shoulder, neck, back, and arm and is intensified during deep inspiration, movement, and coughing), pericardial friction rub, dyspnea, weakness, fatigue, persistent temperature elevation, increase in white blood cell count and sedimentation rate, and increased anxiety level (Ulrich et al., 1994). Precordial pain must be distinguished from the pain of an acute MI.

Detection of pericardial friction rubs is the most common method of diagnosing pericarditis. The friction rub is usually heard best on inspiration with the diaphragm of the stethoscope placed over the second, third, or fourth intercostal space at the sternal border. Friction rubs have been described as grating, scraping, squeaking, or scratching sounds. This rubbing sound results from an increase in fibrous exudate between the two irritated pericardial layers; this condition causes increased friction as the heart beats within the pericardial sac. The pericardial friction rub may be the hallmark of a transmural MI, in which damage to the entire myocardial wall has occurred.

The treatment of patients with pericarditis involves relief of pain, usually through medication (antibiotics, if the causative agent is bacterial in origin, and anti-inflammatory agents, such as indomethacin and ibuprofen) (Dziadulewicz and Shannon-Stone, 1995), and treatment of other systemic symptoms. In some extreme cases in which relief is not obtained or the inflammation is of a lasting nature, a pericardiectomy may be indicated. Complications of untreated pericarditis include pericardial effusion, cardiac tamponade, chronic pericarditis, and constrictive pericarditis.

Endocarditis

Infective endocarditis is an infection of microorganisms circulating in the bloodstream that attach onto an endocardial surface. It is caused by various microbes and frequently involves the heart valves. Bacteria of the genus *Streptococcus* are the organisms most commonly responsible for subacute infective endocarditis. Endocarditis can also be caused by staphylococci, gram-negative bacilli (e.g., *Escherichia coli* and *Klebsiella* species), and fungi (e.g., *Candida* and *Histoplasma* species).

Infectious lesions or vegetations form on the heart valves. These lesions have irregular edges and have been known to have a cauliflower-like appearance. The mitral valve is the most common area to be affected, followed by the aortic valve. The vegetative process can grow to involve the chordae tendineae, the papillary muscles, and the conduction system. Therefore, the patient may experience dysrhythmias or die of heart failure.

Clinical manifestations of endocarditis include fever, chills, night sweats, cough, weight loss, general malaise, weakness, fatigue, headache, musculoskeletal complaints, new murmur, right-sided or left-sided CHF, pericardial friction rub, MI, clubbing of the fingers, positive blood cultures, anemia, and ECG changes. The presenting symptoms are determined by the valve involved, the organism present, and the length of time and extent of growth of the vegetative process. Treatment involves diagnosing the infective agent, treating with the appropriate antibiotics or antifungal agents, and ultimately performing valve replacement surgery in the most serious cases (Durack, 1990).

Dressler's Syndrome (Post–Myocardial Infarction Syndrome)

The post-MI syndrome appears a few weeks or months after infarction and is characterized by protracted or recurrent fever, chest pain of the pleuropericardial type, pericardial friction rub, and left pleural effusion. The cause of Dressler's syndrome is unknown. Treatment with corticosteroids, indomethacin, or aspirin is usually effective (Morris et al., 1990).

MEDICAL INTERVENTIONS

Medical treatment of MI is usually divided into three types: the pharmacological approach, the interventional approach, and the surgical approach.

Pharmacological Approach

The initial approach to treatment of MI generally includes oxygenation, rest, hemodynamic monitoring, and use of pharmacological agents.

Oxygen is important for assisting the myocardial tissue to continue its pumping activity and for repairing the damaged tissue around the site of the infarct. Rest is imperative, and assistance with activities is required until the patient has stabilized. Then, progressive return to daily activity can begin in order to reduce the patient's feelings of fear, anxiety, frustration, and loss of control. Hemodynamic monitoring,

including fluid balance and left ventricle function, is used to determine cardiac function (Riegel, 1993).

Pharmacological agents used in the treatment of MI can be divided into several groups.

Analgesics. These agents are used for pain. Usually, IV morphine or IV meperidine (Demerol) is used.

Nitroglycerin. Intravenous nitroglycerin is often used to increase coronary perfusion because of its vasodilatory effects; it is also used to decrease cardiac pain and limit complications of an acute MI. It is usually started at titrated doses of 5 to 10 μg/min and increased to a total of 50 to 200 μg/min until chest pain is absent, PCWP decreases, and/or systolic blood pressure decreases (Riegel, 1993). Caution should be used in administering NTG to patients with inferior or right ventricular infarcts.

Antiarrhythmics (Table 9–5)

Type IA. These antiarrhythmics are local anesthetic agents with anticholinergic effects and include quinidine, disopyramide (Norpace), procainamide (Pronestyl), encainide, and flecainide.

Type IB. These are local anesthetics without anticholinergic effects and include phenytoin (Dilantin), lidocaine, (Xylocaine), aprindine, tocainide, and mexiletine. Side effects can vary, but particular attention is given to AV block, bradycardia, and hypotension. The most common antiarrhythmic agent used for acute MI and immediately after MI is lidocaine by IV drip, with a loading dose (bolus) of 1 to 1.5 mg/kg IV push, followed by maintenance dose of 2 to 4 mg/min by IV drip.

Type II. These are cardiotonic medications, such as digoxin and other digitalis preparations (e.g., deslanoside [Cedilanid-D], digitoxin).

Type III. These are antiadrenergic drugs, such as beta-adrenergic blockers, which include propranolol, metoprolol, esmolol, atenolol. Beta-blockers reduce ischemic pain. They are indicated for patients with tachycardia and hypertension because they decrease heart rate and blood pressure (Braunwald et al., 1994).

Type IV. These are calcium channel blockers that are indicated for patients who are unable to tolerate adequate doses of nitrates and beta-blockers or who have variant angina (Braunwald et al., 1994).

Thrombolytic Therapy. Other medical interventions are also used during the initial treatment of an acute MI. One common therapy is thrombolytic therapy. Research has shown that occlusion of the coronary vessel does not cause immediate myocardial cell death. Irreversible injury begins within 20 minutes of the vessel occlusion. Within a period of 5 to 6 hours, the irreversible damage begins at the endocardial surface and progresses to the epicardium. The extent and the progression of the injury are determined by the completeness of the occlusion and the presence of collat-

Table 9–5. THE USE AND EFFECTS OF VARIOUS ANTIARRHYTHMIC AGENTS

Agent	Administration	Metabolism and Excretion	Side Effects	Recommended Therapeutic Serum Level (Trough)
Quinidine	po: 200–300 mg every 6 h (used rarely)	Liver—greatest Renal decrease in alkaline urine	Nausea, vomiting, diarrhea, thrombocytopenia, hypotension, ventricular tachycardia	2–6 mg/ml
Procainamide	20–30 mg/min up to 17 mg/kg; then infusion of 1–4 mg/min po: 1 g (SR) every 6h	50% in liver 50% in kidney	Positive antinuclear antibody with lupus-like syndrome, fever, gastrointestinal distress, agranulocytosis, hypotension, psychosis, hallucinations	3–8 mg/ml
Disopyramide	po: 100–200 mg q 6 h or 300 mg (SR) q 12 h	Kidney Liver	Hypotension, heart failure, vomiting, dry mouth, urinary hesitancy, constipation, blurred vision, hypoglycemia	2–3 mg/ml
Lidocaine	IV: loading dose 1–1.5 mg/kg followed by 0.5 mg/kg every 3–5 min to total of 3 mg/kg; then infusion of 2–4 mg/min	Liver	Tremor, agitation, disorientation, seizures, respiratory arrest, AV block with conduction defects	2–6 mg/ml
Phenytoin	IV: 100 mg q 5 min, up to 700 mg po: 200 mg bid after loading dose	Liver	Nystagmus, dizziness, ataxia, gastrointestinal distress, skin rash, megaloblastic anemia, hyperglycemia	10–20 mg/ml
Propranolol	1–3 mg IV push over 2–5 min; may repeat after 2 min to total dose of 1 mg/kg po: 10–30 mg q 6–8 h;	Liver	Heart failure, hypotension, bradycardia, insomnia, bronchospasm, nausea, vomiting, lethargy, dizziness, nightmares, diarrhea	
Bretylium	5–10 mg/kg IV push. Repeat every 5–30 min, up to total of 35 mg/kg; may follow with infusion at 2 mg/min	70–80% unchanged in urine	Hypotension, nausea, vomiting, enlargement of parotid glands	
Verapamil	2.5–5 mg IV push; repeat 5 mg every 15 min to max dose of 30 mg po: 80 mg q 6–8h; may give up to 480 mg/day in divided doses	Liver	Headache, nausea, vomiting, hypotension, heart failure, bradycardia, AV block	
Tocainide	po: 400–800 mg q 8 h	40% unchanged in urine	Similar to lidocaine, pulmonary fibrosis, worsening of dysrhythmias, visual disturbances, nausea, vomiting, anorexia	4–10 µg/ml
Flecainide	po: 100–200 mg q 12 h	86% in urine	Dizziness, visual disturbances, dyspnea, nausea, constipation, exacerbation of heart failures and dysrhythmias, conduction disturbances, tremor	0.2–1.0 µg/ml
Amiodarone	po: 400–600 mg/day in 1–2 doses	Liver	Pulmonary fibrosis, conduction disturbances, liver injury, exacerbation of dysrhythmias, corneal deposits, photosensitivity, thyroid abnormalities, neurologic problems, nausea, vomiting, constipation, bradycardia	1–2.3 mg/l

Data from Shoemaker, W. C. (1989). *Textbook of critical care* (2nd ed.) Philadelphia: W. B. Saunders Co.; American Heart Association. (1994). *Textbook of advanced cardiac life support;* and Wilson, B. A., Shannon, M. T., & Stang, C. L. (1996). *Nurse drug guide.* Stamford, CT: Appleton & Lange.
po = by mouth; bid = twice a day; IM = intramuscularly; q = every; AV = atrioventricular; SR = sustained release.

eral circulation (Riegel, 1993). The goals are to dissolve the lesion that is occluding the coronary artery and to increase blood flow to the myocardium. The patient must be symptomatic for less than 6 hours, have angina for 20 minutes that was unrelieved by NTG, and have an ECG with an ST segment of greater than or equal to 0.2 mV in two or more contiguous ECG leads.

Streptokinase. This agent is a synthetic protein derived from group C beta-hemolytic streptococci that lyses clots by acting on plasminogen. Therefore, streptokinase may cause allergic reactions, especially in patients who have had streptococcal infections and retain high levels of antibodies. The most common reactions are fever and drug rash. Streptokinase is given in a dose of 1.5 million U in 100 ml of saline infused by the IV route over 60 minutes (GUSTO, 1993).

Tissue Plasminogen Activator. Another medical treatment for the MI patient is tissue plasminogen activator (Alteplase, or t-PA), which is a serum protease that affects the lysis of a clot. It was developed from human DNA and is currently manufactured by use of animal tissue culture. Because t-PA is a human protein, no allergic reactions are expected to the medication, and, if necessary, retreatment is possible. Once t-PA binds to fibrin, it can convert clot-bound plasminogen to clot-bound plasmin, producing a clot-specific state rather than a systemic lytic state. The t-PA is given as a 15-mg IV bolus; then 0.75 mg/kg is given over 30 minutes, not to exceed 50 mg. This is followed by 0.5 mg/kg IV over the next hour, not to exceed 35 mg.

Other Therapies Related to t-PA. Chewable aspirin is administered as soon as possible in a dose of greater than or equal to 160 mg, followed by a daily dose of 160 to 325 mg/d (GUSTO, 1993). Heparin is started 4 hours after the administration of either thrombolytic agent, with a 5000-U bolus, then 1000 U/h for 48 hours. The IV infusion is adjusted to 60 to 85 microdrops/minute; if the patient weighs more than 80 kg, the heparin dose is 1200 U/h (GUSTO, 1993).

Studies on the relative effectiveness of streptokinase and t-PA and the roles of IV as compared with subcutaneous heparin as adjunctive therapy in acute MI are pending. The current GUSTO trial was designed to compare new, aggressive thrombolytic strategies with standard thrombolytic regimens in the treatment of acute MI. In 15 countries and 1081 hospitals, 41,021 patients with evolving MI were randomly assigned to four different thrombolytic groups, consisting of the use of

Streptokinase and subcutaneous heparin (group 1)
Streptokinase and IV heparin (group 2)
Accelerated t-PA and IV heparin (group 3)
Combination of streptokinase plus t-PA with IV heparin (group 4)

"Accelerated" refers to the administration of t-PA over a period of 1 1/2 hours, with two thirds of the dose given in the first 30 minutes. The mortality rates in the four treatment groups were as follows: group 1, 7.2%; group 2, 7.4%; group 3, 6.3%; and group 4, 7.0%. These results reflected a 14% lower mortality for accelerated t-PA compared with that of the other treatments. The findings of this large-scale trial indicate that accelerated t-PA given with IV heparin provides a survival benefit over previous standard thrombolytic regimens (GUSTO, 1993).

Thrombolytic therapy is absolutely contraindicated in patients with previous stroke, active bleeding, previous treatment with streptokinase or t-PA, recent trauma or major surgery, or noncompressible vascular punctures (GUSTO, 1993). Severe, uncontrolled hypertension was considered to be a relative contraindication (GUSTO, 1993).

Nursing care of the patient includes identification of suitable patients for IV thrombolytics, thus ensuring as little delay as possible before the therapy (Tootill, 1995) and screening for contraindications are initiated. Next, the nurse secures three vascular access lines and obtains necessary laboratory data. Initial ECG monitoring is documented before the infusion begins, at the end of the infusion, 1 hour from the end of infusion, and every 8 hours for 24 hours. Medications are administered as ordered. Finally, the patient is monitored for complications, including dysrhythmias (premature ventricular contractions, sinus bradycardia, accelerated idioventricular rhythm, or ventricular tachycardia), minor oozing at venipuncture sites and gingival bleeding, reocclusion, or reinfarction (Riegel, 1993).

Interventional Approach

In the early 1980s, Beth Israel Hospital in Boston emerged as one of the forerunners of interventional cardiology. This model of patient care focuses on teamwork. The intervention consists of cardiac catheterization, percutaneous transluminal coronary angioplasty, directional coronary atherectomy, intracoronary stenting, and excimer laser coronary angioplasty (Clark et al., 1994).

Note: Angiotensin-converting enzyme inhibitors reduce the circulating volume of angiotensin II, a potent vasoconstrictor. (Fara, 1993).

Percutaneous Transluminal Coronary Angioplasty. The purpose of PTCA is to compress intracoronary plaque in order to increase blood flow to the myocardium. It is usually the treatment of choice for patients with uncompromised collateral flow, noncalcified lesions, and lesions not present at bifurcations of vessels. In addition, the patient must be a candidate for CABG surgery. The PTCA is performed in the cardiac catheterization laboratory with the operating room on standby. A balloon catheter is inserted in the manner of coronary arteriography, but it is threaded into the occluded coronary artery and is advanced with the use of a guide wire across the lesion. The balloon is inflated under pressure one or several times in order to compress the lesion (Fig. 9–11). Complications from a PTCA are similar to those from a cardiac catheterization and include dissection of the coronary artery, coronary occlusion, MI, bleeding, decreased pulses distal to the procedure site, allergic reaction to the dye, and death (Fleury and Murdaugh, 1993).

Single-vessel disease remains the classic indication for PTCA. This procedure best treats fixed, noncalcified lesions in the proximal two thirds of the coronary circulation that are accessible for dilatation.

Stenosis of the left mainstem artery is considered unacceptable for dilatation (Fleury and Murdaugh, 1993).

Complications. The most common major complication of PTCA is coronary artery dissection, which is reported in approximately 5% of patients; in addition, myocardial ischemia may occur from coronary artery spasm, coronary embolization, or intimal trauma. Associated minor complications include bradycardia, ventricular fibrillation, hypotension, and vascular complications (Fleury and Murdaugh, 1993).

Directional Coronary Atherectomy. Directional coronary atherectomy is an alternative to PTCA. This procedure not only compresses the atherosclerotic plaque but also shaves it off the vessel wall and removes it (Grab, 1992). A candidate for directional coronary atherectomy must have myocardial ischemia that is confirmed by treadmill stress test or angina that is unresponsive to pharmacological agents. Directional coronary atherectomy is not performed on distal le-

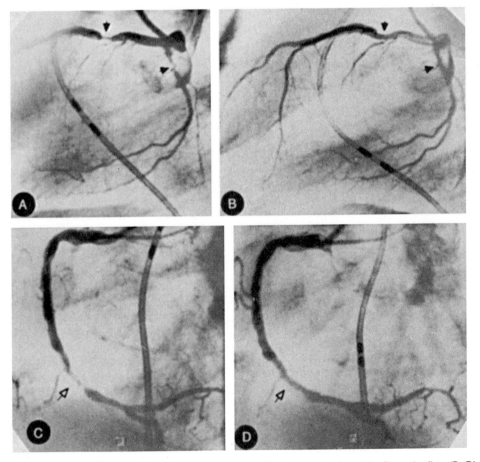

Figure 9–11. Radiographs of patients with triple-vessel disease with images before *(A, C)* and after *(B, D)* angioplasty. (Adapted from Stertzer, S. H., et al. (1989). The setting of coronary angioplasty in multivessel disease: Current status and future directions. *Cardiology Clinics, 7*(4), 773.)

sions or on tortuous or severely calcified vessels. In the catheterization lab, a cardiologist inserts an arterial sheath for catheter placement. The patient's vessel is occluded by inflation of the balloon that anchors the catheter in place. A guide wire is forwarded until the catheter's distal tip reaches the atheroma. After the balloon is inflated, the cutter is advanced, a process that shaves the plaque from the vessel wall. Some devices have a central coaxial guide wire with a flexible shaft that is propelled by an air turbine, of which the distal half is fitted with diamond chips and the proximal half is smooth; the rotational speeds of the device range from 190,000 to 200,000 rpm (Murphy et al., 1994). Debris and tissue fragments are captured in the end of the catheter. Usually, two passes with the cutter are made, but the process may continue until the stenosis is significantly reduced or the cutter fails to shave any more debris from the vessel wall.

Complications. Assessments are performed frequently for complications such as vessel perforation, plaque or air embolism, and acute vessel closure (Grab, 1992). Depending on the type of directional coronary atherectomy performed, vessel perforation can result from too deep a shaving. The most severe complication, acute vessel closure, is caused by arterial spasm, thrombus formation, or vessel dissection.

Intracoronary Stent. Intracoronary stents are tubes that are implanted at the site of stenosis in order to widen the arterial lumen by squeezing atherosclerotic plaque against the artery's walls (as does PTCA). However, the stent can also keep the lumen open by providing structural support (Strimike, 1995). Stent designs differ, but most are springs or slotted or mesh tubes about 15 mm long, with some resembling the spiral bindings used in notebooks. These are tightly wrapped around a balloon catheter, which is inflated in order to implant the stent. The procedure for placing a stent is similar to the procedure in PTCA, in which the patient first undergoes cardiac catheterization and angiography for identification of occlusions in coronary arteries. The balloon catheter bearing the stent is inserted into the coronary artery, and the stent is positioned at the desired site. The balloon is inflated, thereby expanding the stent, which squeezes the atherosclerotic plaque and intimal flaps against the vessel wall. After the balloon is deflated and removed, the stent remains, holding the plaque and other matter in place and providing structural support that keeps the artery from collapsing (Strimike, 1995). Aggressive anticoagulation therapy before, during, and after the procedure is necessary for the prevention of coagulation. Before sheath removal, peripheral perfusion is monitored because the sheath may cause occlusion of the femoral artery. Peripheral pulses, skin color, and temperature are monitored every 30 minutes for the first 2 hours and then hourly for the next 4 hours, then every 2 hours for 8 hours and then every 4 hours. The insertion site is inspected for any oozing or bleeding on the same schedule. After sheath removal, hemostasis is maintained with manual pressure, a C-clamp, or a femoral compression arch. Retroperitoneal bleeding or impaired perfusion may occur after sheath removal. Pain management and proper hydration aid in recovery. Reocclusion most often occurs within 3 to 9 days after stent implantation. Symptoms indicating reocclusion include chest pain, shortness of breath, diaphoresis, and nausea. At times, ECG monitoring is performed until the patient is discharge so that ST-segment changes can be detected (Strimike, 1995).

Excimer Laser Coronary Angioplasty. Excimer laser coronary angioplasty involves the use of a very flexible catheter to treat distal disease in torturous coronary arteries. *Laser* is an acronym for light amplification by stimulated emission of radiation. With excimer lasers, various gases that make up the lasing medium (e.g., neon, xenon, and hydrogen chloride) are unnaturally bound with energy to create excited dimers, which generate laser light when separated. This beam is delivered through a multifiber catheter made of 50 to 100 thin optical or glass fibers arranged around a central lumen that is used for the passage of a guide wire. The ultraviolet energy wavelengths result in photochemical tissue vaporization that dissipates between pulses. This phenomenon allows precise cuts to atheroma, collagen, or calcium without injuring surrounding tissue or causing possible dissection of the arterial wall (Albert, 1994).

Surgical Approach

Surgical approaches used for patients with MI resulting from CAD include coronary revascularization by CABG.

Coronary Artery Bypass Graft. This is a surgical procedure in which the ischemic area or areas of the myocardium are revascularized by implantation of the internal mammary artery or bypassing of the coronary occlusion with a saphenous vein graft. A harvested vessel is anastomosed between the aortic root and a point distal to the obstructing coronary lesion or stenosis (Coleman et al., 1993). The internal mammary artery is usually used on the left anterior descending artery because of the internal mammary artery's long-term patency rate. The indications for CABG are chronic stable angina that is refractory to other therapies, significant left main coronary occlusion (> 50%), triple-vessel CAD, unstable angina pectoris, acute MI, intractable ventricular irritability, left ventricular failure, and failure of PTCA (Coleman et al., 1993).

Coronary artery bypass grafting is performed in the operating room while the patient receives general anesthesia and is intubated. A midsternal, longitudinal incision is made into the chest cavity. The patient is put on cardiopulmonary bypass during the procedure. The coronary arteries are visualized, and a segment of the saphenous vein is grafted or anastomosed to the distal end of the vessel with the proximal end of the graft vessel anastomosed to the aorta. The internal mammary artery can also be used for creating an artery-to-artery graft. Internal mammary revascularization has been shown to have better long-term patency than saphenous vein grafts. It is the preferred graft to lesions of the LAD. The cardiopulmonary bypass is progressively discontinued, chest and mediastinal tubes are inserted, and the chest is closed (Fig. 9–12).

Chest and Mediastinal Tubes. When the chest is opened for heart surgery, the pleural space may be disrupted. If disruption occurs, the accumulation of air or fluid prevents the development of negative pressure necessary for normal respiration. Chest tubes are inserted for the removal of the air or fluid and for the restoration of the normal negative pressure of the pleural space. The tube is connected to an underwater seal drainage apparatus that prevents backflow into the

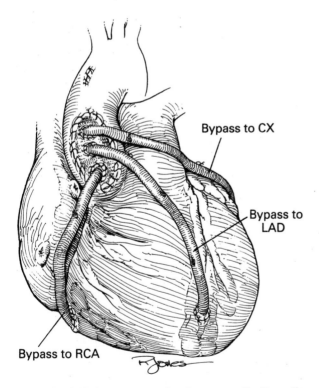

Figure 9–12. Triple coronary artery bypass graft with aortic patch. CX = circumflex; LAD = left anterior descending; RCA = right coronary artery. (Adapted from Cooley, D. A. (1984). *Techniques in cardiac surgery* (2nd ed.). Philadelphia: W. B. Saunders Co.)

pleural space. The tube placed underwater creates a negative pressure. The air or fluid in the chest drains into the apparatus or bottle in an attempt to equalize the negative pressure in the bottle. Air escapes through an air vent in the chest bottle, thereby preventing pressure build-up. Fluid or blood draining from the chest cavity drains into the bottle and, if it drains in large amounts, may necessitate a second collection bottle. Suction may be added to the system to facilitate air removal. The system must remain patent and functioning at all times. Therefore, the chest tube is not to be clamped, or a tension pneumothorax could result. The chest is radiographed so that the correctness of placement can be determined. Once the lungs have adequately reexpanded and negative pressure has been reestablished in the pleural cavity, the chest is radiographed again for final verification of expansion, and the chest tube is removed. An occlusive pressure dressing is applied to the tube insertion site.

Complications. Cardiac tamponade is a complication that must be considered after CABG. Cardiac tamponade is the collection of fluid in the posterior pericardial sac or mediastinal space. The blood returning from the great vessels to the heart and the ejection of blood from the ventricles are obstructed by the fluid collecting in the sac, which compromises cardiac filling. Signs of cardiac tamponade include decreased cardiac output, increased PCWP, decreased arterial pressures, marked decrease in mediastinal tube drainage, mediastinal widening on chest x-ray study, distant heart sounds, narrowing pulse pressure, and decreased ECG voltage (Coleman et al., 1993). This is a life-threatening emergency that requires immediate surgical intervention.

Autotransfusion. This is a procedure that can be used during thoracic and cardiovascular surgery. The patient's own blood is collected, filtered, and reinfused back to the patient in order to minimize use of blood from the blood bank and its potential complications. Regional anticoagulants, such as citrate-phosphate-dextrose, acid-phosphate-dextrose, and heparin, are added to the autotransfusion collection system. The blood may be reinfused to the patient as whole blood or as packed red blood cells. Complications include coagulation problems, hemolysis, air embolus, and sepsis. Autotransfusion can also be performed after open heart surgery through collection of the blood from the mediastinal tubes. Anticoagulation in this instance is not warranted. It is imperative that the reinfusion apparatus remove all the air and filter out all clots from the blood before the blood is returned to the patient.

Intra-aortic Balloon Pump. The use of intra-aortic balloon pump counterpulsation may be seen in the patient who has had an MI, has had severe dysrhythmias or cardiogenic shock (see Chapter 8), and is awaiting surgery, and the patient with acute left ventricular power failure after heart surgery (Fig. 9–13).

Cardiac Transplantation. Cardiac transplantation is a therapeutic option for patients with end-stage dilated cardiomyopathy. Patients with ejection fractions of no more than 25% are offered transplantation in order to prolong survival. Other criteria for patient selection are severe cardiac disease despite tailored medical therapy, no other reasonable surgical option, and upper age limit of 55 to 65 years with the ability to understand and comprehend medical regimen after transplantation and an absence of relative contraindications (Cardin, 1993).

Radiofrequency Catheter Ablation. Radiofrequency catheter ablation is a method of interrupting a supraventricular tachycardia of a dysrhythmia caused by reentry circuit. The objective of catheter ablation is to permanently interrupt electrical conduction or activity in a region of arrhythmogenic cardiac tissue

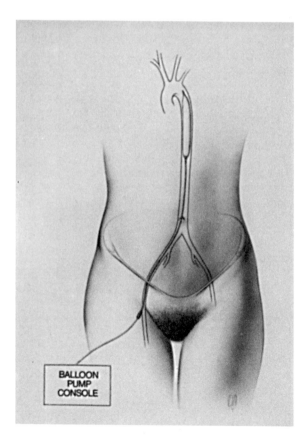

Figure 9–13. Correct positioning of percutaneous intra-aortic balloon pump in descending thoracic aorta. (Adapted from Shoemaker, W. C. (1989). *Textbook of critical care* (2nd ed.). Philadelphia: W. B. Saunders Co.)

(Teplitz, 1994). Radiofrequency catheter ablation is successful in abolishing occurrences of supraventricular tachycardia because it is curative and is performed percutaneously. Indications for radiofrequency catheter ablation include the presence of two conducting pathways, which are in competition with each other, causing reentrant tachycardias. Radiofrequency catheter ablation begins with a diagnostic electrophysiology study. With a catheter positioned at the accessory pathway (and confirmed by AV pathway recording), current passes through the electrical resistance of the cardiac tissue, causing coagulation necrosis in the conduction fibers without destroying the surrounding tissue. After each ablation attempt, the patient is retested until there is no recurrence of the tachycardia (Guaglianone and Tyndall, 1995).

Permanent Pacemakers. When a patient is admitted with an acute MI with the potential for serious bradydysrhythmias as a result of a block in the conducting system of the heart, temporary pacing is instituted. If a block persists beyond the acute phase, a permanent pacemaker is usually implanted.

In the United States, more than 300 types of pacemakers are manufactured by numerous companies. Most pacemakers are multiprogrammable for rates, voltage, sensitivities, stimulus duration, and refractory periods. Many implanted pacemakers are of the ventricular demand type and have the variability to coincide with the patient's changing needs.

Pacemaker functions are described in a code developed in 1987 by the North American Society for Pacing and Electro-physiology. The code is used to denote the capabilities of the pacemaker as programmed for an individual patient. The code originally had three letters, was updated to five, but is more commonly seen with the original three letters denoting the chambers paced, the chamber sensed, and the mode of response (Table 9–6).

The type of pacemaker that stimulates the heart at a constant rate regardless of any present cardiac rhythm is termed *demand*. If it is attached to the atrium, the pacemaker is coded AOO, and if it is applied to the ventricles, it is coded VOO (see Table 9–6 for an explanation of codes). Pacing devices that have the ability to sense as well as respond are classified as *atrial* or *ventricular* pacemakers and are coded AAI, AAT, VVI, and VVT, depending on their placement and inhibiting or triggering activity.

For patients with an acute MI resulting in an AV conduction disturbance, type II AV block, or complete heart block, a pacemaker labeled as an atrial synchronous ventricular pacemaker may be implanted. These are coded VAT and VDD. For patients with bradycardia in addition to an AV conduction disturbance, the pacemaker may be coded DVI, meaning that it senses

Table 9–6. FIVE-POSITION GENERIC (NASPE/BPEG) PACEMAKER CODE

I Chamber Paced	II Chamber Sensed	III Mode of Response	IV Programmable Functions	V Special Tachyarrhythmia Functions
O—None	O—None	O—None	O—None	O—None
A—Atrium	A—Atrium	T—Triggered	P—Simple	P—Pacing
V—Ventricle	V—Ventricle	I—Inhibited	programmable	S—Shock
D—Dual	D—Dual	D—Dual	M—Multiprogrammable	D—Dual
			C—Communicating	
			R—Rate Modulation	

NASPE = North American Society of Pacing and Electrophysiology; BPEG = British Pacing and Electrophysiology Group; NBG–NASPE, BPEG Group.

ventricular activity only but paces both the atria and the ventricles. One of the most current and popular pacing devices used is classified as the universal pacemaker, and it is coded DDD. It has multiple functions. The universal, or fully automatic, pacemaker senses and paces both atria and ventricles and varies the ventricular rate according to the atrial rate. The DDD pacemaker is indicated in patients with complete AV block with or without the sick sinus syndrome.

Most permanent pacemakers use lithium batteries as their power source. These models have a longevity of 8 to 10 years in a system that can be sealed in order to prevent erosion by body fluids and leakage of battery materials. A permanent pacemaker can be inserted in a transvenous mode by use of local anesthesia, with the lead wires traversing through the cephalic vein and the implantation of the device on the right side of the chest. This procedure may be performed in the operating room, but it is commonly performed in the cardiac catheterization laboratory or special procedures area of the radiology department.

Implantable Cardioverter-Defibrillator. The implantable cardioverter-defibrillator (ICD) is an implantable device for detecting and treating ventricular tachycardia or ventricular fibrillation. It is used for patients with one or more sudden cardiac death episodes that are not associated with acute MI or any reversible cause or drug-refractory sustained ventricular tachycardia or ventricular fibrillation (Sirovatka, 1993). It consists of a pulse generator, one or two sensing electrode leads, and an anode and a cathode for cardioversion or defibrillation. The rate-sensing lead consists of a transvenous bipolar lead placed in the right ventricular apex or two myocardial leads screwed onto the left ventricle. The defibrillating lead consists of two patches, one usually placed at the junction of the superior vena cava and the right atrium and the other placed on the left ventricle. Median sternotomy and lateral thoracotomy are the most inva-

sive approaches for device placement and require chest tube drainage. Less invasive procedures, such as subxyphoid or the endocardial system, are often associated with incisional ecchymosis and edema (Sirovatka, 1993).

The ICD comes with an identification card that specifies the heart rate at which shocks occur; this card is given to the patient. This identification card, which also names the manufacturer and model number of the ICD and the telephone numbers of the manufacturer and the primary physician, should be carried with the patient. Bimonthly or quarterly clinic visits are important for the monitoring of ICD function. ICD batteries are predicted to last 2 to 5 years. The nursing care of a patient who is to receive either of these devices, pacemaker or ICD, begins with educating the patient and family in its mechanism of action.

Standard emergency procedures are to be followed with patients who have these devices and suffer cardiovascular collapse. Under no circumstances should cardiopulmonary resuscitation be delayed because the patient has an implanted device. Instead, a magnet may be taped over the generator box in order to temporarily disable the device, and external paddle placement may be modified (Porterfield and Porterfield, 1995). Placement of paddles for these patients is usually anteroposterior rather than sternal-apex.

Third-generation ICDs have backup VVI pacing capabilities. Other advantages and goals for patients with these ICDs include rapid-pacing therapy, improved patient tolerance, prevention of hemodynamic compromise, decreased length of hospital stay, and potential for return to previous lifestyle and activities. ICDs have the ability to terminate ventricular tachycardia via overdrive ventricular pacing, to pace bradycardias, to obtain noninvasive electrophysiological studies via the use of the programmer, monitor gradual increases in rate, to provide lower energy cardioversion, to deliver high-energy shocks as used in defibrillation, and to assist in diagnosis as a result of its memory capabilities (Rasmussen and Mangan, 1994).

Patient and family education about the device includes (Rasmussen and Mangan, 1994)

- Implantable cardioverter-defibrillator/pace-maker function
- Preprocedural teaching
- Response to symptoms
- Diary of events
- Emergency information and plan
- Follow-up care
- Safety measures
- Activities after implantation
- Precautions
- Additional electrophysiological studies
- Replacement procedure
- Family responsibilities
- Patient and family support groups and services

OUTCOMES

Patient outcomes or goals are generalized in order to encompass the wide spectrum of patients who have experienced an MI, uncomplicated or complicated, that requires medical or surgical intervention. The patient will

- Verbalize an absence of chest pain through hemodynamic stability
- Demonstrate stable or improved cardiac output and cardiac index
- Demonstrate reduced anxiety levels
- Along with family and/or support system, demonstrate increased understanding of the disease process and of health management through education and interactive discussion
- Have minimized or absence of complications.

A suggested nursing care plan for the patient with myocardial infarction follows.

Congestive Heart Failure

Left-sided CHF is second only to dysrhythmias as the most common mechanical complication after an MI. In CHF, the pumping capability of the heart is altered, and the metabolic and oxygen needs of the body are affected (Miller, 1994). CHF is most commonly a complication of acute MI, but CHF can also be a complication of CAD or hypertension. Ischemia of the left ventricle can cause the left ventricle not to empty during systole. Diastolic filling increases, and eventually, the volume in the left ventricle is so full that the pressure elevation is reflected backward into the left atrium and pulmonary veins, causing pulmonary congestion (Miller, 1994). CHF is a clinical state

in which the heart is unable to maintain the cardiac output necessary for meeting the body's metabolic demands. In healthy, sedentary subjects between 30 and 80 years of age, resting cardiac output reportedly decreases 1% annually, whereas systolic function is usually preserved (Hixon, 1994). The classic symptomatology of heart failure consists of progressive exertional dyspnea, paroxysmal nocturnal dyspnea, and orthopnea with fatigue, loss of appetite, and organ system dysfunction as the failure advances (Hixon, 1994).

PATHOPHYSIOLOGY

Left-sided heart failure is the inability of the left ventricle to maintain an adequate cardiac output. It is a syndrome or symptom of a physiologically abnormal left ventricle and not a disease process itself. The pathology occurs in a fairly sequential pattern. The left ventricle cannot pump effectively or efficiently, usually as a result of loss of muscle tissue from ischemia (MI). The ineffective pumping action causes a decrease in the cardiac output. The volume of blood remaining in the left ventricle increases after each beat. As this volume builds, it backs up into the left atrium and pulmonary veins and into the lungs. Eventually, fluid accumulates in the lungs and pleural spaces, causing increased pressure in the lungs. Gas exchange (oxygen and carbon dioxide) in the pulmonary system is impaired. The backflow can continue on into the right ventricle and right atrium and into the systemic circulation. This type of failure is known as right-sided failure. As a compensatory mechanism, with an increase in the carbon dioxide levels in the lungs, the respiratory rate increases in order to help eliminate the excess carbon dioxide. This phenomenon causes the heart rate to increase, pumping more blood to the pulmonary tree for the carbon dioxide–oxygen exchange. The increased heart rate results in the pumping of more blood from the systemic circulation into the cardiopulmonary circulation, which is already dangerously overloaded.

Another method of describing CHF is impairment of diastolic and systolic heart functions, a condition that leads to a decrease in cardiac output. As a result, the sympathetic nervous system is activated. This activation

- Produces tachycardia, thereby decreasing preload and contributing to a further decrease in cardiac output
- Causes vasoconstriction, which increases afterload, thereby contributing to a further decrease in cardiac output
- Increases contractility, which increases myocardial oxygen demand, thereby decreasing contractility and possibly decreasing cardiac output

NURSING CARE PLAN FOR THE PATIENT WITH MYOCARDIAL INFARCTION

Nursing Diagnosis	Patient Outcomes	Nursing Interventions
Pain related to myocardial ischemia or necrosis.	Will verbalize absence or relief of chest pain. Will display reduced tension/ relaxed manner.	Determine how client usually responds to pain. Assess description of pain and factors that aggravate pain (e.g., respiration) Implement bed rest; use position of comfort. Provide supplemental oxygen. Administer medications and note response: Analgesics—morphine Nitrates—NTG Beta-blockers—propranolol (Inderal) Calcium channel blockers—nifedipine (Procardia). Monitor blood pressure (BP). Use nonpharmacological pain relief techniques: Train patient in relaxation techniques. Provide quiet, restful environment. Encourage periods of rest and sleep. Organize care to allow for rest periods.
Decreased cardiac output related to loss of myocardial contractility.	Will demonstrate stable or improved cardiac output. Will have cardiac rate, rhythm, and hemodynamic measurements within normal limits. Will have absence of dysrhythmias. Will have absence of pain with activity.	Implement bed rest. Assess and report signs and symptoms of decreased cardiac output, e.g., ↓ BP, ↑ heart rate, ↓ urine output, fatigue, weakness; cool, pale, clammy skin. Monitor BP, apical pulse, temperature, respirations every 2 to 4 hours and as needed. Monitor cardiac rhythm; check strips every 4 to 6 hours and as needed. Administer supplemental oxygen. Auscultate breath sounds every 4 to 6 hours. Auscultate heart sounds every 4 to 6 hours; watch for development of S_3 and S_4. Implement measures to improve cardiac output and reduce cardiac workload. Administer nitrates, beta-blockers, calcium channel blockers, antiarrhythmics, and/or anticoagulants as ordered. Monitor laboratory data: serum enzyme levels—LDH_1-LDH_2 flip, creatine kinase-MB, aspartate transaminase, arterial blood gases, electrolyte levels. Monitor pulmonary artery pressure, pulmonary capillary wedge pressure, central venous pressure. Review 12-lead electrocardiography. Intake and output every 2 to 4 hours. Monitor administration of intravenous fluids. Administer medications and note response: Inotropic—dobutamine (Dobutrex) Nitrates—NTG Diuretics—furosemide (Lasix) Antiarrhythmics—disopyramide (Norpace), procainamide (Pronestyl), lidocaine, phenytoin (Dilantin), propranolol (Inderal), bretylium (Bretylol), verapamil, nifedipine (Procardia), diltiazem (Cardizem) Monitor diet—low fat, low sodium; small, frequent feedings; avoid ice and caffeine. Encourage patient to avoid the Valsalva maneuver—provide laxative or stool softener. Promote rest by providing quiet environment, and balancing activity and rest periods.

Continued on following page

NURSING CARE PLAN FOR THE PATIENT WITH MYOCARDIAL INFARCTION *Continued*

Nursing Diagnosis	Patient Outcomes	Nursing Interventions
Anxiety related to perceived or actual threat of biological integrity.	Will verbalize reduced anxiety level. Will demonstrate effective coping mechanisms. Will participate in treatment and rehabilitation regimen.	Provide comfort and education measures, e.g., provide quiet environment, relaxation techniques; acknowledge feelings of fear; orient patient and support system to procedures and surroundings; answer questions factually; encourage communication. Monitor and minimize contact of patient with anxious family members. Administer sedatives—diazepam (Valium), flurazepam (Dalmane), lorazepam (Ativan). Encourage expression of feelings and anxieties—reassure the patient as appropriate with a calm voice, repeat information frequently.
Knowledge deficit regarding disease process.	Patient and/or support group will demonstrate increased understanding of disease process and health management through interactive discussion. Possible lifestyle changes will be identified in preparation for discharge.	Review patient understanding of his or her cardiac condition. Explain extent of infarct; associated complications; dysrhythmias; angina; post–myocardial infarction syndrome; congestive heart failure; nature of disease process, including risk factors and factors precipitating angina. Explain the importance of rest and of balancing progressive activity with rest. Review importance of controlling existing conditions that aggravate coronary artery disease and inhibit recovery, e.g., hyperlipidemia, hypertension, diabetes. Encourage patient to control weight; lose weight if necessary. Explain importance of using techniques to manage stress. Review importance of physical activity, e.g., walking, jogging, swimming, and when to place limitations and restrictions. Avoid or modify activity after heavy meals, alcohol consumption, emotional stress, extreme temperatures, or temperature change. Encourage independence in self-care. Encourage communication of patient with family and/or support group. Review coping mechanisms for possibility of role change in family group. Review allowances and limitations of sexual activity. Discuss signs and symptoms of myocardial infarction versus angina. Explain importance of calling physician if chest pain lasts more than 20 minutes and is unrelieved by NTG. Review principles of cardiac rehabilitation: Diet; avoid caffeine, tobacco; limit certain foods (eggs, cream, butter, foods high in animal fat); rest after meals. Medication; name, dosage, time, purpose, side effects. Avoid over-the-counter medication until it is cleared by physician. Avoid constipation and straining at stool. Avoid sitting in same position for extended periods of time. Exercise program; at regular intervals, follow prescribed program, incorporate home exercise program. Check with physician regarding resumption of sexual activity, travel, driving. Avoid isometric-type exercise, heavy lifting, and pushing.

Data from Carpenito, L. J: *Handbook of nursing diagnosis 1989–90.* Philadelphia, J. B. Lippincott, 1989; Guzzetta, C. E., and Dossey, B. M.: *Cardiovascular nursing: Bodymind tapestry.* St. Louis, C. V. Mosby, 1984: Johanson, B. C., et al.: *Standards for critical care.* St. Louis, C. V. Mosby, 1988: Moorhouse, M. F., et al.: *Critical care plans: Guidelines for patient care.* Philadelphia, F. A. Davis, 1987.

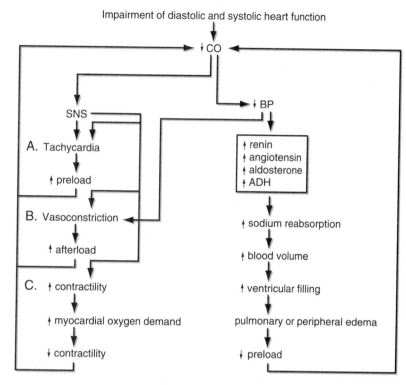

Impairment of diastolic and systolic heart function

Figure 9-14. Coronary artery distribution. CO = cardiac output; BP = blood pressure; SNS = sympathetic nervous system; ADH = antidiuretic hormone.

Simultaneous with the stimulation of the sympathetic nervous system is a decrease in blood pressure, which occurs as a result of a decrease in cardiac output. The kidneys respond to hypotension by increasing renin output, which increases angiotensin to increase aldosterone to increase antidiuretic hormone secretion. This chemical chain of events can lead to vasoconstriction, which, as mentioned previously, increases afterload, thereby decreasing cardiac output. Additionally, sodium reabsorption increases, which in turn increases blood volume, thereby increasing ventricular filling. However, in a patient with impaired diastolic and systolic heart function, signs and symptoms of pulmonary or peripheral edema may manifest, which in turn decreases preload and further compounds an already decreasing cardiac output (Miller, 1994) (Fig. 9-14).

ASSESSMENT

Patient assessment includes the assessment of the cause of both right-sided and left-sided failure, the signs and symptoms, and the precipitating factors as well as diagnostic studies.

Etiology

The causes of CHF include (Miller, 1994)

- Decreased inflow of blood to the heart, such as through hemorrhage or dehydration
- Increased inflow of blood to the heart, such as through excessive administration of IV fluids or sodium and water retention
- Obstructed outflow of blood from heart, such as from damaged valves, narrowed arteries, or hypertension
- Damaged heart muscle, such as from MI or inflammatory processes
- Increased metabolic needs, such as from fever, pregnancy, hyperthyroidism, or chronic anemia (Table 9-7)

Precipitating Factors

Precipitating factors for CHF include MI, dysrhythmias (especially severe tachycardia or bradycardia), severe overexertion, sudden increase in environmental heat or humidity, anemia, thyrotoxicosis, and pregnancy and childbirth.

RESEARCH APPLICATION

Article Reference

Carson, M. M., Barton, D. M., Morrison, C. C., & Tribble, C. G. (1994). Managing pain during mediastinal chest tube removal. *Heart and Lung, 23*(6), 500-505.

Review of Study Methods and Findings

The objective of this study was to compare four analgesic regimens used in preparing patients for chest tube removal. A prospective, randomized, controlled multiple-group comparison of 80 adult patients who underwent heart surgery and who had two mediastinal chest tubes inserted rated pain intensity on a zero- to 100-mm visual analogue scale and described sensations during chest tube removal to six nurses. Before chest tube removal, the subjects were medicated with (1) intravenous morphine sulfate, (2) intravenous morphine and subfascial angiocatheter lidocaine hydrochloride, (3) intravenous morphine and subfascial angiocatheter normal saline solution, or (4) subfascial angiocatheter lidocaine. Mean pain rating scores for groups 1, 2, 3, and 4 were 43.7, 40.9, 36.4, and 38.1, respectively. Analysis of variance showed no significant difference between scores ($P < 0.05$). The percentage of comments rated as ``not bad at all'' or ``not bad'' for groups 1, 2, 3, and 4 were 56%, 83%, 47%, and 75%, respectively. Chi-squared analysis showed a significant difference between ratings ($P < .01$). Ratings of subjects' descriptions of sensations suggested that subfascial lidocaine may be useful in reducing discomfort during chest tube removal.

Brief Critique of Study Strengths/Weaknesses

One of the strengths of the study was that statistical power analysis was performed in order to determine the number of subjects needed in each of the four study groups. Another strength was that the nurses responsible for medication administration and data collection did not know which treatment method was used, nor did the patient. In ad- dition, the nurse administering the medication had no concurrent patient care responsibilities.

A recognized weakness of the study was that eight different physicians were involved in removing chest tubes over the course of the study. It is unknown if a difference existed based on who removed the chest tube. The authors recognized this as a limitation.

The variation in time for removal of chest tubes after analgesics (5 to 15 minutes) may not have been sufficient for the analgesic to work. The onset of action is rapid for morphine and lidocaine but 20 minutes may be required for peak serum concentrations to be reached.

The validity and reliability of the visual analogue scale was reported in the article as established by a variety of techniques; however, the variety of techniques was not reported in this study. In the second instrument, the subjective comments were transcribed verbatim, yet six nurses were then asked to rate the statements by use of five categories. Because pain is subjective and is whatever the patient says it is, the patient's themselves may have been better at giving one of these statements and circling their personal response rather than the method used, which carries the potential of translation error. Investigators noted that some patients did not respond verbally regarding sensation.

Implications of the Study for Nursing Practice

The implications of this study for nursing include encouraging the use of alternate methods for the reduction of pain and anxiety in patients undergoing chest tube removal. Repetition of this study is warranted in order to attempt to control for the variability in personnel who removed the chest tube. The investigators' conclusion is that subfascial lidocaine may be useful in reducing discomfort during chest tube removal.

Table 9–7. CAUSES, SIGNS, AND SYMPTOMS OF RIGHT-SIDED AND LEFT-SIDED HEART FAILURE

Left-Sided Heart Failure	Right-Sided Heart Failure
Specific Causes	
Coronary heart disease	End result of left-sided heart failure
Myocardial infarction	Pulmonary hypertension
Hypertension	Results of right ventricular infarction
Signs and Symptoms	
Anxiety	Dependent edema
Air hunger	Jugular venous distention
Dyspnea/orthopnea	Bounding pulses
Diaphoresis	Oliguria
Crackles/wheezes	Dysrhythmias
Cyanosis	Increased central venous pressure
Increased heart rate	Liver engorgement and tenderness
Elevated pulmonary capillary wedge	Enlarged spleen
pressure (18–25 mm Hg or higher)	Decreased appetite, nausea, vomiting
S_3, and S_4 (gallop)*	
Dysrhythmias	

*In left-sided heart failure, the detection of an S_3 or gallop rhythm is an important early sign. Detection of the S_3 sound and observation of other signs can precipitate early and aggressive management of impending congestive heart failure in order to prevent further problems and complications.

Diagnostic studies that are paramount for the diagnosis and competent treatment of the patient suspected of having CHF include

- A complete history and physical examination incorporating all of the aforementioned assessment measures, signs and symptoms, and precipitating factors.
- Chest x-ray study in order to view the heart size and configuration and to check the lung fields to determine if they are clear or opaque (fluid filled). The procedure can be performed in the radiology department, or if the patient is too unstable, the x-ray study may be portable.
- Increased PCWP or central venous pressure on hemodynamic monitoring. The PCWP reflects left ventricular function; the central venous pressure reflects right ventricle function (see Chapter 5).
- Laboratory studies, specifically ABGs, which may indicate acidosis or alkalosis.
- Liver function test results. The liver can become congested, and may enlarge and become tender, with ascites and/or jaundice becoming noticeable. Liver function is diminished (Chernecky et al., 1993).

NURSING DIAGNOSES

Nursing diagnoses and interventions for the patient with CHF include the following.

Decreased Cardiac Output Related to Decreased Myocardial Contractility

- Administer oxygen.
- Position patient with head of the bed elevated if the patient's blood pressure is stable.
- Administer medications, such as IV dopamine, dobutamine, and amrinone (Inocor) or oral digoxin or digitalis.
- Monitor vital signs and hemodynamic measurements every 15 minutes until the patient is stable; then monitor every hour.
- Monitor urine output every hour.
- Administer vasodilators, such as morphine, nitroprusside, NTG, captopril, hydralazine, and isosorbide, if the patient is normovolemic.
- Administer diuretics as ordered, such as furosemide (Lasix).
- Monitor serum electrolyte levels and ABG results every 6 hours until the patient is stable.
- Administer and monitor the effects of IV fluids, with particular attention paid to recurring signs of CHF.
- Provide quiet environment.
- Provide for periods of uninterrupted sleep.

Decreased Cardiac Output Related to Increased Afterload

- Administer vasodilators, such as nitrates, nitroprusside, hydralazine, minoxidil, and prazosin, as ordered. Vasodilators are used in patients who have had an MI who do not respond to diuretics alone. These agents reduce preload and afterload, improve cardiac output, and relieve myocardial ischemia. Complications include hypotension, tachycardia, reduced cardiac output, and compromised peripheral perfusion (Ulrich et al., 1994).

- Monitor vital signs and hemodynamic measurements every 15 minutes until the patient is stable; then monitor every hour.
- Administer pain medication as needed.
- Provide relaxing environment and encourage sleep.
- Provide sedation as needed.

Impaired Gas Exchange Related to Ventilation-Perfusion Imbalance

- Administer oxygen as ordered.
- Elevate head of bed if patient's blood pressure is stable.
- Monitor ABG results every 4 hours until they are stable.
- Assess breath sounds every 2 hours.
- Instruct patient in deep-breathing techniques.
- Monitor fluid balance, such as through daily weighings and hourly input and output monitoring.
- Monitor hematocrit and hemoglobin values daily for anemia.
- Monitor and treat hyperthermia.
- Provide for rest and sleep.

Risk for Fluid Volume Deficit Related to Excessive Diureses

- Monitor intake and output every hour.
- Monitor patient's response to diuretic.
- Monitor patient's daily weights.
- Instruct patient and family on importance of oral fluid restriction.

Risk for Injury: Dysrhythmias Related to Electrolyte Imbalance

- Monitor electrolyte and acid-base balance.
- Administer potassium as ordered.
- Monitor intake and output.
- Monitor ECG for signs of hypokalemia and hyperkalemia and digitalis toxicity.

Activity Intolerance Related to Generalized Weakness and Imbalance Between Oxygen Supply and Demand

- Maintain oxygen saturation during activities as needed.
- Balance activities with rest periods.
- Encourage independence through assistive devices and energy conservation.

- Monitor response to exercise and gradually increase activity.
- Assist patient as needed while encouraging independence (Ulrich et al., 1994).

INTERVENTIONS

Medical and nursing interventions for the patient with CHF consist of a threefold approach: treatment of the existing symptoms of the crisis situation, prevention of further or expanding complications, and treatment of the underlying cause.

Treatment of existing symptoms includes

1. Improvement pump function through positive inotropic medications (dopamine, dobutamine) and cardiotonics (digoxin).

- Reduction of cardiac workload and oxygen consumption by
- Avoidance of anxiety-provoking situations
- Elevation of head of bed
- Scheduling of rest periods
- Modification of activities of daily living
- Ordering of vasodilators, such as NTG, captopril, and morphine

2. Use of the intra-aortic balloon pump in severe CHF and cardiogenic shock to augment diastole, decrease afterload, and improve perfusion to the coronary arteries and vital organs.

3. Optimization of gas exchange through supplemental oxygen, diuresis, and monitoring of ABGs.

- Control of sodium and water retention
- Diuresis and/or diuretics, such as furosemide, chlorothiazide (Diuril), and bumetanide (Bumex)
- Fluid restriction (oral)
- Careful IV fluid administration
- Low-sodium diet
- Removal of fluid through thoracentesis, paracentesis, dialysis

4. Administration of adequate nutrition through low-calorie, low-residue, bland small feedings.

5. Monitoring of cardiac output and pump function through hemodynamic monitoring measurements (Hixon, 1994; Miller, 1994).

COMPLICATIONS

Complications of CHF can be critical. Interventions must be provided in order to avoid extending the existing conditions or allowing the development of new, life-threatening complications. Two specific complications for which the patient are monitored are pulmonary edema and cardiogenic shock.

Pulmonary Edema

Pulmonary edema is an acute, life-threatening form of CHF. The pulmonary vascular system becomes so full and engorged that fluid seeps out of the vessels into the lung spaces. For example, in an acute MI, when the primary injury is to the left ventricle, thereby decreasing the pumping ability of the left ventricle without compromising the pumping action of the right ventricle, a temporary imbalance results in the output of the two pumps. The right ventricle continues to pump blood into the pulmonary system and the left side of the heart, and the left ventricle has increasing difficulty pumping the blood volume into the systemic circulation. The result is increasing volume and pressure of blood in pulmonary vessels, increasing pressure in pulmonary capillaries, and leaking of fluid into the interstitial spaces of lung tissue.

Pulmonary edema greatly reduces the amount of lung tissue space available for gas exchange and results in clinical symptoms of extreme dyspnea, cyanosis, severe anxiety, diaphoresis, pallor, and blood-tinged, frothy sputum (Miller, 1994). ABG results indicate a severe respiratory acidosis and hypoxemia. Pulmonary edema is treated by improving gas exchange through the administration of oxygen and aminophylline, decreasing intravascular volume by use of diuretics, and decreasing venous return by positioning the patient in a high Fowler's position and administration of IV morphine (which increases venous capacitance), and rotating tourniquets (which are rarely used).

Cardiogenic Shock

Cardiogenic shock is the most acute and ominous form of pump failure. It is the inability of the heart to act as a pump. Shock can be seen after a severe MI, dysrhythmias, CHF, pulmonary embolus, cardiac tamponade, and abdominal aortic aneurysm. Often, the outcome of cardiogenic shock is death (Miller, 1994). Signs and symptoms include increased pulmonary artery pressures, PCWP greater than 18 to 25 mm Hg, decreased cardiac output and cardiac index, decreased blood pressure without evidence of hypovolemia, cyanosis, decreased urine output, decreased or absent pulses, and restlessness and confusion. Patients experiencing cardiogenic shock need to be treated aggressively with vasopressors, such as dopamine, dobutamine, norepinephrine (Levophed), amrinone.

An intra-aortic balloon pump may be used to assist with circulation by decreasing afterload and augmenting diastolic pressure (Fig. 9–15). Often, the patient remains on the pump until surgical intervention can be performed (see Chapter 8).

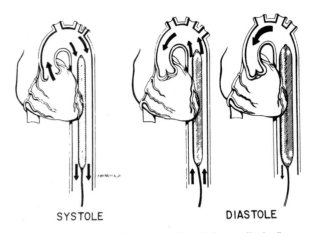

Figure 9–15. Mechanisms of action—intra-aortic balloon pump. Balloon deflates during systole, unloading ventricle; balloon inflates during diastole, increasing coronary perfusion pressure and myocardial oxygen supply. (From Shoemaker, W. C. (1989). *Textbook of critical care* (2nd ed.). Philadelphia: W. B. Saunders Co.)

The medical management program for patients with CHF should also include treating the underlying cause. Once the crisis has passed and the patient is stabilized, the precipitating factor or factors for the complications must be addressed and treated. Treatment may consist of surgical or pharmacological intervention for an MI secondary to CAD, such as CABG, PTCA, and cardiotonic drugs; valve replacement surgery for treatment of long-standing problems, such as valvular diseases secondary to rheumatic heart disease; treatment modalities for pulmonary disorders, such as chronic obstructive pulmonary disease; and management of hypertension (Ulrich et al., 1994).

OUTCOMES

Outcomes for the patient with CHF include

- Cardiac output within normal limits
- Absence of signs and symptoms of decreased cardiac output
- Afterload within normal limits
- Normal ABG results
- Absence of respiratory distress
- Normovolemia and no development of fluid volume deficit
- Absence of dysrhythmias
- Increased level of activity without fatigue, weakness, discomfort, or other abnormal response

Summary

This chapter focused on the care of the patient with alterations in cardiac status. The normal anatomy and physiology of the heart were reviewed, and reasons for deviations from normal were discussed. The pathophysiology of CAD was described, including the potential complications of angina, MI, and CHF. Nursing assessment, diagnosis, interventions and goals, and medical management specific to this population were addressed. The purpose of this chapter was to acquaint the critical care nurse with the problems and pathological conditions most commonly seen in the cardiovascular patient. It is hoped that this chapter provides a basic understanding of the cardiovascular patient that will facilitate sound clinical judgment in the planning of care that is holistic and incorporates a cooperative, interdisciplinary approach.

CRITICAL THINKING QUESTIONS

1. You are preparing to discharge Mrs. Sanchez, aged 62 years, who was admitted for diabetic ketoacidosis, which has been successfully managed. She complains of midsternal chest pressure while you are performing your discharge teaching.
   a. Prioritize your actions at this time.
   b. What assessments will you make to assist in the differential diagnosis of the chest pain?
   c. What history will you obtain from Mrs. Sanchez and/or her chart?
   d. What diagnostic tests do you anticipate?
2. Many patients now come into the hospital the same day as cardiac surgery is performed. Discuss methods for teaching patients effectively given this situation.
3. Discuss your assessments and nursing care for your patient who has just undergone cardiac catheterization/angiography.
4. Mr. Phillips has been hospitalized three times in the past 2 months for chronic CHF. What teaching and interventions can you implement in order to prevent rehospitalization after discharge?

REFERENCES

Albert, N. M. (1994). Laser angioplasty and intracoronary stents: Going beyond the balloon. *AACN Clinical Issues in Critical Care Nursing, 5*(1), 15–20.

American Heart Association (1995). *Heart and stroke facts: 1995 statistical supplement.* Dallas: Author.

American Heart Association (1994a). What is cholesterol-lowering medicine? In *Fighting heart disease and stroke,* 64-9012.

American Heart Association (1994b). What is a heart attack? In *Fighting heart disease and stroke,* 64-9023.

Bogart, D. B., Bogart, M. A., Miller, J. T., Farrar, M. W., Barr, W. K., & Montgomery, M. A. (1995). Femoral artery catheterization complications. *Catheterization for Cardiovascular Diagnosis, 34* (1):8–13.

Braunwald, E., Mark, D. B., Jones, R. H., et al., for the U.S.

Department of Health and Human Services. (1994). *Diagnosing and managing unstable angina: Quick reference guide for clinicians* (AHCPR Publication No. 94-0603). Rockville, MD: Author.

Canobbio, M. (1990). *Cardiovascular disorders.* St. Louis: C. V. Mosby Co.

Cardin, S. (1993). Patients with cardiomyopathies. In J. M. Clochesy, C. Breu, S. Cardin, E. B. Rudy, & A. A. Whittaker (Eds.), *Critical care nursing* (pp. 356–369). Philadelphia: W. B. Saunders Co.

Chernecky, C. C., Krech, R. L., & Berger, B. J. (1993). *Laboratory tests and diagnostic procedures.* Philadelphia: W. B. Saunders Co.

Clark, L. C., Gallagher, S. G., Levesque, M. T., Williams, L. A. S., Brown, C. T., & Silva, J. H. (1994). Planning for collaborative practice: Cardiac interventional medicine. *Nursing Administration Quarterly, 18*(4), 28–32.

Coleman, B., Lavieri, M. C., & Gross, S. (1993). Patients undergoing cardiac surgery. In J. M. Clochesy, C. Breu, S. Cardin, E. B. Rudy, & A. A. Whittaker (Eds.), *Critical care nursing* (pp. 385–436). Philadelphia: W. B. Saunders Co.

Drown, D. J., & Engler, M. M. (1994). New guidelines for blood cholesterol by the National Cholesterol Education Program (NCEP). *Progress in Cardiovascular Nursing, 9*(1), 43–44.

Durack, D. T. (1990). Infective and noninfective endocarditis. In J. W. Hurst, R. C. Schlant, C. E. Rackley, E. H. Sonnenblick, & N. K. Wenger (Eds.), *The Heart* (7th ed., Vol. II.) (pp. 1230–1255). New York: McGraw-Hill Book Co.

Dziadulewicz, L., & Shannon-Stone, M. (1995). Postpericardiotomy syndrome: A complication of cardiac surgery. *AACN Clinical Issues: Advanced Practice in Acute and Critical Care, 6*(3), 464–470.

Expert Panel on Detection, Evaluation, and Treatment of High Blood Cholesterol in Adults. (1993). Summary of the second report of the national cholesterol education program (NCEP) expert panel on detection, evaluation, and treatment of high blood cholesterol in adults (adult treatment panel I) *Journal of the American Medical Association, 269,* 3015–3023.

Fara, A. M. (1993). The role of angiotensin-converting enzyme inhibitors in reducing ventricular remodeling after myocardial infarction. *Journal of Cardiovascular Nursing, 8*(1), 32–48.

Fleury, J., & Murdaugh, C. (1993). Patients with coronary artery disease. In J. M. Clochesy, C. Breu, S. Cardin, E. B. Rudy, & A. A. Whittaker (Eds.), *Critical care nursing* (pp. 257–301). Philadelphia: W. B. Saunders Co.

Frick, M. H., Elo, M. O., Haapa K, et al. (1987). Helsinki Heart Study: Primary-prevention trial with gemfibrozil in middle-aged men with dyslipidemia. *New England Journal of Medicine, 317,* 1237–1245.

Grab, C. J. (1992). The cutting alternative to PTCA. *RN, 55*(7), 22–27.

Guaglianone, D. M., & Tyndall, A. (1995). Comfort issues in patients undergoing radiofrequency catheter ablation. *Critical Care Nurse, 15*(1), 47–50.

GUSTO. (1993). An international randomized trial comparing four thrombolytic strategies for acute myocardial infarction. *New England Journal of Medicine, 329*(10), 673–682.

Hibner, C. S., Moseley, M. J., & Shank, T. (1993). What is transesophageal echocardiography? *American Journal of Roentgenology, 93*(4), 74–80.

Hixon, M. E. (1994). Aging and heart failure. *Progress in Cardiovascular Nursing, 9*(1), 4–12.

Hogan-Miller, E., Rustad, D., Sendelbach, S., & Goldenbery, I. (1995). Effects of three methods of femoral site immobilization on bleeding and comfort after coronary angiogram. *American Journal of Critical Care, 4*(2), 143–148.

Hurst, J. W., & Logue, R. B. (Eds.) (1990). *The heart* (7th ed.). New York: McGraw-Hill Book Co.

Kadota, L. T. (1993). Hemodynamic monitoring. In J. M. Clochesy, C. Breu, S. Cardin, E. B. Rudy, & A. A. Whittaker (Eds.), *Critical care nursing* (pp. 155–182). Philadelphia: W. B. Saunders Co.

Kannel, W. B., Castelli, W. P., Gordon, T., et al. (1987). Serum cholesterol, lipoproteins, and the risk of coronary heart disease: The Framingham study. *Annals of Internal Medicine, 74,* 1–12.

Lipon, K. R., & Carlson, L. R. (1994). Development of a hospital-based cardiovascular risk factor reduction program for the community: Beyond heart disease. *Progress in Cardiovascular Nursing, 9*(2), 16–22.

McCance, K., & Huether, S. (1994). *Pathophysiology.* St. Louis: C. V. Mosby Co.

Miller, M. M. (1994). Current trends in the primary care management of chronic congestive heart failure. *Nurse Practitioner, 19*(5), 64–70.

Morris, D. C., Walter, P. F., & Hurst, J. W. (1990). The recognition and treatment of myocardial infarction and its complications. In J. W. Hurst, R. C. Schlant, C. E. Rackley, E. H. Sonnenblick, & N. K. Wenger (Eds.), *The heart* (7th ed., Vol. I.) (pp. 1054–1078). New York: McGraw-Hill Book Co.

Murphy, M. C., Hansell, H. N., Ward, K., & Shaw, R. E. (1994). Differences in symptoms during and post PTCA versus rotational ablation. *Progress in Cardiovascular Nursing, 9*(2), 4–9.

Porterfield, L. M., & Porterfield, J. G. (1995). Third generation pacemaker-cardioverter-defibrillator: A case study. *Critical Care Nurse, 15*(1), 43–45.

Rasmussen, M. J., & Mangan, D. B. (1994). Third generation anti-tachycardia pacing implantable cardioverter defibrillators. *DCCN, 13*(6), 284–291.

Riegel, B. (1993). Patients with myocardial infarction. In J. M. Clochesy, C. Breu, S. Cardin, E. B. Rudy, & A. A. Whittaker (Eds.), *Critical care nursing* (pp. 302–322). Philadelphia: W. B. Saunders Co.

Shaten, B. J., Kuller, L. H., Neaton, J. D. (1991). Association between baseline risk factors, cigarette smoking, and CHD mortality after 10.5 years: MRFIT research group. *Preventive Medicine, 20*(5), 655–659.

Sirovatka, B. M. (1993). The implantable cardioverter defibrillator: Patient and family education. *DCCN, 12*(6), 328–334.

Skov, P., & Vaska, P. L. (1993). Cardiovascular anatomy and physiology. In J. M. Clochesy, C. Breu, S. Cardin, E. B. Rudy, & A. A. Whittaker (Eds.), *Critical care nursing* (pp. 231–256). Philadelphia: W. B. Saunders Co.

Strimike, C. L. (1995). Caring for a patient with an intracoronary stent. *American Journal of Roentgenology, 95*(1), 40–46.

Teplitz, L. (1994). Transcatheter ablation of tachyarrhythmias: An overview and case studies. *Progress in Cardiovascular Nursing, 9*(3), 16–31.

Thibodeau, G. A. (1990). *Anatomy and physiology* (13th ed.). St. Louis: C. V. Mosby Co.

Tootill, D. M. (1995). Thrombolytic therapy: Nursing strategies for successful patient outcomes. *Progress in Cardiovascular Nursing, 10*(1), 3–12.

Ulrich, S. P., Canale, S. W., & Wendell, S. A. (1994). *Medical-surgical nursing care planning guides* (3rd ed.). Philadelphia: W. B. Saunders Co.

Vander, A., Sherman, J., & Luciano, D. (1990). *Human physiology: The mechanism of body function* (5th ed.). New York: McGraw-Hill Book Co.

Williams, K., & Morton, P. G. (1995). Diagnosis and treatment of acute myocardial infarction. *AACN Clinical Issues: Advanced Practice in Acute and Critical Care, 6*(3), 375–386.

RECOMMENDED READING

Cliff, D. L., & Blazewicz, P. A. (1993). Radiofrequency catheter ablation. Part 1: Pre- and post-procedure nursing responsibilities. *DCCN, 12*(6), 313–318.

Ferguson, J. A. (1992). Pain following coronary artery bypass grafting: An exploration of contributing factors. *Intensive and Critical Care Nursing, 8*(3), 153–162.

Liehr, P., Todd, B., Rossi, M., & Culligan, M. (1992). Effect of venous support on edema and leg pain in patients after coronary artery bypass graft surgery. *Heart and Lung, 21*(1), 6–11.

Papadantonaki, A., Stotts, N. A., & Paulm, S. M. (1994). Comparison of quality of life before and after coronary artery bypass surgery and percutaneous transluminal angioplasty. *Heart and Lung, 23*(1), 45–52.

Vitale, M. B., & Funk, M. (1995). Quality of life in younger persons with an implantable cardioverter defibrillator. *DCCN, 14*(2), 100–111.

C H A P T E R

10

Nervous System Alterations

Jeanette C. Hartshorn, Ph.D., R.N., FAAN
Vicki L. Byers, Ph.D., R.N.

OBJECTIVES

- Describe the pathophysiology, nursing, and medical management of patients with increased intracranial pressure.
- Complete an assessment on a critically ill patient with nervous system injury.
- Describe the pathophysiology, nursing, and medical management of patients with head injury.

- Define current nursing and medical therapy for spinal cord injury.
- Discuss the nursing assessment and care of a critically ill patient with cerebrovascular disease.
- Define the pathophysiology and expected treatment for status epilepticus

---

Introduction

Neurological illness and trauma to the central nervous system are devastating and frequently life-threatening events. These patients have so many unique needs during the acute phase of their illness that caring for them is a challenge for critical care nurses. Nursing care can make a significant difference for both the patient and the family as they adjust to these events.

The brain is important in all aspects of our lives—for consciousness, thinking, problem solving, judgment, memory, language, perceptions, emotions, movements, and autonomic functions. The spinal cord is important because most sensory pathways go through the spinal cord on the way to the brain. Most motor pathways pass through the spinal cord on their journey to the rest of the body, and most reflex activity is accomplished at the spinal cord level. When these structures are damaged, a person's activities are greatly altered. In this chapter, the pathophysiology, assessment, nursing diagnosis, interventions, and outcomes related to increased intracranial pressure, head injury,

spinal cord injury, status epilepticus, and cerebrovascular disease are discussed.

Increased Intracranial Pressure

One of the most commonly encountered problems in the critical care setting is increased intracranial pressure (ICP). Planning for the care of these patients is based on the concepts of volume-pressure relationships, cerebral blood flow (CBF), cerebral edema, cerebrospinal fluid (CSF) changes, and herniation. Patients with increased ICP are dependent on astute and timely nursing assessment and interventions to limit the possible damage from the increased pressure. A plan of care must be developed for each individual patient as his or her responses to environmental changes are noted.

Under normal circumstances, ICP (normal range 0 to 15 mm Hg) fluctuates in response to changes in blood pressure, respiratory cycle, isometric contractions, coughing, and Valsalva's maneuvers (e.g., breath holding, straining). With brain pathology (e.g., head injury, stroke, tumor, hydrocephalus, infection, cerebral edema, hematoma formation, anoxia), an increase in ICP is life threatening.

PATHOPHYSIOLOGY

Increased ICP (16 mm Hg and greater) is a life-threatening event. The rigid cranial vault contains three types of noncompressible contents: semisolid brain, intravascular blood, and CSF (Fig. 10–1). When the volume of any one of these three components increases, one or both of the other components must decrease proportionally, or there will be an increase in ICP (modified Monro-Kellie doctrine).

To compensate for an increased intracranial component, CSF is displaced into the spinal canal or is absorbed into the venous system. In pathological conditions in which additional volume is added, such as an increase in blood volume, cerebral edema, or hemorrhage, these compensatory mechanisms fail, and additional intracranial volume is not tolerated. At this point, the patient begins to display symptoms of increased ICP. Physiologically, the brain is said to lose its ability to compensate, which is demonstrated by an alteration in intracranial compliance.

Intracranial Compliance

Intracranial compliance is a measure of the brain's compensatory mechanisms and demonstrates the effects of volume on pressure. In Figure 10–2, the curve is flat until point A. Adding volume up to this point has very little effect on pressure; the ICP remains stable. This response is known as high compliance; the brain is able to adapt to changes in intracranial volume without a change in pressure (Andrus, 1991; Hickey, 1992). During normal compensation, CSF is

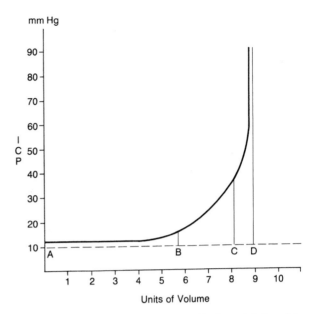

Figure 10–2. Pressure-volume curve. Up to point A, addition of volume has little effect on pressure; after that point, there is a dramatic increase in response to the addition of volume, especially from point B onward. (From Hickey, J. V. (1992). *The clinical practice of neurological neurosurgical nursing* (3rd ed.) (p. 248). Philadelphia: J. B. Lippincott Co.)

displaced into the spinal subarachnoid space, and blood is displaced into the venous sinuses. Nursing measures such as bathing, turning, and suctioning are safe to perform during this interval (Marshall et al., 1990; Hickey, 1992). In Figure 10–2, B on the steep portion of the curve indicates the point at which small changes in volume produce large changes in pressure—when compensatory volume displacement mechanisms are exhausted (low compliance). Patients on the steep portion of this curve can experience large and dangerous increases in ICP with ordinary activities of daily living or nursing care measures that were previously of little consequence (Marshall et al., 1990; Andrus, 1991; Germon, 1994). Patients in this situation must be monitored closely.

Other causes of increased ICP include altered CBF, loss of autoregulation, compression of the venous system, and herniation.

Altered Cerebral Blood Flow

CBF brings oxygen and glucose to the brain for energy production. Waste products are also removed by the blood. When metabolism is increased, the CBF is increased to meet those demands (Marshall et al., 1990). Under pathological situations, CBF can increase

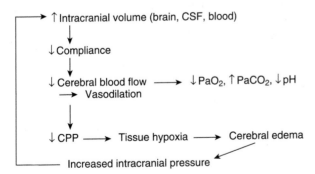

Figure 10–1. Pathophysiology flow diagram—increased intracranial pressure. This process contributes to decreased mentation, impaired motor function, cranial nerve dysfunction, sensory impairment, and autonomic nervous system dysfunction.

to such an extent that it adds to brain bulk and, consequently, ICP (Marshall et al., 1990). Conversely, a decrease in CBF while there is an increase in metabolic activity can render an area ischemic by increasing $PaCO_2$ and causing cerebral edema, contributing to increased ICP (Marshall et al., 1990; Prendergast, 1994).

Cerebral perfusion pressure (CPP) is an estimate of the level of cellular perfusion. It is calculated by subtracting mean ICP from mean systemic arterial blood pressure (MAP). The acceptable range for CPP is 60 to 100 mm Hg. It is important to maintain CPP above 60 mm Hg in order to perfuse the brain with blood. A CPP of 60 mm Hg or lower is considered not only low but potentially life-threatening (Andrus, 1991). When ICP approaches mean systemic arterial pressure, CPP decreases to a point at which autoregulation is impaired and CBF decreases. This decrease in flow will cause ischemia and eventually infarction of cerebral tissue if the situation is not corrected.

Autoregulation

Under normal limits, the cerebral vasculature exhibits pressure and chemical autoregulation. Pressure autoregulation provides a constant blood volume and CPP over a wide range of mean arterial pressures. Pathological states, such as head injury, hemorrhage, or craniotomy, lead to a loss of pressure autoregulation. When autoregulation is lost, hypertension increases CBF and hypotension causes ischemia. Both of these situations cause increased ICP. CPP is a reflection of CBF and can be calculated at the bedside.

The cerebral vessels are also sensitive to chemical autoregulation. A $PaCO_2$ greater than 30 mm Hg and a PaO_2 of 50 mm Hg or less cause the cerebral arteries to vasodilate. $PaCO_2$ is the most potent vasodilator, leading to an increase in CBF, cerebral blood volume, and ICP. Cerebral arteries are less sensitive to changes in PaO_2. The CBF is not affected until the PaO_2 is 50 mm Hg or less. A PaO_2 of 50 mm Hg causes hypoxia and vasodilation of the cerebral vasculature, which increase CBF and ICP (Marshall et al., 1990; Andrus, 1991; Germon, 1994).

Obstructed Venous Outflow

Shunting CSF into the venous system is another way to compensate for an increase in intracranial volume. In pathological states, venous outflow can become obstructed in several ways. Different neck positions (hyperflexion, hyperextension, rotation) compress the jugular vein, inhibit venous return, cause central venous engorgement, and increase ICP. A second mechanism for venous outflow obstruction is transmis-

sion of a high pressure that impairs venous return. Mechanisms that increase intrathoracic or intra-abdominal pressure (e.g., coughing, vomiting, posturing, isometric exercise, Valsalva's maneuver, or positive end-expiratory pressure) produce increased pressure that impairs venous return. When the jugular vein is compressed, venous return is inhibited, resulting in venous engorgement. As venous outflow decreases, an increase in ICP occurs.

Cerebral Edema

Cerebral edema is an increase in the water content of the brain tissue. When cerebral edema occurs as a result of trauma, hemorrhage, tumor, abscess, or ischemia, an increase in ICP occurs. Experimental data suggest that as cerebral edema increases, there is a decrease in CBF prior to an increase in ICP. As CBF decreases, cellular activity is impaired, and signs and symptoms related to neurological dysfunction become apparent.

Cytotoxic and vasogenic edema are two categories of cerebral edema. Cytotoxic edema is characterized by intracellular swelling of neurons, which is most often due to hypoxia and hypo-osmolality. Hypoxia causes decreased adenosine triphosphate production and leads to the failure of the sodium-potassium pump. As the activity of the pump ceases, sodium is not pumped outside the cell, and potassium remains extracellular. In addition, water enters the cell and causes swelling. In cases of acute hypo-osmolality, water moves into the cell by osmosis. Thus, cytotoxic cerebral edema frequently accompanies states of diabetic ketoacidosis.

Vasogenic cerebral edema occurs due to a breakdown of the blood-brain barrier, leading to an increase in the extracellular fluid space. With the breakdown of the blood-brain barrier, osmotically active substances (proteins) leak into the interstitium and draw the water from the vascular system. This results in an increase in extracellular fluid and a consequent increase in ICP. Head injuries, brain tumors, and abscesses are common causes of vasogenic cerebral edema.

Herniation

When a mass effect occurs in the semisolid brain within a compartment, the pressure exerted by this mass is not equally divided, resulting in shifting or herniation of the brain from one compartment of high pressure to one of lower pressure. This causes pressure or traction on certain neurological structures, and an increase in neurological deficits or death can occur.

Herniation syndromes are classified as supraten-

Figure 10–3. Types of herniation. Cross section of a normal brain (left) and a brain with intracranial shifts from supratentorial lesions (right). *(1)* Herniation of the cingulate gyrus under the falx. *(2)* Central herniation causing a downward shift of the cerebral hemispheres, basal ganglia, and diencephalon through the tentorial notch. *(3)* Uncal herniation causing the temporal lobe to pass through the tentorial notch. *(4)* Tonsillar herniation causing the cerebellar tonsils to be displaced through the foramen magnum. (Modified from Plum, F., & Posner, J. (1972). *Diagnosis of stupor and coma* (2nd ed.). Philadelphia: F. A. Davis.)

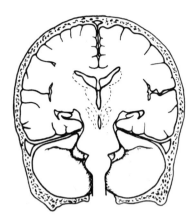
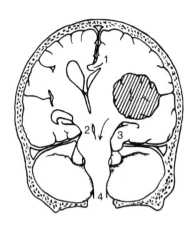

torial (cingulate, central, and uncal herniation) or infratentorial (tonsillar herniation).

Cingulate Herniation. When a unilateral lesion creates a shift of brain tissue of one cerebral hemisphere under the falx cerebri to the other cerebral hemisphere, cingulate herniation occurs (Fig. 10–3). This type of herniation compresses cerebral blood vessels and brain tissue, causing cerebral ischemia, cerebral edema, and increased ICP. Changes in arousal (level of consciousness) and mental status are associated with this type of herniation.

Central Herniation. A downward shift of the cerebral hemispheres, basal ganglia, and diencephalon through the tentorial notch causes central herniation (Morrison, 1990). The supratentorial contents compress vital centers of the brain stem (see Fig. 10–3). Early signs and symptoms include changes in arousal and mental status, increased muscle tone, motor weakness, change in the respiratory pattern (increased yawning, deep sighs, rate changes), small reactive pupils, and bilateral Babinski's reflexes. Late signs and symptoms include decorticate posturing and Cheyne-Stokes respirations.

Uncal Herniation. When a unilateral lesion above the tentorium forces the uncus of the temporal lobe to displace through the tentorial notch, uncal herniation is the result (see Fig. 10–3). The displaced uncus compresses the midbrain, causing dysfunction of the parasympathetic fibers of the ipsilateral third nerve. Signs and symptoms include unilateral pupil dilation, ipsilateral third nerve palsy, and contralateral hemiplegia. Without treatment, the patient becomes unresponsive to the environment and progresses into full coma. In addition, brain stem dysfunction (loss of oculocephalic reflex, fixed midposition pupils, altered respirations) and decerebrate posturing are present.

Tonsillar Herniation. When the cerebellar tonsils are displaced through the foramen magnum, tonsillar herniation results (see Fig. 10–3). This displacement

distorts the brain stem, compresses the medulla, and causes fatal damage to the respiratory and cardiac centers.

Any change in intracranial compliance, CBF, autoregulation, and cerebral edema can potentially cause increased ICP and subsequent herniation.

ASSESSMENT

Nursing Assessment

History and neurological assessment provide needed information about the patient's current condition. Initial and ongoing assessment of a patient with increased ICP provides an active picture of improvement or deterioration and guides therapeutic efforts.

Ideally, the patient is the primary source of the historical data. If the patient is unable to give the history, family or friends should supply information related to symptoms, onset, progression, and chronology of the event. If headache is a presenting symptom, information must be obtained about the location, onset, type of pain, duration, presence of other symptoms, and what makes the headache better or worse. If the patient is admitted secondary to nervous system trauma, specific information concerning the mechanism of injury, immediate posttrauma care, and emergency treatments are needed.

The Glasgow Coma Scale (GCS) is a standardized tool used as a guide in assessing a patient with head injury and increased ICP. The components of this assessment tool are eye opening, verbal response, and motor response (Fig. 10–4). A consistent stimulus—either a verbal command or a painful stimulus—is applied. The responsiveness of the patient is expressed as a number according to the listed criteria. A high number (approaching 15) indicates normal functioning, whereas a low number (approaching 3) suggests impaired functioning. Generally, the actual numbers on

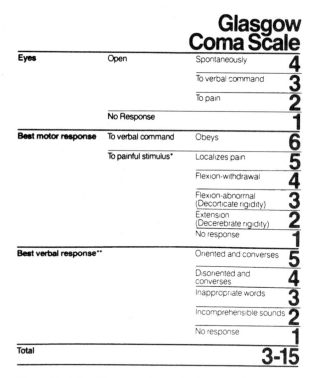

Glasgow Coma Scale

Eyes	Open	Spontaneously	4
		To verbal command	3
		To pain	2
	No Response		1
Best motor response	To verbal command	Obeys	6
	To painful stimulus*	Localizes pain	5
		Flexion-withdrawal	4
		Flexion-abnormal (Decorticate rigidity)	3
		Extension (Decerebrate rigidity)	2
		No response	1
Best verbal response**		Oriented and converses	5
		Disoriented and converses	4
		Inappropriate words	3
		Incomprehensible sounds	2
		No response	1
Total			3-15

Figure 10–4. The Glasgow Coma Scale, which is based on eye opening, verbal responses, and memory responses, is a practical means of monitoring changes in the level of consciousness. Each response is given a number (high for normal and low for impaired responses), and the responsiveness of the patient is expressed as the sum of the figures. The lowest score is 3; the highest is 15. (Modified from Becker, D. P., & Gudeman, S. K. (1989). *Textbook of head injury* (p. 388). Philadelphia, W. B. Saunders Co.)

the scale are less meaningful than the trend of scores. The GCS is a fast way to assess consciousness. Its advantages are its simplicity and universality (Ingersoll and Leyden, 1990). The major disadvantage is that the GCS has limited applicability and does not replace neurological assessment of the specific area of the brain involved.

When performing a neurological assessment, the critical care nurse focuses on mental status, cranial nerve functioning, and motor status. A neurological flow chart and narrative charting are frequently used to provide necessary information.

Mental Status

When assessing a patient's mental status or consciousness, the critical care nurse tests arousal and cognition.

Consciousness. The level of consciousness is evaluated by the patient's response to the environment. The highest level of response is the patient's acknowl-

edgment of the nurse's presence (e.g., appropriate verbal response, gesture of greeting, eye contact). The lowest level is a lack of any response to the environment. Any change in the level of consciousness is an *early* sign of neurological deterioration and is one of the most important aspects of mental status assessment. Once consciousness is established, the nurse assesses the patient's orientation, which is assessed in terms of person, place, and time.

Language Skills. The second component of mental status to be assessed is language skills. If the patient is not intubated, it is important to assess his or her ability to talk, fluency of speech, and word-finding difficulty and whether the speech is spontaneous. An inability to talk is termed expressive aphasia (Dolan, 1991). If the patient is intubated, a similar evaluation is possible by assessing his or her writing skills. A patient with only expressive problems can comprehend language and follow commands.

The next step is to assess the patient's ability to follow verbal commands. The patient may be presented with simple commands that he or she do simple things such as pointing to the clock, pointing to the window, or raising the right arm. Upon successful completion of simple commands, the patient may be presented with a complex command such as raising the right arm and folding a piece of paper. The inability to follow commands is called receptive aphasia (Dolan, 1991). A patient with only receptive problems who is not intubated can speak spontaneously, but the verbal response does not follow the context of the conversation because of the patient's lack of comprehension. A patient's inability to both talk and follow commands is called global aphasia. These simple tests assess the patient's ability to understand information presented to him or her.

Memory. The third component of mental status to be assessed is memory. Short-term memory is assessed by asking the patient to *recall* the names of three words or objects (e.g., chair, clock, blue) after a 3-minute interval. This simple test can be used with an intubated patient by having the patient write down the words on a piece of paper rather than giving a verbal response. Long-term memory is tested by asking questions about the patient's distant past (e.g., birth place, year of birth, year of graduation from school, year of marriage). If the patient is intubated, the patient can write down the answers.

Cranial Nerve Functioning

Knowing the location of the each cranial nerve (Table 10–1) helps localize the lesion in the brain stem and assists the nurse in identifying specific patient problems related to the cranial nerve deficit. Ten of the twelve cranial nerves are located in the brain stem.

Table 10–1. THE 12 CRANIAL NERVES

Cranial Nerve	Name	Major Functions
I	Olfactory	Smell
II	Optic	Vision
III	Oculomotor	Movements of eyes; pupillary constriction and accommodation
IV	Trochlear	Movement of eyes
V	Trigeminal	Muscles of mastication and eardrum tension; general sensations from anterior half of head, including face, nose, mouth, and meninges
VI	Abducens	Movements of eyes
VII	Facial	Muscles of facial expression and tension on ear bones (stapes); lacrimation and salivation; taste
VIII	Auditory	Hearing and equilibrium reception (vestibulocochlear)
IX	Glossopharyngeal	Swallowing; salivation; taste; visceral sensory
X	Vagus	Swallowing movements and laryngeal control; parasympathetics to thoracic and abdominal viscera
XI	Spinal accessory	Movements of head and shoulders
XII	Hypoglossal	Movements of tongue

From Marshall, S. B., Marshall, L. F., Vos, H. R., & Chesnut, R. M. (1990). *Neuroscience critical care.* Philadelphia: W. B. Saunders Co.

On the initial baseline neurological assessment, all cranial nerves are assessed. Subsequent neurological assessments focus on cranial nerves II, III, IV, V, VI, VII, IX, and X, which regulate pupil response, eye movement, and protective mechanisms. Changes in the functioning of these cranial nerves help localize the level of brain stem involvement and identify significant changes in neurological status that require nursing intervention.

Cranial Nerve II. Tests for visual acuity, direct light response, and visual fields assess the function of cranial nerve II. Testing all these functions is important initially, but serial assessments can focus on direct light response and visual acuity only.

Cranial Nerves III, IV, and VI. The third cranial nerve is responsible for the consensual light response, elevation of the eyelids, and eye movement. Cranial nerves III, IV, and VI affect extraocular movements of the eye (Fig. 10–5). When assessing extraocular movements, the nurse should check gaze and note the presence of nystagmus. In an unconscious patient, eye movements are an indication of brain stem activity and are tested by the oculocephalic response (doll's eyes maneuver Fig. 10–6). When the doll's eyes maneuver is intact, the eyes move in the opposite direction when the head is turned. Abnormal responses include movement of the eyes in the same direction as the head or the eyes staying midline when the head is turned. An abnormal response indicates a disruption in the processing of information through the brain stem. Contraindications to performing oculocephalic testing include cervical cord injuries and severely increased ICP. An alternative test—usually performed only by physicians—is the oculovestibular response (ice water

calorics). This also tests for brain stem function but is believed to be more reliable than the oculocephalic response. To test for the oculovestibular response, the head of the patient's bed is elevated 30° and 30 to 50 ml of ice water is quickly injected into the ear. The normal response, indicating an intact brain stem, is for the eyes to move in the direction of the ice water. Any other response is considered abnormal and indicates severe brain stem injury. An abnormal oculovestibular response is an ominous sign.

Examination of the pupils includes checking for size, shape, equality, and light reflex. Normal pupil size, which ranges from 1.5 to 6 mm in diameter, reflects a balance between the sympathetic and parasympathetic innervation. Exact measurement using a millimeter scale (Fig. 10–7) is the most reliable method of determining size and equality. Unequal pupils (anisocoria) normally occur in approximately 10% of the general population. Otherwise, inequality of pupils (greater than 1 mm) is a sign of pathology (e.g., increased ICP, ischemia, herniation, cervical cord trauma).

The light reflexes are tested with a bright penlight in dim surrounding light. The direct light reflex is elicited by approaching the eye from the side with a penlight. The pupil should constrict as a response. The consensual light reflex occurs when the contralateral pupil constricts. The rate of pupillary reaction is an important variable to assess. Reaction rates are generally described as brisk, sluggish, or nonreactive. A change from briskly to sluggishly reactive or from sluggish to nonreactive is extremely important. These often subtle changes may be an indication of increasing ICP, causing a deterioration in neurological status.

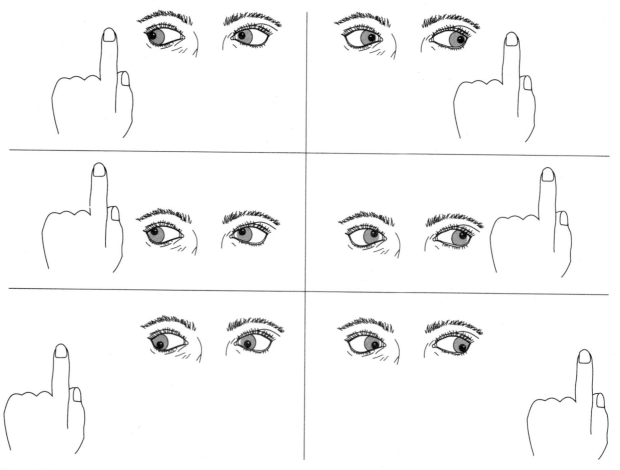

Figure 10–5. Extraocular movements. The patient is instructed to follow the examiner's finger without moving the head from side to side or up and down. (From Simpson, J. F., & Magee, K. R. (1973). *Clinical evaluation of the nervous system* (Fig. 12). Boston: Little, Brown.)

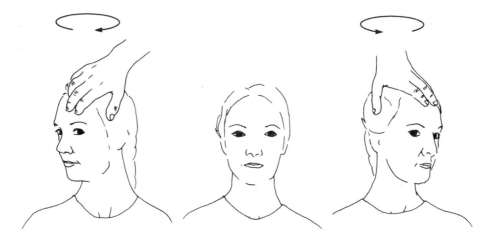

Figure 10–6. Doll's eyes—the eyes move in the opposite direction when the head is turned. The doll's eyes response is absent when the eyes move in the same direction when the head is turned or stay in the midline. (From Mitchell, P., Cammermeyer, M., Ozuna, J., & Woods, N. F. (1984). *Neurological assessment for nursing practice* (Fig. 2–21). Reston, VA: Reston Publishing Co.)

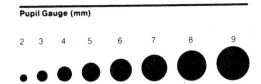

Pupil Gauge (mm)

2   3   4   5   6   7   8   9

Figure 10–7. Pupil gauge in millimeters for measuring pupil size. (From Marshall, S. B., Marshall, L. F., Vos, H. R., & Chesnut, R. M. (1990). *Neuroscience critical care*. Philadelphia: W. B. Saunders Co.)

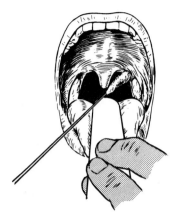

Figure 10–9. The gag reflex. In a conscious patient, ask the patient to say "ah." The examiner observes the rise of the soft palate and the midline uvula. In an unconscious patient, stimulate the posterior pharynx and observe the same response. (From Van Allen, M. W., & Rodnitzky, R. L. (1984). *Pictorial manual of neurologic tests* (2nd ed.) (Fig. 20). Chicago: Year Book.)

Differences between pupils are also important. For example, pressure on the pathway of the oculomotor nerve may cause the ipsilateral pupil (same side as pressure) to be dilated and sluggish or even nonreactive to light, whereas the contralateral pupil (opposite side of pressure) remains normal in size and reactivity.

Cranial Nerves V, IX, and X. Cranial nerves V, IX, and X control the protective reflexes. Testing cranial nerve V determines whether the corneal reflex is intact (Fig. 10–8). Observing for a bilateral blink is one way to test cranial nerve V. When there is an asymmetrical blink, a wisp of cotton is used to touch the cornea. The normal response is blinking in that eye. When this reflex is absent or diminished, the patient is at risk of developing a corneal abrasion.

Testing of cranial nerves IX and X involves the cough, gag, and swallowing reflexes. If the patient is able to follow commands, he or she should be instructed to cough and to swallow. To test the gag reflex, the patient must be asked to open his or her mouth and say "ah." During this maneuver, observe for symmetry; the soft palate rises on both sides, and the uvula is midline. If the patient is unable to follow commands or is unconscious, stimulating the pharyngeal wall elicits a "retching" response (Fig. 10–9). It is important to have the head of the bed elevated 30° with the patient lying on his or her side prior to testing the gag reflex. When these reflexes are diminished or absent, the patient has difficulty handling secretions and oral intake and is at risk of aspiration.

Cranial Nerves VII and XII. To test the facial nerve (cranial nerve VII), the nurse asks the patient to smile, frown, and puff out the cheeks and observes the facial expressions.

Cranial nerve XII moves the tongue and is assessed by asking the patient to stick out his or her tongue and move it from side to side. The nurse is observing for symmetry of movement and inspecting the surface of the tongue for atrophy.

Motor Status

Many centers of the brain are responsible for movement; therefore, motor assessment detects the extent of damage to the motor system. In the assessment of the motor system, the nurse focuses on spontaneous movement of all extremities, muscle strength, muscle tone, coordination, and abnormal postures and reflexes, since muscle groups are assessed for symmetry.

Spontaneous Movement. Spontaneous movement can be assessed by asking the patient to move the extremities on command or by observing while the patient moves around in bed. It is important to notice and document changes in spontaneous movement.

Muscle Strength. Testing generalized muscle strength in a conscious patient consists of the drift test (Fig. 10–10). This test is very sensitive to the subtle changes in strength secondary to neurological deterioration. Lower extremity strength is tested by asking the patient to push his or her feet against the nurse's hands (Fig. 10–11). Patients with brain pathology are

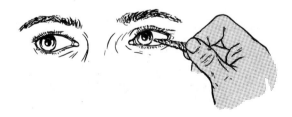

Figure 10–8. Corneal reflex. When spontaneous blinking is absent, the examiner touches a wisp of cotton to the cornea. A normal response is blinking and tearing of the stimulated eye. (From Van Allen, M. W., & Rodnitzky, R. L. (1984). *Pictorial manual of neurologic tests* (2nd ed.) (Fig. 16c). Chicago: Year Book.)

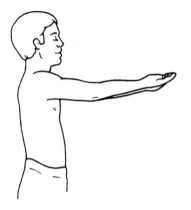

Figure 10–10. Drift test. With the eyes closed, the patient's arms are held straight out in front with the palms up for 20 to 30 seconds. Watch how the patient holds this position. A tendency to drift downward and pronating palms are signs of muscle weakness. (From Hickey, J. V. (1992). *The clinical practice of neurological neurosurgical nursing* (3rd ed.). Philadelphia: J. B. Lippincott Co.)

told to exhale through the mouth during this test to avoid breath holding that could cause increased ICP. Specific muscle groups can be tested by exerting resistance ("push-pull"). It is possible to get an estimate of muscle strength in a patient who inconsistently follows commands or is restless. Trying to push the patient's outstretched arms or legs down is one method of assessing strength informally. Unfortunately, it is not possible to test strength in an unconscious patient.

Muscle Tone. Muscle tone is assessed by taking each extremity through a passive range of motion. Normal muscle tone shows slight resistance to the range of motion. Limp, flabby muscles are characterized by decreased or loss of tone, so there is no resistance to movement. Increased muscle tone is characterized by spasticity and rigidity, resulting in muscle groups' increased resistance to the range of motion.

Coordination of Movement. Coordination of movement is under cerebellar control. It can be assessed by asking the patient to perform rapid alternating movements, to place the finger to the nose, or to run the heel down the shin bilaterally (Fig. 10–12). These tests require the patient to be able to follow verbal commands.

Abnormal Postures and Reflexes. Assessment for abnormal postures and reflexes is important in a brain-injured patient.

Hemiplegia. Early hemiplegia occurs when one side of the patient's body stops moving spontaneously and becomes paretic. This state indicates a cortical lesion and is a sign of further neurological deterioration secondary to a mass effect. The lesion (cerebral edema, hematoma, tumor) is compressing the motor fibers in the motor strip in the frontal lobe. Prolonged compression on motor fibers leads to paralysis.

Decorticate Rigidity. Decorticate rigidity (Fig. 10–13) can be the result of a cortical, subcortical, or diencephalon lesion. Characteristics of this posture are flexion of the upper extremities and extension, with internal rotation of the lower extremities.

Decerebrate Rigidity. Decerebrate posturing is the result of a midbrain or pons lesion. In this posture, the patient's jaws are clenched, extremities are in full extension, feet are in plantar extension, forearms are pronated, and wrists and fingers are flexed (see Fig. 10–13). Both decerebrate and decorticate posturing can occur in response to noxious stimuli such as suctioning or pain.

Bilateral Flaccidity. In bilateral flaccidity, there is no response to noxious stimuli (see Fig. 10–13).

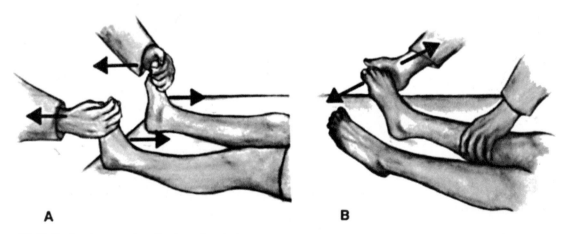

A   **B**

Figure 10–11. Testing lower extremity strength. *(A)* Testing for dorsiflexion. *(B)* Testing for plantarflexion. (From Hickey, J. V. (1992). *The clinical practice of neurological neurosurgical nursing* (3rd ed.) (p. 80). Philadelphia: J. B. Lippincott Co.)

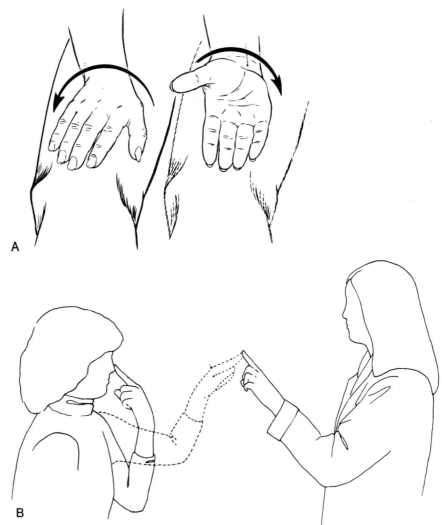

Figure 10–12. Tests for coordination. *(A)* Alternating movements. *(B)* Finger-to-nose test. A normal response is accurate, rapid, and coordinated. (*A* from Van Allen, M. W., & Rodnitsky, R. L. (1984). *Pictorial manual of neurologic tests* (2nd ed.) (Fig. 27a). Chicago: Year Book; *B* from Mitchell, P., Cammermeyer, M., Ozuna, J., & Woods, N. F. (1984). *Neurological assessment for nursing practice* (Fig. 2–10). Reston, VA: Reston Publishing Co.)

Babinski's Reflex. The major pathological deep tendon reflex is Babinski's reflex (Fig. 10–14). This reflex is assessed during the initial baseline assessment and periodically thereafter. In an adult, the presence of a Babinski's reflex is a sign of an upper motor neuron lesion and damage to the corticospinal tract.

All these assessments provide a complete neurological evaluation of a critically ill patient. The nurse reassesses the neurological parameters every 1 to 2 hours. Table 10–2 contains the components of an hourly assessment for a patient with increased ICP, head injury, or cerebrovascular accident (CVA).

Vital Signs

Changes in vital signs appear late in the course of neurological dysfunction. Patients with neurological dysfunction are managed to limit extreme fluctuations in vital signs, since fluctuations can increase damage. Hyperthermia causes an increase in the metabolic demands of neurons, whereas extreme hypothermia leads to cardiac dysrhythmias. Respiratory changes correlate with lesions at various levels of injury; therefore, changes in respiratory rate, rhythm, and depth are important. Pulse and blood pressure changes are unreliable as part of the overall assessment. Both of these changes occur late in the course of increased ICP. Cushing's reflex is another late sign of increased ICP and consists of a widening pulse pressure (systolic pressure rises faster than diastolic pressure) and bradycardia.

It is essential that the nurse recognize that a patient may experience severe damage by the time vital sign changes occur.

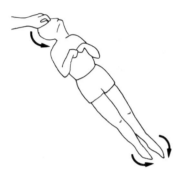

Bilateral Decortication
___(Abnormal Flexion)___

Arms flexed
Wrists flexed
Legs extended

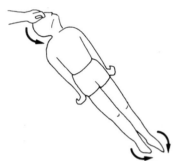

Bilateral Decerebration
___(Extension)___

Arms extended
External rotation of wrists
Legs extended
Internal rotation of feet

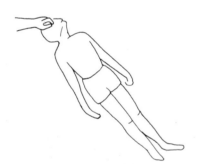

Bilateral Flaccidity

No response in any extremity to
noxious stimuli
Note: Spinal cord injury must be
ruled out as cause of flaccidity
before patient is considered
brain dead.

Figure 10–13. Abnormal postures.
(From Marshall, S. B., Marshall, L. F.,
Vos, H. R., & Chesnut, R. M. (1990).
Neuroscience critical care. Philadel-
phia: W. B. Saunders Co.)

Table 10–2. COMPONENTS OF THE HOURLY NEUROLOGICAL ASSESSMENT FOR PATIENTS WITH INCREASED INTRACRANIAL PRESSURE, HEAD INJURY, OR CEREBROVASCULAR ACCIDENT

Mental Status	Focal Motor	Pupils	Brain Stem/Cranial Nerves
Glasgow Coma Scale Assesses level of consciousness, expressive language, ability to follow commands	Move all extremities Strength all extremities (compares right and left sides) Motor response (Glasgow Coma Scale)	Size Shape Reaction to light (direct and consensual) Extraocular movements	Corneal reflex Present—immediate blinking bilaterally Diminished—blinking asymmetrically Absent—no blinking Doll's eyes (unconscious patient—no spinal fracture) Cough, gag, swallow reflex Observe for excessive drooling Observe for cough/swallow reflex

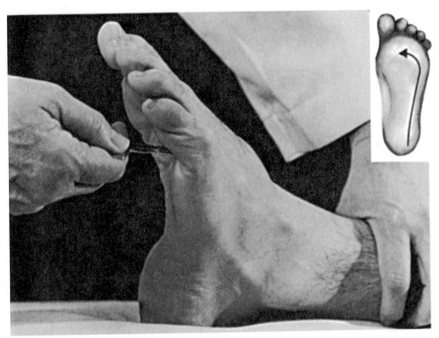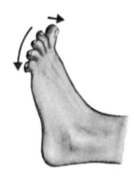

Figure 10–14. Babinski's reflex. With a moderately sharp object, such as a key, stroke the lateral aspect of the sole from the heel to the ball of the foot, curving medially across the ball. Use the lightest stimulus that provokes a response. Note movement of the toes, normally flexion. Dorsiflexion of the great toe with fanning of the other toes indicates upper motor neuron disease. (From Bates, B. (1991). *Guide to physical examination* (p. 537). Philadelphia: J. B. Lippincott Co.)

Monitoring Techniques

Other assessment parameters for a patient with increased ICP include ICP, arterial, and hemodynamic monitoring.

ICP Monitoring. The use of ICP monitoring is controversial; therefore, the benefits of its use must outweigh the associated risk of morbidity.

ICP can be measured continuously via intraparenchymal, intraventricular, subarachnoid, and epidural catheters (Fig. 10–15). ICP monitoring is indicated when ICP rises to 20 mm Hg. The mean ICP reading is taken at the end of the respiratory cycle and before inspiration. There are four types of ICP monitoring devices: intraparenchymal probe, intraventricular catheter, epidural probe, and subarachnoid bolt.

Intraparenchymal Fiberoptic Probe. The intraparenchymal fiberoptic probe (see Fig. 10–15A) is inserted into nondominant brain tissue. This device measures brain tissue pressure. The probe is connected to a monitor that has an analog reading and can interface with a monitor to visualize a waveform. The quality of the waveform and pressure readings is similar to that achieved with the intraventricular catheter. There are several advantages of this fiberoptic system: easy insertion; minimal trauma to tissue because of its small diameter (French); location of the transducer in the tip

of the probe, so there is no concern about the level of the transducer; and a lower incidence of infection because it is not an air- or fluid-filled system (Germon, 1994). The major disadvantage of this system is that the fiberoptic probe is fragile and can break, in which case a new fiberoptic probe must be inserted. A second disadvantage is the expense of the equipment.

Intraventricular Catheter. The intraventricular catheter is inserted into the lateral ventricle of the nondominant cerebral hemisphere. The catheter is connected by a stopcock to fluid-filled pressure tubing attached to a transducer (see Fig. 10–15B) that is positioned at the level of the foramen of Monro (middle of the ear as a reference point). The major advantages of this system include accurate CSF pressure readings, therapeutic draining of CSF, and withdrawal of CSF for laboratory analysis (Germon, 1994). Disadvantages of this system include the risk of infection, unnecessary loss of CSF, and difficult insertion if the ventricles are small or displaced.

Epidural Probe. The epidural probe is placed between the skull and the dura mater in the epidural space (see Fig. 10–15C). Advantages of this monitoring system include the ability to monitor ICP without tearing the dura mater, thereby reducing the risk of intracerebral infection. The major disadvantage is inaccurate pressure readings at high ICP levels.

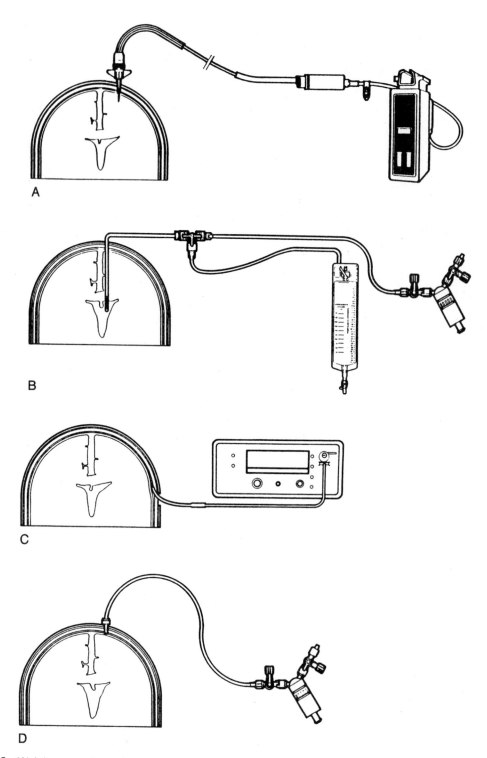

Figure 10–15. (A) Intraparenchymal monitoring system. (B) Intraventricular monitoring system. (C) Epidural monitoring system. (D) Subdural monitoring system. (Courtesy of Camino Laboratories, San Diego, CA.)

Subarachnoid Bolt. The fourth intracranial pressure system is the subarachnoid bolt, placed in the subarachnoid space (see Fig. 10–15D). Advantages of this system include accuracy of CSF pressure measurement and ease of insertion. Major disadvantages include the frequent irrigations needed to maintain the system's patency and an increased risk of infection.

Intraventricular and subarachnoid systems are maintained as closed systems to avoid contamination and infection. Another important consideration is maintaining the transducer at the level of the foramen of Monro. In addition to leveling the transducer, zero balancing and keeping bubbles out of the tubing enhance the accuracy of the readings.

Waveform Monitoring. All types of monitoring systems allow nurses to observe an ICP waveform pattern. There are three types of waveforms (Fig. 10–16).

A waves (plateau waves) are waves between 50 and 100 mm Hg. These waves are associated with advanced intracranial hypertension. A waves generally last 15 to 20 minutes, and the nurse needs to obtain a strip chart of trends to identify A waves. The waveform does not change on the monitor, it just shows a rise in ICP for an extended period of time. B waves less than 50 mm Hg correspond to respirations. B waves may serve as a warning to the nurse of the *potential* risk of increased ICP and impairment of intracranial compliance (Marshall et al., 1990). C waves are small waves (16 to 20 mm Hg) that correlate with changes in blood pressure and respirations. C waves lack clinical significance.

In assessing ICP, the nurse utilizes information about waveforms and potential changes to ensure patient safety (see Fig. 10–16).

Hemodynamic Monitoring. Hemodynamic monitoring allows direct measurement of pulmonary artery and other pressures. These measurements are important for fluid management and overall management of the cardiovascular system. For a detailed discussion related to this type of monitoring, see Chapter 4.

Monitoring Cerebral Oxygenation. A promising technology being used in a few medical centers today is the monitoring of jugular bulb oxygen saturation ($S_{jb}O_2$). Taking blood samples from the jugular bulb allows the nurse to monitor cerebral metabolic usage (Bell et al., 1994; Prendergast, 1994). Using jugular bulb blood oxygen saturation along with systemic oxygen consumption is an indirect method of measuring the brain's oxygen use. The use of the jugular bulb catheter also detects hyperfusion, which leads to increased ICP (Bell et al., 1994). Fiberoptic catheters are being used to monitor jugular bulb oxygen saturation on a continuous basis without having to draw frequent blood samples.

Arterial Monitoring. Accurate assessment of arterial pressure is essential because it has a dramatic effect on ICP. Therefore, continuous monitoring of oxygen saturation via pulse oximetry or arterial pressure monitoring is frequently used for a patient with increased ICP. Arterial blood gas analysis to track the pH, PaO_2, $PaCO_2$, and O_2 saturation is also important, because these substances have a significant effect on the cerebral vasculature.

Bedside Electroencephalographic (EEG) Monitoring. Continuous bedside EEG monitoring is used

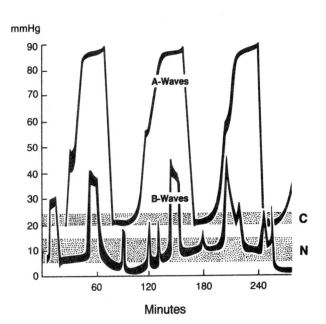

Figure 10–16. Intracranial pressure waveforms. Waveforms reflect pressure in mm Hg and time in minutes. Two abnormal waveforms are depicted, including A waves and B waves. A waves reflect intracranial pressure in the range of 50 to 100 mm Hg. They have a duration of 5 to 20 minutes or longer. Because their waveforms have a distinctive plateau, they are referred to as "plateau" waves. B waves occur as sharp, peaked (sawtooth pattern) rhythmic oscillations, which may reach a peak pressure of 50 mm Hg. They have a duration of 0.5 to 2.0 minutes. N refers to "normal" intracranial pressure waveforms and reflects a pressure within the range of 0 to 15 mm Hg. C refers to the pressure waveform for C waves, which are usually rapid, rhythmic waves with an amplitude of about 20 mm Hg. They occur every 4 to 8 minutes. (From Dolan, J. T. (Ed.) (1991). *Critical care nursing: Clinical management through the nursing process* (p. 93). Philadelphia: F. A. Davis.)

to provide a recording of electrical activity in the brain. The continuous EEG allows for recording, trending, and using evoked potentials to correlate with ICP monitoring. By observing electrical activity in conjunction with ICP monitoring, one can take a more individualized approach related to cerebral perfusion and compliance.

Transcranial Doppler Monitoring. Transcranial Doppler is a noninvasive technology that allows for the indirect monitoring of CBF and is done at the bedside. Like the EEG, the information about CBF is correlated with ICP monitoring and patient activities.

Evoked Potential Monitoring. Evoked potentials are another noninvasive way of applying specific sensory stimuli and recording the minute electrical potentials created. Each potential is recorded and stored in a computer, and an average curve is calculated. The two common types of evoked potentials used in a critical care setting are brain stem auditory evoked potentials and somatosensory evoked potentials. Brainstem auditory evoked potentials are used to evaluate brain stem function and can be conducted on a conscious or unconscious patient, or even during an operation. Somatosensory evoked potentials measure peripheral nerve responses and can be helpful in evaluating spinal cord function.

These technological modalities allow the patient's progress to be followed at the bedside. They allow the practitioner to assess the effect that an ICP value or a treatment intervention is having on a patient with increased precision and accuracy, enabling a more individualized intervention.

Medical Assessment

The initial baseline laboratory tests obtained in a patient with increased ICP are:

- Arterial blood gases and continuous oxygen saturation
- Complete blood count, with an emphasis on red blood cells, hematocrit, and hemoglobin
- Coagulation profile (prothrombin time, partial thromboplastin time, platelet count)
- Electrolytes, blood urea nitrogen, creatinine, liver functions, and serum osmolality
- Urinalysis and urine osmolality

The ongoing laboratory tests obtained in a patient with increased ICP are:

- Arterial blood gases and continuous oxygen saturation
- Hematocrit and hemoglobin
- Electrolytes, blood urea nitrogen, creatinine, and serum osmolality

The x-ray studies and other diagnostic tests performed on a patient with increased ICP include:

- Computed tomography (CT) scan
- Skull x-ray studies
- EEG
- CBF studies
- Cerebral angiography

NURSING DIAGNOSES

Nursing diagnoses appropriate for a patient experiencing increased ICP are:

- Decreased adaptive capacity related to neurological illness or trauma
- Risk for altered cerebral tissue perfusion related to increased ICP, decreased CBF, hypertension or hypotension
- Risk for ineffective breathing pattern or impaired gas exchange related to underlying neurological and respiratory problems
- Ineffective airway clearance related to cranial nerve impairment, obstruction in respiratory system, respiratory infection, and underlying neurological problem
- Risk for fluid volume deficit related to underlying neurological problem and treatment of increased ICP
- Altered nutrition (less than body requirements) related to a hypermetabolic state following trauma or surgery
- Impaired physical mobility related to injury to the motor pathways in the brain
- Risk for infection related to invasive techniques and steroid therapy
- Altered thought processes related to increased ICP and structural damage ischemia
- Self-care deficit: activities of daily living related to the neurological deficits
- Risk for injury related to impaired mobility, memory, or judgment; decreased attention span; and impulsiveness
- Ineffective family coping related to the patient's neurological deficits

INTERVENTIONS

Nursing Interventions

Objectives of nursing management for a patient with increased ICP incorporate the following:

- Maintaining a normal ICP
- Maintaining adequate CBF that is well oxygenated
- Maintaining fluid and electrolyte balance

- Minimizing the hypermetabolic state, muscle wasting, and weight loss
- Preventing the hazards of immobility
- Preventing infections
- Minimizing impaired thought processes
- Protecting from injury
- Promoting self-care
- Promoting effective family coping

Refer to the Nursing Care Plan for the Patient with Increased ICP, Head Injury, or CVA for a detailed description of specific nursing interventions.

General Nursing Care

For the last 20 years, nurse researchers have identified some nursing activities (e.g., suctioning, head positioning, repositioning, and hygiene measures) that are associated with increases in ICP (Andrus, 1991; Crosby and Parsons, 1992; Brucia et al., 1992; Kerr et al., 1993; Rising, 1993; Prendergast, 1994). The ICP response to nursing activities is an individual patient response that depends on the patient's position on the volume-pressure curve.

Head and body position is an important factor in minimizing increased ICP. Elevating the head of the bed 15° to 30° and keeping the head in a neutral position in relation to the body facilitate venous drainage and decrease the risk of venous obstruction. When the head is turned 45°, increases in ICP can occur. This is because the jugular vein becomes obstructed and venous drainage is impeded. Extreme hip flexion also causes elevation in ICP. Extreme hip flexion causes an increase in intra-abdominal and intrathoracic pressure and results in increased ICP.

Frequently, patients with increased ICP are fluid restricted. The goal of fluid restriction is to maintain intravascular volume without adding free water. An increase in free water (extracellular fluid excess) would increase cerebral edema and further increase ICP. Strict measurement of intake and output is required. When osmotic and loop diuretics are used, it is critical to monitor fluid and electrolyte status. Hypokalemia is common after mannitol therapy. This electrolyte imbalance is corrected with a potassium supplement. An elevation of serum osmolarity can occur with osmotic diuretic use. Hyperosmolarity can result in renal failure, neurological deterioration, and death if it is not corrected. Other factors leading to fluid and electrolyte imbalance are diabetes insipidus (DI) and the syndrome of inappropriate antidiuretic hormone (SIADH) secretion; either can occur with brain injury.

The development of DI and SIADH in a critically ill neurological patient presents a threat to the body's water and electrolyte balance. Antidiuretic hormone (ADH; arginine vasopressin) plays a major role in this balance by decreasing the amount of water excreted by the kidneys. ADH is the renal control of plasma osmolality.

ADH Physiology. ADH has very potent vasoconstrictive properties. It is manufactured in the anterior hypothalamus, stored in the posterior pituitary gland, released when plasma osmolality increases (normal range is 280 to 295 mOsm/kg), and inhibited when plasma osmolality decreases below 280 mOsm/kg. Osmoreceptors are located in the anterior hypothalamus and detect changes in the sodium ion concentration of the extracellular fluid; they are stimulated when serum osmolality increases. When the hypothalamus is stimulated to secrete ADH, the osmoreceptors are also stimulated, and the thirst center in the lateral hypothalamus is stimulated. From the thirst center, signals are sent to the cerebral cortex, and an alert adult becomes thirsty and drinks fluid.

Diabetes Insipidus. DI is a condition that occurs when impaired ADH synthesis, release, or renal resistance to ADH causes loss of water through a dilute, hypo-osmolar urine, despite plasma and extracellular hyperosmolality (Bell, 1994; Buonocore and Robinson, 1993). The two types of DI are central (neurological cause) and nephrogenic. DI can be a temporary or a permanent condition.

Central DI. Central DI occurs when there is absent or diminished circulating ADH from damaged neural pathways or structures (i.e., hypothalamus or pituitary gland). Therefore, the problem is with the production, synthesis, or release of ADH. As a result of an inadequate circulating ADH, massive free water loss occurs, causing serum sodium and plasma osmolality levels to rise. Central DI can show a triphasic pattern. In the initial phase there is polyuria from several hours to 2 days; in the second phase there is uncontrolled ADH release with oliguria; the last phase consists of polyuria.

Nephrogenic DI. This type of DI occurs when the renal collection ducts and distal tubules are unresponsive to ADH. ADH is produced, synthesized, and released; the kidneys fail to respond to ADH to conserve water.

Clinical Presentation. The hallmark sign of DI is polyuria, with urinary volumes of 2 to 15 L/day independent of fluid intake (Bell, 1994). Consecutive urine outputs of 200 ml or greater for 2 hours should be reported to the physician. The appearance of the urine is pale and dilute. There is a decreased urine osmolality (100 to 200 mOsm/kg) and low specific gravity in the range of 1.001 to 1.005 (Bell, 1994; Buonocore and Robinson, 1993).

A second sign on presentation is hypernatremia (greater than 145 mEq/L). The hypernatremia is a

NURSING CARE PLAN FOR THE PATIENT WITH INCREASED INTRACRANIAL PRESSURE, HEAD INJURY, OR CEREBROVASCULAR ACCIDENT

Nursing Diagnosis	Patient Outcomes	Nursing Interventions
Decreased adaptive capacity (intracranial) related to neurological illness/trauma.	Intracranial pressure (ICP) at rest will be within the range of 0–15 mm Hg. Cerebral perfusion pressure (CPP) will be maintained at >60 mm Hg. CPP = MAP − ICP. Temperature 38°C. Patient is awake and exhibits appropriate responses to the environment. Absence of headaches. ABGs within normal limits (WNL).	Neurological assessments every hour. Notify physician of changes. Maintain airway. Monitor ICP measurements continuously; record and report changes in readings. Notify if CPP ≤60 mm Hg. Elevate HOB 30–45°. Monitor response to all nursing activities for increases in ICP. Maintain head in neutral position. Avoid extreme hip flexion, isometric exercises, straining with stool, breath-holding episodes. Fluid restriction as ordered (range 80–100 ml/h). Do not suction for more than 15 sec at a time. Hyperoxygenate with suctioning (pre and post). Maintain quiet environment. Space nursing activities to avoid cumulative effect. Monitor fluid and electrolyte status. Monitor electrolytes, Hgb and Hct, BUN, creatinine. Record I&O. Administer medications as ordered (steroids, diuretics, anticonvulsants). Monitor side effects of medications. Maintain temp at 38°C using hypothermia blanket, antipyretics. Monitor ABGs.
Risk for altered tissue perfusion (cerebral) related to increased ICP, decreased cerebral blood flow, hypertension/hypotension.	Mean arterial pressure range 63–124 mm Hg. Systolic BP 100–140 mm Hg. Diastolic range 60–90 mm Hg. Stable vital signs. Urine output ≥30 ml/h. Hgb/Hct, WNL. Normal sinus rhythm. CVP 3–10 mm Hg. PCWP 5–15 mm Hg. Improved neurological status, especially level of consciousness. ABGs WNL. No complications of therapy.	Neurological assessment every hour. Monitor BP and pulse every hour or as ordered. Monitor correlation between BP and neurological status. Monitor respiratory status. Monitor ECG pattern continuously. CVP and PAP as ordered. Hourly urine outputs. Specific gravity every 2 h. Check for hematuria. Assess for signs of bleeding from chest, abdomen, pelvis, extremities. Control scalp bleeding by compression. Administer volume expanders (albumin, Plasmanate, blood products). Calm, quiet environment. Administer medications as ordered. Monitor effects of medications (antihypertensive agents, heparin, warfarin, antifibrinolytic agents). Administer medications for vasospasm (calcium channel blockers, steroid therapy, fibrinolytic agents.

NURSING CARE PLAN FOR THE PATIENT WITH INCREASED INTRACRANIAL PRESSURE, HEAD INJURY, OR CEREBROVASCULAR ACCIDENT *Continued*

Nursing Diagnosis	Patient Outcomes	Nursing Interventions
		Minimize restlessness and agitation. Monitor electrolytes, Hgb/Hct, serum osmolality, ABGs.
Risk for ineffective breathing pattern or impaired gas exchange related to underlying neurological and respiratory problems.	Maintain airway. Vital capacity 60–75 ml/kg. ABGs WNL. O_2 saturation WNL 96%. Breath sounds bilaterally.	Monitor temperature, report if abnormal. Monitor respiratory rate and rhythm. Assess breath sounds every hour for 72 h then prn. Observe for anxiety, restlessness, trouble breathing. Assist with clearing secretions with suctioning.
Ineffective airway clearance related to cranial nerve impairment, obstruction in respiratory system, and underlying neurological problem.	CXR WNL. No atelectasis/pneumonia. Temp WNL. No dyspnea, tachypnea. No restlessness or anxiety. Free from mucous plugs.	Maintain patency of endotracheal tube or tracheostomy tube. Observe for tolerance for turning. Chest physiotherapy. Administer antibiotics as ordered. Monitor O_2 saturation with arterial live or pulse oximeter. Administer O_2 as needed. Gradually decrease ventilatory assistance. Assess for fatigue.
Fluid volume deficit related to fluid restriction, diuretics, GI suction, DI, and SIADH.	Urine output >30 ml/h <200 ml/h. Good skin turgor. Maintain admission weight. Electrolytes, BUN, creatinine, Hct, WNL. Serum osmolality <320 mOsm. Normal sinus rhythm on rhythmic strip. Normothermic. Moist mucous membranes.	Assess skin and mucous membranes every 2 h. Foley catheter for strict I&O. Report urine outputs <30 ml/h or >200 ml/h every 2 h. Weigh daily. Monitor lab results: electrolytes, BUN, creatinine, Hct, Hgb, serum osmolality. Monitor ECG. Monitor temperature every 2 h.
Altered nutrition (less than body requirements) related to the hypermetabolic state.	Maintenance of admission weight. Absence of vomiting. Absence of abdominal distention. Bowel sounds present and active. Absence of impaction. Absorbing tube feeding. Serum proteins and albumin WNL. Positive nitrogen balance.	Early nutritional support (enteral or parenteral). Auscultate bowel sounds prior to intermittent NG tube feeding and p.r.n. Palpate abdomen for distention. Sump or NG tube on low continuous suction for abdominal distention. Daily weights. Monitor electrolytes, BUN, creatinine, Hct, Hgb, serum proteins. Check for gastric tube residual when tube feedings are initiated. Aseptic technique when manipulating central lines. Do not infuse other fluids through line used for enteral nutrition. Assess abdomen distention. Record bowel evacuation. Metamucil for diarrhea per order. I&O.

Continued on following page

NURSING CARE PLAN FOR THE PATIENT WITH INCREASED INTRACRANIAL PRESSURE, HEAD INJURY, OR CEREBROVASCULAR ACCIDENT *Continued*

Nursing Diagnosis	Patient Outcomes	Nursing Interventions
Impaired physical mobility related to increased ICP, head injury, CVA.	Intact motor and sensory function on unaffected side. Absence of edema. Absence of thrombosis. Absence of atelectasis. Absence of skin breakdown.	Neurological assessment. Change positions every 2 h (unless contraindicated by ICP). Skin assessment. Range-of-motion of extremities prevent footdrop (i.e., high-top tennis shoes on 2 h, off 2 h, footboard). Monitor for local swelling, calf measurement. Monitor color, temp, tenderness/pain over veins. Antiembolism stockings. Apply moist heat to area as ordered. Anticoagulant therapy as ordered. Monitor PT, PTT, Hct, Hgb, platelets. Normal CXR. Breath sounds present.
Potential for infection related to invasive techniques and steroid therapy.	Afebrile. WBC WNL. Negative cultures.	Wash hands prior to contact with patient. Aseptic technique when performing invasive procedures and working with patients, catheters, tubes. Discontinue invasive lines, catheters ASAP. Use gloves when performing nursing activities. Minimize patient exposure to infected staff/visitors. Monitor results of CBC. Obtain cultures. Monitor vital signs. Assess vital signs, body fluids, skin for signs and symptoms of infection and report abnormalities. Keep ICP and hemodynamic monitor devices a closed system. Administer antibiotics as ordered.
Altered thought processes related to increased ICP.	Appropriate behavior patterns. Appropriate verbalizations. Minimal memory impairments.	Explain nursing activities prior to initiation. Orient to person, place, time: use clocks and calendars in patient room to help orient. Avoid sensory overload. Allow for frequent rest periods. Provide a structured environment. Continuity of staff taking care of patient. Place call light, water, tissues within reach. Identify objects by name. Involve significant other in care and goal setting. Identify behaviors occurring as a result of inaccurate thoughts and document these behaviors. Teach patient, family, significant other strategies to deal with altered behaviors. Speak slowly, using concrete thoughts and allowing adequate response time from patient.

NURSING CARE PLAN FOR THE PATIENT WITH INCREASED INTRACRANIAL PRESSURE, HEAD INJURY, OR CEREBROVASCULAR ACCIDENT Continued

Nursing Diagnosis	Patient Outcomes	Nursing Interventions
Self-care deficit in activities of daily living (ADLs) related to the neurological problem.	Perform self-care activities without a change in vital signs or ICP.	Assist patient as necessary. Monitor energy requirements and expenditure for self-care activity. Assess activity tolerance (monitor heart rate). Assist in positioning patient for ADLs. Keep objects within easy reach of patient. Schedule frequent rest periods.
Risk for injury related to impaired mobility, memory/judgment, decreased attention span, and impulsiveness.	No falling. No bruising from use of physical restraints. Patient asks for assistance when needed.	Identify certain behaviors that may increase risk for injury: restless, agitated, impulsive, short attention span. Assess judgment and decision-making ability. Remove clutter from environment. Examine environment for potential risks.
Ineffective family coping related to the neurological problem.	Verbalizes need for more information related to disease process or particular situation. Discuss changes in patient/family as a result of neurological problem. Demonstrates understanding of information given. Decreased anxiety. Significant other participates in care of patient. Verbalizes feelings to nurses/other family members.	Assess areas in which a knowledge deficit exists. Provide adequate and correct information to patient/family. Discuss usual reactions to neurological problem: stress, anxiety, inattention, depression, dependency. Assess prior coping skills and try to enhance those skills in dealing with current situation. Provide information on routine care, hospital routines and services. Assist family members to recognize roles to maintain family integrity. Involve family members in care of patient. Encourage the use of additional support systems—friends, clergy, professional health care providers.

Data from Kim, M. J., et al. (1987). *Pocket guide to nursing diagnoses* (2nd ed.). St. Louis: C. V. Mosby; and Marshall, S. B., Marshall, L. F., Vos, H. R., & Chesnut, R. M. (1990). *Neuroscience critical care.* Philadelphia: W. B. Saunders Co.

result of the hyperosmolar state due to the free water loss. Hypernatremia can lead to lethargy, seizures, and coma if it is not corrected. With nephrogenic DI, the patient also has hypokalemia or hypercalcemia (Bell, 1994).

The patient may also present with dehydration and hypovolemia, especially if he or she cannot perceive thirst, cannot drink fluids, or is behind on intravenous (IV) fluid replacement. Signs and symptoms associated with dehydration and hypovolemia are tachycardia, orthostatic hypotension, poor skin turgor, dry mucous membranes, thick secretions, and sunken eyes. Hypovolemia can result in hemodynamic instability, complicating the underlying problem.

If the patient is alert, extreme thirst is reported. The patient wants to drink massive amounts of fluid, which leads to polyuria. With alert patients who can drink fluids, dehydration is rarely a problem. Hypernatremia and hyperosmolality will result if the patient cannot respond to thirst, does not sense thirst, or has such tremendous fluid requirements that he or she cannot drink enough fluid to compensate the fluid loss. In these patients, IV dextrose in water corrects the hypernatremia and hyperosmolality.

Treatment of DI. An important aspect of treatment is assessing and following the trends of intake and output, urine specific gravity, urine osmolality, serum electrolytes (focusing on sodium), and plasma osmolality and observing for dehydration and performing frequent neurological checks. It is also important to know which patients are at risk for developing DI.

The maintenance of fluid and electrolytes is critical in acute DI to minimize further neurological deterioration, dehydration, and perfusion to vital organs. Replacement of hypotonic fluid (5% dextrose in water) is titrated to cover urinary loss and insensible fluid loss. A hypotonic solution is preferred over saline solution unless there is a concurrent circulatory failure or severe hypernatremia. Strict intake and output as well as daily weights help monitor fluid balance. Serial urine and serum lab tests, strict intake and output, and daily weights and physical assessment monitor the patient's progress and response to treatment.

Pharmacological Management of DI. For central DI, exogenous ADH is administered. During the acute management of central DI, aqueous arginine vasopressin is used to control free water loss. This agent is a short-acting drug with antidiuretic and pressor effects and a prompt onset of action. After intramuscular or subcutaneous administration, its antidiuretic activity lasts 2 to 8 hours. This agent has a very short half-life of 5 to 30 minutes. The usual adult dose is 5 to 10 U every 8 to 12 hours (Bell, 1994). The side effects relate to vasoconstrictive effects (cardiac) and water overload. This drug is used with extreme caution in patients with a cardiac history.

A long-acting ADH preparation used for the ongoing management of DI is desmopressin (DDAVP). This drug is 10 to 100 times as potent as arginine vasopressin and has negligible pressor effects. The onset of action is 1 hour, and its antidiuretic effect lasts 8 to 24 hours. DDAVP is usually given intranasally but can be given intravenously, intramuscularly, or subcutaneously. The parenteral dose is 0.5 to 1 ml (2 to 4 µg) in two divided doses. The intranasal dose is 0.1 to 0.4 ml (10 to 40 µg) in a single or divided doses (Bell, 1994). The side effects of DDAVP relate to water overload (hyponatremia, weight gain, headache, listlessness, peripheral edema).

Nephrogenic DI is treated with water replacement and restriction of dietary sodium and protein intake. The administration of a thiazide diuretic produces a mild hypovolemia. ADH preparations do not help in nephrogenic DI.

SIADH. SIADH is a condition in which too much ADH is produced or secreted despite a low serum osmolality, hyponatremia, and an increase in extracellular fluid volume. There is a failure of the feedback loop that regulates the release and inhibition of ADH. There are a variety of causes of SIADH, including malignancies (bronchogenic carcinoma), central nervous system disorders (brain tumor, head trauma, CVA), nonmalignant pulmonary conditions (tuberculosis, lung abscess, bacterial pneumonia), the immediate postoperative period, and certain drugs (barbiturates, morphine, anesthetics, carbamazepine).

Clinical Presentation. SIADH causes the patient to manifest signs and symptoms associated with water retention (weight gain), hyponatremia (less than 135 mEq/L), and hypo-osmolality (less than 280 mOsm/kg). The urine output is low and very concentrated, with urine osmolality over 100 mOsm/kg (Batcheller, 1994). Patients with SIADH do not present with signs of intravascular volume depletion (e.g., tachycardia, orthostatic hypotension) or peripheral edema.

Neurological deficits are caused by two things: cerebral edema because of the breakdown in the intracellular-extracellular osmotic gradient, causing water to shift into brain cells; or hyponatremia, leading to altered mental status, headache, and seizures.

Treatment. Medical treatment is aimed at relieving the water retention and hyponatremia, and fluid restriction is the key. Water intake should not exceed urinary output and insensible fluid loss (i.e., 1000 cc/day). With fluid restriction, the serum sodium increases, and there is a gradual weight loss. Fluid restriction is difficult for the patient because of the feeling of being thirsty, so the fluid should be spread out over a 24-hour period.

The second aspect of treatment is correcting the acute hyponatremia (fall of serum sodium less than 120 mEq/L in less than 48 hours). Aggressive treatment consists of using a hypertonic IV solution (e.g., 3% sodium chloride) with an infusion pump. The patient must be closely monitored for hypernatremia. The rate of administering the 3% sodium chloride solution is 1 to 2 ml/kg/hr to raise the serum sodium no faster than 1 to 2 mEq/L/hr (Batcheller, 1994). Loop diuretics may also be administered, but electrolytes must be closely monitored.

Chronic hyponatremia (fall in serum sodium longer than 48 hours) is managed with fluid restriction. If fluid restriction is unsuccessful, the next step is to administer drugs that reduce ADH secretion (e.g., phenytoin) or decrease renal responsiveness to ADH (e.g., lithium or demeclocycline). Use of these drugs requires monitoring of renal function because of nephrotoxicity.

Nursing Implications. Monitoring intake and output, urine specific gravity, daily weights, and pulmonary pressures is an important part of treatment. Fluid restriction is uncomfortable for many patients, so frequent mouth care, oral rinses without swallowing, use of chilled beverages, and sucking on hard candy (if the patient is able) are pleasing to patients and help them through a difficult aspect of treatment. Mouthwashes with an alcohol base and lemon or glycerine swabs should be avoided due to the drying effect on mucous membranes.

Assessment of body systems is very important, since SIADH can effect multiple systems. Assessment of the gastrointestinal (GI) tract is important, because gastric motility is decreased in SIADH, and constipation is a potential problem. Tap water or saline enemas are to be avoided, because they can contribute to water intoxication due to water absorption through the intestines. Nasogastric and enteral tubes should be irrigated with normal saline instead of water to minimize the free water intake. IV fluids for mixing antibiotics should not be diluted with 5% dextrose in water or other hypotonic fluid.

Hyperthermia increases the metabolic demand of brain cells, causing an increase in CBF and increased ICP. Therefore, the body temperature should not exceed 38°C. Patients with neurological injury affecting the hypothalamus are particularly prone to temperature fluctuations. Often, they respond directly to environmental temperatures. Therefore, the environmental temperature is kept cool for their safety.

Medical (Nonsurgical) Interventions

The first task of the physician is to decrease ICP and then identify the cause. Once the cause is discovered, treatment is centered on permanently decreasing the high ICP, maintaining the airway, providing ventilation and oxygenation, maintaining CPP, and decreasing the metabolic demands placed on the injured brain. Many of these medical interventions are used individually or in combination.

Medical treatment of increased ICP usually includes hyperventilation, osmotic and loop diuretics, positioning, fluid restriction, corticosteroids, oxygenation, maintaining blood pressure, and decreasing the metabolic demand of injured brain cells.

Hyperventilation. Acute hyperventilation decreases $PaCO_2$, causing vasoconstriction of the cerebral arteries, reducing CBF, and decreasing ICP. Using hyperventilation over a long period of time is controversial and may not reduce ICP significantly (Marshall et al., 1990; Prendergast, 1994). However, physicians may utilize the technique by setting the ventilator at a rate that produces hyperventilation. In addition, the patient can be hyperventilated using the manual button

on the ventilator or periodically hyperventilating by using a bag-valve device. $PaCO_2$ is generally maintained at 30 mm Hg.

Diuretic Therapy. Osmotic diuretics (mannitol 20%) draw water from normal brain cells to the plasma, thereby decreasing ICP. The effects of decreasing ICP and increasing CPP occur within 20 minutes of infusion. Side effects of osmotic diuretics include hypotension, electrolyte disturbance, and rebound ICP. The nurse must observe for rebound ICP. Osmotic diuretics are contraindicated in patients with renal disease. Since osmotic diuretics are not metabolized, the drug is excreted unchanged in the urine and therefore affects specific gravity.

Loop diuretics (furosemide, ethacrynic acid) decrease ICP by removing sodium and water from injured brain cells. These agents also decrease CSF formation.

Corticosteroids. The use of corticosteroids for reducing ICP is controversial. Corticosteroids reduce cerebral edema associated with brain tumors, but studies are inconsistent in reporting the value of corticosteroids to reduce ICP in other intracranial conditions. Corticosteroids reduce CSF production as well as stabilize the blood-brain barrier and cell membranes, and these actions improve overall neuronal function. The most commonly prescribed corticosteroid is dexamethasone (Decadron). The major side effects include muscle weakness, fluid retention, GI hemorrhage, nausea, abdominal distension, increased appetite, poor wound healing, and thrombocytopenia. The GI side effects may be prevented by using an H_2 receptor antagonist agent (cimetidine, nizatidine) and antacids (Marshall et al., 1990). Once the patient has been treated with corticosteroids, the drug must be carefully weaned. Abrupt withdrawal of steroids generally leads to a metabolic crisis (Cushing's crisis).

Oxygenation. Patency of the airway is important for any patient and is no less important for a patient with increased ICP. Without oxygen, the brain cannot meet metabolic demands, and the resultant hypoxia can lead to the death of neurons. For many patients with increased ICP, short-term management of the airway is accomplished by an endotracheal tube. Long-term management entails the use of a tracheostomy tube.

Blood Pressure Management. Blood pressure must be carefully controlled in a patient with increased ICP, because hypotension causes a decrease in CBF, which leads to cerebral ischemia. Hypertension (greater than 160 mm Hg systolic) worsens cerebral edema and leads to ischemia by compressing cerebral vessels. Mean systolic blood pressures greater than 160 mm Hg can be lowered by using labetalol or propranolol. These beta-blockers decrease the ongoing catecholamine release from the sympathetic stimulation associated with neurological injury. The goal is to keep a patient with increased ICP normotensive and have a CPP in the range of 60 to 70 mm Hg (Ropper and Rockoff, 1988). These "high" systolic pressures are needed to achieve an adequate CPP when increased ICP is present. Some antihypertensive agents (nitroprusside, hydrazine) and some calcium channel blockers (verapamil, nifedipine) cause cerebral vasodilatation. This vasodilatation increases CBF and causes increased ICP. The use of these vasodilators and calcium channel blockers is avoided in patients with poor intracranial compliance.

Reducing Metabolic Demands. Seizure activity is another factor that raises the metabolic rate, increases CBF, expends oxygen, depletes energy stores, and causes increased ICP. Ischemia develops when flow cannot meet metabolic demands. Seizures can be controlled with phenytoin (Dilantin) 15 to 18 mg/kg IV (loading dose). It is important not to exceed 50 mg/min in order to avoid the cardiotoxic effects of this drug. A 5- to 10-mg IV bolus of diazepam (Valium) at a rate of 2 mg/min can also be given to stop the seizures. If these measures fail and the patient is intubated, a neuromuscular blocker (pancuronium bromide [Pavulon]) can be used.

Other pharmacological agents used to decrease the metabolic demand and blunt environmental stimuli include morphine sulfate (small IV bolus or continuous dose 2 to 8 mg/hr), sedatives, muscle relaxants, and barbiturates. If barbiturates are used, the patient is intubated with mechanical ventilation, and arterial and intracranial pressures are monitored. Either thiopental (short-term use) or pentobarbital (long-term use) is effective in reducing the metabolic demand on injured brain cells. Major side effects of barbiturate therapy are hypotension and myocardial instability. Table 10–9 outlines other nursing parameters associated with administering drugs.

Surgical Interventions

Surgical intervention may be required to remove the source of a mass or lesion causing the increased ICP. This involves the removal of infarcted areas and hematomas (epidural, subdural, or intracerebral). Removing the clot eliminates the mass lesion, decreases the brain component within the skull, and decreases cerebral edema around the area of the clot. Such surgical measures contribute to decreasing ICP.

PATIENT OUTCOMES

Patient outcomes for increased ICP are focused on maintaining ICP within the normal range (0 to 15 mm Hg), maintaining the airway, and promoting adequate oxygenation and CPP. Other patient outcomes are directed at maintaining fluid and electrolyte balance, preventing nutritional problems, preventing the hazards of immobility, and helping the family cope.

Family members of a critically ill neurological patient are different from family members of patients without neurological deficits. Neurological injury (especially head trauma) often occurs without warning and may be severe. This often places the family in a state of disequilibrium. Adding further stress on the family is the fact that the patient has suffered an insult to the nervous system (especially the brain) and may respond inappropriately or uncharacteristically or not be able to respond at all to the family. Neurological insults to the brain or spinal cord cause uncertainty related to the patient's physical and mental outcomes. The personality and mental changes associated with brain insults can be devastating to the family. In Engli and Kirsivali-Farmer's (1993) study, family members indicated that information concerning their relatives' condition, prognosis, and treatment was a priority. Nurses often fulfill these information needs, because physicians are not always available at the bedside. By providing information to family members, nurses give them psychosocial support and reduce their anxiety (see Nursing Care Plan for the Patient with Increased ICP, Head Injury, or CVA).

Head Injury

Head injury is a common occurrence in the United States. Trauma is the leading cause of death between the ages of 1 and 44, with approximately 500,000 incidents of head injury every year (Doberstein et al., 1993). Severe head injury represents 10% of this figure, and mortality from head injury prior to hospitalization is considerable.

PATHOPHYSIOLOGY

When head injury occurs, it can damage the scalp, skull, and brain and its pathways, meninges, cranial nerves, and intracranial vessels (Fig. 10–17). The head injury can be open or closed. With an open head injury, the scalp is torn or a fracture extends into the sinuses or middle ear. The meninges can also be penetrated. A closed head injury occurs when there is no break in the scalp. Acceleration-deceleration is a common mechanism for head injury. With this injury, the movement of the head follows a straight line, and the moving head (acceleration) hits a stationary object (deceleration). Rotation or a twisting of the brain within the cranial vault adds to the insult, and the

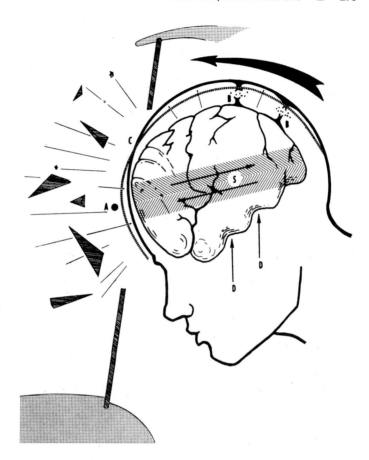

Figure 10–17. Closed blunt injury. Skull molding occurs at the site of impact. *(A)* Stippled line, preinjury contour. *(C)* Solid line, contour moments after impact, with inbending at *(A)* and outbending at the vertex. *(B)* Subdural veins torn as brain rotates forward. *(S)* Shearing strains throughout the brain. *(D)* Direct trauma to inferior temporal and frontal lobes over floors of the middle and anterior fossae. (From Eliasson, S. G., Prensky, A. L., & Hardin, W. B. (1978). *Neurological pathophysiology* (2nd ed.) (Fig. 9–5). New York: Oxford University Press.)

extent of head injury can range from mild to severe (Fig. 10–18).

Scalp Lacerations

Scalp lacerations are common in head injury and can be associated with skull fracture. The scalp offers some resistance to compression and absorbs mild blows by distributing forces over the entire area of the scalp. Highly violent blows, however, do penetrate the scalp. In addition, the scalp is very vascular and can be the source of significant blood loss, which is difficult to stop. Once bleeding is stopped, it is important to clip the hair around the laceration. The wound is cleansed, débrided, inspected, and palpated for a depressed skull fracture. Inattention to these details can lead to infection.

Skull Fractures

The skull is composed of three layers that add stability and act as shock absorbers. The skull also has high compressive strength and is somewhat elastic. Following impact, the skull is compressed, and there is an inbending of the skull at the point of impact and an outbending at the vertex. The area of outbending of tensile stresses creates a fracture line that moves toward the base of the skull.

There are several types of skull fractures following head injury: linear, depressed, and basilar.

Linear Skull Fracture

Linear skull fracture is the most common type. This fracture is uneventful unless there is an extension of the fracture to the orbit or sinus or across a vessel. When there is extension of the fracture, the patient is admitted for observation of signs of intracranial bleeding.

Depressed Skull Fracture

A depressed skull fracture occurs when the outer table of the skull is depressed below the inner table of the surrounding intact skull. The dura may be intact, bruised, or torn. If the dura is torn, there is direct communication between the brain and the environment, and meningitis can occur. In addition, the com-

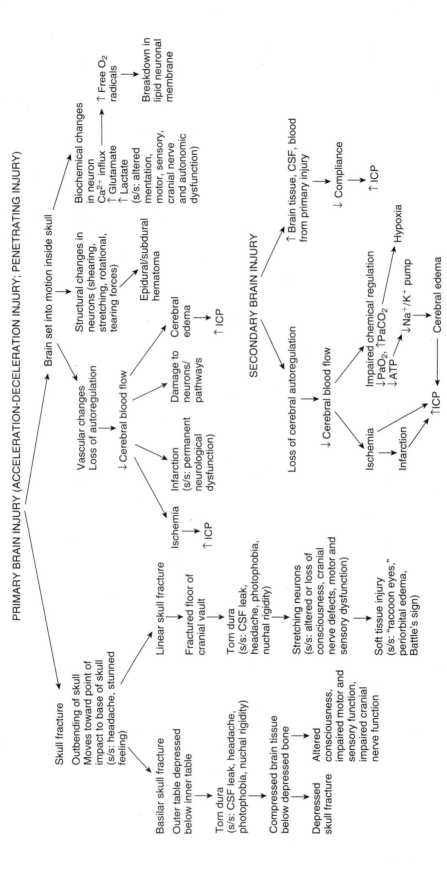

Figure 10-18. Pathophysiology flow diagram—head injury.

pressed and bruised brain beneath the depressed bone is the source of focal neurological deficit and may become an epileptogenic focal area. Mechanisms of closed head injury, along with associated signs and symptoms, are listed in Table 10–3.

Basilar Skull Fracture

A basilar skull fracture occurs at the base of the cranial vault and can extend into the anterior, middle, and posterior fossae. This type of fracture is difficult to confirm on a radiograph and is diagnosed by clinical presentation of the patient (see Table 10–3). Dural tears are very common with a basilar skull fracture and may lead to meningitis. Drainage of CSF from the nose (rhinorrhea), postnasal drainage, or drainage of CSF from the ear (otorrhea) may be indicative of a dural tear that allows a CSF leak. It is important to allow the CSF to flow freely. Nothing should be placed in the nose or ear, although small bandages can be used to collect the drainage. The patient is also instructed not to blow his or her nose. If needed, suction catheters, nasogastric tubes, and endotracheal tubes should be inserted through the mouth rather than the nose. If CSF is suspected to be present in drainage, a sample in a plain test tube is sent to the laboratory for analysis. Glucose test strips may not differentiate between CSF rhinorrhea and rhinorrhea from the respiratory tract. Cranial nerves and the internal carotid artery passing through the skull floor can also be damaged in association with the injury.

Brain Injury

Brain injury from head injury is classified as primary and secondary brain injury.

Primary Brain Injury

Primary brain injury is the direct injury that occurs to the brain from an impact. With impact, the semisolid brain moves around inside the skull. The area under the direct impact is injured (coup injury). Injury to adjacent poles occurs from the movement of the brain inside the skull (contrecoup injury). The stretching, shearing, rotational, and tearing forces that result from impact cause an interruption of normal neuronal pathways and early vasogenic edema.

On a cellular level, following a direct injury, there is a series of biochemical events that contribute to the overproduction of free oxygen radicals (molecules or atoms that contain an unpaired electron in their outermost orbit, creating a lot of reactivity with other molecules), breaking down the lipid neuronal cell membrane and causing early neuronal deterioration (Siesjo,

1993; Prendergast, 1994). In addition, there is a loss of cellular calcium homeostasis, liberation of glutamate, and cellular acidosis. The patient shows signs or symptoms of neuronal deterioration and is unstable neurologically.

Concussion, contusion, penetrating injuries, hematomas, and intracerebral hemorrhage are all types of primary brain injury (see Table 10–3). Concussion represents a mild form of head injury, whereas contusion, penetrating injuries, hematomas, and hemorrhage constitute severe head injuries.

Concussion. Concussion occurs when there is a mechanical force of short duration applied to the skull. This injury results in the temporary failure of impulse conduction. The neurological deficits are reversible and generally mild. Patients may lose consciousness for a few seconds at the time of injury, but lasting effects are not common.

Contusion. Contusion is the result of coup and contrecoup injuries, accompanied by bruising and generalized hemorrhage into brain tissue. Traumatic laceration of the cortical surface associated with contrecoup injuries may be greater than those seen directly under the point of impact. Signs and symptoms are variable (see Table 10–3).

Diffuse Axonal Injury. Diffuse axonal injury is the result of coup and contrecoup injuries, accompanied by generalized shearing of brain tissue. Traumatic laceration of the cortical surface associated with contrecoup injuries may be greater than that seen directly under the point of impact. Signs and symptoms are variable (see Table 10–3). This type of injury causes damage to the axonal pathways in the brain.

Penetrating Injury. Penetrating injuries are the result of low- or high-velocity forces such as gunshots, knives, or sharp objects. With this type of injury, there is a deep laceration of brain tissue and possible damage to the ventricular system. A low-velocity (stabbing) injury is limited to the track of entry, and the greatest concern is bleeding and infection. A high-velocity (gunshot) injury causes extensive damage because of the entry of bone fragments at the site. In addition, because bullets spin irregularly, they create many paths and shock waves that cause extensive brain damage.

A more global injury is diffuse axonal involvement. With this injury, there is widespread white matter axonal damage secondary to tearing and shearing forces. This type of injury is associated with disruption of axons in the cerebral hemispheres, diencephalon, and brain stem. Clinically, these patients show no, or only minimal, signs of recovery.

Hematoma

Epidural Hematoma. Collection of blood in the space between the inner table of the skull and the dura causes an epidural hematoma (Fig. 10–19). Many such

Table 10-3. MECHANISMS OF CLOSED HEAD INJURY WITH ASSOCIATED SIGNS/SYMPTOMS

Injury	Signs and Symptoms
Skull Fractures (Deformation of Skull, Secondary to Impact)	
Linear: Starts at outbended area, moves toward point of impact and to base of skull	Swelling, redness, bruising, tenderness on scalp, scalp laceration
Depressed: Outer table depressed below the inner table, associated with torn dura, and brain beneath depressed bone is bruised	Palpation of depressed area in contour of skull; CSF leak from nose, ear, postnasal; scalp bruising, tenderness, laceration
Basilar: Fracture is the anterior, middle, and/or posterior fossa along the floor of the cranial vault, dura is torn	
Anterior Fossa Fracture	Raccoon or panda eyes, periorbital edema, CSF leak nose, nasal congestion, cranial nerve deficits
Middle Fossa Facture	CSF leak ear, hematympanum, battle sign, decreased hearing, cranial nerve deficits
Posterior Fossa Fracture	Bruising base of the neck, cranial nerve deficits
Cellular Injuries to Brain Cells (Interruption of Normal Connections, Neurons, Pathways; Biochemical Changes Secondary to Stretching, Shearing, Rotational and Shearing Forces Associated with Impact)	
Focal Injuries: Concussion, contusion, avulsion	
Concussion: Altered level of consciousness (LOC), confusion, disorientation, retrograde amnesia	
Contusion: Injury can be to the area directly beneath impact (coup) or injury can be to the brain's poles (contrecoup); since these areas are prone to bleeding and swelling, they act as an intracranial expanding mass	Altered LOC, retrograde amnesia, motor deficits (weakness to paralysis), restlessness, combative, confusion, speech disturbances, cranial nerve dysfunction, decorticate and decerebrate posturing, abnormal breathing patterns, coma
Penetrating Injuries: Injury is caused by deep laceration of brain tissue, damage to the ventricular system	
Low Velocity: Stab wound—injury is caused by deep laceration of brain tissue, damage to the ventricular system	
High Velocity: Gunshot wound—extensive injury because of the entry of many bone fragments at the site, bullets spin irregularly creating many paths, increasing the brain damage, and shock waves cause brain disruption	
Diffuse Brain Injury: Tearing of axons and myelin sheaths, secondary to generalized movement of brain from impact—prolonged coma, cranial nerve deficits, motor deficits	
Secondary Injury: Caused by increased ICP, cerebral edema, herniation, ischemia, hypoxia; these situations complicate intracerebral bleeds, focal and penetrating injuries	Prolonged coma, cranial nerve deficits, motor deficits
Intracerebral Bleeds (Cerebral Vessels Are Broken or Sheared Off Secondary to Impact)	
Epidural: Tearing of an artery from a skull fracture, brisk bleeding and rapid accumulation in the epidural space	Onset short period of LOC then lucid, then confusion, irritability, headache, deterioration LOC, motor, CN
Subdural: Tearing of bridging cortical veins—blood accumulates in the space between the dura and arachnoid	Acute and subacute—depressed LOC, pupil and extraocular movement changes, motor changes; headache, *chronic* personality changes, gait problems
Subarachnoid: Bleeding into the subarachnoid space from the rupture of a traumatic aneurysm; altered LOC, headache, nuchal rigidity, photophobia	
Intraventricular: Bleeding to the ventricles; altered LOC, cranial nerve dysfunction, motor changes	
Intracerebral: Bleeding into brain tissue, producing necrosis	Similar to focal injuries

Nervous System Alterations ■ 297

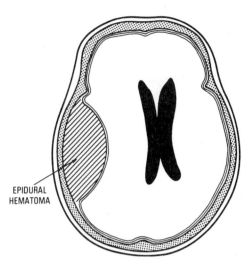

Figure 10–19. Epidural hematoma. (From Marshall, S. B., Marshall, L. F., Vos, H. R., & Chesnut, R. M. (1990). *Neuroscience critical care*. Philadelphia: W. B. Saunders Co.)

hematomas are associated with a linear fracture of the temporal bone and result from the tearing of the middle meningeal artery. Arterial blood accumulates rapidly in this space. The patient usually experiences a lucid period prior to neurological deterioration. The lucid period can last for a few hours to 48 hours (Hickey, 1992). Pupils are fixed and dilated on the side of the lesion.

Subdural Hematoma. Collection of blood in the subdural space causes a subdural hematoma (Fig. 10–20). It occurs when a surface vein is torn around the vertex. Subdural hematomas occur at all ages. In infants, they occur as a result of birth trauma; in the elderly, a subdural hematoma is most frequently the result of a fall. There are three kinds of subdural hematomas: acute, subacute, and chronic.

Acute subdural hematoma occur within 48 hours of an injury (Hickey, 1992). This type of hematoma is seen in deceleration injuries and is associated with contusions. Subacute hematomas occur from 2 days to 2 weeks after an injury (Hickey, 1992). Onset of symptoms is much slower, and the symptoms are subtle. Prognosis is good for this kind of hematoma. Chronic subdural hematomas occur as a result of a low-velocity impact. They occur 2 weeks to several months after an injury. In the elderly, these hematomas can be bilateral. The elderly incur subdural hematomas because the normal aging process results in balance and coordination deficits, which makes them prone to falling. Chronic subdural hematoma is also attributed to alcohol abuse. Signs and symptoms of subdural hematomas are discussed in Table 10–3.

Intracerebral Hemorrhage. An intracerebral hemorrhage is a large hemorrhage into brain tissue that creates a mass lesion. This lesion can occur anywhere in the brain. Signs and symptoms vary with this kind of lesion (see Table 10–3).

Secondary Brain Injury

Secondary brain injury complicates the situation following a primary brain injury and is the result of hypoxia, hypotension, anemia, hypercarbia, uncontrolled increased ICP, cerebral edema, hypermetabolic state, infection, and fluid and electrolyte imbalance. All these complications are caused by primary head injury and involve uncontrolled increased ICP and altered CBF. These insults add to the degree and extent of cellular dysfunction following head injury. All these insults can increase brain damage and affect functional recovery.

ASSESSMENT

Nursing Assessment

The GCS is used as a guide in assessing a head-injured patient. In addition, the assessment of a patient must be supplemented with the neurological examination discussed in the previous section. Assessment should be specific to the area of the brain involved. If a patient has a brain stem injury, in addition to the GCS, the nurse assesses cranial nerves and respiratory rate and rhythm. All findings are documented with a description of the patient's behavior.

Another area for assessment is the respiratory

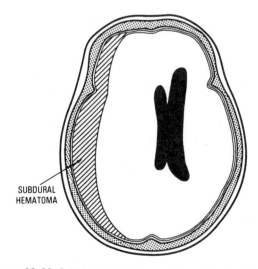

Figure 10–20. Subdural hematoma. (From Marshall, S. B., Marshall, L. F., Vos, H. R., & Chesnut, R. M. (1990). *Neuroscience critical care*. Philadelphia: W. B. Saunders Co.)

status. A high percentage of severely head-injured patients arrive at the hospital hypoxic. A PaO_2 below 50 mm Hg causes vasodilatation of cerebral vessels, increased CBF, and increased ICP. This hypoxia can further compromise the patient's progress.

Medical Assessment

Prompt and aggressive medical treatment is beneficial for a head-injured patient. Medical assessment is based on the neurological examination, which includes reflex testing, ICP and hemodynamic monitoring, and respiratory assessment. A head-injured patient requires the same laboratory studies and diagnostic studies as a patient with increased ICP.

NURSING DIAGNOSES

The same nursing diagnoses are necessary for a head-injured patient and a patient with increased ICP (see Nursing Care Plan for the Patient with Increased ICP, Head Injury, or CVA). These diagnoses cover both primary and secondary head injuries.

INTERVENTIONS

Nursing Interventions

The nursing interventions are the same as those for patients with increased ICP (see Nursing Care Plan for the Patient with Increased ICP, Head Injury, or CVA). An important consideration for nursing intervention is the sequence and timing of these activities. When the patient is having episodes of increased ICP, it is important to control the patient's environment and activities to minimize stimuli that contribute to the increased ICP. A thorough assessment assists the nurse in determining how to proceed with nursing care without jeopardizing the patient's status. For example, a patient with a severe head injury and excessively high ICP requires careful control of all activities. Thus, he or she requires rest periods after each nursing intervention to allow the ICP to return to normal.

Medical (Nonsurgical) Interventions

The nonsurgical treatment of a patient with a head injury is the same as for a patient with increased ICP. The emphasis is on reducing ICP, maintaining the airway, providing oxygenation, maintaining cerebral perfusion, and preventing secondary head injury.

Surgical Interventions

A variety of surgical procedures exist for head-injured patients. For a patient with a depressed skull fracture, elevation of the fracture may be needed, depending on the nature of the fracture. Surgical removal of an epidural, subdural, or intracerebral hematoma may be performed to prevent a mass lesion from causing a shift in brain tissue or herniation, thereby minimizing neurological deterioration of the patient. Penetrating wounds to the skull and brain may necessitate a craniotomy to explore the pathway of the missile, repair laceration of intracranial vessels and brain tissue, remove bone fragments, and, in the case of a gunshot wound, retrieve the bullet.

Postoperative care is directed at maintaining normal ICP, cerebral tissue perfusion, and airway; preventing fluid and electrolyte imbalance and complications from immobility; avoiding nutritional deficits; and reducing the incidence of infection. A postcraniotomy patient needs to have the craniotomy dressing assessed for drainage (color and amount) and fluid accumulation under the skin flap. Once the dressing is removed, the incision is assessed for swelling, redness, drainage, and tenderness. Individuals with penetrating wounds to the brain are at high risk for the development of not only infections but also brain abscesses.

PATIENT OUTCOMES

With diligent nursing and medical care, a head-injured patient should have a positive outcome. Outcomes for head-injured patients are as favorable as they are for patients with increased ICP (see Nursing Care Plan for the Patient with Increased ICP, Head Injury, or CVA).

Spinal Cord Injury

There are approximately 200,000 people in the United States with spinal cord injury (SCI). Each year, there are 10,000 to 12,000 additional victims who sustain SCI. Most of these individuals are men under 40 years of age. The causes of SCI are motor vehicle accidents, falls, sports injuries, missile injuries, and diving accidents. It is not uncommon to see head injury in association with SCI; therefore, SCI should be considered as a possibility in all unconscious patients.

PATHOPHYSIOLOGY

An SCI occurs when there is some type of sudden force exerted on the vertebral column, resulting in damage to the spinal cord. A series of responses result from this injury (Fig. 10–21). There is altered autonomic function, leading to cardiovascular instability. The loss of sympathetic input (spinal nerves T1–L1) creates bradycardia, hypotension, venous stasis, and

SPINAL CORD INJURY

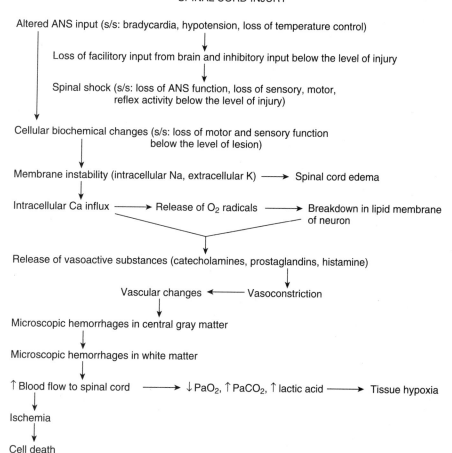

Figure 10–21. Pathophysiology flow diagram—spinal cord injury.

loss of temperature control (spinal shock). Spinal shock is the temporary loss of autonomic, sensory, and motor functions below the level of the lesion and is secondary to the loss of facilitory input from the brain and inhibitory input below the level of the injury. A sign of the termination of spinal shock is the return of reflex activity below the level of the lesion. Another response to injury is an inflammatory reaction that creates cord edema. Cord edema compresses spinal cord tissue as well as cord blood vessels. Cord edema can ascend or descend from the level of injury.

The injury itself creates a series of biochemical changes. Potassium is lost from inside the cell to the extracellular compartment. There is also a calcium influx inside the cell that leads to the lipid membrane breakdown of neurons. Free oxygen radicals are increased, which potentiates further breakdown of cell membranes. This results in free fatty acids. There is a release of vasoactive substances (norepinephrine, histamine, dopamine, glutamate, dynorphin, prostaglan-

din) as a result of these biochemical changes. This event leads to vasoconstriction of the blood vessels, decrease in tissue O_2, a buildup of lactic acid, and ischemia. If the ischemia is not reversed, axonal degeneration and conduction failure of the neuron occur. Eventually, there is cell death and permanent loss of function. This process also occurs with head injury.

The final response to SCI is vascular change. Instantly after injury, there are microscopic hemorrhages in the central gray matter of the spinal cord. After several hours, these hemorrhages invade the surrounding white matter, cord blood flow is decreased, and ischemia results. If the ischemia is not reversed, neuronal cell death occurs.

SCI can result in a complete or incomplete lesion. A complete lesion causes total loss of motor and sensory functions below the level of injury. An incomplete lesion results in the sparing of motor and sensory functions below the level of injury (Fig. 10–22). Most patients with an incomplete lesion show a mixed pat-

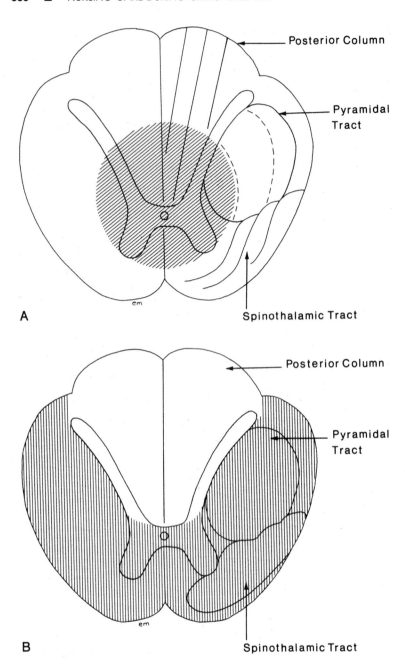

Figure 10–22. Incomplete spinal cord injuries. *(A)* Central cord syndrome. Damage to the structures of the cervical cord gray matter and the pyramidal tract. More loss in the upper extremities. *(B)* Anterior spinal cord syndrome. Damage to the anterior horn cells and the spinothalamic tract. Deficits are loss of motor function and pain and temperature sensation below the level of the lesion.

tern of motor and sensory functions rather than a classic syndrome.

ASSESSMENT

Nursing Assessment

Airway and Respiratory Status

Assessment of the airway and respiratory status is the first assessment priority. The higher the level of

SCI, the greater the functional impairment is. Respiratory problems are frequently associated with SCI. Ineffective breathing patterns are commonly caused by paralysis of the diaphragm or intercostal muscles and by chest trauma. Therefore, the lungs must be auscultated for the presence of breath sounds in all areas, as well as for the presence of adventitious sound. Observing the respiratory rate and the rhythm and depth of respiration is also important. Signs of respiratory distress include excessive retraction of accessory neck

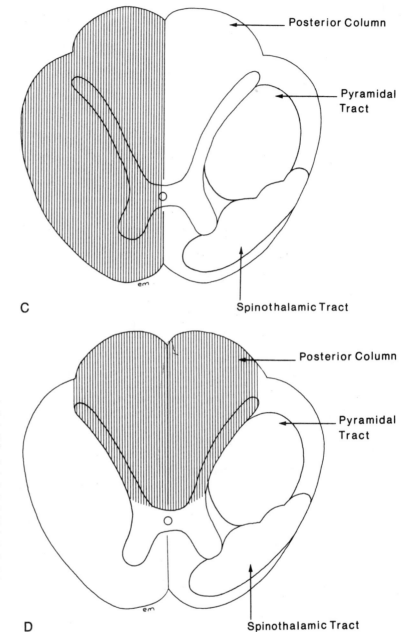

Posterior Column

Pyramidal Tract

Spinothalamic Tract

C

Posterior Column

Pyramidal Tract

Spinothalamic Tract

D

Figure 10–22. *Continued (C)* Brown-Sequard syndrome. Hemisection of the spinal cord results in loss of motor function and touch, pressure, and position sense ipsilateral to the lesion and loss of pain and temperature sensation on the contralateral side of the body. This lateral disparity results because the spinothalamic tracts (pain and temperature) cross at the spinal level, whereas the dorsal columns and the corticospinal tracts decussate in the medulla. *(D)* Dorsal column syndrome. Damage is to the dorsal column pathway. The deficit is loss of touch, vibration, and position sense below the level of injury. Motor function is preserved. (From Marshall, S. B., Marshall, L. F., Vos, H. R., & Chesnut, R. M. (1990). *Neuroscience critical care.* Philadelphia: W. B. Saunders Co.)

muscles with respiratory effort, paradoxical expansion of the abdominal wall with inspiration, and cyanosis. Baseline arterial blood gases collected when the patient arrives in the unit provide important information about the actual exchange of gases within the lung.

Patients with high cervical fractures (C1–C5) with spinal cord involvement can experience hypoventilation with or without sleep apnea. This hypoventilation syndrome starts with vague complaints of the patient's experiencing air hunger and drowsiness with sighing respirations. When the patient is questioned, he or she is anxious, disoriented, or confused. Although the patient appears anxious, it is important not to sedate the patient, because the drug will worsen hypoventilation and the patient may experience respiratory arrest as he or she drops off to sleep. If the patient is awakened prior to the respiratory arrest, normal breathing occurs. This hypoventilation syndrome occurs be-

Table 10–4. SPINAL NERVE INNERVATION OF MAJOR MUSCLE GROUPS

Spinal Nerve	Muscle Group Movement	Assessment Technique
C4–C5	Shoulder abduction	Shrug shoulders against downward pressure of examiner's hands
C5–C6	Elbow flexion (biceps)	Arm is pulled up from resting position against resistance
C7	Elbow extension (triceps)	From the flexed position, arm is straightened out against resistance
C7	Thumb-index pinch	Index finger is held firmly to thumb against resistance to pull apart
C8	Hand grasp	Hand grasp strength is evaluated
L2–L4	Hip flexion	Leg is lifted from bed against resistance
L5–S1	Knee flexion	Knee is flexed against resistance
L2–L4	Knee extension	From flexed position, knee is extended against resistance
L5	Foot dorsiflexion	Foot pulled up toward nose against resistance
S1	Foot plantar flexion	Foot pushed down (stepping on the gas) against resistance

From Marshall, S. B., Marshall, L. F., Vos, H. R., & Chesnut, R. M. (1990). *Neuroscience critical care*. Philadelphia: W. B. Saunders Co.

cause of the decreased sensitivity of the respiratory drive to carbon dioxide and mechanical factors such as immobilization. The hypoventilation syndrome usually lasts for the first 10 days after injury, and mechanical ventilation at night is the treatment of choice. Oxygen is administered cautiously in those patients dependent on the hypoxic drive for breathing.

Respiratory impairment varies with the level of injury and the type of injury (complete or incomplete). Patients with a complete lesion at vertebral levels C1–C4 usually experience total loss of respiratory function. Patients with complete lesions at vertebral levels C1–C3 are ventilator dependent. Patients with complete lesions at vertebral levels C4–C5 experience phrenic nerve damage and are candidates for phrenic nerve pacers. Individuals with complete SCIs below vertebra C5 have intact diaphragmatic breathing without intercostal and abdominal muscle function. Individuals with complete lesions from vertebral levels T1–L2 experience varying amounts of intercostal and abdominal muscle loss. Respiratory impairment results from the dysfunction or loss of the diaphragm, intercostals, and abdominal muscles. Individuals with incomplete spinal cord lesions present with varying degrees of respiratory impairment, depending on the level of the lesion and whether the motor system is impaired.

Neurological Assessment

Once airway and respiratory assessment is complete, the neurological examination follows. If the patient also has a head injury, all components of the neurological examination are performed, as described in the section on increased ICP. For a patient with an SCI, comprehensive motor, reflex, and sensory assessments are done.

Motor and Reflex Assessments

An assessment of the spinal nerve innervation of major muscle groups is important for determining the level of injury to the motor system (Table 10–4). A grading of muscle strength is also part of the motor assessment (Table 10–5), because it offers a basis for comparative assessment throughout the course of treatment. The grading of muscle strength is based on the ability to move muscle groups, hold a position against gravity, and maintain that position against the nurse's resistance to the muscle groups. By observing or asking the patient to move his or her right arm, the nurse establishes the patient's ability to move the right arm, which is rated a 1 on the scale. When the patient holds his or her right arm extended in front of him or her with palms up and maintains the position for 6 seconds, the patient is rated a 3 on the scale. The last step is for the nurse to apply resistance to the muscles when the patient has his or her right arm extended in front of him or her ("I am going to push your right arm down, so try to prevent me from doing that"). If the patient has difficulty resisting the examiner, the rating is a 4; if the patient maintains the position with resistance, the rating is 5.

Table 10–5. MOTOR STRENGTH GRADING SCALE

Score	Motor Function
0	None
1	Trace
2	Not greater than gravity
3	Greater than gravity
4	Slight weakness
5	Normal

From Marshall, S. B., Marshall, L. F., Vos, H. R., & Chesnut, R. M. (1990). *Neuroscience critical care*. Philadelphia: W. B. Saunders Co.

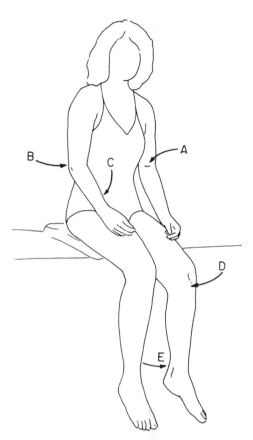

Figure 10–23. Deep tendon reflexes. *(A)* Biceps. *(B)* Triceps. *(C)* Brachioradialis. *(D)* Patellar. *(E)* Achilles. (From Mitchell, P., Cammermeyer, M., Ozuna, J., & Woods, N. F. (1984). *Neurological assessment for nursing practice* (Fig. 2–16). Reston, VA: Reston Publishing Co.)

Superficial and deep tendon reflexes should also be included in the motor assessment (Fig. 10–23). Reflex testing assists in establishing the level of SCI, and the return of deep tendon reflexes below the level of injury signals the end of spinal shock.

Deep tendon reflexes are obtained by a brisk tapping of a reflex hammer on the tendons of a muscle group (see Fig. 10–23). The response is contraction of the stimulated muscle group. Deep tendon reflexes are graded according to the response elicited (0, no reflex; 1, hypoactive; 2, normal; 3, hyperactive).

Superficial reflexes are cutaneous sensations over the abdomen and groin area. They are elicited by scratching the surface of the area.

Sensory Assessment

Sensory assessment is performed to determine superficial response to pinprick (sharp, dull, hyperesthesia, absent), position sense, and temperature. The sensory dermatomes are the segmental distribution of sensation (Fig. 10–24). The areas of sensation on the skin are supplied by one spinal segment. For example, the ability to sense a superficial pinprick on the lateral forearm, thumb, and index finger tests the innervation by dermatome C6. While undergoing sensory testing, the patient is instructed to close his or her eyes. Position sense is determined by having the nurse grasp the patient's thumb or big toe and move the digit up or down or leave it in a neutral position. The patient is asked to identify the pattern of movement. Temperature is assessed by filling up one test tube with hot water and another test tube with cold water. The patient is asked to identify the sensation when the test tube touches the skin. Table 10–6 outlines the components of the hourly assessment for an SCI patient without a head injury, and Table 10–7 lists those for a patient with both an SCI and a head injury.

Hemodynamic Assessment

Another important consideration is hemodynamic instability. The patient needs continuous hemodynamic monitoring during the acute period following the injury to assist in early recognition of hemodynamic instability. The usual hemodynamic response in injuries above the C5 level is a decrease or loss of sympathetic innervation, causing vasodilatation, decreased venous return, and hypotension. The patient's vasomotor response returns over the course of a couple of months. Bradycardia is common and is due to the loss of

Table 10–6. COMPONENTS OF THE HOURLY NEUROLOGICAL ASSESSMENT FOR PATIENTS WITH SPINAL CORD INJURY WITHOUT HEAD INJURY

Motor	Sensation
Respirations 　Rate, rhythm, respiratory 　　effort Assess movement/strength 　bilaterally 　Shrug shoulders 　Elbow flexion 　Elbow extension 　Bending wrists 　Touching thumb to 　　index finger 　Hand grasp 　Lift leg off the bed 　Bend knee 　Extend knee 　Pull feet up 　Push feet down	Pinprick (sharp, dull) 　All surfaces of the 　　body Position sense Temperature 　All surfaces of the 　　body

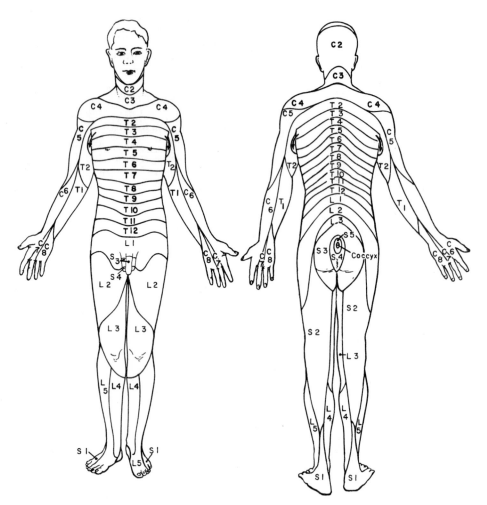

Figure 10–24. Sensory dermatomes. Cutaneous distribution of spinal nerves. (From Marshall, S. B., Marshall, L. F., Vos, H. R., & Chesnut, R. M. (1990). *Neuroscience critical care*. Philadelphia: W. B. Saunders Co.)

sympathetic outflow; it is aggravated by hypothermia and hypoxia. The patient is therefore at risk for a vasovagal response when suctioned, which leads to hypoxia and vagal stimulation. This reflex is prevented by preoxygenating the patient prior to suctioning (Alspach, 1991).

Venous stasis occurs as a result of loss of vasomotor tone and paralysis. This stasis increases the risk of thrombosis in the legs and pelvis.

A patient with high-level SCI (above C5) also has trouble regulating body temperature. The level of injury interrupts the pathway between the hypothalamus and the blood vessels, causing body temperature to rise and fall according to the environmental temperature.

GI Tract Assessment

The GI tract is another area to assess in an SCI patient. The loss of autonomic tone causes abdominal distension and paralytic ileus. A nasogastric tube for decompression is inserted until bowel sounds return. Gastric dilatation interferes with diaphragmatic functions, causing hypoventilation and fatigue while breathing. Stress ulcers can occur due to vagus-stimulated gastric acid production. Steroid therapy is part of acute management, but it also irritates the gastric mucosa, leading to additional GI problems. A thorough nutritional assessment is important, because the injury leads to a hypermetabolic state.

Bowel and Bladder Assessment

Bowel and bladder atony occurs during spinal shock. The bladder does not contract, and the detrusor muscle does not open due to the paralysis. Urinary retention is a common problem, and a Foley catheter during spinal shock is the treatment of choice. The

Table 10–7. COMPONENTS OF THE HOURLY NEUROLOGICAL ASSESSMENT FOR PATIENTS WITH SPINAL CORD AND HEAD INJURY

Mental Status	Motor	Pupils	Brain Stem/Cranial Nerves	Sensation

Glasgow Coma Scale Assesses level of consciousness, expressive language, ability to follow commands	Respirations
	  Rate, rhythm, respiratory effort
	Assess movement/ strength bilaterally
	Shrug shoulders
	Elbow flexion
	Elbow extension
	Bending wrists
	Touching thumb to index finger
	Hand grasp
	Lift leg off the bed
	Bend knee
	Extend knee
	Pull feet up
	Push feet down
		Size
		Shape
		Reaction to light (direct and consensual)
		Extraocular movements
			Corneal reflex
			  Present—immediate blinking bilaterally
			  Diminished—blinking asymmetrically
			  Absent—no blinking
			Doll's eyes (unconscious patient—no spinal fracture)
			Cough, gag, swallow reflex
			Observe for excessive drooling
			Observe for cough/ swallow reflex
				Pinprick (sharp, dull)
				  All surfaces of the body
				Position sense
				Temperature
				  All surfaces of the body

bowel does not have peristaltic movement secondary to SCI. This loss of peristaltic movement places the patient at risk for a paralytic ileus. During the first 72 hours after SCI, the placement of a nasogastric tube on low constant suction decompresses the bowel. Once bowel sounds return, flatus and a decrease in gastric output or a bowel movement removes the danger of an ileus. After this, a bowel program is initiated. This program consists of bisacodyl suppositories or enemas every other day, stool softeners, and digital stimulation to stimulate reflex colonic activity (Marshall et al., 1990).

Autonomic Dysreflexia

Autonomic dysreflexia (hyperreflexia) occurs after spinal shock has ceased and can be an ongoing problem for an SCI patient with a lesion above T6. Autonomic dysreflexia is characterized by an exaggerated response of the sympathetic nervous system to a variety of stimuli (e.g., draft in the room, kinked Foley catheter, bladder distention, bowel impaction, routine bowel or bladder procedures). This exaggerated response by the sympathetic nervous system results from the lack of input from the brain due to the blockage of the SCI. Common signs and symptoms are sudden, severe, pounding headache; elevated, uncontrolled blood pressure; bradycardia; nasal congestion; profuse sweating above the level of the lesion; flushing of the face and neck; and anxiety. Blood pressure can rise to a dangerous or fatal level, making autonomic dysreflexia an emergency situation. Treatment is directed

at finding and removing the cause (external or internal stimuli) of the exaggerated response. Once the cause has been located and removed, the symptoms quickly disappear. Until that time, autonomic dysreflexia should be considered a severe medical emergency.

Skin Assessment

Inspection of the skin should be part of the assessment. Because of impaired circulation and immobility, an SCI patient is at risk for skin breakdown. The skin around the halo or tong pins should be inspected and pin care should be performed every 8 hours. The assessment includes observing the site for redness, swelling, drainage, and pain. Inspecting areas under the halo brace for signs of skin breakdown is also important.

Psychological Assessment

A psychological assessment is important during the acute period of injury. Initially, the patient is concerned with surviving the injury and does not realize the extent of his or her injury or disability. The patient's perceptions are also impaired by medications and the physiological effects of injury. As the patient gains insight into the situation, it is important for the nurse to include the patient in planning his or her care and to give the patient choices about that care, because feelings of powerlessness are common (Richmond et al., 1992). Family members also go through a similar experience. First there is shock related to the injury itself and the seriousness of the patient's condition. During this time, the family needs support and answers to their questions.

Medical Assessment

Common baseline laboratory studies include chemical profile, complete blood count, prothrombin time, partial thromboplastin time, platelet count, and arterial blood gases.

Common diagnostic studies to confirm the extent of vertebral injury and SCI include anteroposterior and lateral spine x-ray studies, chest x-ray studies, CT scan, magnetic resonance imaging (MRI), myelography, and somatosensory–cortical evoked potentials. The latter are performed to see whether sensory pathways between the site of stimulation and the site of recording are intact. This test requires tactile stimulation to elicit a response.

NURSING DIAGNOSES

Nursing diagnoses appropriate for a patient with SCI are:

- Altered impaired physical mobility related to SCI
- Ineffective breathing pattern or ineffective cough related to impaired diaphragm, poor chest excursion, diaphragm or intercostal muscle fatigue, autonomic nervous system (ANS) instability
- Altered tissue perfusion related to cardiovascular instability (spinal shock)
- Ineffective thermoregulation (poikilothermy) related to loss of sympathetic innervation
- Altered nutrition (less than body requirements) related to paralytic ileus from SCI, stress ulcers from stress response and therapy, hypermetabolic state
- Impaired physical mobility related to SCI
- Risk for fluid volume excess related to paralytic ileus, gastric suction, fluid overload
- Altered urinary elimination related to atonic bladder, upper neuron lesion
- Bowel incontinence related to SCI
- Chronic pain related to spasticity, bladder spasms, dysesthesia from SCI
- Self-care deficit related to impaired mobility
- Powerlessness related to SCI and ineffective coping mechanism
- Body image disturbance related to SCI

INTERVENTIONS

Nursing Interventions

Nursing interventions are focused on maintaining stabilization of the spinal alignment, maintaining the airway and respiratory status, and preventing complications associated with immobility and the SCI (see Nursing Care Plan for the Patient with Spinal Cord Injury).

Medical Interventions

Maintaining a patent airway and respiratory function is the first aspect of treatment. If the patient is having difficulty sustaining his or her own respiration, mechanical ventilation is the treatment of choice.

Stabilization of the fracture or dislocation to bring about spinal alignment and prevent further neurological deterioration is accomplished by skeletal traction—a halo brace or tongs (Fig. 10–25). If tongs are used initially to stabilize the spine, the amount of weight is controversial. Usually 10 pounds of traction is used initially, building up to 80 pounds maximally. The halo brace offers many advantages, such as easy access to the neck for diagnostic procedures and surgery, early mobilization, and ambulation. For both types of skeletal traction, pin care and skin assessment over pressure areas are important nursing interventions.

Maintaining perfusion pressure of the spinal cord is the next focus of medical therapy. Since the goal is to maintain blood pressure within normal limits, using volume expanders is a preferred option in treatment. A pulmonary artery catheter is used to determine the need for fluids.

Glucocorticoids have been used in the treatment of SCI for many years. The current controversy over the use of these drugs relates to the correct dosage needed to reverse the effects of SCI. As a result of a landmark study, National Acute Spinal Cord Injury Study 2, high-dose methylprednisolone is administered within 8 hours of SCI. The dosing regimen is initiated with a bolus of 30 mg/kg over 15 minutes, followed by a continuous IV infusion of 5.4 mg/kg/hr over 23 hours to maintain plasma levels to effect lipid peroxidation (Deglin, 1997; Nayduch et al., 1994; Nolan, 1994).

To prevent thrombus formation and pulmonary embolism, prophylactic anticoagulant therapy is initiated during the acute aspect of SCI, as well as the use of antiembolic hose or pulsatile hose.

PATIENT OUTCOMES

During the past 20 years, functional outcomes for SCI patients have been discouraging. With advances

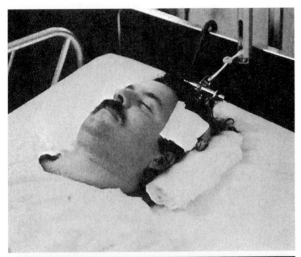

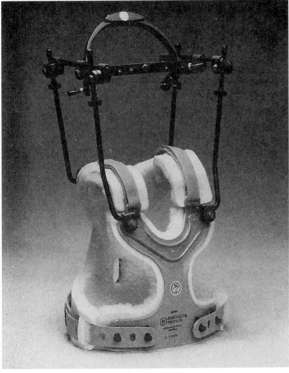

Figure 10–25. Skeletal traction with Crutchfield tongs. (From Hickey, J. V. (1992). *Clinical practice of neurological neurosurgical nursing* (3rd ed.) (p. 400). Philadelphia: J. B. Lippincott Co.)

in neuroscience research, a better understanding of the pathophysiology of SCI, better treatment options, more skilled nursing care, and better rehabilitation opportunities, the future for SCI patients will be brighter. (See Nursing Care Plan for the Patient with Spinal Cord Injury.)

Acute Cerebrovascular Disease

Although cerebrovascular disease is the third leading cause of death (500,000 people a year) in the United States, over the last 20 years, there has been a decline in mortality resulting from CVA. Some factors responsible for this decline are improved control of blood pressure with antihypertensive medications, low-sodium and low-fat diets, and a decrease in cigarette smoking. CVA is a broad term that covers a variety of intracranial vascular problems, which are usually found in the older population.

The critical care nurse encounters patients with intracranial hemorrhage more frequently than those with other kinds of cerebrovascular disorders. A patient with an occlusive stroke is seldom admitted to the critical care unit unless there is extensive neurological damage or decreased ventilatory ability.

PATHOPHYSIOLOGY

The mechanisms underlying CVA are due to atherosclerosis (thrombosis, embolism) or bleeding (hypertensive hemorrhage, aneurysm, arteriovenous malformation [AVM]) of a cerebral vessel.

Blockage in a cerebral vessel results in a decrease in CBF secondary to the blocked portion of the artery, and ischemia results. Along with ischemia, there is inadequate oxygen delivery to brain cells, inadequate CO_2 removal, increased intracellular lactic acid production, decreased adenosine triphosphate, and disruption of the blood-brain barrier.

The underlying cause of a blocked artery is a thrombus or an embolus. Atherosclerosis, the most frequent cause of thrombotic disease, results in plaque at bifurcations and curves in arteries. An embolus occurs when the plaque fragments, breaks off, and travels to the brain. When this plaque lodges in a cerebral artery, CBF is decreased. Cardiac sources of cerebral emboli (atrial fibrillation, rheumatic heart disease, acute myocardial infarction, endocarditis, mitral valve prolapse, and valve prosthesis) are of paramount importance when planning treatment. In these cases, it is important to treat the cardiac as well as the neurological problem.

When a cerebral vessel ruptures, the result is a hemorrhagic CVA. The major types of hemorrhagic events are lacunar infarcts and bleeding into the subarachnoid space (e.g., ruptured aneurysm, AVM).

Chronic hypertension causes fibrinoid necrosis of the very small cerebral arteries, thereby reducing the tensile strength in the vessel wall. This weakness causes the artery to leak, and blood escapes into brain tissue. The characteristic locations of lacunar infarcts

NURSING CARE PLAN FOR THE PATIENT WITH SPINAL CORD INJURY

Nursing Diagnosis	Patient Outcomes	Nursing Interventions
Impaired physical mobility related to SCI.	Vertebral alignment maintained. Preservation of neurological function at initial SCI level.	Maintain halo or tong traction or other device for immobilization. Neurological assessments—motor, reflex, and sensory functions. Report ascending lesion or progression of deficits from baseline. Safe use of special beds for turning. Explain immobilization to patient and get his or her cooperation. Pin care every 8 h. If skeletal traction slips or accidentally removed, maintain head in a neutral position. Turning, lifting, transferring patient use 5 people with 1 person at head stabilizing neck, guiding traction.
Ineffective breathing pattern or ineffective cough related to impaired diaphragm, poor chest excursion, diaphragm/ intercostal muscle fatigue, PE, ANS instability.	Maintain airway. Vital capacity 60–75 ml/kg. ABG within normal limits (WNL). O_2 saturation WNL 96%. Breath sounds bilaterally. CXR WNL. No atelectasis/pneumonia. Temp WNL. No dyspnea, tachypnea. No restlessness or anxiety.	Monitor temperature. Monitor respiratory rate and rhythm. Assess breath sounds every hour for 72 h. Observe for anxiety, restlessness, or statements related to ``not getting enough air,'' ``trouble breathing.'' Assist in clearing secretions with suctioning or Quad coughing. Encourage deep breathing and use of incentive spirometer. Maintain patency of endotracheal or tracheostomy tube (for intubation, fiberoptic laryngoscopy or jaw thrust is used). Observe tolerance for turning on special frames or beds. Chest physiotherapy. Administer antibiotics as ordered. Monitor O_2 saturation. Administer O_2 as needed. Gradually decrease ventilatory assistance.
Altered tissue perfusion related to cardiovascular instability (spinal shock).	Hemodynamic monitoring WNL. Urine output ≥30 ml/h. VS stable. Normal sinus rhythm. BP WNL.	Monitor BP, pulse, respirations, temp every hour for 72 h or as ordered. Record I&O hourly. Use antiembolism stockings. Administer medications and volume expanders as ordered. Monitor lab values CBC, Hgb, Hct, BUN, creatinine, electrolytes.
Altered body temperature (poikilothermy) related to loss of sympathetic innervation.	Maintain temperature at 37°C.	Adjust environmental temperature to 75°F. Correlate environmental temperature to body temperature. Avoid the use of many blankets on patient. For hyperthermia, check environmental temperature, use cooling blanket and antipyretics when ordered.

NURSING CARE PLAN FOR THE PATIENT WITH SPINAL CORD INJURY *Continued*

Nursing Diagnosis	Patient Outcomes	Nursing Interventions
Altered nutrition (less than body requirements) related to paralytic ileus from SCI, stress ulcers from stress response and therapy, hypermetabolic state.	Bowel sounds present. Absence of abdominal distension. Absence of vomiting. Potassium WNL. Absence of T-wave depression. Gastric secretions and stool negative for occult blood. Maintain gastric pH ≥3. Hct and Hgb WNL. Maintain admission weight. Return of bowel movements and flatus.	Use of NG tube on low suction to prevent abdominal distention/possible aspiration. Daily weights with bed scales. Measure abdominal girth every 8 h for 72 h. NPO until bowel sounds present. Nutritional assessment. Parenteral nutrition if ordered. When bowel sounds return, advance diet slowly, give clear liquids in small amounts, and increase as tolerated. Monitor serum albumin and proteins initially and every 3 days thereafter. Monitor gastric pH; report if <3. Administer antacids, H_2 receptor blockers. Monitor Hct and Hgb. Sudden unexplained shoulder pain can be referred pain from GI tract. Start bowel program when bowel sounds return. Record bowel movement pattern.
Impaired physical mobility related to SCI.	Intact skin. Calves and thighs symmetrical. Absence of lower extremity (LE) edema. No signs of pulmonary embolism. Verbalizes importance of reposition. Adequate nutritional status.	Turn at least every 2 h; use special bed, foam mattress, or air mattress. Assess extremities for change in color, size, temperature. Measure calf and thighs on admission and daily; report changes in circumference to physician. Passive range of motion to LE qid. Apply antiembolism stockings. Remove antiembolism stockings every 8 h for 30 min and assess legs. Administer heparin 5000 U SC every 12 h or as ordered. Monitor PTT as long as heparin ordered; report abnormal results. Inspect skin and give skin care every 2 h. Avoid skin wetness from perspiration, stool, urine. Assess skin under halo brace or other braces. Teach patient the importance of skin care and frequent repositioning.
Risk for fluid volume excess related to paralytic ileus, gastric suction, fluid overload.	Electrolytes WNL. Balanced I&O. CXR WNL. Maintain admission weight.	Record I&O, specific gravity every 8 h. Monitor daily electrolytes; report abnormalities to physician. Assess breath sounds. Administer IV fluids. Daily weights.

Continued on following page

NURSING CARE PLAN FOR THE PATIENT WITH SPINAL CORD INJURY Continued

Nursing Diagnosis	Patient Outcomes	Nursing Interventions
Altered urinary elimination related to atonic bladder, upper motor neuron lesion.	Output consistent with intake. Absence of bladder distention. Normal temperature. BUN, creatinine, WNL. No residual urine after catheter DC. Negative urine cultures. Clear urine. No bladder spasms. WBC WNL.	Indwelling catheter initially during spinal shock. Hourly urinary output. Catheter care tid. Avoid using a large-size Foley catheter. Intermittent catheterization following spinal shock. Acidify the urine—vitamin C, cranberry juice, apple juice. Urinalysis daily for 72 h then weekly. Keep drainage bag off the floor and lower than the abdomen. Monitor urine pH; maintain <5.8. Monitor WBC and report abnormalities.
Chronic pain related to spasticity, bladder spasms, dysesthesia from SCI.	Understands abnormal sensations/loss. No skin breakdown. No reports of bladder spasms. No reports of spasticity. Temperature WNL.	Assess pain/discomfort. Turn patient every hour. Monitor temperature. Report abnormal temperature to physician. Protect anesthetic areas. Utilize visual imagery/biofeedback, distraction. Administer analgesics that do not cause respiratory depression.
Self-care deficits related to impaired mobility.	Performs self-care activities within ability of SCI.	Help identify which activities patient can perform. Offer encouragement throughout activity. Involve family in care. Allow patient to make decisions related to ADLs. Obtain physical and occupational therapy consultations.
Powerlessness related to SCI.	Verbalizes increased control over activities.	Encourage patient to talk about feelings about self and illness. Include the patient in planning care. Allow patient to make choices related to ADLs. Display sensitivity toward events that could cause powerlessness. Obtain patient views prior to providing information/directions. Encourage patient to ask questions.

Data from Kim, M. J., et al. (1987). *Pocket guide to nursing diagnoses* (2nd ed.). St. Louis: C. V. Mosby; and Marshall, S. B., Marshall, L. F., Vos, H. R., & Chesnut, R. M. (1990). *Neuroscience critical care*. Philadelphia: W. B. Saunders Co.

are the basal ganglia, subcortical white matter, thalamus, cerebellum, and brain stem.

A ruptured cerebral aneurysm is a common cause of subarachnoid hemorrhage (SAH). A portion of a cerebral artery that has an aneurysm presents as a bulging balloonlike area with a thin dome. Cerebral aneurysms occur at the bifurcation of large arteries at the base of the brain (circle of Willis) and rupture into the subarachnoid space of the basal cisterns. Occasionally, cerebral aneurysms rupture into the ventricular system or into brain tissue. When the aneurysm forms, a weakness in the arterial wall allows the development of the dome and neck of the aneurysm. Rupture usually takes place at the dome. After rupture into the subarachnoid space, autoregulation is impaired. SAH secondary to a ruptured cerebral aneurysm is associated with a high morbidity and mortality. Most patients with cerebral aneurysms are asymptomatic prior to rupture.

Prior to rupture, a cerebral aneurysm can mimic a mass lesion and compress brain tissue, cranial nerves, and blood vessels. Immediately following the rupture, there is bleeding into adjacent tissue, and increased ICP may be focal (near the aneurysm) or global. CBF is altered by increased ICP and impaired autoregulation. This altered CBF causes a gradual ischemia. If the vessel does not seal off following the rupture, the ICP will equal the systemic arterial pressure and reduce CPP.

Following the aneurysm's rupture, the patient can also experience cardiac dysrhythmias, rebleeding, hydrocephalus, seizures, and vasospasm. The neurological injury can also be related to these events.

Cardiac dysrhythmia occurs as a result of stimulation of the sympathetic nervous system. Cardiac dysrhythmias can cause a transient loss of consciousness following acute aneurysm rupture. In addition to cardiac dysrhythmias, increased sympathetic tone also causes a high incidence of large T waves, prolonged QT intervals, and ST abnormalities.

Another problem following the initial aneurysm rupture is rebleeding prior to surgical clipping of the aneurysm. The mechanism causing rebleeding is an increased tension on the aneurysm wall. The increase in tension is due to hypertension and a sudden decrease in pressure around the aneurysm. Rebleeding can also occur from normal breakdown of the clot in 7 to 10 days following the initial bleed. If the patient is neurologically stable, he or she will undergo surgery early in the course of this problem. If the patient is unstable, aminocaproic acid is administered to prevent the clot from breaking down.

An SAH can impair the circulation and reabsorption of CSF. A blood clot can obstruct the flow in the ventricular system, causing an obstructive hydrocephalus. As blood enters the subarachnoid space, an inflammatory response is triggered. This inflammatory response can cause fibrosis and thickening of the arachnoid villi, which inhibits reabsorption. This inhibition of reabsorption of CSF causes communicating hydrocephalus. Both obstructive and communicating hydrocephalus cause increased ICP.

Another potential problem following a ruptured aneurysm is seizures. Seizures increase the metabolic demand and oxygen requirements of brain cells. Seizures occurring within the first 12 hours following rupture are attributed to increased ICP. After the initial 12 hours but before surgical clipping of the aneurysm, seizures are associated with rebleeding of the aneurysm. Because of the potential danger of the effects of seizures, most patients are given phenytoin to prevent seizures from occurring.

Cerebral vasospasm is a narrowing of arteries adjacent to the aneurysm, which results in ischemia and infarction of brain tissue if it is unresolved. The usual period for vasospasm to occur is 4 to 14 days after the rupture. The exact mechanism for vasospasm is unknown, but some factors that contribute to vasospasm are structural changes in the adjacent cerebral arteries, denervation of adjacent arteries, generation of oxygen free radicals, and release of vasoactive substances (serotonin, catecholamines, prostaglandins, oxyhemoglobin) that initiate vasospasm, an inflammatory response, and calcium influx.

AVMs of the brain are composed of tangled, dilated vessels that form an abnormal communication network between the arterial and venous systems. Arterial blood is directly shunted into the venous system without a capillary network. The size and location of AVMs vary, but they all cause varying degrees of ischemia, scarring of brain tissue, abnormal tissue development, compression, hemorrhage, hydrocephalus, and cardiac decompensation. AVMs are the leading cause of SAH and ventricular hemorrhage in young people.

ASSESSMENT

Nursing Assessment

As with patients with increased ICP and head injury, history and neurological assessment are very important. Mental status, cranial nerve functioning, and motor status are included in the assessment.

Since hemodynamic instability is common with acute CVA, assessments of the airway, blood pressure, pulse, respiration, and fluid and electrolyte status are also priorities. A patient with CVA generally has ICP, hemodynamic status, and cardiac function monitored. Assessing functional status in relation to the normal ranges of each of these parameters is also part of the assessment.

Patients who undergo cerebral angiography need to have a baseline neurological assessment both before and after the procedure. The puncture site is inspected for hematoma or bleeding and is immobilized for 6 to 8 hours to prevent bleeding. When the femoral site is used, circulatory checks are performed bilaterally, including femoral and pedal pulses as well as color and temperature of the extremity.

Since there are a variety of medications used for occlusive and hemorrhagic CVA, assessing the patient for side effects of medications is part of the nursing assessment.

Medical Assessment

The initial baseline laboratory tests obtained in a CVA patient are:

- Complete blood count (red blood cells, hemoglobin, hematocrit, platelet count)
- Sedimentation rate
- Blood urea nitrogen, creatinine, electrolytes, and serum osmolality
- Fibrinogen levels (SAH)
- Urinalysis and urine osmolality

Diagnostic tests that are performed to confirm the diagnosis of CVA include:

- Chest x-ray studies (cardiac contour, pulmonary AVM)
- CT scan of the brain (ischemia, hemorrhage)
- MRI (sensitive to the presence and extent of ischemia)
- Doppler carotid studies (middle cerebral artery stenosis or occlusion)
- Transcranial Doppler
- Digital subtraction angiography (detects carotid occlusion and information about vertebral arteries)
- Angiography (defines shallow ulcerated plaques, stenosis, mural thrombus, dissections, multiple lesions, aneurysms, AVMs; reveals poor blood flow, collateral flow)
- Lumbar puncture (performed if CT scan does not demonstrate SAH, mass lesion, or obstructive hydrocephalus; diagnostic for SAH)

NURSING DIAGNOSES

A patient with CVA has similar nursing diagnoses as a patient with increased ICP and head injury. Refer to the Nursing Care Plan for the Patient with Increased ICP, Head Injury, or CVA for the specific nursing diagnoses.

INTERVENTIONS

Nursing Interventions

For a patient with CVA due to blockage, the nursing interventions are neurological assessment, administration of medications (i.e., anticoagulants, streptokinase, antihypertensive agents), observation for side effects of medications, and maintenance of hemodynamic stability. Because the risk of hemorrhage into an ischemic area is present in a hypertensive patient, blood pressure is reduced slowly, with the goal of preventing an intracerebral hemorrhage, but not low enough to cause ischemia. It is important to keep the CPP in the range of 60 to 70 mm Hg (Ropper and Kennedy, 1988). To prevent vasospasm, the blood pressure is maintained at an elevated level (systolic 160 to 170 mm Hg).

A patient with a hemorrhagic CVA presents the nurse with many challenges. When arterial blood enters the subarachnoid space, its presence is irritating to the meninges. If conscious, the patient may complain of a severe headache, experience photophobia, and have a stiff neck. These signs of meningeal irritation are common following a subarachnoid bleed. This patient may also experience increased ICP, alteration in CBF, hemodynamic instability, vasospasm, rebleeding, and hydrocephalus. A variety of medications are used with these patients, depending on the cause of the bleeding. Possible medications are hypertensive agents, volume expanders, calcium channel blockers, steroids, mild sedatives, osmotic diuretics, and antifibrinolytic and anticonvulsant agents.

Important interventions for a patient with SAH are a quiet environment, bed rest, and few visitors. Dimming the room lights and turning down the volume of the patient's monitors can be beneficial in reducing noxious stimuli.

The interventions for CVA patients are similar to those for patients with increased ICP and head injury (see Nursing Care Plan for the Patient with Increased ICP, Head Injury, or CVA).

Medical (Nonsurgical) Interventions for Occlusive CVA

Quick, aggressive treatment of CVA is the current theme of medical treatment. The goal for management of CVA is maintaining CBF to limit infarct size and to prevent ischemia that leads to cell death.

For a patient with an occlusive CVA, the medical treatment is to improve blood flow to impaired, poorly perfused areas of the brain, reestablish perfusion, and minimize reperfusion injury.

Improving blood flow to poorly perfused areas is accomplished by maintaining adequate tissue oxygenation. Hypoxia can be avoided by attending to airway obstruction, hypoventilation, aspiration, and atelectasis.

Reperfusion is directed at reversing the areas of ischemia around the infarct, where damaged cells can heal. Medical management includes hypervolemic hemodilution, normovolemic hemodilution, and thrombolytics. Hypervolemic hemodilution (using dextran, albumin, plasma protein fraction) increases intravascular volume, reduces blood viscosity, and decreases hematocrit and platelet aggregation. Hemodynamic monitoring must be used in these patients. The use of hypervolemic hemodilution is controversial and is generally not recommended because the clinical benefit has not been established (Adams et al., 1994). If this treatment is used, caution is advised in patients with cerebral edema and in those prone to fluid overload (Whitney, 1994). Normovolemic hemodilution (using crystalloids, 20% albumin) with hemodynamic monitoring is recommended. This approach reduces blood viscosity and maintains intravascular volume (Wityk and Stern, 1994).

Thrombolytic therapy (tissue plasminogen activator [tPA]) is used to lyse the clot and restore CBF. A disadvantage of thrombolytic therapy is the risk of cerebral hemorrhage.

Anticoagulation therapy (e.g., heparin, heparinoids, aspirin, warfarin) has been the therapy of choice for years in the treatment of ischemic stroke. These drugs work when there is injury to the vessel wall. They interfere with clot formation. The value of heparin in acute ischemic stroke is currently being challenged, and heparin use remains a matter of preference of the treating physician (Adams et al., 1994).

Therapy is also directed toward minimizing reperfusion injury. Many of these new therapies are in clinical trials across the country. At the time of reperfusion, the ischemic tissues develop a relative anaerobic state. This state is associated with oxidation and free radical formation, calcium influx across the cell membrane, and release of excitatory amino acids (glutamate). Medical therapy is directed at protecting neurons from further damage. Antioxidants (e.g., tirilazad) are used to inhibit lipid peroxidation by oxygen free radicals. It is also possible that tirilazad protects the microcirculation.

Calcium enters ischemic neurons, causing further damage to the neuron. Therefore, calcium antagonists (e.g., nimodipine) are given to block calcium from entering the neuron. The calcium antagonist also produces vasodilatation, improving CBF.

When excitatory amino acids (glutamate) are released, there is stimulation on the N-methyl-D-aspartate (NMDA) receptors. The activation of these receptors causes calcium, sodium, chloride, and water to cross the cell membrane, causing neuronal death. Blocking the receptor site by using a glutamate antagonist (e.g., dextromethorphan, dextrorphan, CNS 1102) halts the chain of events associated with receptor activation (Wityk and Stern, 1994; Whitney, 1994).

Surgical Interventions for Occlusive CVA

Carotid endarterectomy is performed to remove plaque from the cervical internal carotid artery (see Fig. 10–26). During the first 24 hours after surgery, fluctuating blood pressure can occur. The most common fluctuation is hypotension with bradycardia, which might require treatment with a vasopressor agent. Hypertension has also been associated with cerebral hemorrhage. Other complications from this surgery are neck hematoma and myocardial infarction.

Another surgical procedure is the extracranial-intracranial bypass, which is controversial. This procedure theoretically increases CBF to areas that are surgically inaccessible by bypassing occluded parts of the circulation. An external artery is grafted to an intracranial artery. In randomized trials of this surgical procedure, the desired effect of increasing CBF was not produced, and indications for the bypass must be revisited (Bronstein et al., 1991).

Medical Interventions for Hemorrhagic CVA

Time is a critical factor in hemorrhagic CVA. Treatment is based on the size, extent, and location of the bleeding. The goal is to stop the bleeding and to prevent the resulting brain damage. The patient's level of consciousness is the single factor that guides treatment decisions. When a patient arrives at the hospital awake and responsive to the environment and continues to maintain an intact mental status, medical treatment is the first choice. However, when a patient is admitted with, or develops, deterioration in mental status, he or she may be a surgical candidate, especially if there are large areas of hemorrhage or hemispheric bleeding.

Intracerebral hemorrhage caused by hypertension is treated by reducing the blood pressure gradually. Usually the goal is to maintain the systolic pressure at 160 mm Hg or the mean pressure below 110 mm Hg in a conscious patient. Examples of agents used for reducing the blood pressure are nitroglycerin, nitroprusside, and labetalol. Other therapies are directed toward minimizing increased ICP, cerebral edema, and hydrocephalus. For large hematomas and brain stem hematomas, surgical evacuation of the clot is necessary.

SAH secondary to a ruptured aneurysm or AVM requires medical and surgical interventions. Early medical treatment is aggressive and is aimed toward preventing complications associated with rebleeding of the aneurysm and vasospasm. Rebleeding can lead to significant morbidity and mortality. Signs and symptoms of rebleeding are change in the level of consciousness, sudden severe headache associated with nausea and vomiting, and any new neurological deficits. Treatment is centered around maintenance of systolic blood pressure around 150 mm Hg. Antifibrinolytics (e.g., aminocaproic acid) may be initiated to prevent lysis of the clot surrounding the aneurysmal rupture. Aminocaproic acid is usually given intravenously by continuous infusion at a rate of 30 to 60 g/day for up to 3 weeks (Hickey, 1992). It is not given to a patient who is at risk for vasospasm. Other medical interventions are directed toward minimizing cerebral

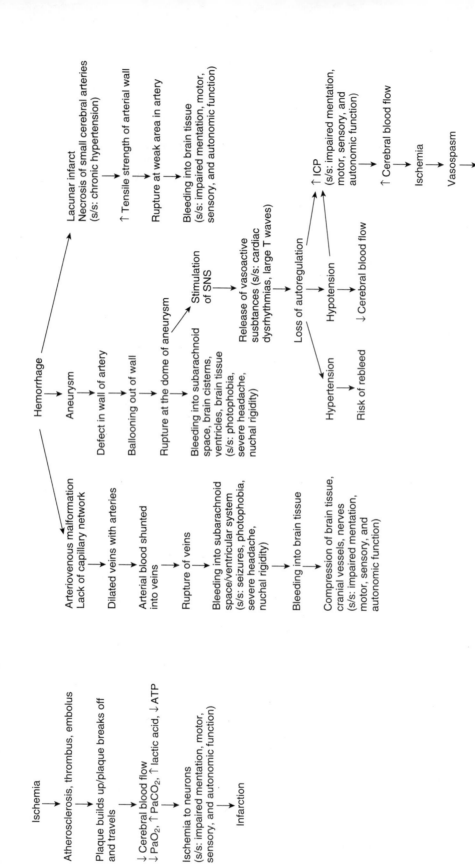

Figure 10-26. Pathophysiology flow diagram—stroke.

edema, hypertension, increased ICP, hydrocephalus, and seizures.

Precautions directed at preventing an aneurysm rebleed involve mainly control of the environment. The patient's environment must be calm, quiet, and free from situations that would cause emotional upset. If the patient has photophobia, the room lights should be dimmed to minimize the associated headache. Visitors are kept to a minimum during this acute period. A mild sedative and nonnarcotic analgesics for headache are given as needed. The other aspect of treatment is minimizing increased ICP to prevent rebleeding. Head and body positioning, prevention of strain, and isometric exercises are important components of therapy. A stool softener is ordered to prevent straining. The patient may be instructed not to assist in turning from side to side in bed.

Vasospasm is the narrowing of a cerebral blood vessel that leads to a decrease in cerebral perfusion and ischemia. A variety of techniques are used to treat vasospasm. The exact mechanism for vasospasm is unknown, but a contributing factor is the breakdown of blood by-products (e.g., prostaglandins, serotonin, catecholamines) that trigger vasospasm (Counsell et al., 1995). The mainstay of treatment is drug therapy, but there is no commonly accepted protocol. Volume expansion (albumin, plasma protein fraction [Plasmanate]) is one such therapy. While hypervolemic hemodilution is being used, the patient is monitored with a pulmonary artery catheter. Volume expansion maintains intravascular volume, and catecholamines are not released, thereby preventing vasoconstriction of cerebral arteries. This therapy is directed at minimizing cerebral ischemia. Other modes of therapy include the administration of calcium channel blockers (e.g., nimodipine), hypertensive agents, steroids (methylprednisolone, dexamethasone), osmotic and loop diuretics (mannitol, furosemide [Lasix]), and anticonvulsants (phenytoin, phenobarbital, valproic acid).

Surgical Interventions for Hemorrhagic CVA

Surgical intervention for an intracerebral hematoma is dependent on the size, extent, and location of the hematoma. The surgical procedure is directed at removing the hematoma and necrotic tissue in the area.

Surgery for a cerebral aneurysm consists of occlusion of the neck of the aneurysm (using a ligature or metal clip), reinforcement of the sac (wrapping the sac with muscle, fibrin foam, or solidifying polymer), or proximal ligation of a feeding vessel. If the neck of the aneurysm is narrow, using a ligature or metal clip is desirable. When the neck of the aneurysm is too broad, reinforcing the aneurysmal sac is the goal of

surgery. Proximal ligation may be preferred when the aneurysm is of the internal carotid artery. The disadvantage of this procedure is decreased CBF to certain parts of the brain. The trend is to stabilize the patient early and take him or her to surgery early (within hours of the rupture). The timing of the surgery is important for an acceptable neurological outcome. The goal is to operate when there is minimal neurological dysfunction and before any episodes of rebleeding or vasospasm.

Hemorrhage from an AVM is a low-pressure bleed, and the mortality from such a hemorrhage is lower than that from a ruptured aneurysm. The rebleeding rate is also much lower than that of an aneurysm. Surgery for removal of an AVM is done either as a single step or in multiple stages. Postoperatively, the major problem is breakthrough bleeding from cauterized vessels. Rapid increases in blood pressure during recovery from anesthesia are to be avoided.

PATIENT OUTCOMES

Patient outcomes for CVA include maintaining CBF and minimizing complications associated with ischemia, cerebral edema, increased ICP, hydrocephalus, rebleeding, vasospasm, and seizures. The outcomes of patients with CVA are identical to the outcomes of patients with increased ICP and head injury (see Nursing Care Plan for the Patient with Increased ICP, Head Injury, and CVA).

Status Epilepticus

A seizure can be a sequela of a wide variety of neurological disorders and systemic diseases. A seizure is an abnormal electrical discharge in the brain that is a symptom of central nervous system irritability. Abnormalities can occur in the motor, sensory, or autonomic nervous systems. Seizures consist of repetitive depolarization of hyperactive, hypersensitive cells at a rate of 300 to 1000 per second. When seizures occur in close proximity to each other, they have the potential to lead to a life-threatening situation, referred to as status epilepticus (SE).

PATHOPHYSIOLOGY

Status epilepticus can occur with any seizure type (Fig. 10–27). The international classification of seizures is presented in Table 10–8. SE is said to exist when seizures repeat frequently enough so that brain function does not return to normal between attacks. Specifically, SE is present when seizure activity lasts for 30 minutes or consciousness is not regained be-

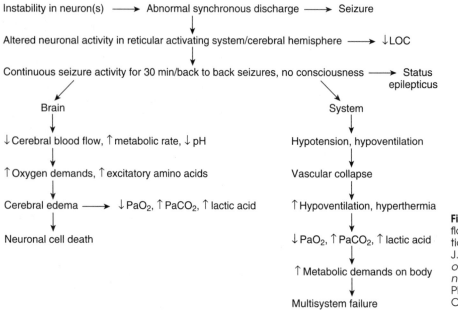

Instability in neuron(s) ⟶ Abnormal synchronous discharge ⟶ Seizure

Altered neuronal activity in reticular activating system/cerebral hemisphere ⟶ ↓LOC

Continuous seizure activity for 30 min/back to back seizures, no consciousness ⟶ Status epilepticus

Brain

↓Cerebral blood flow, ↑metabolic rate, ↓pH

↑Oxygen demands, ↑excitatory amino acids

Cerebral edema ⟶ ↓PaO$_2$, ↑PaCO$_2$, ↑lactic acid

Neuronal cell death

System

Hypotension, hypoventilation

Vascular collapse

↑Hypoventilation, hyperthermia

↓PaO$_2$, ↑PaCO$_2$, ↑lactic acid

↑Metabolic demands on body

Multisystem failure

Figure 10–27. Pathophysiology flow diagram—status epilepticus. (Modified from Hickey, J. V. (1992). *Clinical practice of neurological neurosurgical nursing* (3rd ed.) (Fig. 12–4). Philadelphia: J. B. Lippincott Co.)

tween seizures. SE is present in the case of partial seizures when the episode lasts 30 minutes or longer. It has been estimated that between 50,000 and 60,000 individuals experience SE each year (Shepherd, 1994). SE is more likely to occur with tonic-clonic seizures that have a specific causative factor than with seizures of an idiopathic nature.

The most frequent precipitating factor in SE is irregular intake of anticonvulsants, withdrawal from habitual use of alcohol or sedative drugs, electrolyte imbalance, azotemia, head trauma, and brain tumor.

During SE, metabolism and brain energy requirements may be five times greater than normal. When seizures are prolonged, calcium, prostaglandins, and various diglycerides accumulate in the nerve cells. This leads to cerebral edema and eventually nerve cell death (Shepherd, 1994). The pathological changes occurring from SE follow the pattern of cerebral hypoxia or severe hypoglycemia, although the precise mechanism is not known (Shepherd, 1994).

In the tonic phase of SE, adequate oxygenation may be precluded by the tonic fixation of the chest wall and the obstruction of the airway by the glottis. In addition to these mechanical causes, there are two other deterrents to adequate ventilation. First, neurogenic pulmonary edema may be triggered by the massive autonomic discharges that occur. This may be associated with excessive bronchial secretions and bronchial constriction. Second, respiratory centers in the brain stem may be affected by the abnormal neuronal discharge (Shepherd, 1994).

A seizure's effects on the sympathetic nervous system can lead to serum epinephrine and norepinephrine levels that are high enough to cause cardiac arrhythmias (Burnstine et al., 1990; Shepherd, 1994). Hypoxia and acidosis may also contribute to arrhythmias. In the initial stages, CBF is increased, along with systemic blood pressure.

The autonomic dysfunction also causes hyperpyrexia, excessive sweating, and vomiting that leads to dehydration and electrolyte loss. Initial hyperglycemia is probably a result of the increased release of epinephrine and activation of hepatic gluconeogenesis (Shepherd, 1994). As the seizure continues, energy stores are depleted, leading to hypoglycemia, an increase in the metabolism of lactic acid, and eventually cytotoxic cerebral edema.

The mortality rate of SE in adults ranges from 6 to 10% (Shepherd, 1994). Death is more likely to occur when there is an underlying neurological disease responsible for the condition and may result from the seizure or from the acute illness that precipitated the seizure. Generalized seizures that last for as little as 30 to 45 minutes result in neuronal necrosis in the areas of the basal ganglia, hippocampus, and neocortex, even with adequate oxygenation. This may result in permanent neurological deficits. To avoid permanent neurological dysfunction such as hemiparesis or chronic impairment of recent memory, even focal SE and nonconvulsive SE require prompt treatment (Shepherd, 1994).

Additionally, SE may lead to other systemic complications. Renal failure may result from rhabdomyolysis and acute myoglobinuria. These may also cause

Table 10–8. INTERNATIONAL CLASSIFICATION OF EPILEPTIC SEIZURES

I. Partial or focal seizures
  A. Elementary
    1. Motor symptoms
    2. Sensory symptoms
    3. Autonomic symptoms
    4. Mixed symptoms
  B. Complex (temporal lobe or psychomotor)
    1. Impaired consciousness only
    2. Cognitive symptoms
    3. Affective symptoms
    4. Psychosensory symptoms
    5. Psychomotor symptoms
  C. Partial seizure that secondarily generalizes

II. Generalized seizures (without focal onset)
  A. Tonic-clonic (grand mal)
  B. Status epilepticus
  C. Absence attacks (petit mal)
  D. Tonic
  E. Clonic
  F. Myoclonic
  G. Atonic
  H. Akinetic

III. Unclassified (incomplete data)

Reproduced by permission from Rudy, E. B. (1984). *Advanced neurological and neurosurgical nursing.* St. Louis: C. V. Mosby; adapted from Gastaut, H. (1970). *Epilepsia, 11,* 102.

hyperkalemia and acute intravascular coagulation (Shepherd, 1994). Prolonged clonic-tonic seizure activity leads to many systemic effects. Changes occur in the cardiovascular system because of increased demands from repeated skeletal muscle activity. Initially, tachycardia is present to increase cardiac output. Hypertension occurs to increase CBF to meet the metabolic demands of O_2 and glucose for neurons. As the seizure activity continues, more stimulation of the vagus nerve occurs, resulting in bradycardia. Cardiac dysrhythmias result from hyperkalemia (increased muscle activity), metabolic acidosis, and decreased respirations during SE.

Due to the excessive muscle activity from prolonged skeletal muscle contraction and traumatic injury during SE, a disintegration of striated muscle fibers occurs. Myoglobinuria results from this muscle damage and may lead to renal failure.

ASSESSMENT

Nursing Assessment

Nursing assessment during SE incorporates neurological, respiratory, and cardiovascular assessment. Characteristics of the seizure and the neurological state between seizures are important aspects for the nurse to monitor and record. Documentation of the length of time and pattern of the seizure is necessary. Automatisms and head and eye deviation need to be noted. Assessment of respirations and monitoring of arterial blood gases are needed to ensure the adequacy of oxygenation. Because autonomic changes can result in pulmonary edema, it is imperative to note the onset of fine basilar crackles. Because SE may precipitate arrhythmias, cardiac monitoring and assessment are required.

Medical Assessment

Laboratory studies for a patient with SE include electrocardiogram (ECG), serum electrolytes, serum medication levels, and blood and urine toxicology screens. Cardiac enzymes and arterial blood gases assist in assessing the effect of the seizure on other body systems. Continuous cardiac monitoring needs to be in place prior to the administration of IV medications (Burnstine et al., 1990).

Appropriate radiological studies are needed to rule out a space-occupying lesion that may be responsible for the episode of SE. These may include CT and MRI. Additional studies may be appropriate to rule out injury.

NURSING DIAGNOSES

Nursing diagnoses appropriate for a patient experiencing status epilepticus are:

- Risk for altered tissue perfusion (cerebral) related to the seizure activity
- Risk for ineffective breathing pattern or impaired gas exchange related to the seizure activity
- Risk for ineffective airway clearance related to underlying neurological problem and seizure activity
- Risk for fluid volume excess related to underlying neurological problem, SE, and drug therapy
- Risk for injury related to underlying neurological problems and/or seizure activity
- Altered thought processes related to the postictal state
- Impaired verbal communication related to the postictal state
- Self-esteem disturbance related to seizure activity
- Risk for ineffective family coping related to seizure activity

RESEARCH APPLICATION

Article Reference

Schinner, K. M., Chisholm, A. H., Grap, M. J., Siva, P., Hallinan, M., & LaVoice-Hawkins, A. M. (1995). Effects of auditory stimuli on intracranial pressure and cerebral perfusion pressure in traumatic brain injury. *Journal of Neuroscience Nursing, 27*(6), 348–354.

Study Overview

The purpose of this study was to determine the effect of auditory stimulation on intracranial pressure (ICP) and cerebral perfusion pressure (CPP) in traumatic brain-injured patients. Past research has shown that auditory stimulation, such as voices or conversations, may affect the ICP. Data about exactly what effect auditory stimulation has on ICP have been conflicting. Variables that have been studied include type and content of auditory stimulation, conversation about the patient, conversation unrelated to the patient, music, and normal environmental noise. Studies have also considered the response of patients at various levels of consciousness.

A total of 15 patients with severe brain injury (Glasgow Coma Scale score between 3 and 8) were enrolled in this study. Each had a ventricular catheter in place and a radial arterial line for systolic, diastolic, and mean arterial pressure measurements. Each subject received three treatments—earplugs, a music tape, and a tape of intensive care unit environmental noise—applied in a computer-generated random order. The tapes delivered sound at 70 decibels. Each intervention lasted 15 minutes. ICP and CPP were recorded at a 30-second resolution time through a bedside computer.

Results

There were no statistical or clinically significant changes in ICP or CPP with any auditory intervention. The authors suggest that either the type of auditory stimulation used in these studies does not affect the patient enough to elicit a physiological response or the patient does not hear or process the type of auditory stimulation used.

Strengths and Weaknesses

This is a well-designed study that attempted to control several variables affecting ICP. Several weaknesses can be identified: small sample size ($n = 15$), length of interventions (15 minutes may not be adequate to achieve a response), and severely injured subjects (those at a different point in recovery—e.g., Glasgow Coma Scale score > 8—may respond differently).

Practice Implications

The clinical instincts of practicing nurses suggest that patients respond to auditory stimulation even in a comatose state. Although this particular study does not support that clinical instinct, other studies do. This area of research has produced conflicting results, and this study has added to the conflict. Although this study revealed no effect of auditory stimulation on ICP and CPP, the subjects had very deep levels of coma. Other studies involving subjects with higher Glasgow Coma Scale scores, indicating a "lighter" level of coma, reported patient responses. Therefore, practicing nurses should continue to provide auditory input to patients and monitor their response.

INTERVENTIONS

Nursing Interventions

Objectives of nursing management during SE need to incorporate the following:

- Maintaining a patent airway
- Providing adequate oxygenation
- Maintaining vascular access for the administration of medications
- Maintaining seizure precautions

A patent airway is facilitated by the use of an endotracheal tube or nasal airway. This also assists in removing secretions that collect in the oropharynx. Supplemental oxygen is used to improve oxygenation. Suction equipment needs to be readily available to assist with airway clearance. Poor gas exchange during SE or as a result of respiratory depression from medications may necessitate intubation to provide adequate oxygenation. A nasogastric tube with intermittent suction is needed to ensure that the airway is not compromised by aspiration.

Vascular access must be maintained to provide a route for the administration of medication. The specific medication given depends on the physician's preference and the type of seizure.

Seizure precautions are continued during SE. This includes padding the side rails on the patient's bed and making sure that the bed has full-length side rails. The bed needs to remain in a low position with side rails up except when direct nursing care is being given. Do not try to insert padded tongue blades between the tonically clenched teeth of a patient undergoing a seizure. Patients have inadvertently been injured from aspirating teeth that were loosened during attempts to forcefully insert a padded tongue blade between their teeth. First a neuromuscular blocker is used, and then an oral airway is inserted.

Medical Interventions

SE needs to be stopped within 20 minutes. No consensus has been reached as to the drug of choice, because no ideal drug exists (Treiman, 1993). For tonic-clonic seizures, either diazepam (Valium) or lorazepam (Ativan) is given in an IV bolus for rapid control of SE (Shepherd, 1994). Diazepam has a rapid onset and is given at a rate of 2 mg/min, for a total dose of 30 mg. Diazepam does not mix with other solutions and is administered at the IV port closest to the catheter. Lorazepam is given to adults as an IV bolus 0.1 mg/kg at a rate of 1 to 2 mg/min, up to 10 mg (Shepherd, 1994). Lorazepam has a longer duration of action than diazepam and is the drug of choice.

Phenytoin is also given during SE and requires a loading dose that may require 20 minutes to administer. The drug is given in a loading dose of 20 mg/kg, no faster than 40 to 50 mg/min. Phenytoin mixes only with normal saline; however, it is stable in solution for only 20 minutes, making it impractical for IV piggyback administration. It may be given as a push after clearing the line with saline or slowly pushed with normal saline running.

Phenobarbital is also used intravenously in SE. The loading dose of phenobarbital in adults is 20 mg/kg at an infusion rate of 60 to 100 mg/min (Shepherd, 1994). Because of the potential for respiratory depression, it is not recommended for use with diazepam.

General anesthesia may be initiated with artificial respirations and cardiorespiratory monitoring if SE has not been terminated within 60 minutes. General anesthesia can be achieved in the critical care setting with low-dose continuous-drip IV pentobarbital therapy. Patients should be assessed for evidence of hemodynamic instability. Treatment of such a patient should include control of metabolic disturbances (Shepherd, 1994). Refer to Table 10–9 for drug therapy.

PATIENT OUTCOMES

Patient outcomes for SE are focused on protection during the life-threatening episode and prevention of recurrence. The first outcome is that the patient maintains an adequate breathing and cardiovascular pattern. Second, the patient does not experience any injury related to the seizure activity. Finally, the patient demonstrates knowledge of the disease process, including precipitating factors, medication routines, and side effects of medications.

CRITICAL THINKING QUESTIONS

1. You are caring for Tim Smith, who has suffered a closed head injury from a motor vehicle accident. He has an intraventricular catheter for continuous measurement of intracranial pressure (ICP). His ICP has been stable at 13 mm Hg for the past 4 hours. The alarm on the monitor sounds because his ICP is now 20 mm Hg. What are your priority assessments and interventions at this time?
2. Many nurses believe that visiting should be restricted for neurological patients, especially those with head injuries. What assessments can you make to determine whether family visits are helpful or harmful to your patient?
3. What interventions can you teach families to assist in the care and rehabilitation of patients with prolonged unconsciousness after a head injury or cranial surgery?
4. Barry Brown is an 18-year-old patient who was admitted in generalized convulsive status epilepticus. While receiving anticonvulsant therapy, he also received several doses of mannitol and dexamethasone. Why?

Table 10–9. DRUG THERAPY IN PATIENTS WITH INCREASED INTRACRANIAL PRESSURE, HEAD INJURY, CEREBROVASCULAR ACCIDENT, SPINAL CORD INJURY, OR STATUS EPILEPTICUS

Drug	Actions/Uses	Dosage/Route	Side Effects	Nursing Implications
Mannitol (20%)	Draws water from normal brain cells into plasma; reduces ICP; increases CPP	1.5–2 g/kg initial IV over 30 to 60 min, then 0.25–0.5 g/kg IV every 3–5 hr depending on ICP, CPP, serum osmolarity	Hypotension, dehydration, electrolyte imbalance, tachycardia, rebound edema	1–2 hr neurological assessments; monitor ICP, CPP, serum osmolarity; hourly I&O; daily weights, monitor electrolytes, monitor ABGs, VS
Furosemide (Lasix)	Renal tubular diuretic; reduces cerebral edema by drawing sodium and water out of injured neurons; decreases CSF production	20–80 mg IV (dose may be increased as ordered), max. dose, 600 mg/24 hr *or* 1 mg/kg IV bolus every 6–12 hr (Becker and Gudeman, 1989)	Ototoxicity, polyuria, electrolyte disturbances, gastric irritation, muscle cramps, hypotension	Same as above
Dexamethasone (Decadron)	Steroid that has a stabilizing effect on cell membrane and prevents destructive effect of free O₂ radicals; decreases inflammation by suppressing white cells	6–20 mg IV initially, then 4–6 mg every 6 hr IV	Flushing, sweating, hypotension, tachycardia, thrombocytopenia, weakness, nausea, diarrhea, GI irritation/hemorrhage, fluid retention, poor wound healing, weight gain	Decreases effects of anticoagulants, anticonvulsants, antidiabetic agents; increases effects of digitalis; monitor glucose, potassium, daily weights; monitor VS; causes edema; taper drug prior to discontinuing
Cimetidine	Inhibits histamine at the H₂ receptor sites, inhibiting gastric acid secretion; decreases GI irritation to stress response following neurological injury and steroid use	300 mg in 50 ml 0.9% NaCl every 6–8 hr	Diarrhea, increases BUN, creatinine, thrombocytopenia; increases prothrombin time, bradycardia	Increases toxicity of phenytoin, lidocaine, procainamide; antacids decrease action of cimetidine; give slowly IV—can cause bradycardia

Drug	Action/Use	Dosage/Administration	Side Effects	Nursing Considerations
Labetalol (Normodyne)	Beta-blocker that is nonselecting; decreases blood pressure	200 mg in 200 ml 0.9% NS at 2 mg/min IV; repeat every 6–8 hr as needed or 20 mg/over 2 min IV bolus; may repeat 20–80 mg every 10 min not to exceed 300 mg (Skidmore-Roth, 1988)	Hypotension, bradycardia, CHF, ventricular dysrhythmias, drowsiness, lethargy, nausea, tinnitis, wheezing	Cimetidine increases hypotension; increases hypoglycemia; hourly I&O; daily weights; monitor BP, pulse; taper drug if long-term use
Phenytoin (Dilantin)	Inhibits the spread of seizures; status epilepticus	For status epilepticus, 15–20 mg/kg IV (or 100- to 250-mg bolus). Additional 100–150 mg IV in 30 min; can be diluted in NS. Do not give faster than 50 mg/min	Bradycardia, hypotension nystagmus/ataxia—dose-related gingival hyperplasia, blood dyscrasias; rash	Slow rate down if bradycardia or cardiac dysrhythmias occur; monitor ECG and BP; monitor lab; monitor respiratory status
Diazepam (Valium)	Depresses subcortical areas of CNS; status epilepticus	5–10 mg initially; may be repeated at 10- to 15-min intervals up to a maximum of 30 mg, rate of administration not to exceed 5 mg/min	Respiratory depression, hypotension, drowsiness, dry mouth	Monitor respiratory status; administer IV bolus in a large vein
Lorazepam (Ativan)	Same as diazepam	0.5 mg/kg IV to total of 4 mg IV; two additional doses of 0.5 mg/kg may be given every 10 to 15 min if needed; dilute with equal volume of sterile water, NS, or 5% D/W	Respiratory depression, hypotension, drowsiness	Same as diazepam
Pentobarbital	Sedation: barbiturate metabolism and energy requirements; may prevent peroxidation of lipid components of cell membrane; used for refractory increased ICP and refractory status epilepticus	For increased ICP, 3–5 mg/kg IV in boluses of 50–100 mg doses monitoring ICP—loading dose; hourly maintenance doses of 100–200 mg (1–2 mg/kg) For status epilepticus, 2–8 mg/kg IV loading dose; maintenance dose 1–3 mg/kg/hr IV	Hypotension (at time of bolus), myocardial depression; respiratory depression	Monitor ICP (goal is to decrease ICP to 15–20 mm Hg), monitor CPP; monitor vital signs and hemodynamic status, response of individual patients is variable; each one must be monitored closely

Data from Hodgson, B. B., Kizior, R. J., & Kingdon, R. T. (1996). *Nurse's drug handbook 1996*. Philadelphia: W. B. Saunders Co.; and Booker M. F., & Ignativicius, D. D. (1996). *Infusion therapy techniques* (2nd ed.). Philadelphia: W. B. Saunders Co.

REFERENCES

Adams, H. P., Brott, T. G., & Crowell, R. M. (1994). Guidelines for the management of patients with acute ischemic stroke: A statement for healthcare professionals from a special writing group of the Stroke Council, American Heart Association. *Circulation, 90*(3), 1588–1601.

Alspach, J. G. (1991). *AACN core curriculum for critical care nursing* (4th ed.). Philadelphia: W. B. Saunders Co.

Andrus, C. (1991). Intracranial pressure: Dynamics and nursing management. *Journal of Neuroscience Nursing, 23*(2), 85–91.

Batcheller, J. (1994). Syndrome of inappropriate antidiuretic hormone secretion. *Critical Care Nursing Clinics of North America, 6*(4), 687–692.

Becker, D. P., & Gudeman, S. K. (1989). *Textbook of head injury.* Philadelphia: W. B. Saunders Co.

Bell, S. D., Guyer, D., Snyder, M. A., et al. (1994). Cerebral hemodynamics: Monitoring arteriojugular oxygen content differences. *Journal of Neuroscience Nursing, 26*(5), 270.

Bell, T. N. (1994). Diabetes insipidus. *Critical Care Nursing Clinics of North America, 6*(4), 675–685.

Bronstein, K. S., Popovich, J. M., & Stewart-Amidei, C. (1991). *Promoting stroke recovery.* St. Louis: Mosby Year Book.

Brucia, J. J., Owens, D. C., & Rudy, E. B. (1992). The effects of lidocaine on intracranial hypertension. *Journal of Neuroscience Nursing, 24*(4), 205–214.

Buonocore, C. M., & Robinson, A. G. (1993). The diagnosis and management of diabetes insipidus during medical emergencies. *Endocrinology and Metabolism Clinics of North America, 22*(2), 411–423.

Burnstine, T. H., Lesser, R. P., & Hanley, D. F. (1990). Cardiorespiratory abnormalities. *Critical Care Report, 1*(1), 39–42.

Counsell, C., Gilbert, M., & Snively, C. (1995). Nimodipine: A drug therapy for treatment of vasospasm. *Journal of Neuroscience Nursing, 27*(1), 53–55.

Crosby, L. J., & Parsons, L. C. (1992). Cerebrovascular response of closed head-injured patients to a standardized endotracheal tube suctioning and manual hyperventilation procedure. *Journal of Neuroscience Nursing, 24*(1), 40–49.

Deglin JH: Davis' drug guide for nurses (5th ed.) (1997). Philadelphia: F. A. Davis.

Doberstein, C. E., Hovda, D. A., & Becker, D. P. (1993). Clinical considerations in the reduction of secondary brain injury. *Annals of Emergency Medicine, 22*(6), 993–997.

Dolan, J. T. (Ed.) (1991). *Critical care nursing: Clinical management through the nursing process.* Philadelphia: F. A. Davis, p. 93.

Engli, M., & Kirsivali-Farmer, K. (1993). Needs of family members of critically ill patients with and without acute brain injury. *Journal of Neuroscience Nursing, 25*(2), 78–85.

Germon, K. (1994). Intracranial pressure monitoring in the 1990s. *Critical Care Nurse Quarterly, 17*(1), 21–32.

Hickey, J. V. (1992). *The clinical practice of neurological and neurosurgical nursing* (3rd ed.). Philadelphia: J. B. Lippincott Co.

Ingersoll, G. L., & Leyden, D. B. (1990). The Glasgow Coma Scale for patients with head injuries. *Critical Care Nurse, 7*(5), 26–32.

Kerr, M. E., Rudy, E. B., Brucia, J., et al. (1993). Head-injured adults: Recommendations for endotracheal suctioning. *Journal of Neuroscience Nursing, 25*(2), 86–91.

Marshall, S. B., Marshall, L. F., Vos, H. R., et al. (1990). *Neuroscience critical care.* Philadelphia: W. B. Saunders Co.

Morrison, C. A. M. (1990). Brain herniation syndromes. *Critical Care Nurse, 7*(5), 34–38.

Nayduch, D., Lee, A., & Butler, D. (1994). High-dose methylprednisolone after acute spinal cord injury. *Critical Care Nurse, 14*(4); 69–72, 77–78.

Nolan, S. (1994). Current trends in the management of acute spinal cord injury. *Critical Care Nurse, 17*(1), 64–78.

Prendergast, V. (1994). Current trends in research and treatment of intracranial hypertension. *Critical Care Nurse Quarterly, 17*(1), 1–8.

Richmond, T. S., Metcalf, J., Daly, M., et al. (1992). Powerlessness in acute spinal cord injury patients: A descriptive study. *Journal of Neuroscience Nursing, 24*(3), 146–152.

Rising, C. J. (1993). The relationship of selected nursing activities to ICP. *Journal of Neuroscience Nursing, 25*(5), 302–308.

Ropper A. H., & Kennedy S. F. (Eds.) (1988). *Neurological and neurosurgical intensive care* (2nd ed.) Rockville, MD: Aspen, pp. 9–21.

Ropper A. H., & Rockoff, M. A. (1988). *Neurological and neurosurgical intensive care.* Rockville, MD: Aspen, pp. 24–25.

Shepherd, S. M. (1994). Management of status epilepticus. *Emergency Medicine Clinics of North America, 12*(4), 941–961.

Siesjo, B. K. (1993). Basic mechanisms of traumatic brain damage. *Annals of Emergency Medicine, 22*(6), 959.

Treiman, D. M. (1993). *Current treatment strategies in selected situation epilepsy. Epilepsia 34*(S5): S17–S23.

Whitney, F. (1994). Drug therapy for acute stroke. *Journal of Neuroscience Nursing, 26*(2), 111–117.

Wityk, R. J., & Stern, B. J. (1994). Ischemic stroke: Today and tomorrow. *Critical Care Medicine, 22*(8), 1278–1293.

RECOMMENDED READINGS

Borgeat, A., Wilder-Smith, O. H. G., Jallon, P., & Suter, P. M. (1994). Protocol in the management of refractory status epilepticus: A case report. *Intensive Care Medicine, 20*, 148–149.

German, K. (1988). Interpretation of ICP pulse waves to determine intracerebral compliance. *Journal of Neuroscience Nursing, 20*(6), 344–351.

Hummel, S. K. (1989). Cerebral vasospasm: Current concepts of pathogenesis and treatment. *Journal of Neuroscience Nursing, 21*(4), 216–225.

Leppik, I. E. (Ed.) (1990). Status epilepticus in perspective. *Neurology, 40*(5) (Suppl. 2), 1–51.

MacDonald, E. (1989). Aneurysmal subarachnoid hemorrhage. *Journal of Neuroscience Nursing, 21*(5), 313–321.

Mahon-Darby, J., Ketchik-Renshaw, B., Richmond, T. S., & Gates, E. M. (1988). Powerlessness in cervical spinal cord injury patients. *Dimensions of Critical Care Nursing, 7*(6), 346–355.

Manifold, S. L. (1990). Aneurysmal SAH: Cerebral vasospasm and early repair. *Critical Care Nurse, 10*(8), 62–69.

Palmer, M., & Wyness, M. A. (1988). Positioning and handling: Important considerations in the care of the severely head-injured patient. *Journal of Neuroscience Nursing, 20*(1), 42–49.

Pollack-Latham, C. L. (1990). Intracranial pressure monitoring: Part I. Physiological principles. *Critical Care Nurse, 7*(5), 40–51.

Pollack-Latham, C. L. (1990). Intracranial pressure monitoring: Part II. Patient care. *Critical Care Nurse, 7*(6), 53–72.

Rosner, M. J., Rosner, S. D., & Johnson, A. H. (1995). Cerebral perfusion pressure: Management protocol and clinical results. *Journal of Neurosurgery, 83*, 949–962.

Rutledge, B. (1989). Aneurysm wrapping: Principles application. *Journal of Neuroscience Nursing, 21*(6), 370–374.

Schinner, K. M., Chisholm, A. N., Grap, M. J., Siva, P., Hallinan, M., & LaVoice-Hawkins, A. M. (1995). Effects of auditory stimuli on intracranial pressure and cerebral perfusion pressure in traumatic brain injury. *Journal of Neuroscience Nursing, 27*(6), 348–354.

Scholtes, F. B., Reiner, W. O., & Meinardi, H. (1994). Generalized convulsive status epilepticus: Causes, therapy, and outcome in 36 patients. *Epilepsia, 35*(5), 1104–1112.

Shepherd, S. M. (1994). Management of status epilepticus. *Emergency Medicine Clinics of North America, 12*(4), 941–961.

Teasdale, G. M. (1995). Head injury. *Journal of Neurology, Neurosurgery, and Psychiatry, 58*, 526–539.

11

Acute Respiratory Failure

Susan Zorb, M.S.N., R.N., CCRN, ANP
Phyllis A. Enfanto, M.S., R.N., CCRN

OBJECTIVES

- Describe the pathophysiology of acute respiratory failure.
- Compare the etiology, pathophysiology, assessment, nursing diagnoses, interventions, and outcomes for adult respiratory distress syndrome, acute

respiratory failure in the patient with chronic obstructive pulmonary disease, and pulmonary embolus.
- Formulate a plan of care for the patient with adult respiratory distress syndrome.

Introduction

Acute respiratory failure may occur in many settings. It may be the patient's primary problem, or it may be a complicating factor in other conditions. This chapter reviews the pathophysiology of acute respiratory failure as well as several common causes and the nursing care involved in the treatment of these patients.

Respiratory Failure

DEFINITION

Respiratory failure is defined as an impairment of oxygen uptake, carbon dioxide elimination, or a combination of the two (Luce et al., 1984). No absolute values that define respiratory failure exist for partial pressures of arterial oxygen (PaO_2) or carbon dioxide ($PaCO_2$). However, in the general population, a PaO_2 of less than 60 mm Hg or a $PaCO_2$ of greater than 50 mm Hg is generally thought to be indicative of respiratory failure. Respiratory failure can be the result of failure of arterial oxygenation or failure of ventilation. It is divided into acute, which occurs rap-

idly with little time for bodily compensation, and chronic, which develops over time and allows the body's compensatory defenses to activate.

Acute respiratory failure and chronic respiratory failure are not mutually exclusive. Acute respiratory failure, which is the subject of this chapter, may occur in a person who has chronic respiratory failure who develops a sudden respiratory infection or is exposed to other types of stressors.

PATHOPHYSIOLOGY

Failure of Oxygenation

Failure of oxygenation is present when the PaO_2 cannot be adequately maintained. Five generally accepted mechanisms of reduced arterial oxygen concentrations (hypoxemia) exist: (1) hypoventilation, (2) intrapulmonary shunting, (3) ventilation-perfusion mismatching, (4) diffusion defects, and (5) decreased barometric pressure (Ahrens, 1989a) (Fig. 11–1). All of these mechanisms may contribute to the failure of oxygenation associated with acute respiratory failure. The least common mechanism, decreased barometric pressure, which occurs at high altitudes, is not ad-

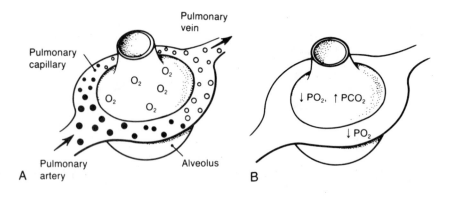

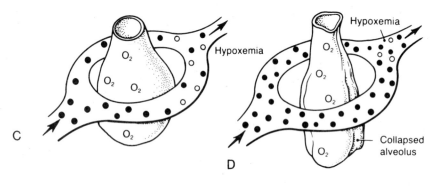

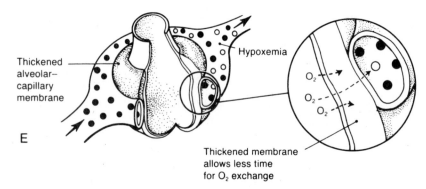

Figure 11–1. The four physiological causes of hypoxemia. *(A)*, A normal alveolar-capillary unit. Unoxygenated blood *(filled circles)* in the pulmonary capillary obtains O_2 from the alveolus. Oxygenated blood *(open circles)* leaves via the pulmonary veins. *(B)*, Hypoventilation results in an increased PCO_2 and decreased PO_2. *(C)*, Ventilation/perfusion mismatch resulting from poor alveolar ventilation; hypoxemia results. *(D)*, Right-to-left shunt. Hypoxemia results from many disorders, all of which lead to collapsed alveoli. *(E)*, Diffusion defect. The diffusion of O_2 across the alveolar-capillary membrane is decreased when the membrane is thickened or filled with fluid. (From Yee, B. H., & Zorb, S. L. (1985). *Cardiac critical care nursing* (p. 109). Boston: Little, Brown & Co.)

dressed in this text. In addition, other conditions, such as decreased cardiac output (CO) and low hemoglobin level, may result in tissue hypoxia.

Hypoventilation. In the normal lung, the partial pressure of alveolar oxygen (PAO_2) is approximately equal to the PaO_2. Alveolar ventilation refers to the amount of gas that enters the alveoli per minute. If the alveolar ventilation is reduced because of hypoventilation, the PAO_2 and the PaO_2 are reduced. Factors that lead to hypoventilation include drugs, such as morphine sulfate and other central nervous system depres-

sants, and neurological disorders that cause a decrease in the rate or depth of respirations. The hypoxemia associated with hypoventilation can be successfully treated with supplemental oxygen administration (West, 1990). Hypoventilation also produces an increase in the alveolar carbon dioxide level because the carbon dioxide that is produced in the tissues is delivered to the lungs but is not released from the body. This build-up of carbon dioxide in the alveoli further contributes to the reduced PaO_2 (West, 1990).

Intrapulmonary Shunting. In a perfectly functioning lung, the PaO_2 exactly equals the PAO_2; however, this is never the case. Normally, a small amount of blood returns to the left side of the heart without engaging in alveolar gas exchange. This blood is referred to as the *physiological shunt*. If, in addition to the normal shunt, more blood returns to the left side of the heart without being oxygenated, a decrease in the PaO_2 occurs. This condition exists when areas of the lung that are being inadequately ventilated are being adequately perfused (see Fig. 11–1). The blood, therefore, is shunted past the lung and returns unoxygenated to the left side of the heart. This intrapulmonary shunting is referred to as Q_s/Q_t disturbances. Q_s denotes the amount of shunted flow, and Q_t denotes the total amount of flow.

As the shunt increases, the PaO_2 continues to decrease. This cause of hypoxemia cannot be effectively treated by increasing the fraction of inspired oxygen (FiO_2), because the unventilated alveolar units do not receive any of the enriched air. Clinically, several methods for estimating the size of the shunt exist (Ahrens, 1989a). All of the methods are accurate about 70% of the time.

The most easily understood method for estimating a shunt is the calculation of the arterial/alveolar ratio (a/A ratio). In this method, the actual PAO_2 is compared with what the PAO_2 should be at a certain FiO_2. The alveolar oxygen tension is calculated by use of the following alveolar air equation:

$$PAO_2 = FiO_2 (P_B - PH_2O) - PaCO_2/r$$

where

FiO_2 = fraction of inspired oxygen
P_B = barometric pressure (760 mm Hg at sea level)
PH_2O = water vapor pressure (47 mm Hg at sea level)
$PaCO_2$ = pressure of arterial carbon dioxide
r = respiratory quotient (usually 0.8)
PAO_2 = 0.21 (760 − 47) − 45/0.8
PAO_2 = 93.5
a/A = 50/93.5
a/A = 0.53

If the patient is breathing room air (FiO_2 = 0.21) and has a PaO_2 of 50 mm Hg and a $PaCO_2$ of 45 mm Hg, the a/A ratio is 0.53. A normal a/A ratio is 0.75, but any value greater than 0.60 may be clinically acceptable (Ahrens, 1989a). Use of the a/A ratio enables the clinician to assess the patient's response to therapy and to select the most appropriate FiO_2.

Ventilation/Perfusion Mismatching. The rate of ventilation (V) usually equals the rate of perfusion (Q), resulting in a ventilation/perfusion ($\dot{V}/\dot{Q}$) ratio of 1. If ventilation exceeds blood flow, the $\dot{V}/\dot{Q}$ ratio is greater than 1; if ventilation is less than blood flow, the $\dot{V}/\dot{Q}$ ratio is less than 1. In respiratory failure, $\dot{V}/\dot{Q}$ mismatching is the most common cause of hypoxemia. At any given moment, the lung has various $\dot{V}/\dot{Q}$ ratios; one region may be better ventilated and another better perfused. In the failing lung, a reduction in the ventilation to a region may occur as a result of increased secretions that obstruct the airway or as a result of bronchospasms. If there is partial ventilation of the alveoli involved, the hypoxemia caused by this $\dot{V}/\dot{Q}$ mismatch responds somewhat to an increase in FiO_2. If perfusion is reduced to an area that has normal ventilation, as in pulmonary emboli, the dead space (V_{DS}) increases in relation to the tidal volume (V_T). The effect of this $\dot{V}/\dot{Q}$ mismatch is discussed under failure of ventilation.

Diffusion Defects. The distance between the alveoli and the pulmonary capillaries is usually only one or two cells thick. This narrowness of space facilitates efficient diffusion of oxygen and carbon dioxide across the cell membrane. In respiratory failure, the distance between the alveoli and the capillaries may be increased by the addition of fluid into the interstitial space (see Fig. 11–1). Changes in capillary perfusion pressure as well as leaking of plasma proteins into the interstitial space and destruction of the capillary membrane contribute to the build-up of fluids around the alveolus (Ahrens, 1989b). Fibrotic changes in the lung tissue itself may also contribute to a reduction in the diffusion capacity of the lung. As this capacity is reduced, PaO_2 is the first parameter affected, and hypoxemia results. Because carbon dioxide is more readily diffusible than oxygen, hypercapnia is a later-occurring sign of diffusion defect.

Low Cardiac Output. Adequate oxygenation depends on a balance between oxygen supply and demand. Normal oxygen transport is between 600 and 1000 ml/min (Rutherford, 1989b). The major determinant of oxygen supply is CO, as indicated by the formula for normal oxygen transport:

$$CaO_2 \times CO \times 10$$

where CaO_2 = arterial oxygen content.

Cardiac output is the product of heart rate times stroke volume. If the CO decreases, less blood is delivered to the tissues. In order to maintain aerobic metabolism, the tissues must extract increasing amounts of oxygen from the blood. When this increase in extraction can no longer compensate for the decreased CO, anaerobic metabolism takes over. This phenomenon results in a build-up of lactic acids, which further depresses the myocardium and results in an even lower CO. The patient exhibits a low PaO_2 as well as a low mixed venous oxygen saturation. This reduction in mixed venous oxygen saturation reflects the increased extraction of oxygen at the tissue level. This reduction in oxygenation is seen in patients with reduced CO with or without concomitant pulmonary disease.

Low Hemoglobin Level. Most oxygen is transported to the tissues bound to hemoglobin. Each gram of hemoglobin can carry 1.34 ml of oxygen when all of its oxygen bonding sites are completely filled. The term *oxygen saturation* refers to the percent of oxygen bonding sites on each hemoglobin molecule that are filled with oxygen. For example, a hemoglobin molecule with half of its bonding sites filled is said to be 50% saturated. When a normal person is breathing room air, his or her hemoglobin is about 95% saturated. Factors such as fever and acidosis reduce the hemoglobin affinity for oxygen and make it easier to unload the oxygen to the tissues. If a patient's hemoglobin level is less than normal, oxygen supply to the tissues may be impaired, and tissue hypoxia may occur.

Tissue Hypoxia. In acute respiratory failure, tissue hypoxia causes the damage. As previously mentioned, anaerobic metabolism occurs when the tissues can no longer obtain adequate oxygen to meet their metabolic needs. Anaerobic metabolism is inefficient and results in the build-up of lactic acids. The point at which anaerobic metabolism begins to occur is not known and may vary with different organ systems. The effects of tissue hypoxia vary with the severity of the hypoxia.

Initially, mild central nervous system changes, such as changes in visual acuity, impaired mental performance, and hyperventilation, may be seen. As the hypoxia increases, changes may be seen in multiple organ systems. The patient may have a headache, a change in the level of consciousness, convulsions, and permanent brain damage. Tachycardia and mild hypertension may be the initial signs in the cardiovascular system, followed by bradycardia, hypotension, and failure as the hypoxia worsens. Renal involvement produces a decrease in urine output with sodium retention and proteinuria. Pulmonary hypertension occurs as a result of vasoconstriction in response to alveolar hypoxia. Treatment for respiratory failure is discussed in each section.

Failure of Ventilation

The partial pressure of arterial carbon dioxide is the index used in the evaluation of ventilation. When $PaCO_2$ is increased (hypercapnia), ventilation is reduced. When $PaCO_2$ is reduced (hypocapnia), ventilation is increased. Hypoventilation and $\dot{V}/\dot{Q}$ mis-

matching are the two mechanisms responsible for hypercapnia.

Hypoventilation. Hypoventilation is the cause of respiratory failure that occurs in patients with neuromuscular disorders, drug overdoses, and chest wall abnormalities (see Fig. 11–1). In hypoventilation, carbon dioxide accumulates in the alveoli and is not blown off. Respiratory acidosis occurs rapidly before renal compensation can occur. Mechanical ventilation may be necessary for support of the patient until the initial cause of the hypoventilation can be corrected.

Ventilation/Perfusion Mismatching. Because the upper and lower airways do not play a part in gas exchange, the volume of inspired gas that fills these structures is referred to as dead space. This dead space is normally 25 to 30% of the inspired volume.

A major mechanism for changes in $PaCO_2$ is an alteration in the amount of dead space in relation to the entire tidal volume (V_D/V_T). The amount of dead space in the lung increases when perfusion is reduced to an area that is ventilated because that area no longer participates in gas exchange. A change in the V_D/V_T ratio must be accompanied by an increase in minute ventilation in order for the $PaCO_2$ to remain normal. If the V_D/V_T increases without an accompanying change in minute ventilation, then the $PaCO_2$ increases.

Hypercapnia greatly increases cerebral blood flow and may result in headache, increased cerebrospinal fluid pressure, and papilledema. The patient may appear restless and may demonstrate slurred speech, mood swings, and a depressed level of consciousness.

Acute Respiratory Failure in Adult Respiratory Distress Syndrome

DEFINITION

Adult respiratory distress syndrome (ARDS) is a form of noncardiogenic pulmonary edema that can occur as a result of a variety of lung insults. (Some texts now refer to ARDS as acute respiratory distress syndrome.) It is a major cause of respiratory failure in patients with previously healthy lungs. After a lung insult, the permeability of the alveolar capillary membrane increases. This phenomenon is characterized by severe dyspnea, hypoxemia, and diffuse bilateral infiltrations on chest x-ray study. The pathophysiological changes are similar to those that occur in the respiratory distress syndrome of the newborn.

The signs, symptoms, and pathophysiology that occur with ARDS were first described as a clinical syndrome in adults by Ashbaugh et al. in 1967. This term quickly replaced the many others that were previously used to describe similar physical findings. These synonyms are presented in Table 11–1.

Table 11-1. SYNONYMS FOR ADULT RESPIRATORY DISTRESS SYNDROME

Adult hyaline membrane disease
Congestive atelectasis
Da Nang lung
High-permeability pulmonary edema
Liver lung
Noncardiogenic pulmonary edema
Postperfusion lung
Posttraumatic pulmonary insufficiency
Posttraumatic wet lung
Pump lung
Respirator lung
Shock lung
White lung

ETIOLOGY

Although the signs, symptoms, and pathophysiology are the same, many potential causes have been implicated in the development or worsening of ARDS (Table 11-2). The most frequently identified risk fac-

Table 11-2. POSSIBLE CAUSES FOR ADULT RESPIRATORY DISTRESS SYNDROME

Anaphylaxis
Aspiration of gastric contents
Cardiopulmonary bypass
Diffuse pneumonia
Disseminated intravascular coagulation
Drug overdose
Eclampsia
Fat embolism
Fractures, especially of the pelvis or long bones
Goodpasture's syndrome
High altitude
Idiopathic
Idiosyncratic drug reaction
Increased intracranial pressure
Leukemia
Multiple transfusions
Multisystem trauma
Near-drowning
Neurogenic pulmonary edema
Oxygen toxicity
Pancreatitis
Paraquat toxicity
Prolonged mechanical ventilation
Pulmonary contusion
Radiation
Sepsis
Smoke or irritant gas inhalation
Surface burns
Thrombotic thrombocytopenic purpura
Uremia
Venous air embolism

tors or potential causes are sepsis, aspiration of gastric contents, and massive trauma (Vollman, 1994).

The mortality rate for patients diagnosed with ARDS is 60 to 70% (Chillcott and Sheridan, 1995; Willms et al., 1994). Of those patients who recover, about 85% return to near-normal pulmonary function within 1 year.

The etiology of ARDS is most important in the planning of collaborative interventions to attain successful patient outcomes. Although treatment plans may be similar because of the overall problems with oxygenation and fluid balance, all of the possible underlying causes should be considered. This careful consideration guides the therapy and can improve the patient's chance of a successful outcome.

PATHOPHYSIOLOGY

Regardless of the cause of ARDS, the initial injury to the lung results in pulmonary hypoperfusion, which disrupts the lung's normal function by damaging the alveolar or vascular epithelium (Fig. 11-2). The resulting tissue hypoxia then leads to lactic acidosis and release of vasoactive substances. Platelet and leukocyte aggregation also occur, serotonin is released, and embolization and occlusion of the pulmonary microcirculation occur as a result of intravascular clotting. Dead space also increases. Each of these three factors results in an increase in the permeability of the alveolar-capillary membrane, thereby allowing fluid to gradually leak into the interstitial space and alveoli, causing pulmonary edema and alveolar collapse.

The edema, accompanied by a decrease in capillary perfusion, also results in a decrease in the production of surfactant owing to injury to the type II pneumocytes. The alveoli become more unstable and collapse unless they are filled with fluid. Gas exchange is impaired, and hypoxemia develops because the alveoli are either filled with fluid or collapsed.

Fluid continues to leak into the interstitial spaces, resulting in interstitial edema, compression, further collapse of alveoli, and overall decrease in lung volume. These changes are exhibited by hypoxemia and a decrease in functional residual capacity. These as well as the other changes result in an overall decrease in lung compliance and an increased work of breathing. The decrease in compliance is compounded by pulmonary vasoconstriction and bronchoconstriction caused by the release of arachidonic acid metabolites (Vollman, 1994).

The alveoli continue to receive blood flow, even though they are not receiving adequate ventilation; this blood flow results in intrapulmonary shunting. These changes along with the increase in wasted ventilation result in an overall $\dot{V}/\dot{Q}$ mismatch and hypoxemia.

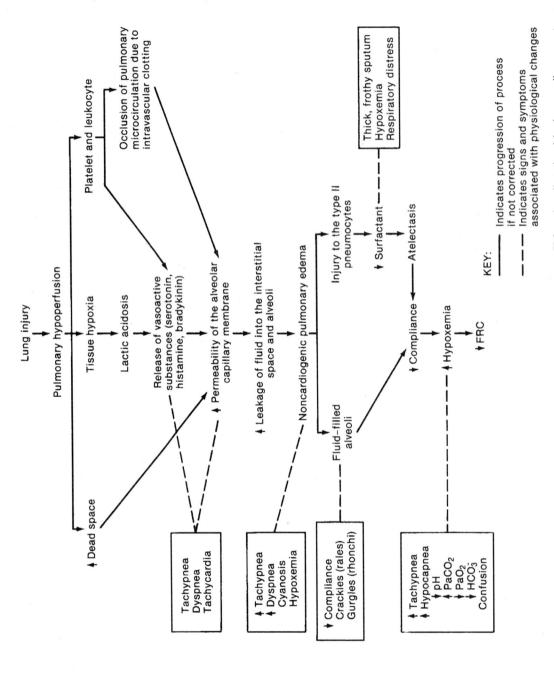

Figure 11-2. Pathophysiology of adult respiratory distress syndrome. FRC = functional residual capacity.

Clinically, the patient hyperventilates in an attempt to increase the PaO_2. The result of the tachypnea is hypocapnia, increased airway resistance, increased oxygen consumption, and decreased compliance.

The resulting pulmonary dysfunction is compounded by a reflex increase in CO and minute ventilation in an attempt to compensate for the hypoxemia. The venous return increases as a result of the increased inspiratory effort needed to open the alveoli. Fluid continues to leak through the damaged capillary membranes into the interstitial spaces, and compliance is further impaired.

High levels of oxygen are often required for the maintenance of adequate tissue perfusion despite the $\dot{V}/\dot{Q}$ mismatch. When levels of oxygen greater than 50% are utilized for extended periods of time, oxygen toxicity may result. This situation further compounds matters because progression of oxygen toxicity leads to damage to the alveoli and aggravation of the symptoms already present as a result of ARDS. Initial symptoms include tracheobronchitis, cough, inspiratory pain, and dyspnea.

ASSESSMENT

Early assessment and diagnosis of ARDS guide the caregivers to institute appropriate therapies and decrease the chance that the initial changes are compounded by the inappropriate use of oxygen, fluids, mechanical ventilation, and drugs. Symptoms of ARDS may not be present until 6 to 48 hours after the initial insult to the lung, and the critical care nurse is often the first to detect the early warning signs (Table 11–3).

One of the initial signs of ARDS is restlessness and changes in the patient's behavior. These changes can include mood swings, disorientation, and change in level of consciousness. Other early warning signs are dyspnea and hyperventilation with normal breath

---

Table 11–3. EARLY WARNING SIGNS OF ADULT RESPIRATORY DISTRESS SYNDROME

Restlessness
Change in patient's behavior, e.g., mood swings, disorientation, or change in the level of consciousness
Dyspnea
Hyperventilation with normal breath sounds
Cough
Respiratory alkalosis
Increased peak inspiratory pressures
Normal chest x-ray study
Tachycardia
Increased temperature

Table 11–4. LATE SIGNS OF ADULT RESPIRATORY DISTRESS SYNDROME

Decreased PaO_2
Severe dyspnea
Grunting with respirations
Decreased $PaCO_2$ with respiratory alkalosis
Intercostal and suprasternal retractions
Hypocapnia and hypoxemia
Tachycardia
Pallor
Cyanosis
Metabolic acidosis
Adventitious breath sounds—crackles, rhonchi, or bronchial breath sounds
Chest x-ray study showing bilateral patchy infiltrates
Decreased functional residual capacity
Increased peak inspiratory pressures

PaO_2 = partial pressure of arterial oxygen; $PaCO_2$ = partial pressure of arterial carbon dioxide.

---

sounds. The dyspnea may not be evident in an otherwise young healthy patient, because he or she can easily double and triple minute ventilation at rest.

Patients may also exhibit a cough accompanied by respiratory alkalosis. If the patient is mechanically ventilated, the critical care nurse observes an increase in peak inspiratory pressures. This finding is an indication of the decrease in compliance. Pulse and temperature may be increased, and chest x-ray studies are usually normal. These early warning signs should alert the health team members to search for potential causes of lung injury.

As the process progresses and the PaO_2 decreases, dyspnea becomes severe, and the patient may grunt with respirations (Table 11–4). The $PaCO_2$ continues to decrease, resulting in respiratory alkalosis without an improvement in oxygenation. Intercostal and suprasternal retractions are present on physical examination. Hypocapnia and hypoxemia do not respond to increasing levels of oxygen. Tachycardia, pallor, and cyanosis are present.

The respiratory alkalosis is accompanied by a metabolic acidosis that is caused by lactic acid buildup. The presence of this condition can be confirmed by serum lactate level determinations. As the ARDS progresses, the nurse hears crackles, rhonchi, and bronchial breath sounds on auscultation. A chest x-ray study shows bilateral patchy infiltrates, which progress to what is often referred to as "white lung."

Pulmonary mechanics show a decrease in lung volumes, especially functional residual capacity, and a decrease in static and dynamic compliance. As the patient's condition deteriorates, peak inspiratory pressures on the ventilator continue to rise. Pulmonary artery pressure (PAP), pulmonary capillary wedge pressure (PCWP), and CO can be normal, but if they are abnormal, these results help to guide treatment.

Assessment of a patient with ARDS should be collaborative. A key clinical finding that is often diagnostic of ARDS is a lung insult followed by respiratory distress with profound dyspnea, tachypnea, and hypoxemia that does not respond to oxygen therapy. Once the condition is diagnosed, important assessment data that are used to guide treatment include hemodynamic measurements, arterial blood gases (ABGs), mixed venous blood gases, breath sounds, serial chest x-ray studies, fluid and electrolyte values, metabolic and nutritional needs, and psychosocial needs of the patient and family.

NURSING DIAGNOSES

Several nursing diagnoses must be addressed in the care of a patient with ARDS. Addressing these diagnoses assists the nurse in meeting the major goals of therapy. These goals include (1) increasing delivery of oxygen to the tissues, (2) decreasing overall oxygen consumption, (3) supplying adequate nutrition in order to meet the metabolic demands of the patient, (4) maintaining fluid and electrolyte balance, and (5) providing support to the patient and family.

To meet these goals, the critical care nurse should devise a plan of care by addressing the following nursing diagnoses:

- Ineffective breathing pattern related to increased alveolar capillary permeability and decreased lung compliance, as indicated by dyspnea, cough, tachypnea, use of accessory muscles, and abnormal ABG results.
- Impaired gas exchange related to increased alveolar capillary membrane changes, decreased surfactant, and embolization and occlusion of the pulmonary microcirculation, as indicated by hypoxemia, restlessness, and increased $\dot{V}/\dot{Q}$ mismatch.
- Risk for infection related to illness and invasive procedures, as indicated by increased temperatures; warm, flushed skin; and increased white blood cell count.
- Fluid volume excess related to excess fluid intake, as indicated by an intake greater than the output, increased PCWP, and weight gain.
- Altered nutrition (less than body requirements) related to increased metabolic demands and decreased ability to take in food as a result of infection, trauma, and mechanical ventilation, as indicated by calorie counts that do not meet metabolic demands.

- Risk for impaired skin integrity related to bed rest and inadequate nutrition.
- Altered tissue perfusion (cardiopulmonary) related to microembolization of the pulmonary vasculature, decreased surfactant, and increased permeability of the alveolar-capillary membrane, as indicated by atelectasis, pulmonary infiltrates, hypoxemia, and increased $\dot{V}/\dot{Q}$ mismatch.
- Altered tissue perfusion (peripheral) related to vasoconstriction and hypoxemia, as indicated by cold extremities, peripheral cyanosis, and abnormal mixed venous blood gas results.
- Risk for anxiety related to inability to speak, situational crises, uncertainty, and lack of control, as indicated by increased heart rate, blood pressure, and respiratory rate; increased muscle tension; and inappropriate behaviors.
- Risk for ineffective family coping related to knowledge deficits of family members that result from inadequate information and uncertain outcome, as indicated by verbalization of fears.
- Activity intolerance related to hypoxia, as indicated by inability to perform self-care functions.

INTERVENTIONS

Interventions for a patient with ARDS should be collaborative and should have common goals. Whether the consideration is oxygenation, nutrition, or family support, the outcomes are more easily reached when a collaborative approach is taken. The main factors to address in the care of a patient with ARDS are oxygenation, maintenance of fluid and electrolyte balance, maintenance of adequate nutrition, and provision of psychosocial support.

Oxygenation

The first intervention used for the relief of hypoxemia is the use of supplemental oxygen. Patients with ARDS usually require intubation and mechanical ventilation. In order to achieve the desired PaO_2, the physician may initially use a high tidal volume. As the patient deteriorates and requires an FiO_2 of greater than 50%, the physician often adds positive end-expiratory pressure (PEEP) in an attempt to improve oxygenation. Such improvement occurs by provision of a positive airway pressure throughout the cycle that reexpands collapsed alveoli and increases functional residual capacity. The anticipated result is greater oxygenation at a lower FiO_2.

Some patients remain hypoxic despite these interventions. The critical care nurse may observe that the patient continues to try to hyperventilate despite undergoing mechanical ventilation, a phenomenon often referred to as "bucking" the ventilator. The patient tries to exhale during the inspiratory phase of the ventilator, and the result is a worsening of the hypoxemic state. The patient may be treated with sedatives in order to decrease anxiety and the work of breathing. If this measure is not effective, neuromuscular blocking agents may be used in order to paralyze the skeletal muscles and allow the ventilator to completely control the work of breathing.

An arterial line and a pulmonary artery catheter are needed for monitoring of the patient's hemodynamic status, blood pressure, and ABGs. The critical care nurse collects these data, and the nurse and the physician analyze the data and make alterations in therapy.

Cardiac output, and subsequently blood pressure, are important parameters for the critical care nurse to monitor in a patient receiving ventilator support with PEEP. The increase in pleural pressure caused by the PEEP may result in a decrease in venous return and a subsequent decrease in CO and blood pressure, causing a paradoxical decrease in oxygen delivery.

A decrease in CO may be critical in an already compromised patient with hypotension. Nursing interventions aimed at promoting venous return include elevating the foot of the bed 10° to 20° and providing passive range-of-motion exercises. Urine output should also be monitored closely, and the physician should be notified if it drops to less than 30 ml/h.

Peripheral circulation needs to be assessed and monitored closely, especially if the patient is on vasopressors. Signs of compromise include cold extremities, decreased or absent pulse, pallor, and cyanosis. The PEEP may need to be adjusted, along with tidal volume and FiO_2, in order to supply adequate tissue oxygenation. The adjustments are often determined by assessing samples of both arterial and mixed venous blood gases.

Frequent repositioning and good pulmonary hygiene are nursing interventions that assist in decreasing the occurrence of atelectasis and pooling of secretions in the lungs. Repositioning also decreases the occurrence of skin breakdown. Any increases in oxygenation that result from position changes should be assessed. If lung disease is unilateral, improved gas exchange may be seen by placing the patient in the lateral position with the good lung down. This position allows greater blood flow to the better-functioning lung.

In addition to maximizing oxygen delivery to the tissues, the critical care nurse must work collaboratively with the physician to decrease oxygen consumption. This includes implementing measures to make the febrile patient normothermic, such as antipyretics,

tepid baths, and a cooling blanket, if necessary. Activities are spaced out, and substantial periods of rest are provided. The patient's comfort is considered, including whether or not he or she is having any pain. Signs of pain or discomfort include tachycardia, restlessness, guarding, and decreased attention span. Analgesics and comfort measures are indicated if such behaviors are present.

Maintenance of Fluid and Electrolyte Balance

A second area of treatment that must be addressed is fluid and electrolyte balance. Careful assessment and treatment are paramount because the large volumes of fluid used for the maintenance of intravascular volume and the treatment of hypotension may worsen the pulmonary edema when it leaks through the alveolar capillary membrane. Intake and output, along with PCWP or PAD, must be monitored closely. Initially, PCWP and PAD may be normal or low. Intravenous fluid may be required, with the goal being the maintenance of the lowest PCWP and PAD needed for the provision of adequate CO and tissue perfusion. Clinically, this is assessed by blood pressure, blood urea nitrogen level, serum creatinine, mixed venous blood gas results, and level of consciousness.

Controversy exists regarding the use of crystalloids or colloids in the treatment of patients with ARDS. Colloids have been used in an attempt to increase oncotic pressure within the vascular space, but because of the increased capillary permeability in ARDS, the proteins can leak into the interstitial tissues and further compound the problem. Crystalloids are often chosen in the initial stages of treatment for ARDS when fluids are needed for the maintenance of CO. The critical care nurse must inform the physician if the PCWP begins to increase because this situation is usually treated with fluid restriction and diuretics.

Maintenance of Adequate Nutrition

The nutritional needs of the critically ill patient with ARDS must also be addressed because the caloric requirements of such patients increase 1.5 to 2.0 times that of normal (Murphy and Conforti, 1993). Many factors, such as stress, sepsis, trauma, and use of mechanical ventilation, contribute to this increase in caloric requirements. If the nutritional requirements are not met, respiratory muscle function is impaired as a result of the negative nitrogen balance, and weaning is not possible. Unless aspiration is a major risk, enteral nutrition is preferred because it carries fewer overall complications than parenteral nutrition.

Provision of Psychosocial Support

As with all patients in a critical care setting, the health team members must always remember to provide a warm, nurturing environment in which the patient and family can feel safe. The onset of ARDS and its long recovery phase result in stress and anxiety for both the patient and the family. The patient may also experience feelings of isolation because of the length of the recovery phase.

All health care team members should take the time to sensitively explain procedures, equipment, changes in the patient's condition, and outcomes to patients and families. The patient should be allowed to participate in the planning of care as much as possible and should feel comfortable verbalizing fears and questions to the staff. In the intubated patient, communication is impaired, which may increase the patient's sense of isolation. The isolation and accompanying depression can often be minimized by allowing frequent visits from families and friends while still providing adequate rest periods for the patient. Personal items from home, such as photographs of loved ones, may also assist the critical care nurse to meet the patient's psychosocial needs.

Other Therapies

The physician may elect to provide other forms of treatment in addition to those discussed earlier. In the presence of actual or presumed infection, many ARDS patients receive antibiotic therapy. Although still controversial, corticosteroid therapy is sometimes used in order to assist the patient with an anti-inflammatory process during this period of stress. These agents also stabilize the capillary and cell membranes, enhance surfactant production, and decrease platelet aggregation (Vollman, 1994). Although these properties are desired, they may also predispose the patient to infection. The advantages of therapy must be weighed against the disadvantages in each case.

Additional therapies for the treatment of ARDS include surfactant replacement and extracorporeal carbon dioxide removal. These innovative therapies have shown early promise in the reduction of mortality (Sinski and Corbo, 1994; Chillcott and Sheridan, 1995).

OUTCOMES

For each patient with ARDS, the therapies and interventions are chosen based on the individual's clinical data. Therapies can be altered, changed, or discontinued, depending on the patient's response. In each situation, health team members are working with patients and families to reach common goals. The expected patient outcomes for a patient with ARDS include the following:

- Effective breathing pattern and adequate gas exchange without mechanical ventilation
- Adequate oxygenation to the organs and peripheral tissues
- Decreased oxygen consumption
- Normothermia (body temperature)
- Absence of infection
- Optimal fluid balance
- Adequate nutrition to effectively meet metabolic demands
- Intact skin
- Minimal damage to lung tissues
- Stable blood pressure and CO
- Reduction or elimination of anxiety, fears, and social isolation
- Gradual increase in activity back to baseline without signs of tachypnea, dyspnea or abnormal ABG results

A review of the care of the patient with ARDS can be found in the nursing care plan.

Acute Respiratory Failure in Chronic Obstructive Pulmonary Disease

DEFINITION

Chronic obstructive pulmonary disease (COPD) refers to a group of disorders that result in obstruction of airflow in the lungs. These disorders include asthma, emphysema, and chronic bronchitis. Generally, COPD is marked by a gradual decline in the patient's lung function. However, acute respiratory failure can occur at any time in the patient with COPD. These patients normally have little respiratory reserve, and any condition that causes increased work of breathing, worsened $\dot{V}/\dot{Q}$ mismatching, or increased secretions and bronchoconstriction may result in acute respiratory failure.

PATHOPHYSIOLOGY

The abnormality associated with COPD is obstruction to airflow. This obstruction may be caused by several factors, some of which are reversible and others of which are fixed.

Asthma

Asthma is a reversible airway obstruction caused by bronchospasm. This bronchospasm results in air

NURSING CARE PLAN FOR A PATIENT WITH ACUTE RESPIRATORY FAILURE DUE TO ADULT RESPIRATORY DISTRESS SYNDROME

Nursing Diagnosis	Patient Outcomes	Nursing Interventions
Ineffective breathing pattern related to increased alveolar-capillary permeability and decreased lung compliance, as indicated by dyspnea, cough, tachypnea, use of accessory muscles, and abnormal arterial blood gas (ABG) results.	Airflow will be maximized. Respiratory distress will be absent. Respirations will be unlabored at rate of 12–18 breaths/ min. ABGs will be within normal limits (WNL).	Assess and document respiratory status every 1 to 2 h, including breathing pattern, rate, depth, and rhythm. Assess chest expansion, use of accessory muscles, and breath sounds. Position in semi-Fowler's position or that in which breathing pattern is most comfortable. Administer medications to increase airflow as ordered; evaluate their effectiveness; may include such drugs as isoetharine hydrochloride (Bronkosol) and metaproterenol sulfate (Alupent). Administer anti-inflammatories as ordered; may include corticosteroids, e.g., methylprednisolone. Give oxygen therapy or maintain mechanical ventilation as indicated. Monitor for dyspnea and signs of increasing respiratory distress. Assist with activities designed to conserve energy. Provide patient with adequate periods of rest. Monitor arterial blood gases. If patient is febrile, administer antipyretics as ordered in order to decrease temperature and, therefore, oxygen consumption.
Impaired gas exchange related to increased alveolar-capillary membrane changes, decreased surfactant, and embolization and occlusion of the pulmonary microcirculation, as indicated by hypoxemia, restlessness, and increased ventilation/perfusion ($\dot{V}/\dot{Q}$) mismatch.	Gas exchange will be adequate. ABGs will be WNL.	Assess for hypoxemia and hypercapnea. Assess for restlessness or change in the level of consciousness. Position for maximal gas exchange; if only right lung is affected, position with left lung down in order to improve gas exchange. Provide supplemental oxygen as needed or maintain mechanical ventilation as indicated. Encourage coughing and deep breathing. Use paralysis and sedation as ordered in order to maintain optimal gas exchange. Provide good pulmonary hygiene as needed. Monitor ABG results. Provide frequent periods of rest.
Altered tissue perfusion (cardiopulmonary) related to microembolization of the pulmonary vasculature, decreased surfactant, and increased permeability of the alveolar capillary membrane, as indicated by atelectasis, pulmonary infiltrates, hypoxemia, and increased $\dot{V}/\dot{Q}$ mismatch.	Tissue perfusion to the cardiopulmonary system will be adequate. Respirations will be unlabored. Heart rate and rhythm will be WNL. Breath sounds will be normal. Blood pressure and cardiac output will be WNL. Chest pain will be absent.	Monitor and document vital signs. Monitor central venous pressure, pulmonary artery pressure, pulmonary capillary wedge pressure (PCWP), and cardiac output. Monitor respiratory rate and pattern and breath sounds. Maintain on a cardiac monitor and document any dysrhythmias. Assess electrocardiogram for ischemia. Monitor heart sounds. Maintain oxygen therapy. Institute measures to promote venous return, e.g., raising the foot of the bed if patient becomes hypotensive. Assess any chest pain and institute measures to relieve it. Maintain vasopressors as ordered in order to maintain blood pressure.

Continued on following page

NURSING CARE PLAN FOR A PATIENT WITH ACUTE RESPIRATORY FAILURE DUE TO ADULT RESPIRATORY DISTRESS SYNDROME *Continued*

Nursing Diagnosis	Patient Outcomes	Nursing Interventions
Altered nutrition (less than body requirements) related to increased metabolic demands and decreased ability to eat owing to infection, trauma, and mechanical ventilation, as indicated by calorie counts that do not meet the metabolic demands.	Decrease in metabolic demands as condition improves. Calorie counts indicative of nutritional requirements is being met. No weight loss. Laboratory results WNL.	If patient is able to take food by mouth, provide frequent small meals that are high in proteins and calories. Increase usual caloric intake by 1.5–2.0 times normal. If patient is mechanically ventilated, provide enteral or parenteral nutrition as ordered. If enteral feedings are used, elevate the head of the bed and monitor gastric residual every 2 h. If parenteral nutrition is used maintain strict aseptic technique when caring for the lines and administering total parenteral nutrition. Monitor daily weights. Maintain calorie counts.
Risk for infection related to illness and invasive procedures, as indicated by elevated temperatures, warm, flushed skin, and increased white blood cell (WBC) count.	Temperature will be normothermic. White blood cell count will be WNL. Infection will be absent.	Monitor temperature every 4 h, more frequently if elevated. Monitor WBC; notify physician if WBC count is elevated. Reposition at least every 2 h to assist with mobilization of secretions. Provide good pulmonary hygiene. Assess central line and intravenous site for signs of infection: redness, swelling, and drainage. Use aseptic technique with all invasive procedures and dressing changes. Change dressings per protocol, and as needed if they become soiled.
Fluid volume excess related to excess fluid intake, as indicated by intake greater than output, elevated pulmonary capillary wedge pressure (PCWP), crackles, and weight gain.	Body weight will be WNL. Intake and output will be balanced. Electrolyte levels will be WNL. PCWP will be in the range of 8–12 mm Hg. Breath sounds will be clear.	Weigh patient daily. Monitor intake and output. Maintain fluid restriction if ordered. Administer diuretics if ordered. Assess for peripheral edema. Monitor serum electrolytes; replace as ordered. Monitor blood urea nitrogen (BUN) and creatinine levels. Measure urine specifiic gravity every shift and as needed. Monitor PCWP every hour and as needed. Administer inotropic and vasodilating medications as ordered. Assess breath sounds every 2 h and as needed. Maintain oxygen therapy as ordered. Monitor ABGs.
Risk for impaired skin integrity related to bed rest and inadequate nutrition.	Skin will remain intact. Perfusion to all areas of the body will be maximized. Nutritional status will be optimized.	Assess every shift for areas of skin breakdown. Keep skin clean and dry. Apply protective creams. Reposition patient every 1–2 h. If unable to turn patient owing to hemodynamic instability, place on specialized bed (e.g., air mattress, water mattress). Massage all bony prominences and around all reddened areas with each position change. Assist with active and passive range-of-motion exercises. Monitor loboratory values that may have an effect on skin, and report all abnormalities to physician: albumin, hematocrit and hemoglobin, uric acid, BUN, bilirubin, ABGs. Collaborate with physician and dietitian in planning dietary intake, whether it be oral or parenteral.

NURSING CARE PLAN FOR A PATIENT WITH ACUTE RESPIRATORY FAILURE DUE TO ADULT RESPIRATORY DISTRESS SYNDROME *Continued*

Nursing Diagnosis	Patient Outcomes	Nursing Interventions
		Plan diet that has adequate intake of proteins, fluids, and calories. Monitor and assess calorie counts.
Altered tissue perfusion (peripheral) related to vasoconstriction and hypoxemia, as indicated by cold extremities, peripheral cyanosis, and abnormal mixed venous blood results.	Tissue perfusion and cellular oxygenation of the peripheral system will be adequate. Oxygen consumption will be decreased. Hypoxemia and vasoconstriction will be minimized. Mixed venous blood gases will have an oxygen saturation >70%	Monitor and document vital signs. Assess quality of arterial pulses. Assess skin temperature, color, and texture. Assist with active and passive range-of-motion exercises. Maintain oxygen therapy. Reposition frequently and assess for increases in oxygenation; if only one lung is affected, oxygenation may improve if patient is positioned laterally with good lung down. Monitor temperature; if it is elevated, institute measures to return it to normal. Assess vasoconstrictive effects of medications. Avoid long period of pressure to extremities. Assess mixed venous blood gases.
Risk for anxiety related to inability to speak, situational crises, uncertainty, and lack of control, as indicated by an elevated heart rate, blood pressure, and respiratory rate, increased muscle tension, and inappropriate behaviors.	Vital signs will be WNL. Muscle tension will be reduced; patient will remain relaxed. Anxiety will be reduced, and patient will not exhibit inappropriate behaviors, e.g., anger, fear, withdrawal, and regression.	Monitor for signs of anxiety: increased heart rate, blood pressure, and respiratory rate, muscle tension, inappropriate behaviors. Develop trusting relationship with the patient by using calm, consistent, and reliable behaviors. Always introduce yourself and all unfamiliar faces to the patient, and explain why they are there. Thoroughly explain all procedures and happenings to the patient. Avoid conflicts with the patient. Provide nurturing environment and increase attention to the patient as indicated. Allow the patient some control over decision making, if possible. Do not reinforce inappropriate behaviors. Attempt to structure environment in providing consistent caregivers and decreased stimulation. Teach relaxation techniques, e.g., the use of slow rhythmic breathing during stressful periods. Administer sedatives as ordered if indicated. Allow frequent family visits to decrease isolation.
Risk for ineffective family coping related to knowledge deficits of family members owing to inadequate information and uncertain outcome, as indicated by verbalization of fears.	Family integrity will be maintained. Family members will verbalize educational needs. Family members will verbalize fears and feel comfortable asking questions related to patient's prognosis. Family members will work together in making decisions for their loved one when necessary.	Assess family unit and coping behaviors. Establish healthy relationship with the family. Assist family to identify roles to maintain family integrity. Assist family members to verbalize distress. Sensitively explain procedures, equipment, changes in the patient's condition, and outcomes to family members. Always allow time for family members to ask questions and verbalize fears. Inform family of resources available to them, such as chaplain and psychiatric liaison. Assist family to prioritize their needs. Provide conferences with family and health care providers to supply information, be supportive, and allow family to see that all members of health care team are working together to provide the best quality and continuity of care for their loved one.

trapping, prolonged expiration, $\dot{V}/\dot{Q}$ mismatching with an increased intrapulmonary shunt, and cough that produces thick, tenacious sputum. The bronchial airways are hyperactive and respond to both intrinsic stimuli, such as emotions and sympathetic and parasympathetic balance, and extrinsic stimuli, such as various antigens and airway irritants. In addition to the bronchospasm, bronchial wall edema and increased mucus secretion add to the amount of obstruction.

The lungs become overinflated and stiff, which increases the work of breathing and results in hyperventilation and decreased $PaCO_2$. Status asthmaticus occurs when the bronchoconstriction is no longer responsive to bronchodilator therapy, and acute respiratory failure ensues. The patient experiences fatigue from the severe dyspnea, cough, and increased work of breathing. Hypercapnia and acidosis develop, and CO decreases as a result of a decreased venous return that is related to the increased intrathoracic pressures. Dehydration resulting from hyperventilation and reduced oral intake may further impair CO and contribute to circulatory collapse.

Emphysema

Emphysema is a nonreversible obstructive disease characterized by the destruction of the alveolar walls and connective tissue with loss of elastic recoil. As a result of this tissue destruction, the terminal airways collapse during expiration, and secretions are retained, leading to increased infections. $\dot{V}/\dot{Q}$ mismatching occurs as a result of gas trapping and generalized pulmonary artery constriction. Diffusion is reduced because of the reduction of alveolar surface area. This situation results in chronic hypercapnia. Cor pulmonale may occur as the right ventricle dilates and hypertrophies in response to the increased PAP. Acute respiratory failure may occur when infection develops or when other bodily stressors, such as surgery or shock, place demands on the pulmonary system.

The emphysematous patient is often a man in his mid-50s who complains of increasing shortness of breath for the past several years with no cough or a nonproductive cough. He may have had recent weight loss. His chest is overexpanded, and he appears to puff as he breathes, despite ABG results that may be within normal limits. The normal appearance of the arterial blood (pink), coupled with the presence of shortness of breath, leads to the name of "pink-puffers."

Chronic Bronchitis

Chronic bronchitis is defined as a productive cough for at least 3 consecutive months documented for at least 2 consecutive years. Chronic bronchitis results from an increase in the number of mucus-secreting glands accompanied by swelling, inflammation, and hypertrophy of the mucosal layer of the bronchial tree. In addition, thick, tenacious mucus clogs the airway. Areas of cilia are also destroyed, contributing to the patient's inability to clear the increased mucus.

In the early stages, chronic bronchitis is reversible by reducing exposure to causative agents, such as cigarette smoke and air pollutants. As the disease progresses, however, the changes in the airways become irreversible. As in other types of obstructive disorders, expiration is prolonged. Air trapping and hypercapnia occur, and cor pulmonale is usually present. As in emphysema, anything that increases the work of breathing may result in acute respiratory failure. Because of the constant presence of thick, tenacious sputum in these patients, they are especially prone to the development of a superimposed respiratory infection.

The patient with chronic bronchitis is often a man in his mid-40s with the cough history previously described for emphysema. He may report increasing dyspnea on exertion and reduced exercise tolerance. He often has cyanosis and signs of fluid retention, such as ankle edema and neck vein distention. His ABG determinations may reveal hypoxia and carbon dioxide retention. The patient with chronic bronchitis is often referred to as a "blue bloater" because the appearance of the arterial blood is poor and because the patient appears bloated with edema.

ASSESSMENT

Regardless of the specific underlying pathophysiology, the patient with COPD is at risk for the development of respiratory failure and requires constant close assessment. Dyspnea and hyperventilation are early signs of respiratory failure in the patient with chronic pulmonary disease. However, these classic symptoms may be part of the patient's baseline respiratory status. The critical care nurse must obtain an accurate assessment of the patient's usual respiratory status so that subtle changes are not missed.

Worsening cough, increased sputum production, or change in the character of the sputum may signal the development of a respiratory infection that could produce profound respiratory failure. Wheezing indicates narrowing of the airways from bronchospasm. The patient is more comfortable in the upright position and may show retraction of the intercostal muscles with inspiration. Tachycardia and hypotension may result from reduced CO.

Pulmonary function studies show a marked reduction in expiratory flow. Functional residual capacity is increased as a result of air trapping. Crackles may be heard throughout the lung fields. The chest x-ray study shows the flat low diaphragm that is characteristic of patients with COPD.

Arterial blood gases are a sensitive monitor for the patient's status. It is extremely important for the critical care nurse to know the patient's baseline levels because the person with COPD may have chronically abnormal ABG results. In the patient with asthma, ABG results are often normal except during an acute attack, when the $PaCO_2$ may decrease because of hyperventilation. In this instance, a return to a normal $PaCO_2$ in the face of an ongoing episode may be an early sign of impending failure. Hypercapnia is a late-occurring, ominous sign. The patient with COPD who chronically retains carbon dioxide may have baseline ABG results that show a normal pH and a PaO_2 and $PaCO_2$ in the range of 50 to 59 mm Hg. When acute failure ensues, the $PaCO_2$ increases, and the PaO_2 may decrease further, resulting in tissue hypoxia and acidosis (Grossbach, 1994).

Because ABG determinations are invasive and require frequent blood sampling, other methods are being developed for the constant monitoring of the patient's oxygenation and ventilation. Pulse oximetry measures the oxygen saturation of the hemoglobin molecule and provides the clinician with a practical noninvasive method of assessing oxygenation (Rutherford, 1989b). In the ventilated patient, exhaled gas can be analyzed for carbon dioxide content, thereby providing an assessment of ventilation (St. John, 1989). Both of these techniques may be used for the patient with COPD who has developed acute respiratory failure. Interpretation of the data, however, must take into account the patient's previously impaired respiratory function.

NURSING DIAGNOSES

The nursing diagnoses and outcomes for the patient with chronic pulmonary disease who develops acute respiratory failure include all of the diagnoses previously discussed in the section on ARDS. In addition, the following nursing diagnosis pertains to a patient with COPD:

- Decisional conflict (personal health) related to whether or not the patient should be intubated during an acute event because of the uncertainty of the outcome of weaning ·

INTERVENTIONS

The goals of therapy in this group of patients are to sustain them during this episode of acute failure and to return them to their previous level of functioning.

In many cases, achieving this goal is not possible, and each episode of acute failure leaves the patient with chronically diminished function. The most important intervention is adequate body positioning. This intervention is aimed at both preventing and treating respiratory problems (Grossbach, 1994). Frequent repositioning fosters the mobilization of secretions and prevents the development of atelectasis and pneumonia.

Postural drainage may be useful but is often contraindicated in patients with compromised CO. Adequate hydration is important for the loosening of secretions and the maintenance of adequate blood volume. Infections are treated with appropriate antibiotics. Bronchodilators, such as theophylline, are used in order to counteract the bronchospastic component.

Oxygen therapy is judiciously prescribed, and its effects are carefully monitored. Patients who normally retain carbon dioxide breathe as a result of their hypoxic drive. If the PaO_2 is rapidly increased, the hypoxic drive is eliminated, and the patient stops breathing. Therefore, low-flow oxygen therapy is initially tried. The patient's response to this therapy is evaluated, and changes are made accordingly. The goal of therapy is to achieve a PaO_2 that provides adequate tissue oxygenation while enabling the patient to continue to breathe unassisted.

Intubation and mechanical ventilation in this patient population are the therapies of last resort. Every effort is made to avoid intubating the patient with COPD because the risk of complications is high, and the long-term prognosis is often poor. Menzies et al. (1989) found that of 95 patients with COPD complicated by acute respiratory failure that necessitated ventilation, 59 were dead within 1 year, and 23 were never successfully weaned from the ventilator. However, intubation allows for optimal pulmonary toilet and clearing of secretions, and mechanical ventilation reduces the work of breathing. If the process that precipitated the acute respiratory failure can be successfully treated, the patient with COPD has a good chance of being weaned from the ventilator and returning to previous activities.

Acute Respiratory Failure Resulting from a Pulmonary Embolism

DEFINITION

A pulmonary embolism (PE) is the blockage of a pulmonary artery from a thrombus that usually arises from the systemic veins and results in obstruction of blood flow to the lung tissue. It is a fairly common complication of hospitalization. The sites of origin for these thrombi are usually the deep veins in the lower extremities of the body, mainly the calf, plantar, and femoral veins. They can also originate from the right side of the heart and the pelvis. The thrombi break off and travel through the venous system into the right side of the heart and out to the lungs.

A PE can be acute or massive, and partial or complete. Acute thromboembolism is usually characterized by the presence of many small emboli lodged in the distal branches of the pulmonary artery, causing a partial occlusion. A massive PE occurs when the thrombus is lodged in a major branch of the pulmonary artery, causing a complete blockage of one or both of the major pulmonary arteries. The more massive the PE, the more grave the prognosis.

ETIOLOGY

The three main mechanisms, often referred to as Virchow's triad, that favor the development of a venous thrombi are (1) venous stasis, or a reduction in blood flow; (2) the presence of a disease state that may alter the coagulability of blood; and (3) damage to the vessel walls. Specific causes of PE that fall under these three categories are listed in Table 11–5. Both a hypercoagulable state and venous wall damage contribute to the development of a thrombus but may not alone cause a thromboembolism. They are seen in conjunction with other factors that result in stasis.

PATHOPHYSIOLOGY

Once a thrombus is formed in the venous system, it can easily be dislodged by activities such as standing. Once dislodged, the thrombus travels up to the heart, through the right atrium and ventricle, and out into the pulmonary artery. Large clots may lodge in a major pulmonary vessel, and smaller ones often travel to the distal branches of the pulmonary artery vasculature. The result in both cases is the obstruction of blood flow to the pulmonary system. The hemodynamic changes that occur result in alterations in both the cardiac and the pulmonary systems.

As emboli lodge in the distal vessels, and even the larger vessels, blood flow to the alveoli beyond that occlusion is eliminated. The result is a lack of perfusion to ventilated alveoli, an increase in dead space, a $\dot{V}/\dot{Q}$ mismatch, and a decrease in carbon dioxide tension in the embolized lung zone. Gas exchange cannot occur, and hypocarbia results. The hypocarbia affects the bronchial smooth muscle by causing bronchoconstriction, increased pulmonary resistance, and decreased compliance.

Pneumoconstriction in the terminal airways of the nonperfused lung zones results in alveolar shrinking

Table 11–5. ETIOLOGIC FACTORS IN THE DEVELOPMENT OF PULMONARY THROMBOEMBOLISM

Venous stasis
Prolonged bed rest
Immobility
Obesity
Decreased cardiac output resulting from
  Prolonged surgical procedure
  Atrial fibrillation
  Congestive heart failure (CHF)
  Myocardial infarction
Pregnancy
Chronic obstructive airway disease
Postoperative state
Advanced age

Disease states and altered coagulability
Hip fractures
Malignancy
Hematologic disorders
Use of contraceptives (estrogens increase coagulability and platelet aggregation)
Postoperative period (resulting from abrupt discontinuation of anticoagulant therapy)
Pregnancy
Antithrombin III deficiency
Chronic CHF or atrial fibrillation
Thromboembolism
Dehydration

Vessel wall damage
Venostasis
Trauma
Sepsis
Burns
Venous punctures
Atherosclerosis

and decreased wasted ventilation. Although this is a protective mechanism to shunt inspired air to the functioning alveoli, the result is an increase in the work of breathing for the critically ill patient.

The reduction in blood flow to the alveoli also results in hypoxia for the type II pneumocytes, which are responsible for the production of surfactant. Although the effects are not seen for 24 to 48 hours, the decrease in surfactant results in an unequal gas distribution, an increase in the work of breathing, and a stiffening and collapse of the alveoli. Ventilation is then shifted away from these units.

Atelectasis and shunting may also occur as a result of the release of serotonin from the platelets that surround the clot. The result is peripheral airway constriction, which often involves functioning alveoli. In this situation, perfusion with inadequate ventilation occurs. This along with the other causes of $\dot{V}/\dot{Q}$ mismatch is manifested by arterial hypoxemia.

Pulmonary hypertension also contributes to the increased shunting that occurs with a PE. Pulmonary hypertension usually occurs when greater than 50% of the functional cross-sectional area of the pulmonary vascular bed is occluded. Hemodynamically, the critical care nurse observes an increase in pulmonary vascular resistance, PAP, and right ventricular work. The PAP continues to increase as the pulmonary vascular resistance increases. Pulmonary hypertension is often distinguished by a mean PAP of greater than 15 mm Hg.

As the PAP increases, the patient exhibits signs of breathlessness. In order to maintain CO despite the increased resistance, the right ventricle continues to increase its work until it reaches maximum function. A normal right ventricle is able to increase its mean pressure approximately 35 to 40 mm Hg. If the pulmonary obstruction continues beyond the limits of the right ventricle, the right ventricle fails. Clinically, the patient exhibits a decrease in CO, syncope, and a shock state. This situation may be compounded by the release of reflex humoral factors, such as serotonin, that constrict blood vessels and further increase the pulmonary pressure.

Pulmonary hypertension and the release of humoral agents stimulate the juxtapulmonary capillary receptors (J receptors) that are located in the alveolar wall. The patient exhibits dyspnea and tachypnea, or rapid shallow breathing. These are classic signs in patients with a PE (Von Ruden, 1995).

One potential outcome for a patient with a PE is pulmonary infarction. This complication is most likely to occur in a patient with some underlying cardiopulmonary abnormality, including lung disease and congestive heart failure, that has already impaired pulmonary circulation. Clinically, alveolar hemorrhage, consolidation, and tissue necrosis are present in these patients that may be complicated by lung abscesses, pleural effusion, or pleuritic-type pain.

The overall prognosis after a PE depends on two main factors. The first is whether or not any underlying cardiopulmonary problem preceded the PE, and the second is the extent of the pulmonary vascular circulation that is occluded by the thrombus.

ASSESSMENT

Most critically ill patients have several of the risk factors associated with a PE; therefore, the critical care nurse should be astutely aware of the signs and symptoms of a PE. Some of the most common signs and symptoms are dyspnea, cough, diaphoresis, hemoptysis, pleuritic pain, syncope, apprehension, fever, palpitations, and leg or calf pain. A patient can present with all or none of these symptoms. Most frequently,

however, patients present with a sudden onset of dyspnea or breathlessness.

The critical care nurse questions the patient about current symptoms and obtains an accurate medical and surgical history, in addition to information about the patient's chief complaint. The dyspnea should be described, including type of onset (acute or gradual), whether it is transient or prolonged, and whether it occurs with activity or at rest. Chest pain should also be described, including location and radiation; character; frequency; and influence of respiration, position, movement, activity, and cough.

Past medical and surgical history is particularly important, especially if it unveils the presence of any of the potential causes or a prior history of emboli. Other factors that may be important in the medical history are listed in Table 11–6.

The dyspnea and other symptoms may be transient or prolonged and may vary in severity, depending on the extent of the PE. It is often precipitated by physical exertion, such as walking. When greater than 50 to 60% of the pulmonary vascular tree is obstructed, the patient may have substernal chest pain as a result of the pulmonary hypertension. A pleuritic pain that is greatest with inspiration and decreases when the patient is upright may indicate pulmonary infarction. Lightheadedness and syncope occur with a massive PE as a result of the right ventricular failure.

On physical examination, signs of tachycardia may be present that can also be transient. In the presence of pulmonary hypertension, an increased intensity of the pulmonary S_2 heart sound may exist. Other possible cardiovascular symptoms that the critical care nurse should assess for include distended neck veins, murmur of the tricuspid and pulmonic regurgitation, and atrial or ventricular gallop on inspiration. If right ventricular failure has occurred, the patient has arterial hypotension along with peripheral vasoconstriction and central cyanosis. The 12-lead electrocardiogram (ECG) may show nonspecific ST changes.

When tachypnea is present, the critical care nurse

Table 11–6. MEDICAL HISTORY THAT IS IMPORTANT IN THE DIAGNOSIS OF PULMONARY THROMBOEMBOLISM

History of heart, lung, or blood disease
Recent surgery, trauma, or bed rest
Long car trip
Pregnancy or use of birth control pills
Varicose veins
Recent increase in weight
Use of constricting undergarments
Occupation that requires prolonged standing

carefully assesses the patient's breath sounds. Initially, no changes in breath sounds may occur, or breath sounds may be decreased. This may be accompanied by mild rales or wheezing if underlying bronchial disease is present. In the presence of a pulmonary infarction, the nurse's assessment might reveal a cough with hemoptysis along with a pleural effusion and a friction rub. Such a patient often also experiences pleuritic pain and exhibits splinting on inspiration.

Along with a complete cardiopulmonary assessment, the critical care nurse observes the affect of the patient. Signs of apprehension are indicative of a possible PE. The nurse also assesses and documents any edema, peripheral or central cyanosis, and the patient's position in bed. If a PE is suspected, further assessment includes searching for indicators of the presence of phlebitis, including tenderness, warmth, erythema, a cordlike vein, and a positive Homans' sign.

Along with the patient's history and physical examination, the physician involved in the case orders several laboratory and diagnostic tests in order to make a differential diagnosis. If clinical symptoms suggest a possible PE, the physician may order a complete blood count; determinations of electrolyte levels, enzyme levels, and ABGs; a chest x-ray study; and an ECG. Leukocytosis with an increased sedimentation rate and increased lactate dehydrogenase and aspartate transaminase levels indicates the presence of a pulmonary infarction. Electrolyte levels may show signs of dehydration. ABG results may reveal hypoxemia, hypocarbia, and respiratory alkalosis. All of these findings may be altered in a patient with underlying pulmonary disease.

A chest x-ray study may be nondiagnostic or may have subtle changes, including an elevated hemidiaphragm on the side of the embolus, an enlarged pulmonary artery, an unexplained density, a decreased visualization of lung fields, or a pleural effusion. Changes in the ECG usually do not occur unless massive embolization is present. Possible ECG changes include enlarged P waves, ST-segment depression, peaked or inverted T waves, and right-axis deviation. Dysrhythmias, such as paroxysmal atrial tachycardia and atrial fibrillation, may also be present.

The next diagnostic test is a lung scan, although an abnormality is not always a specific diagnostic finding. Any pulmonary or cardiac disease that affects lung function may also cause an abnormality. If the perfusion abnormality is more localized to a lobe or a segment, the probability of a PE is increased. Negative perfusion scan results do, however, rule out PE (*Chest*, 1995).

A ventilation scan is performed next in order to assess the distribution of gas in the alveoli. If abnormalities of ventilation occur in the same areas as abnormalities of perfusion, and if the chest x-ray study is normal, then a $\dot{V}/\dot{Q}$ mismatch is present that results from an underlying lung disorder. The likelihood of a PE increases if ventilation is normal in areas where a perfusion defect is present. If the diagnosis continues to be questionable, then the physician orders a pulmonary angiogram.

A pulmonary angiogram is an invasive procedure in which a right-sided heart catheterization must be performed. It is diagnostic for PE. A radiopaque dye is injected into the pulmonary artery, and flow is disrupted in areas where a defect or embolism is present.

NURSING DIAGNOSES

Several nursing diagnoses can be identified by the critical care nurse planning the nursing care for a patient with a PE. Addressing these goals assists the health team members to meet the major goals of therapy. These goals include (1) prevention of any further decrease in the delivery of oxygen to the tissues, (2) provision of cardiopulmonary support, (3) maintenance of fluid balance, and (4) provision of support to the patient and family.

To meet these goals, the critical care nurse should develop the plan of care by addressing the following nursing diagnoses:

- Activity intolerance related to hypoxia, as indicated by tachypnea, dyspnea, and abnormal ABG results.
- Anxiety related to uncertain outcome, as indicated by apprehension and nervousness.
- Decreased CO related to increased pulmonary vascular resistance and right ventricular failure, as indicated by jugular vein distention, cyanosis, hypotension, cold, clammy skin, decreased urine output, and dyspnea.
- Risk for ineffective family coping related to knowledge deficit of family members owing to inadequate information and uncertain outcome, as indicated by verbalization of fears.
- Impaired gas exchange related to decreased perfusion of alveoli and atelectasis, as indicated by dyspnea, tachypnea, hypoxemia, $\dot{V}/\dot{Q}$ mismatch, and abnormal ABG results.
- Risk for fluid volume excess related to increased pulmonary vascular resistance, as indicated by jugular vein distention, S_3 gallop, edema, liver enlargement, and atrial dysrhythmias.
- Risk for injury related to coagulopathy caused by anticoagulant therapy, as indicated by excessive bleeding, easy bruising, and abnormal hematocrit and hemoglobin values.

- Risk for pain related to decreased blood flow to the area resulting from thrombophlebitis, as indicated by splinting with inspiration, shallow breathing, tachycardia, and complaints of pain.
- Altered tissue perfusion (cardiopulmonary) related to the interruption in the arterial flow of the pulmonary system resulting from the thromboembolism, as indicated by dyspnea, tachypnea, tachycardia, abnormal breath sounds, cyanosis, pain, hypotension, ECG changes, and dysrhythmias.

INTERVENTIONS

In the case of a PE, the best therapy is prevention. Several prophylactic nursing interventions can be instituted in the hospitalized patient that may decrease the chance of PE development. Early postoperative ambulation, or in cases in which such ambulation is not possible, use of pneumatic boots that provide intermittent compression of the lower extremities increase venous flow. Walking schedules along with active and passive range-of-motion exercises also increase circulation in the critically ill.

Other nursing interventions that may reduce the risk of PE include not adjusting the knee section of the patient's bed and avoiding the use of pillows below the knees. Proper application of elastic bandages and elastic stockings is also essential. The patient should be instructed not to cross his or her legs and to make frequent position changes in order to promote circulation when sitting for long periods.

The presence of atrial dysrhythmias and signs of a deep vein thrombosis are important indicators of a potential PE that should be assessed by the critical care nurse on an ongoing basis. Signs of thrombophlebitis, such as pain on dorsiflexion of the foot, redness, swelling, warmth, tenderness, and low-grade fevers, should be documented in the nurse's note and reported to the physician.

Most critically ill patients fall into a high-risk category for PE and are often treated prophylactically. Treatment includes the use of low-dose heparin, aspirin, dipyridamole, and dextran (Handler and Feied, 1995).

Once a PE has occurred, the interventions are collaborative and focus on the common goals of alleviation of symptoms, support of cardiopulmonary function, prevention of further spread of the clot, maintenance of fluid balance and nutrition, management of pain, and management of hypoxemia. Regardless of the factor addressed, the actual treatment depends on the degree of dysfunction caused by the PE.

Assessment by the critical care nurse includes searching for signs and symptoms of hypoxia and hypoxemia. One of the earliest signs of hypoxemia is restlessness. The presence of this early indicator should alert the critical care nurse to perform a more detailed evaluation before instituting nursing interventions. This evaluation includes assessing for a respiratory rate of greater than 20 breaths/min, pallor, nasal flaring, retractions of intercostal spaces, splinting, asymmetrical lung expansion, and cyanosis. Auscultation may reveal a friction rub, diminished breath sounds, crackles, rhonchi, or wheezes.

The goals of the treatment of hypoxemia include relieving breathlessness, improving oxygen delivery, and preserving respiratory function. Nursing interventions include monitoring ABG results for evidence of hypoxia and hypocarbia and administering oxygen therapy, with a doctor's order, as needed. The severity of the PE dictates the mode of oxygen delivery, including the use of a nasal cannula or a face mask. If secretions are also interfering with respiratory function, the critical care nurse focuses on providing good bronchial hygiene, which includes assisting the patient to cough and take a deep breath at least every 2 hours. Postural drainage and chest physical therapy may also be needed.

Other nursing interventions that assist in the support of pulmonary function include placing the patient in a semi-Fowler's position and administering narcotics as ordered that alleviate any associated pain as well as decrease vasospasms. The end result is an overall decrease in pulmonary vascular resistance. In more severe cases, intubation and mechanical ventilation with PEEP may be necessary for the maintenance of adequate tissue perfusion. Cardiac monitoring is also important because patients are at increased risk for dysrhythmias that may need to be treated.

Accurate monitoring of intake and output is another important intervention performed by the critical care nurse. Owing to the loss in surfactant and the resultant change in the permeability of the alveolar membrane, an increase in interstitial edema and pulmonary congestion occurs. The increase in pulmonary vascular resistance also contributes to congestive heart failure because of the increase in the workload of the right ventricle. It is therefore imperative that the critical care nurse assess the patient for signs of congestive heart failure and pulmonary edema. Some of the indicators include jugular vein distention, peripheral edema, crackles, dysrhythmias, and increasing tachypnea.

In addition to being aware of the potential for congestive heart failure, the critical care nurse should also assess the patient for signs of shock. If the PE extends, it can result in obstruction of a major portion of the pulmonary vascular system. Clinically, the critical care nurse observes a severe tachycardia, followed by a decrease in CO and blood pressure.

Accompanying signs and symptoms include inferior wall ECG changes, a right bundle branch block pattern, atrial dysrhythmias, and flipped T waves in the precordial leads. The nurse also monitors and documents central venous pressure; PAP; urine output; peripheral pulses; level of consciousness; and skin temperature, color, and moisture. In some cases, right and left ventricular failure, decreased CO, and decreased renal tissue perfusion occur. If these problems are not corrected, organ failure and death result.

Collaborative interventions should be directed at alleviating the pain associated with a PE. The pain is often pleuritic and is caused by a decrease in oxygen. It becomes more severe with deep breathing and coughing. Because these are two important activities, the patient may require a narcotic analgesic. Decreasing the patient's activity conserves oxygen. If the patient also complains of calf pain that results from a concurrent deep vein thrombosis, the critical care nurse can apply heat to the area for added comfort.

The severe dyspnea exhibited by a patient with a PE may interfere with his or her ability to consume a regular diet. The critical care nurse can be creative in providing better conditions in order to improve the patient's nutritional status. Smaller, more frequent meals, including food brought from home, may be helpful. If the patient's respiratory function is significantly improved after respiratory treatments, it may be better to provide meals after the treatments. Calorie counts should be maintained for documentation of nutrition. The nurse should consult a dietitian for meal planning as needed.

The physician can choose to treat the patient medically, surgically, or both. In addition to oxygen therapy for the maintenance of a PaO$_2$ of greater than 60 mm Hg, analgesics are ordered for the relief of pain. In the presence of congestive heart failure and cardiac failure, the physician may use diuretics, such as furosemide (Lasix) and digoxin. When CO is impaired, vasopressor and inotropic agents are used.

Oxygen and heparin therapy are considered the drugs of choice for the reduction of morbidity and mortality in the patient with a PE (Handler and Feied, 1995). Before initiating the treatment, the physician orders determinations of prothrombin time and partial thromboplastin time. The intravenous loading dose of heparin varies from 2000 to 10,000 U, followed by a continuous infusion that is usually begun at about 1000 U/h. This hourly dose is increased or decreased, depending on subsequent partial thromboplastin times. Optimal anticoagulation is obtained with a partial thromboplastin time that is 2.0 to 2.5 times that of normal.

Heparin therapy is continued for 7 to 14 days. Usually, at around day 4 or 5 of heparin therapy,

warfarin (Coumadin) therapy is begun. This oral anticoagulant often takes 4 to 6 days to reach therapeutic levels. Therapeutic levels are determined by serum prothrombin times. Optimum therapy reveals a prothrombin time of 1.5 to 2.0 times that of normal.

Because adequate heparin therapy only prevents further spread of the clot, many physicians may choose to use a thrombolytic agent in patients with a massive PE with severe hemodynamic compromise. Thrombolytics can dissolve the clot and rapidly restore hemodynamic stability. Thrombolytic therapy is begun during an acute event as soon as a diagnosis is made. The most frequently used thrombolytics are streptokinase and urokinase. When administration of these drugs is discontinued, heparin therapy follows. Two drawbacks of thrombolytic therapy are the cost and the increased risk of bleeding that results from breakdown of beneficial thrombi and destruction of the clot that was repairing the break in a vascular membrane.

Surgical intervention may be necessary for some patients, including those in whom anticoagulants and thrombolytics are contraindicated, those who do not respond to medical treatment, those who are having life-threatening complications, and often those who have greater than 50% obstruction. Surgical procedures include an embolectomy, ligation of the inferior vena cava, and transvenous placement of a vena caval umbrella.

OUTCOMES

For each patient with a PE, the interventions chosen depend on the current clinical presentation as well as on the medical and surgical histories. Treatments are also adjusted based on the patient's response. Certainly, prevention is the best therapy. In each situation, health team members work together with the patient to meet common goals and to return the patient to an optimal state of health. The expected outcomes for a patient with a PE include the following:

- Gradual increase in activity, back to baseline without signs of tachypnea, dyspnea, or abnormal ABG results.
- No signs of apprehension and nervousness and vital signs within normal limits.
- Stable fluid balance, with a urine output greater than 50 ml/h.
- Stable blood pressure, CO, PAP, and central venous pressure.
- Stable cardiac rhythm, without signs of tachycardia, ECG changes, or dysrhythmias.
- Family members' verbalizing fears and feeling comfortable asking questions related to patient's prognosis.

RESEARCH APPLICATION

Article Reference

Chlan, L. L. (1995). Psychophysiologic responses of mechanically ventilated patients to music: A pilot study. *American Journal of Critical Care, 4*(3), 233-238.

Objective

To examine selected psychophysiological responses of mechanically ventilated patients to music.

Methods

A two-group experimental design with pretest, posttest, and repeated measures was used. Twenty mechanically ventilated patients were randomly assigned to a music-listening group or to a nonmusic (headphones only) group. Data on physiologically dependent measures (heart rate and rhythm, respiratory rate, systolic and diastolic blood pressures, oxygen saturation, and airway) were collected at timed intervals. Psychological data were collected before and after intervention by use of the Profile of Mood States.

Results

As determined by repeated-measures analysis of variance, results for heart rate and respiratory rate over time within groups and between groups were significant. Between-group differences were significant for respi-

ratory rate. Significant differences were found via *t*-test for the music group's Profile of Mood States scores. No adverse cardiovascular responses were noted for either group.

Conclusions

Data indicated that music listening decreased heart rate, respiratory rate, and Profile of Mood States scores, indicating relaxation and mood improvement.

Critique

Using mechanically ventilated patients to study the effects of music therapy enables the investigator to apply previous research to a large portion of the intensive care unit population—the patient receiving ventilation. This is a pilot study with a small sample size, a characteristic that limits its generalizability. In addition, the potential effects of medications on the measured variables were not examined. When this study is replicated, attention should be paid to matching subjects for their medications—especially sedatives.

Implications

Music therapy is a nonpharmacological approach to reducing the stress response that can be safely used in mechanically ventilated patients without fear of untoward effects. Nurses should add this therapy to their repertoire of independent interventions in providing holistic care to these patients.

- Adequate oxygen delivery to the tissues.
- Normal respiratory function, including no use of accessory muscles.
- Normal breath sounds.
- Partial pressure of arterial oxygen of greater than 80%.
- No peripheral or sacral edema.
- No further extension of clot.
- Prothrombin time and partial thromboplastin time within therapeutic range.
- Relief of pain.
- Adequate tissue perfusion and cellular oxygenation of the peripheral system.

Summary

Acute respiratory failure is a disorder that can affect all segments of the population from young trauma victims to elderly people with long-standing pulmonary disease. Patients in the critical care areas are at high risk for acute respiratory failure related to ARDS and pulmonary emboli. The critical care nurse must be constantly alert to signs of impending failure. Changes in respiratory rate and character, breath sounds, and blood gases must be closely evaluated. Frequent position changes, good pulmonary toilet, and careful attention to the nutritional status all contribute to the successful maintenance of a patient's respiratory system and to the prevention of acute respiratory failure.

CRITICAL THINKING QUESTIONS

1. John Doe is a 42-year-old homeless man brought to the emergency department with a decreased level of consciousness. You note an alcohol odor on his breath. The physician orders ABG determinations. The results are as follows:

   pH, 7.29; PaO_2, 42 mm Hg; arterial oxygen saturation (SaO_2), 78%; $PaCO_2$, 60 mm Hg; bicarbonate (HCO_3), 24 mEq/L
   a. What is your interpretation of these ABGs?
   b. What are possible causes of these ABGs?

2. Your 80-kg patient with ARDS is experiencing worsening hypoxemia. He is currently mechanically ventilated with the following settings:

   V_T, 800 ml; FiO_2, 0.60; intermittent mandatory ventilation, 8 breaths/min; PEEP, 5 cm H_2O; total respiratory rate, 16 breaths/min with a spontaneous V_T of 50 ml and an SaO_2 of 88%. What changes would you expect in his ventilatory management?

3. Mr. C, aged 27 years, is hospitalized after fracturing his femur in a snow-skiing accident. Two days after admission, he has a cough, low-grade fever, tachycardia, and dyspnea. His oxygen saturation begins to decrease.
   a. What are possible causes for Mr. C's symptoms?
   b. What interventions do you anticipate?

4. Mrs. D, aged 84 years, comes to the hospital with a fever and acute respiratory failure. She is intubated and placed on mechanical ventilation in the assist/control mode at a rate of 16 breaths/min. She has a 90 pack year history of smoking.
   a. What are possible causes for Mrs. D's respiratory failure?
   b. What were her likely ABGs before intubation?
   c. What are primary interventions for assisting Mrs. D to return to her optimal health status?
   d. How would you discuss Mrs. D's smoking during your patient teaching?

REFERENCES

Ahrens, T. (1989a). Blood gas assessment of intrapulmonary shunting and deadspace. *Critical Care Nursing Clinics of North America, 1*(4), 641–648.

Ahrens, T. (1989b). Extravascular lung water concepts in clinical application. *Critical Care Nursing Clinics of North America, 1*(4), 681–688.

Ashbaugh, D. G., Bigelow, D. B., Petty, T. L., & Levine, B. E. (1967). Acute respiratory distress in adults. *Lancet, 2*, 319–323.

Chillcott, S., & Sheridan, P. S. (1995). ECCO2: An experimental approach to treating ARDS. *Critical Care Nurse, 15*(2), 50–56.

Grossbach, I. (1994). The COPD patient in acute respiratory failure. *Critical Care Nurse, 14*(12), 32–38.

Handler, J. A., & Feied, C. F. (1995). Acute pulmonary embolism: Aggressive therapy with anticoagulants and thrombolytics. *Postgraduate Medicine, 97*(1), 61–62, 65–68.

Huffman, M. H. (1983). Acute care of the patient with a pulmonary embolism due to venous thromboemboli. *Critical Care Nurse, 3*(2), 70–73.

(1995). Invasive and noninvasive diagnosis of pulmonary embolism: Preliminary results of the prospective investigative study of acute pulmonary embolism diagnosis. *Chest, 107*(Suppl. 1), 33S–38S.

Luce, J. M., Tyler, M. L., & Pierson, D. J. (1984). *Intensive respiratory care*. Philadelphia: W. B. Saunders Co.

Menzies, R., Gibbons, W., & Goldberg, P. (1989). Determinants of weaning and survival among patients with COPD who require mechanical ventilation for acute respiratory failure. *Chest, 95*, 398–405.

Murphy, L. M., & Conforti, C. G. (1993). Nutritional support of the cardiopulmonary patient. *Critical Care Nursing Clinics of North America, 5*(1), 57–64.

Rutherford, K. A. (1989a). Advances in the treatment of oxygenation disturbances. *Critical Care Nursing Clinics of North America, 1*(4), 659–668.

Rutherford, K. A. (1989b). Principles and application of oximetry. *Critical Care Nursing Clinics of North America, 1*(4), 649–657.

St. John, R. E. (1989). Exhaled gas analysis: Technical and clinical aspects of capnography and oxygen consumption. *Critical Care Nursing Clinics of North America, 1*(4), 669–680.

Sinski, A., & Corbo, J. (1994). Surfactant replacement in adults and children with ARDS: An effective therapy? *Critical Care Nurse, 14*(12), 54–59.

Vollman, K. M. (1994). Adult respiratory distress syndrome mediators on the run. *Critical Care Nursing Clinics of North America, 6*(2), 341–358.

Von Ruden, K. T., & Harris, J. R. (1995). Pulmonary dysfunction related to immobility in the trauma patient. *AACN Clinical Issues: Advanced Practice in Acute and Critical Care, 6*(2), 212–228.

West, J. B. (1990). *Respiratory physiology: The essentials* (4th ed.). Baltimore: Williams & Wilkins.

Willms, D., Nield, M., & Gocka, I. (1994). Adult respiratory distress syndrome: Outcome in a community hospital. *American Journal of Critical Care, 3*(5), 337–341.

RECOMMENDED READINGS

Byers, J. F., & Noll, M. L. (1995). Chronotherapy in acutely ill patients with respiratory disorders. Part I: Respiratory chronobiology and chronopathology. *AACN Clinical Issues, 6,* 316–322.

Byers, J. F., & Noll, M. L. (1995). Chronotherapy in acutely ill patients with respiratory disorders. Part II: Application of chrono-pharmacology in patient care. *AACN Clinical Issues, 6,* 323–332.

Dantzker, D. R., MacIntyre, N. R., & Bakow, E. D. (Eds.) (1995). *Comprehensive respiratory care.* Philadelphia: W.B. Saunders Co.

Dirkes, S., Dickindon, S., & Valentine, J. (1992). Acute respiratory failure and ECMO. *Critical Care Nurse, 12*(7), 39–47.

Ecklund, M. M. (1995). Optimizing the flow of care for prevention and treatment of deep vein thrombosis and pulmonary embolism. *AACN Clinical Issues: Advanced Practice in Acute and Critical Care, 6,* 588–601.

Hamner, J. (1995). Challenging diagnosis: Adult respiratory distress syndrome. *Critical Care Nurse 15*(5), 46–51.

Jones, M. A. (1991). ARDS revisited: New ways to look at an old enemy. *Nursing 24*(12), 34–43.

Kersten, L. D. (1989). *Comprehensive respiratory nursing: A decision making approach.* Philadelphia: W. B. Saunders Co.

Kuhn, M. A. (1994). Multiple trauma with respiratory distress. *Critical Care Nurse, 14*(2), 68-72, 77–80.

Noll, M. L. (Ed.). (1990). Respiratory care in adults. *AACN Clinical Issues in Critical Care Nursing, 1*(2), 237–326.

Zorb, S. L., & Stevens, J. B. (1990). Contemporary bioethical issues in critical care. *Critical Care Nursing Clinics of North America, 2*(3), 515–526.

C H A P T E R

12

Acute Renal Failure

Janet Goshorn, M.S.N., R.N., CCRN

OBJECTIVES

- Review the anatomy and physiology of the renal system.
- Describe the pathophysiology of the three categories of acute renal failure.
- Identify the systemic manifestations of acute renal failure.
- Describe the methods for assessing the renal system, including physical

assessment, interpretation of serum and urine laboratory values, and radiological diagnostic tests.
- Develop a patient-centered plan of care for the patient with acute renal failure.
- Discuss the nursing assessment and care of the patient receiving dialysis or continuous renal replacement therapy.

Introduction

The renal system is the primary regulator of the body's internal environment and is thus essential to the maintenance of life. With sudden cessation of renal function, the body is incapable of maintaining a stable internal environment, thereby disrupting all body systems. Acute renal failure occurs in 2 to 5% of patients admitted to a general medical-surgical unit and in up to 23% of critical care patients (Feest et al., 1993). It occasionally occurs in otherwise healthy individuals, but it usually strikes the already critically ill patient, increasing the complexity of the situation and compromising the patient's ability to adapt to the other body system changes.

Despite the advanced treatments available, acute renal failure is still associated with significant morbidity and 50% mortality (Finn, 1993). Indeed, mortality rates have not significantly improved over the past 20 years, making prevention of acute renal failure a high priority for all health care professionals. Nursing can play a pivotal role in promoting positive outcomes in patients with acute renal failure. Recognition of high-risk patients, preventive measures, sharp assessment

skills, and supportive nursing care are fundamental to ensuring delivery of high-quality care to these challenging and complex patients.

For a better understanding of the pathophysiology of acute renal failure and the systemic manifestations seen, a brief review of renal anatomy and the numerous physiological functions of the kidneys is necessary.

Review of Renal Anatomy and Physiology

The kidneys are a pair of highly vascularized bean-shaped organs that are located retroperitoneally on each side of the vertebral column, adjacent to the first and second lumbar vertebrae. The right kidney sits slightly lower than the left kidney because the liver lies above it. An adrenal gland sits on top of each kidney and is responsible for the production of aldosterone, a hormone that influences sodium and water balance. Each kidney is divided into two regions: an outer region, called the cortex, and an inner region, called the medulla.

The nephron is the basic functional unit of the

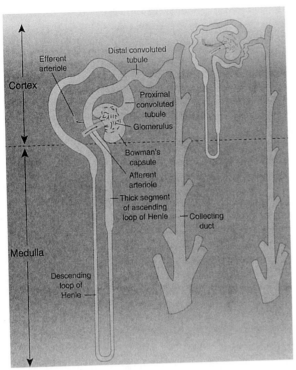

Figure 12–1. Anatomy of the nephron, the functional unit of the kidney. (From Ignatavicius, D. D., Workman, M. L., & Mishler, M. A. (1995). *Medical-surgical nursing: A nursing process approach* (2nd ed.) (p. 2014). Philadelphia: W. B. Saunders Co.)

kidney. A nephron is composed of a renal corpuscle (glomerulus and Bowman's capsule) and a tubular structure, as depicted in Figure 12–1. Approximately 1 to 3 million nephrons exist per kidney. About 85% of these nephrons are found in the cortex of the kidney and have short loops of Henle. The remaining 15% of nephrons are called juxtamedullary nephrons because of their location just outside of the medulla (Tische and Madsen, 1996). Juxtamedullary nephrons have long loops of Henle and, along with the vasa recta (long capillary loops), are primarily responsible for concentration of urine.

The kidneys receive approximately 20 to 25% of the cardiac output, which computes to 1200 ml of blood per minute. Blood enters the kidneys through the renal artery, travels through a series of arterial branches, and reaches the glomerulus by way of the afferent arteriole ("afferent" means to carry toward). Blood leaves the glomerulus through the efferent arteriole ("efferent" means to carry away from), which then divides into two extensive capillary networks called the peritubular capillaries and the vasa recta. The capillaries then rejoin to form venous branches by which blood eventually exits the kidney via the renal

vein. The glomerulus is a cluster of minute blood vessels that filter blood. The glomerular walls are composed of three layers: the endothelium, the basement membrane, and the epithelium. The epithelium of the glomerulus is continuous with the inner layer of Bowman's capsule, the sac that surrounds the glomerulus. Bowman's capsule is the entry site for filtrate leaving the glomerulus (Chmielewski, 1992).

The kidneys perform numerous functions that are essential for the maintenance of a stable internal environment. The following text provides a brief overview of key roles the kidneys perform in maintaining homeostasis. Table 12–1 provides a complete listing of kidney functions.

REGULATION OF FLUID AND ELECTROLYTES AND EXCRETION OF WASTE PRODUCTS

As blood flows through each glomerulus, water, electrolytes, and waste products are filtered out of the blood, across the glomerular membrane and into Bowman's capsule, forming what is known as *filtrate*. The glomerular capillary membrane is extremely permeable (approximately 100 times more permeable than other capillaries). It acts as a high-efficiency sieve and normally allows only substances with a certain molecular weight to cross. Red blood cells, albumin, and globulin are too large to pass through the glomerular membrane. Normal glomerular filtrate is basically protein-free and contains electrolytes, including sodium, chloride, and phosphate, and nitrogenous waste products, such as creatinine, urea, and uric acid, in amounts similar to those in plasma (Holechek, 1992).

Glomerular filtration occurs as a result of a pressure gradient, which is the difference between the forces that favor filtration and the pressures that oppose filtration. Generally, the capillary hydrostatic pressure favors glomerular filtration, whereas the colloid osmotic pressure and the hydrostatic pressure in Bowman's capsule oppose filtration (Fig. 12–2). Under normal conditions, the capillary hydrostatic pressure is greater than the two opposing forces, and glomerular filtration occurs.

Table 12–1. FUNCTIONS OF THE KIDNEY

Regulation of fluid volume
Regulation of electrolyte balance
Regulation of acid-base balance
Regulation of blood pressure
Excretion of nitrogenous waste products
Regulation of erythropoiesis
Metabolism of vitamin D
Synthesis of prostaglandin

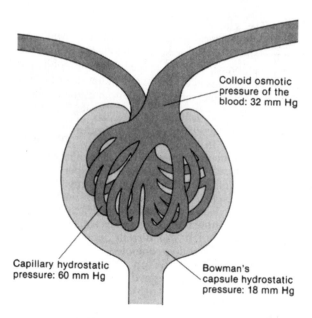

NET FILTRATION PRESSURE
60 − 32 − 18 = 10 mm Hg

Figure 12–2. Average pressures involved in filtration from the glomerular capillaries. (From Clochesy, J. M., Breu, C., Cardin, S., Ruby, E. B., & Whittaker, A. A. (1993). *Critical care nursing.* Philadelphia: W. B. Saunders Co.)

At a normal glomerular filtration rate (GFR) of 125 ml/min, the kidneys produce 180 L of filtrate a day. As the filtrate passes through the various components of the nephron's tubules, 99% is reabsorbed into the peritubular capillaries or vasa recta. *Reabsorption* is the movement of substances from the filtrate back into the capillaries. A second process that occurs in the tubules is *secretion,* or the movement of substances from the peritubular capillaries into the tubular network. Various electrolytes are reabsorbed or secreted at numerous points along the tubules, thus helping regulate the electrolyte composition of the internal environment (Fig. 12–3). Aldosterone and antidiuretic hormone play a role in water reabsorption in the distal convoluted tubule and collecting duct. Eventually, the remaining filtrate (1% of the original 180 L/d) is excreted as urine, for an average urine output of 1 to 2 L/d.

REGULATION OF ACID-BASE BALANCE

The kidneys help maintain acid-base equilibrium in three ways: reabsorption of filtered bicarbonate, production of new bicarbonate, and excretion of small amounts of hydrogen ions (acid) buffered by phosphates and ammonia (Felver, 1995). The tubular cells

are capable of generating ammonia in order to help with excretion of hydrogen ions. This ability of the kidney to assist with ammonia production and excretion of hydrogen ions (in exchange for sodium) is the predominant adaptive response by the kidney when the patient is acidotic. When alkalosis is present, increased amounts of bicarbonate are excreted in the urine, causing the serum pH to return toward normal.

REGULATION OF BLOOD PRESSURE

Specialized cells in the afferent and efferent arterioles and the distal convoluted tubule are collectively known as the juxtaglomerular apparatus. These cells are responsible for the production of a hormone called renin, which plays a role in blood pressure regulation. Renin is released whenever blood flow through the afferent and efferent arterioles decreases. A decrease in the sodium ion concentration of the blood flowing past the specialized cells also stimulates the release of renin. Renin activates the renin-angiotensin-aldosterone cascade, as depicted in Figure 12–4, which ultimately results in angiotensin II production. Angiotensin II causes vasoconstriction and release of aldosterone from the adrenal glands, thereby raising blood pressure and flow and increasing sodium and water reabsorption in the distal tubule and collecting ducts.

Pathophysiology of Acute Renal Failure

Definition

Acute renal failure is the sudden deterioration of renal function, resulting in retention of nitrogenous waste products (azotemia). It is usually accompanied by oliguria (urine output < 400 ml/24 hours), although roughly 30 to 50% of patients (Brady et al., 1996) are nonoliguric and have a urine output of greater than 400 ml/24 hours. Individuals with nonoliguric acute renal failure may even excrete 2 to 4 L of fluid in 24 hours, but the fluid is deficient in the solutes and waste products that compose normal urine. Anuria (urine output < 100 ml/24 hours) is less commonly seen in acute renal failure.

Etiology

Numerous clinical conditions can precipitate acute renal failure. In general, the causes of acute renal failure are classified into three categories: prerenal, postrenal, and intrinsic (parenchymal), depending on where the precipitating factor exerts its pathophysio-

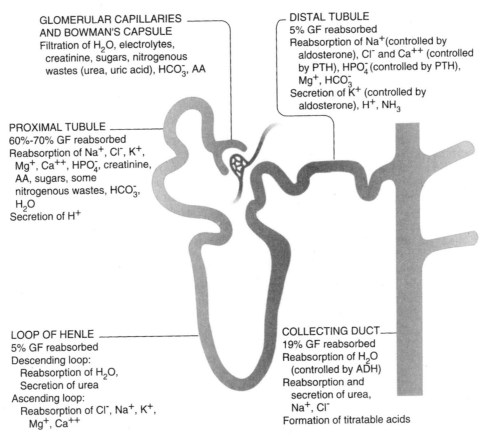

GLOMERULAR CAPILLARIES
AND BOWMAN'S CAPSULE
Filtration of H_2O, electrolytes,
creatinine, sugars, nitrogenous
wastes (urea, uric acid), HCO_3^-, AA

DISTAL TUBULE
5% GF reabsorbed
Reabsorption of Na^+(controlled by
aldosterone), Cl^- and Ca^{++} (controlled
by PTH), HPO_4^- (controlled by PTH),
Mg^+, HCO_3^-
Secretion of K^+ (controlled by
aldosterone), H^+, NH_3

PROXIMAL TUBULE
60%-70% GF reabsorbed
Reabsorption of Na^+, Cl^-, K^+,
Mg^+, Ca^{++}, HPO_4^-, creatinine,
AA, sugars, some
nitrogenous wastes, HCO_3^-,
H_2O
Secretion of H^+

LOOP OF HENLE
5% GF reabsorbed
Descending loop:
    Reabsorption of H_2O,
    Secretion of urea
Ascending loop:
    Reabsorption of Cl^-, Na^+, K^+,
    Mg^+, Ca^{++}

COLLECTING DUCT
19% GF reabsorbed
Reabsorption of H_2O
    (controlled by ADH)
Reabsorption and
    secretion of urea,
    Na^+, Cl^-
Formation of titratable acids

Figure 12-3. Major functions of the nephron. AA = amino acid; ADH = antidiuretic hormone; CA^{++} = calcium ion; Cl^- = chloride ion; GF = glomerular filtrate; H^+ = hydrogen ion; HCO_3^- = bicarbonate; H_2O = water; HPO_4^- = phosphate; K^+ = potassium ion; Mg^+ = magnesium ion; Na^+ = sodium ion; NH_3 = ammonia; PTH = parathyroid hormone. (From Copstead, L. (1995). *Perspective on pathophysiology* (p. 558). Philadelphia: W. B. Saunders Co.)

logical effect on the kidney. Table 12–2 depicts the percentage of patients with acute renal failure according to cause.

Conditions that produce acute renal failure by interfering with renal perfusion are classified as *prerenal*. Prerenal azotemia is the most common cause of acute renal failure (Brady et al., 1996). Prerenal azotemia is usually caused by fluid volume loss, extracellular fluid volume sequestration (third spacing), inadequate cardiac output, or vasoconstriction of the renal blood vessels. Precipitating causes of prerenal azotemia are listed in Table 12–3. All of these conditions reduce the glomerular perfusion and the GFR and hence hypoperfuse the kidney. For example, abdominal aortic aneurysm repair can cause hypoperfusion of the kidneys as a result of blood lost during the procedure or clamping of the aorta in the repair of the aneurysm.

In prerenal azotemia, the body attempts to normalize renal perfusion by reabsorbing sodium and water. If adequate blood flow is restored to the kidney,

normal renal function resumes. However, prolonged or severe prerenal azotemia can progress to intrinsic renal damage, acute tubular necrosis (ATN), or acute cortical necrosis. Therefore, implementation of preventive measures, recognition of the condition, and prompt treatment of prerenal failure are extremely important.

Acute renal failure resulting from obstruction of the flow of urine is classified as *postrenal* azotemia or obstructive renal failure. Obstruction can occur at any point along the urinary system (Table 12–4). In postrenal azotemia, increased intratubular pressure results in a decrease in the GFR and in abnormal nephron function. Postrenal azotemia usually reverses rapidly once the obstruction is removed.

Acute Tubular Necrosis

Finally, conditions that produce acute renal failure by directly acting on functioning kidney tissue are

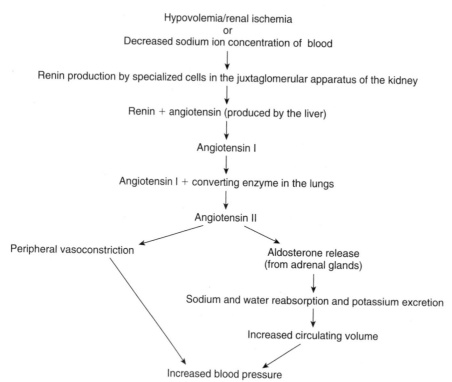

Figure 12–4. Renin-angiotensin mechanism.

classified as *intrinsic* (also known as intrarenal or parenchymal). Intrinsic azotemia can be caused by problems with either the glomerulus or the renal tubules. The most common cause of intrinsic azotemia is ATN. ATN may occur after prolonged ischemia, exposure to nephrotoxic substances, or a combination of these. Ischemic ATN usually occurs when perfusion to the kidney is significantly reduced. Some patients have ATN after only several minutes of hypotension or hypovolemia, whereas others can tolerate hours of

renal ischemia without having any tubular damage. Severe vasoconstriction and ischemia damage the glomerular basement membrane and tubular epithelium, predominately the proximal tubule. When the glomerular basement membrane is damaged, it cannot completely regenerate. The tubular epithelium often regenerates in an indiscriminate manner, leading to obstruction at the damaged sites. Nephrotoxic agents (particularly aminoglycosides and radiographic contrast materials) can also damage the tubular epithelium

Table 12–2. CLASSIFICATION AND MAJOR DISEASE CATEGORIES CAUSING ACUTE RENAL FAILURE

Disease Category	% of Patients with Acute Renal Failure
Prerenal azotemia caused by acute renal hypoperfusion	55–60
Intrinsic renal azotemia caused by acute diseases of renal parenchyma	35–40
Diseases involving large renal vessels	
Diseases of small renal vessels and glomeruli	
Acute injury to renal tubules mediated by ischemia or toxins*	
Acute diseases of the tubulointerstitium	
Postrenal azotemia caused by acute obstruction of urinary collecting system	≤5

From Brady, H., Brenner, B., Lieberthal, W. (1996). Acute renal failure. In B. Brenner (Ed.), *Brenner and Rector's the kidney* (5th ed., Vol. II) (pp. 1200–1252). Philadelphia: W.B. Saunders Co.
*Accounts for more than 90% of cases in the intrinsic renal azotemia category.

Table 12–3. CAUSES OF PRERENAL AZOTEMIA

Volume Depletion	Vasodilation	Impaired Cardiac Performance	Miscellaneous

Hemorrhage
  Trauma
  Surgery
  Postpartum period
	Sepsis
	
	Anaphylaxis
		Congestive heart failure
		
		Myocardial infarction
			Angiotensin-converting enzyme inhibitors in renal artery stenosis

Gastrointestinal loss
  Diarrhea
  Nasogastric suction
  Vomiting
	Drugs
	  Antihypertensives
	  Afterload reducers
	  Anesthesia
		Cardiogenic shock
		
		Dysrhythmias
		
		Pulmonary embolism
			Inhibition of prostaglandins by nonsteroidal anti-inflammatory drug use during renal hypoperfusion

Renal loss
  Diuretics
  Osmotic diuresis
  Diabetes insipidus
		Pulmonary hypertension
		
		Positive-pressure ventilation
			Renal vasoconstriction
			  Norepinephrine
			  Ergotamine
			  Hypercalcemia

Volume shifts
  Burns
  Ileus
  Pancreatitis
  Peritonitis
  Hypoalbuminemia
		Pericardial tamponade	

but do not destroy the basement membrane. Acute renal failure does not occur in all patients who receive nephrotoxic agents; however, predisposing factors, such as advanced age, diabetes mellitus, and dehydration, appear to enhance susceptibility to intrinsic damage (Llach, 1993). Patients with nephrotoxic ATN often have a good chance of complete recovery from their renal failure. Other causes of intrinsic azotemia are listed in Table 12–5.

Pathophysiology

An assortment of theories have been proposed to explain the oliguria that most often accompanies ATN (Brady et al., 1996). Five mechanisms are discussed: (1) increased renal vasoconstriction, (2) cellular edema, (3) decreased glomerular capillary permeabil-

Table 12–4. CAUSES OF POSTRENAL AZOTEMIA

Benign prostatic hypertrophy
Blood clots
Renal stones or crystals
Tumors
Postoperative edema
Drugs
  Tricyclic antidepressants
  Ganglionic blocking agents
Foley catheter obstruction
Ligation of ureter during surgery

ity, (4) intratubular obstruction, and (5) back leak of glomerular filtrate. Any or all of these mechanisms may be operative in any patient at any specific point in time in order to produce the oliguria. Figure 12–5 is a schematic of mechanisms that may play a role in the ATN cascade.

The ischemic episode activates the renin-angiotensin system, which produces increased renal vasoconstriction and decreased glomerular capillary pressure, both of which decrease GFR. The decreased GFR and renal blood flow lead to tubular dysfunction, which not only produces oliguria but also results in further increases in renal vasoconstriction that continue to perpetuate the dysfunction.

When the tubules are damaged, necrotic endothelial cells and other cellular debris accumulate and can obstruct the lumen of the tubule. This intratubular obstruction increases the intratubular pressure, which decreases the GFR and leads to tubular dysfunction and oliguria. In addition, the tubular damage usually produces alterations in the tubular structure that permit the glomerular filtrate to leak out of the tubular lumen and back into the plasma. This back leak of filtrate is a component of the tubular dysfunction that results in oliguria.

The ischemic episode also results in decreased energy supplies, such as adenosine triphosphate (ATP). Without ATP, the sodium-potassium adenosine triphosphatase (ATPase) of the cell membrane can no longer pump sodium out of the cell or accumulate potassium. Chloride enters the cell as depolarization occurs, and

Table 12–5. CAUSES OF INTRINSIC AZOTEMIA

Glomerular, Vascular, or Hematologic Problem

Glomerulonephritis (poststreptococcal)
Vasculitis
Malignant hypertension
Systemic lupus erythematosus
Hemolytic uremic syndrome
Disseminated intravascular coagulation
Scleroderma
Bacterial endocarditis
Toxemia of pregnancy
Thrombosis of renal artery or vein

Tubular Problem (Acute Tubular Necrosis or Acute Interstitial Nephritis)

Ischemia
  Any of the prerenal azotemia causes (see Table 12–3)
  Hypotension from any cause
  Hypovolemia from any cause
  Obstetric complications (hemorrhage, abruptio placentae, placenta previa)
Nephrotoxic agents
  Drugs: aminoglycosides, amphotericin B, penicillins, acyclovir, vancomycin, pentamidine, rifampin, cisplatin,
    cyclosporine, ifosfamide, methotrexate, nonsteroidal anti-inflammatory drugs, cephalosporins
  Radiocontrast dyes
  Endogenous substances: transfusion reaction causing hemoglobinuria, tumor lysis syndrome, rhabdomyolysis (caused
    by trauma, crush injuries, alcohol or drug abuse, heat stroke, status epilepticus, thyroid storm, strenuous exercise
    beyond usual capabilities)
Miscellaneous: heavy metals (mercury, arsenic), paraquat, snake bites, organic solvents (ethylene glycol, toluene,
  carbon tetrachloride), pesticides, fungicides

the result is an increase in cellular solutes that facilitate cellular edema. Cellular edema further decreases renal blood flow and GFR, damages the tubules, and ultimately leads to tubular dysfunction and oliguria.

The insult to the nephron that occurs as a result of nephrotoxic substances, such as heavy metals, contrast media, and pharmacological agents, is one of direct tubular damage. The nephrotoxic agent destroys component parts of the tubule, resulting in intratubular obstruction and back leak of glomerular filtrate. The end result is tubular dysfunction and often oliguria. The nephrotoxic agent may accumulate in the renal cortex and may not cause renal failure for days (Swan and Bennett, 1991).

Course

The individual with ATN progresses through three phases of the disease process: the initiation phase, the maintenance phase, and the recovery phase (Brady et al., 1996).

Initiation Phase. The initiation phase is the period of time that elapses from the occurrence of the precipitating event to the beginning of the change in urine output. This phase usually spans several hours to 2 days, during which time the normal renal processes begin to deteriorate, but actual intrinsic renal damage is not yet established. The patient cannot compensate for the diminished renal function and exhibits significant clinical signs and symptoms that reflect the chemical imbalances in the internal environment. ATN is potentially reversible during the initiation phase.

Maintenance Phase. During this phase, intrinsic renal damage is well established, and GFR stabilizes at approximately 5 to 10 ml/min. Urine volume is usually at its lowest point during the maintenance phase. This phase usually lasts 8 to 14 days, but it may last as long as 1 to 11 months. The longer a patient remains in this stage, the slower the recovery and the greater the chance of permanent renal damage. Complications resulting from uremia, including hyperkalemia and infection, usually arise during this phase.

Recovery Phase. This phase is the period during which the renal tissue recovers and repairs itself. A gradual increase in urine output and an improvement in laboratory values occur. Some patients may have a large diuresis during this phase that is caused by (1) salt and water accumulation in extracellular spaces that results from inability of the renal tubules to regulate sodium and water, (2) osmotic diuresis that results from retained waste products, or (3) diuretics given to speed up salt and water excretion. However, with early and aggressive use of dialytic therapy, many patients are maintained in a relatively "dry" or volume-

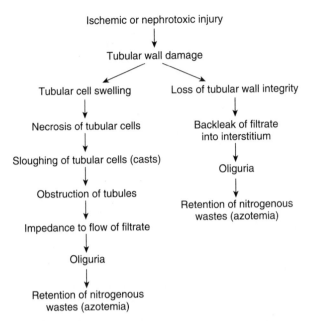

Ischemic or nephrotoxic injury

Tubular wall damage

Tubular cell swelling / Loss of tubular wall integrity

Necrosis of tubular cells

Sloughing of tubular cells (casts)

Obstruction of tubules

Impedance to flow of filtrate

Oliguria

Retention of nitrogenous wastes (azotemia)

Backleak of filtrate into interstitium

Oliguria

Retention of nitrogenous wastes (azotemia)

Figure 12–5. Proposed mechanisms of acute tubular necrosis cascade.

depleted state and do not experience a large post-ATN diuresis. Recovery may take as long as 4 to 6 months.

Acute tubular necrosis is irreversible in about 5% of patients, who must undergo long-term renal replacement therapy or transplantation. Most patients, however, recover sufficient renal function to lead normal lives, although approximately 50% have subclinical defects in their GFR and urinary concentrating abilities. Elderly patients and those with previously existing renal diseases are at increased risk for developing some degree of residual impairment. An additional 5% of patients have progressive renal deterioration after their initial recovery (Brady et al., 1996). Patients who have experienced one episode of ATN are at increased risk for repeated episodes of ATN if these patients are exposed to nephrotoxins or ischemia.

Assessment

PATIENT HISTORY

Many aspects of the patient history are important to keep in mind in discussions of the renal system. Many patients do not volunteer essential parts of the history unless they are asked specific questions. Renal-related symptoms that a patient reports can provide valuable clues that assist the clinician in focusing the assessment in order to obtain essential data. Table 12–6 presents a list of the renal-related symptoms and

their correlated potential pathologies. The history can also provide clues to medical conditions that can predispose the patient to acute renal failure, including diabetes mellitus, hypertension, and any hereditary disorders, such as polycystic disease. Recent exposure to potential nephrotoxins, such as insecticides, should also be evaluated. The medical record should be carefully examined in order to elicit any risk factors, such as hypotensive episodes, exposure to potential nephrotoxins, and any surgical or radiographic procedures performed. Current and admission body weight, as well as intake and output information are evaluated.

VITAL SIGNS

Changes in blood pressure are common in acute renal failure. Patients with prerenal azotemia may be hypotensive and tachycardic as a result of volume deficits. Intrinsic azotemia, particularly if associated with oliguria, often causes hypertension. Patients may hyperventilate as the lungs attempt to compensate for the metabolic acidosis often seen in acute renal failure. Body temperature may be decreased (as a result of the antipyretic effect of an increased blood urea nitrogen [BUN] level), normal, or increased (as a result of infection) (Brady et al., 1996).

MEDICATION HISTORY

The clinician normally documents all prescribed and nonprescribed medications and their patterns and frequencies of ingestion by the patient. This informa-

Table 12–6. RENAL-RELATED SYMPTOMS AND THEIR POTENTIAL PATHOLOGIES

Symptom	Potential Pathology
Dysuria	Infection
Dribbling	Prostatic enlargement
	Strictures
Edema	Renal failure
Frequency	Infection
Hematuria	Trauma
	Glomerular membrane disease
Hesitancy	Prostatic enlargement
Incontinence	Infection
	Prolapsed uterus
Nocturia	Infection
	Increased fluid intake
Oliguria	Insufficient fluids
	Renal failure
Proteinuria	Glomerular membrane disease
Pyuria	Infection
Renal colic	Calculi
	Infection
Urinary urgency	Prostatic disease

tion is extremely important in assessing the possibility that a nephrotoxic insult has occurred as the result of the chronic use or abuse of pharmacological agents. The most common offenders are antibiotics, such as aminoglycosides, penicillins, amphotericin B, cephalosporins, tetracyclines, and sulfonamides. Nonoliguric renal failure is seen in 10 to 30% of patients who receive aminoglycosides, even when blood levels are therapeutic (Brady et al., 1996). Symptoms of acute renal failure are usually seen about 1 to 2 weeks after exposure. Because of this delay, the patient must be questioned about any recent medical therapy (clinic or emergency room visits) for which an aminoglycoside might have been prescribed. Nephrotoxicity is noted in more than 80% of patients receiving amphotericin B, especially if cumulative doses exceed 1 g (Swan and Bennett, 1993). Nonsteroidal anti-inflammatory agents are also a common cause of nephrotoxicity (Llach, 1993).

PHYSICAL ASSESSMENT

The patient's general appearance is assessed for signs of uremia, such as malaise, fatigue, disorientation, and drowsiness. The skin is assessed for color, texture, bruising, petechiae, or edema. The patient's hydration status should also be carefully assessed. Skin turgor, mucous membranes, breath sounds, presence of edema, neck vein distension, body weight, and vital signs (blood pressure and heart rate) are all key indicators of fluid balance. An oliguric patient with weight loss, tachycardia, hypotension, dry mucous membranes, flat neck veins, and poor skin turgor may be volume depleted (prerenal cause). Weight gain, edema, distended neck veins, and hypertension in the presence of oliguria suggest an intrinsic cause. Table 12–7 lists other signs and symptoms that may be seen in patients with acute renal failure.

EVALUATION OF LABORATORY VALUES

Because the renal system is the primary regulator of the internal environment of the body, any alteration in its function is rapidly evident in the serum and urine laboratory values. Serum laboratory values of a patient with acute renal failure are usually monitored at least daily, whereas urinary laboratory values are checked much less frequently. The clinician assesses the laboratory values for deviations from normal and expected changes for an individual with acute renal failure. Tables 12–8 and 12–9 list normal values and the anticipated values for an individual with intrinsic acute renal failure.

Assessment of the urine is extremely valuable in the evaluation of acute renal failure. The best measure of renal function is urinary creatinine clearance. Creatinine is a metabolic byproduct of creatine and phosphocreatine in the muscles. Because individuals do not usually alter muscle mass rapidly, the levels of creatinine produced by the body remain relatively stable. Because of this stability, creatinine levels rapidly reflect changes in renal function.

For accurate determinations of the creatinine clearance, the nurse and patient must rigidly adhere to the following procedure:

1. The patient empties his or her bladder, the exact time is recorded, and the specimen is discarded.
2. All urine for the next 24 hours is saved.
3. Exactly 24 hours after the start of the procedure, the patient voids again, and the specimen is saved.
4. Serum creatinine level is assessed at the end of 24 hours.
5. All the urine that was saved is sent to laboratory for testing.

Urinary creatinine clearance is calculated by use of the following formula:

$$U_c \times V/P_c = C_{cr}$$

where U_c = concentration of creatinine in the urine
V = volume of urine per unit of time
P_c = concentration of creatinine in the plasma
C_{cr} = creatinine clearance

Creatinine clearance is an estimate of GFR and is measured in milliliters per minute. Thus, given the following set of patient data:

$$U_c = 175 \text{ mg}/100 \text{ ml}$$
$$V = 288 \text{ ml}/24 \text{ hours}$$
$$P_c = 17.5 \text{ mg}/100 \text{ ml}$$

the patient's creatinine clearance would be calculated as

$$\frac{175 \text{ mg}/100 \text{ ml} \times 288/1440 \text{ min}/24 \text{ h}}{17.5 \text{ mg}/100 \text{ ml}} = 2 \text{ ml/min}$$

Because a normal creatinine clearance is about 125 ml/min, the clinician would recognize this patient's creatinine clearance as being consistent with renal dysfunction.

If no urine is available for a creatinine clearance determination, the following formula is used to determine the creatinine clearance from a serum creatinine value:

$$C_{cr} = \frac{(140 - \text{age in years}) (\text{lean body weight in kilograms})}{72 \times \text{serum creatinine (mg/dl)}}$$

Table 12–7. THE SYSTEMIC MANIFESTATIONS OF ACUTE RENAL FAILURE

System	Manifestation	Pathophysiological Manifestation
Cardiovascular	Fluid overload Congestive heart failure Pulmonary edema	↓ Excretion of fluids Fluid overload and hypertension Fluid overload ↑ Pulmonary capillary permeability Left ventricular dysfunction
	Dysrhythmias	Electrolyte imbalances (especially hyperkalemia, hypocalcemia, and variations in sodium)
	Peripheral or systemic edema	↑ Hydrostatic pressure from fluid overload Right ventricular dysfunction
	Hypertension	Fluid overload ↑ Sodium retention Inappropriate activation of the renin-angiotensin system
Hematological	Anemia	↓ Erythropoietin secretion Loss of RBCs through GI tract, mucous membranes, or dialysis ↓ RBC survival time resulting from uremic toxins Uremic toxins' interference with folic acid secretion
	Alterations in coagulation	Platelet dysfunction resulting from uremic toxins
	Increased susceptibility to infection	↓ Neutrophil phagocytosis and chemotaxis resulting from uremic toxins
	Electrolyte imbalances	↓ Excretion
	Metabolic acidosis	↓ Hydrogen ion excretion ↓ Sodium ion reabsorption ↓ Bicarbonate ion reabsorption and generation ↓ Excretion of phosphate salts or titratable acids ↓ Ammonia synthesis and ammonium excretion
Respiratory	Pneumonia	Thick, tenacious sputum resulting from decreased oral intake Weak, lethargic with depressed cough reflex resulting from uremia Decreased pulmonary macrophage activity
	Pulmonary edema	Fluid overload Left ventricular dysfunction Increased capillary permeability
Gastrointestinal	Anorexia, nausea and vomiting	Uremic toxins Decomposition of urea in GI tract, releasing ammonia that irritates mucosa
	Stomatitis and uremic halitosis	Uremic toxins Decomposition of urea in oral cavity, releasing ammonia
	Gastritis and bleeding	Uremic toxins Decomposition of urea in gut, releasing ammonia that irritates mucosa, causing ulcerations Increased capillary fragility
Neuromuscular	Drowsiness, confusion, irritability, and coma	Uremic toxins produce a uremic encephalopathy Metabolic acidosis
	Tremors, twitching, and convulsions	Electrolyte imbalances Uremic toxins produce a uremic encephalopathy ↓ Nerve conduction resulting from uremic toxins
Psychosocial	Decreased mentation, decreased concentration, and altered perceptions (even to point of frank psychosis)	Uremic toxins that produce a uremic encephalopathy Electrolyte imbalances Metabolic acidosis Tendency to develop cerebral edema

Table continued on following page

Table 12–7. THE SYSTEMIC MANIFESTATIONS OF ACUTE RENAL FAILURE *Continued*

System	Manifestation	Pathophysiological Manifestation
Integumentary	Pallor	Uremic anemia
	Yellowness	Retained urochrome pigment excretion through skin
	Dryness	↓ Secretions from oil and sweat glands resulting from uremic toxins
	Pruritus	Dry skin Calcium and/or phosphate deposit in skin
	Purpura and ecchymosis	Uremic toxins' effect on nerve endings ↑ Capillary fragility Platelet dysfunction
	Uremic frost (seen only in terminal or critically ill patients)	Urea or urate crystal excretion
Endocrine	Glucose intolerance (usually not clinically significant)	Peripheral insensitivity to insulin resulting from uremia Prolonged insulin half-life resulting from renal metabolism
Skeletal	Hypocalcemia	Hyperphosphatemia resulting from ↓ excretion ↓ GI absorption resulting from ↓ renal conversion of vitamin D Deposition of calcium phosphate crystals in soft tissues

RBC = red blood cells.

For female patients, the aforementioned calculated result is then multiplied by 0.85 (Shuler et al., 1996).

In lieu of using creatinine clearance for the evaluation of renal function, the next best measure is serum creatinine level, followed by serum BUN level. Of these two values, BUN level is the least reflective of renal function because BUN level can be influenced by many extrarenal factors (Table 12–10). The relationship between BUN and creatinine, known as the BUN/creatinine ratio, also provides useful information.

Table 12–8. NORMAL SERUM LABORATORY VALUES AND VARIATIONS SEEN IN INTRINSIC ACUTE RENAL FAILURE

Parameter	Normal Values	Variation in Acute Renal Failure
Sodium	136–146 mEq/L	Increases or varies
Potassium	3.5–5.5 mEq/L	Increases
Chloride	96–106 mEq/L	Increases or varies
Blood urea nitrogen	9–20 mg/dl	Increases
Creatinine	0.7–1.5 mg/dl	Increases
Calcium	8.5–10.5 mg/dl 4.5–5.8 mEq/L	Decreases
Phosphorus	2.0–4.5 mg/dl 1.0–1.5 mEq/L	Increases
Uric acid	2.5–6.0 mg/dl	Increases
Carbon dioxide–combining power	24–28 mEq/L	Decreases
Magnesium	1.6–2.2 mEq/L	Increases or normal
Osmolality	280–295 mOsm/kg H_2O	Increases or varies
Hematocrit	40–50%	Decreases
Hemoglobin	12–16 g/dl	Decreases

Table 12–9. NORMAL URINE LABORATORY VALUES AND VARIATIONS SEEN IN INTRINSIC ACUTE RENAL FAILURE

Parameter	Normal Values	Variation in Acute Renal Failure
Amount	0.6–1.5 L/d	Decreases
Specific gravity	1.003–1.030	Fixed at 1.010 or less
pH	4.5–7	Increases
Glucose	0 mg/dl	Normal
Protein	<20 mg/dl or <0.2 g/L	Normal (can vary)
Creatinine	14–26 mg/kg/d	Decreases
Osmolality	50–1400 mOsm/L	Decreases
Sodium	40–80 mEq/d	Increases in oliguria; can vary in non-oliguria
Potassium	23–123 mEq/d (intake dependent)	Decreases
Chloride	80–120 mEq/L/d	Decreases
Calcium	100–250 mg/d	Decreases
Phosphorus	0.4–1.3 g/d	Decreases
Magnesium	5–16 mEq/d	Decreases
Urea	300–600 mmol/d	Decreases

Table 12–10. EXTRARENAL CAUSES OF AN ELEVATED BLOOD UREA NITROGEN LEVEL

Dehydration	Corticosteroids
Excessive protein intake	Infections and fever
Starvation	Surgery and trauma
Blood in the gut	

The normal BUN/creatinine ratio is 10:1 to 20:1 (e.g., BUN level, 20 mg, and creatinine level, 1.0 mg). If this ratio is greater than 20:1 (e.g., BUN level, 60 mg, and creatinine level, 1.0 mg), problems other than renal failure are probably the cause. In prerenal azotemia, an increased BUN/creatinine ratio is typically noted, whereas a normal ratio is present in intrinsic azotemia (Stark, 1994). The same extrarenal causes of an elevated BUN level may cause an elevated BUN/creatinine ratio (see Table 12–10).

Analysis of urinary sediment and electrolyte levels is extremely helpful in distinguishing between prerenal azotemia, intrinsic azotemia, and postrenal azotemia. Urine should be inspected for the presence of cells, casts, and crystals. In prerenal conditions, the urine typically has no cells but may contain hyaline casts (Chernecky et al., 1993). Casts are cylinder-shaped bodies that form when proteins precipitate in the distal tubules and collecting ducts. Postrenal azotemia may present with stones, crystals, sediment, bacteria, and clots from the obstruction. In intrinsic azotemia, granular casts and tubule epithelial cell casts are often seen. Microscopic hematuria and a small amount of protein (< 1 g/dl) may also be seen with intrinsic renal failure. Casts are not absolutely necessary for a diagnosis of intrinsic failure, because they may be absent in 20 to 30% of patients with ischemic or nephrotoxic azotemia (Brady et al., 1996).

Urine electrolyte levels can also be used to help discriminate between prerenal and intrinsic azotemia. The nurse must obtain urine samples for electrolyte determinations before diuretics are administered because these drugs alter the urine results for up to 24 hours.

Random urine electrolyte samplings are sometimes used to help differentiate between categories of acute renal failure. Urinary sodium concentrations of less than 10 mEq/L are seen in prerenal conditions as the kidneys attempt to conserve sodium and water in order to compensate for the hypoperfusion state. On the other hand, urine sodium concentrations are greater than 20 Meq/L with intrinsic azotemia as a result of impaired reabsorption in the diseased tubules (Llach, 1993).

Urine specific gravity and osmolality have a limited role in the diagnosis of acute renal failure, especially in the elderly population because the body's ability to concentrate urine decreases with age. In general, prerenal conditions cause a concentrated urine (high specific gravity and osmolality), whereas intrinsic azotemia causes a dilute urine (low specific gravity and osmolality).

The volume of urine output is not a good indicator of renal function. Patients with nonoliguric acute renal failure excrete large volumes of fluid with little solute. These patients still have renal dysfunction and azotemia, even though they excrete large volumes of fluid.

NONINVASIVE DIAGNOSTIC PROCEDURES

Measurement of intake and output and daily weights are two vital procedures performed by the nurse who is caring for patients with acute renal failure. Accuracy is extremely important. Appropriate measuring devices rather than clinician "guess-timations" must be used for the measurement of urine. For example, a urine meter or some other type of accurate measuring device is used if the patient has an indwelling catheter. Daily weights are one of the most useful noninvasive diagnostic tools available for clinicians (Llach, 1993). Daily weights can be used to validate intake and output measurements. Body weight and intake and output measurements may vary somewhat, but if the clinician recalls that about 500 ml are in 1 pound and factors the patient's insensible loss (normally about 800 ml/24 hours) into the process, the two measurements should closely coincide (Baer and Lancaster, 1992). Daily weights should be obtained at the same time each day by use of the same scale. Many critical care beds have built-in scales, which have simplified the procedure. When the patient is weighed, the nurse ensures that the scale is properly calibrated and that the same amount of bed linens and pillows is weighed with the patient each time.

Other noninvasive diagnostic procedures used to assess the renal system are radiography of the kidneys, ureters, and bladder and renal ultrasonography. These tests reveal information regarding the size, shape, and position of the kidneys. They may be performed before any invasive diagnostic procedures are conducted.

INVASIVE DIAGNOSTIC PROCEDURES

The invasive diagnostic procedures that are used for the assessment of the renal system include intravenous pyelography, computed tomography, renal angiography, renal scanning, and renal biopsy. These procedures are summarized in Table 12–11. For all of

Table 12–11. INVASIVE DIAGNOSTIC PROCEDURES FOR ASSESSING THE RENAL SYSTEM

Procedure	Purpose	Potential Problems
Intravenous pyelography	To visualize the renal parenchyma, calyces, pelves, ureters, and bladder in order to obtain information regarding size, shape, position, and function of the kidneys.	Hypersensitivity reaction to contrast medium Acute renal failure Postinjection hematoma
Computed tomography	To visualize the renal parenchyma in order to obtain data regarding the size, shape, and presence of lesions, cysts, masses, calculi, obstructions, congenital anomalies, and abnormal accumulations of fluid.	Hypersensitivity reaction to contrast medium (if used) Postinjection hematoma
Renal angiography	To visualize the arterial tree, capillaries, and venous drainage of the kidneys in order to obtain data regarding the presence of tumors, cysts, stenosis, infarction, aneurysms, hematomas, lacerations, and abscesses.	Hypersensitivity reaction to contrast medium Hemorrhage or hematoma at the catheter insertion site Acute renal failure
Renal scanning	To determine renal function by visualizing the appearance and disappearance of the radioisotopes within the kidney. It also provides some anatomical information.	Hypersensitivity reaction from contrast medium Postinjection hematoma
Renal biopsy	To obtain data for making a histological diagnosis in order to determine the extent of the pathology, the appropriate therapy, and the possible prognosis.	Hemorrhage Postbiopsy hematoma

these diagnostic procedures, the clinician implements the following general interventions:

- Explain the procedure to the patient, emphasizing the patient's responsibilities during the procedure.
- Reinforce the explanations that have been previously provided by other health care personnel concerning the procedure.
- Determine whether the patient has any allergies to contrast media and notify the physician if an allergy is present.
- Carry out any preparatory activities required for the procedure, such as administration of special diet, bowel preparations, laboratory testing, insertion of intravenous access, and completion of consent forms.
- Provide appropriate fluids to assist the individual in maintaining an adequate hydration state before and after the procedure.
- Provide emotional support to the patient before, during, and after the procedure.
- Assist with the procedure whenever possible or necessary.
- Monitor the patient for any complications after the procedure.
- Document the patient's response to the procedure.

Systemic Manifestations of Acute Renal Failure

One of the facts about patients with acute renal failure that makes caring for them such a challenge is that every body system is affected by the dysfunctional renal system. Table 12–7 summarizes the systemic manifestations of acute renal failure according to body system and also lists the pathophysiological mechanisms that underlie a specific manifestation.

CARDIOVASCULAR SYSTEM

Volume overload is a common occurrence in the individual with acute renal failure. It is primarily caused by fluid and sodium retention. Clinically, the patient may have mild hypertension, bibasilar crackles, peripheral edema, congestive heart failure, or pulmonary edema. Hypertension that is moderate or severe suggests other diagnoses, such as renal artery stenosis. Electrolyte imbalances can result in dysrhythmias. The volume overload problem is especially difficult to handle because these patients often need blood transfusions, numerous intravenous medications, and parenteral nutrition.

HEMATOLOGICAL SYSTEM

The increased susceptibility to infection presents a major problem for the already compromised patient with acute renal failure. Not only is the patient less able to combat infection, he or she now requires numerous, repeated invasive procedures for maintaining and sustaining life, and these procedures increase the risk of infection. Infection is the most common complication of acute renal failure, occurring in 50 to 90% of all cases; it is responsible for up to 75% of all deaths (Brady et al., 1996). These patients are particularly susceptible to pneumonia and urinary tract and wound infections (Llach, 1993).

Anemia can develop rapidly in acute renal failure, but it is usually mild. It has various causes, including bleeding, hemolysis, decreased erythropoietin production, hemodilution, and decreased erythrocyte survival time. The patient may present clinically with pallor, weakness, fatigue, shortness of breath, and chest pain.

Electrolyte imbalances are another commonly encountered condition, especially during oliguric acute renal failure. Table 12–12 summarizes the most commonly encountered electrolyte imbalances in acute renal failure. Electrolyte imbalances must be monitored closely and treated aggressively because they can result in cardiac arrest.

RESPIRATORY SYSTEM

The patient with acute renal failure is at risk for respiratory system dysfunction because uremia impairs the normal immune response of the lungs and suppresses the cough reflex. Sputum becomes thick and tenacious, and along with the depressed cough reflex, places the patient at risk for pneumonia. If oliguria is present, volume overload may result in pulmonary edema.

GASTROINTESTINAL SYSTEM

Anorexia, nausea, and vomiting commonly occur in patients with acute renal failure and may result in insufficient caloric intake and increased catabolism. The more catabolic the individual becomes, the more body tissues are broken down for energy, resulting in increased accumulation of nitrogenous waste products.

In addition, the stomatitis associated with acute renal failure often contributes to increasing tissue catabolism by inhibiting the patient's ability to ingest food substances. The stomatitis is often so painful that the patient cannot tolerate the contact of liquids or solids against the oral mucosa.

The gastrointestinal bleeding that occurs as a result of uremia is an oozing of blood rather than a full-blown hemorrhagic state. The gastrointestinal bleeding accelerates the uremic process. As the gastrointestinal bleeding continues, some of the blood is reabsorbed and metabolized by the body. Because blood is a protein, its metabolism further increases the amount of unexcretable nitrogenous waste products in the body and adds to the patient's already uremic state.

Table 12–12. COMMON ELECTROLYTE IMBALANCES SEEN IN ACUTE RENAL FAILURE

Electrolyte Imbalance	Etiology	Clinical Manifestations
Hyperkalemia	↓ Renal excretion of K^+, excessive intake of K^+, acidosis and catabolism	ECG changes: tall tented T waves, increased PR interval, widening QRS (sine wave), complete heart block, asystole, ventricular fibrillation, muscle weakness, abdominal cramps, diarrhea
Hyponatremia	Fluid retention, oliguria	Nausea and vomiting, headache, fatigue, lethargy, confusion, coma, seizures, diarrhea
Hypocalcemia	↓ Renal excretion of PO_4^+, ↓ renal synthesis of vitamin D	Parasthesias, tetany, seizures, cramps, laryngospasm, positive Chvostek's sign, positive Trousseau's sign
Hyperphosphatemia	↓ Renal excretion of PO_4^+	Same signs as hypocalcemia
Hypermagnesemia	↓ Renal excretion of Mg^{2+}	Lethargy, somnolence, coma, hypotension, hypoventilation, flaccid muscles, weak-to-absent deep tendon reflexes, prolonged PR interval and QT interval, bradycardia, heart blocks

K^+ = potassium ion; PO_4 = phosphate ion; Mg^{2+} = magnesium ion; ECG = electrocardiogram.

NEUROMUSCULAR SYSTEM

Definite evidence demonstrated by electroencephalography indicates that uremic patients have altered brain wave patterns, both in the frequency and the amplitude of the waveforms. Thus, it appears that some uremic toxins pass through the blood-brain barrier. Alterations in neurological function may also occur secondary to cerebral edema associated with fluid overload and uremia. The patient may exhibit changes in mental status that range from lethargy to coma. Other neurological manifestations include seizures, diminished coordination, tremors, and asterixis.

PSYCHOSOCIAL SYSTEM

Uremic patients have significant alterations in their mental processes and therefore often respond more slowly to questions and directives, forget instructions quickly, are disoriented, and view invasive procedures as extremely threatening. Stupor, convulsions, and coma may develop if aggressive treatment is not initiated.

INTEGUMENTARY SYSTEM

The yellowness of the skin that uremic patients develop is caused by the retention and excretion of urochrome pigment through the skin. Urochrome pigment is what normally gives urine its yellow coloration. When the patient is not excreting much urine, the pigment accumulates and seeks other excretory pathways. Uremic yellowness differs from the accompanying hepatic dysfunction in two ways: it is a duller yellow color, and it does not affect the sclerae of the eyes.

Nursing Diagnoses

Nursing care of the patient with acute renal failure is complex. Multiple nursing diagnoses must be dealt with in these often critically ill patients. The nurse formulates a plan of care that addresses the following nursing diagnoses (see Nursing Care Plan):

- Fluid Volume Excess related to sodium and water retention and excess intake.
- Risk for infection related to depressed immune response secondary to uremia and impaired skin integrity.
- Altered nutrition (less than body requirements) related to uremia, altered oral mucous membranes, and dietary restrictions.
- Risk for anxiety related to diagnosis, treatment plan, prognosis, and unfamiliar environment.

- Knowledge deficit related to disease process and therapeutic regimen.

Collaborative Interventions

Treatment of patients with acute renal failure requires close collaboration between all involved health care personnel. Basic management goals include correction of the primary disorder causing the renal dysfunction; prevention of infection; treatment of fluid, electrolyte, and acid-base imbalances; maintenance of the patient in an anabolic state; and treatment of uremic symptoms. The primary interventions depend on whether the cause of the problem is prerenal, postrenal, or intrinsic.

MANAGEMENT OF PRERENAL AZOTEMIA

Prerenal azotemia is usually reversible if renal perfusion is quickly restored; therefore, early recognition and prompt treatment are essential. However, prevention of prerenal conditions is just as important as early recognition and aggressive management. Prompt replacement of extracellular fluids, as well as aggressive treatment of sepsis and cardiogenic shock, may help prevent prerenal azotemia.

Hypovolemia is treated in various ways, depending on the cause. Blood loss necessitates transfusions, whereas burns, pancreatitis, and peritonitis are usually treated with isotonic solutions, such as normal saline. Hypovolemia resulting from large urine or gastrointestinal losses often requires the administration of a hypotonic solution, such as 0.45% saline. Patients suffering from cardiac instability usually require positive inotropic agents, antiarrhythmic agents, preload and/or afterload reducers, or intra-aortic balloon pumping. Hypovolemia from intense vasodilation may require vasoconstrictors, isotonic fluid replacement, blood pressure support, and antibiotics (if the patient is septic) until the underlying problem has resolved. Invasive hemodynamic monitoring with a pulmonary artery catheter is extremely valuable in the management of fluid balance.

MANAGEMENT OF POSTRENAL AZOTEMIA

Postrenal obstruction should be suspected whenever a patient has an unexpected decrease in urine volume. Postrenal conditions are usually resolved with the insertion of an indwelling bladder catheter, either transurethral or suprapubic. Occasionally, a ureteral stent may need to be placed if the obstruction is caused by calculi or carcinoma.

MANAGEMENT OF INTRINSIC AZOTEMIA

Common interventions for the patient with intrinsic azotemia include drug therapy, such as with diuretics and dopamine; dietary management, such as protein and electrolyte restrictions; management of fluid and electrolyte imbalances; and dialysis and continuous renal replacement therapies (CRRTs). Attention should also be given to preventive measures, in light of the high mortality rate associated with intrinsic azotemia, especially ATN.

Considering the detrimental impact of acute renal failure, nurses should implement measures to prevent this disorder. In general, maintenance of cardiovascular function and adequate intravascular volume are the two key goals in the prevention of intrinsic azotemia. Primary measures include

1. Maintaining an adequate hydration state for the patient, especially before surgery and before excretion urography studies
2. Maintaining renal perfusion by administering the following agents:
   a. Vasoactive agents that increase renal blood flow, such as low doses of dopamine, acetylcholine, isoproterenol, kinins, prostaglandins, and calcium antagonists
   b. Volume expanders, such as saline and mannitol
   c. Loop-acting diuretics
3. Monitoring the duration, dosage, and combinations of antibiotics administered to the patient, weighing the risk/benefit ratio carefully, and considering nontoxic alternatives (Anderson, 1993; Swan and Bennett, 1991).

Prevention of infection is paramount in patients with acute renal failure because infection is the leading cause of death in these patients. Indwelling urinary catheters should not automatically be placed in patients with acute renal failure, because they increase the risk of infection. In addition, most patients remain oliguric for 8 to 14 days (Llach, 1993; Stark, 1992). If catheterization is necessary, intermittent catheterization is preferable (Baer, 1992). Strict aseptic technique with all intravenous lines (central and peripheral), including temporary access devices used for dialysis, is also of extreme importance, both at the time of insertion and during daily maintenance.

DRUG THERAPY

Diuretics

The use of diuretic therapy, especially the osmotic and loop diuretics, in the treatment of patients with acute renal failure is controversial. Diuretics are used to convert oliguria to a nonoliguric state (urine output > 400 ml/d). This conversion has been found to be beneficial for several reasons. In general, nonoliguric patients are easier to treat because they require less hemodialysis and have a shortened disease course and a more rapid recovery (Brady et al., 1996; Stark, 1992). Both osmotic and loop diuretics may be effective in decreasing the insult to the kidney *if* they are administered within 4 to 8 hours of the onset of the oliguria (Swan and Bennett, 1991; Dolleris, 1992). The hypothesis is that the diuretics increase renal blood flow, GFR, and intratubular pressure while decreasing tubular obstruction and dysfunction. The problem with using diuretics is that they may indeed only increase urine flow without affecting GFR or tubular function and may thus compromise an already insulted renal system.

If diuretic therapy is implemented, either an osmotic agent or a loop-acting diuretic is generally used. None of the other categories of diuretic agents, including the mercurials, thiazides, carbonic anhydrase inhibitors, and potassium sparing agents, increase GFR and renal blood flow. In addition, only the loop-acting agents are effective for patients with renal dysfunction who have GFRs of less than 20 ml/min (Swan and Bennett, 1991). Thus, most types of diuretic agents are ineffective for the treatment of patients with acute renal failure, and their administration should be discontinued in order to prevent complications. Hypovolemia should be corrected before any diuretics are administered. Table 12–13 summarizes the major types of diuretics used in acute renal failure.

Dopamine

The role of dopamine, like that of diuretics, in acute renal failure is controversial. Dopamine in low doses (1 to 3 μg/kg/min) increases renal blood flow and GFR by stimulating the dopaminergic receptors in the kidney (Dolleris, 1992). Sodium excretion is increased as a result of the enhanced blood flow. Renal responses to dopamine, however, are variable; therefore, the role of dopamine in the management of acute renal failure has yet to be definitively established. However, the use of dopamine immediately at the onset of acute renal failure (in the initiation phase) may avert further damage and help maintain urine output. In addition, the concurrent use of dopamine and furosemide early in the course of acute renal failure may be beneficial. The effects of furosemide are augmented by the dual administration of dopamine, thereby promoting diuresis and sodium excretion (Llach, 1993; Shuler et al., 1996).

Miscellaneous Agents

Numerous drugs have been studied in order to determine their effectiveness in diminishing the injury

Table 12–13. MAJOR TYPES OF DIURETICS USED IN ACUTE RENAL FAILURE

Type of Diuretic	Dosage/Route	Mechanism of Action	Common Side Effects	Comments
Osmotic Mannitol	IV: 50–100 g of a 15–20% solution over 90–120 min	Inhibits renal tubular reabsorption of sodium and chloride; ↑ osmosis into proximal tubule; ↑ GFR and volume expansion	Dry mouth; thirst	Store at room temperature. If crystals seen, warm in hot water and shake well; cool to body temperature before giving. Use a filter for infusion >20% concentration
Loop agents Furosemide (Lasix)	Oral: 20–80 mg/d; may ↑ in 20- to 40-mg increments q 6–8 h; maximum dose: 600 mg IV: 20–40 mg; may ↑ in 20-mg increments no sooner than 2 h after last dose	Enhances excretion of sodium and chloride at the ascending limb of the loop of Henle Dilates renal arteries	Electrolyte imbalances Hypokalemia Hyponatremia GI problems Nausea Cramping Diarrhea Constipation	Give IV furosemide slowly over at least several minutes; give 4 mg/min in renal insufficiency.
Bumetanide (Bumex)	Oral: 0.5–2 mg daily; maximum dose: 10 mg/d IV: 0.5–1 mg; may repeat at 2- to 3-h intervals; maximum dose: 10 mg qd			
Ethacrynic acid (Edecrin)	Oral: 50–100 mg/d; may ↑ in 25- to 50-mg increments until therapeutic response is achieved IV: 0.5–1 mg/kg or 50 mg for the average adult; single IV dose not to exceed 100 mg			

GFR = glomerular filtration rate; GI = gastrointestinal; IV = intravenous.

caused by acute renal failure and therefore in hastening the recovery. None, however, has consistently proved effective. Many of these drugs attempted to improve renal blood flow (prostaglandin E, bradykinin); replenish ATP levels by replenishing the precursors for rapid ATP formation (ATP-MgCl$_2$); prevent accumulation of intracellular calcium, which occurs in ischemic azotemia (calcium channel blockers); or stimulate renal cell regeneration (amino acid infusions, epidermal growth factor, growth hormone). Many of the aforementioned drugs, as well as numerous others, have shown beneficial results in experimental models but have had inconsistent results in the clinical setting. Studies are currently being conducted using atrial natriuretic factor and human growth factor in the prevention and treat-

ment of acute renal failure. It is thought that atrial natriuretic factor prevents the intense vasoconstriction induced by angiotensin II, and that growth factors speed up renal cell regeneration (Wagener et al., 1995).

Drug Therapy Considerations

Drug therapy for the patient with acute renal failure poses a challenge because about two thirds of all drugs or their metabolites are eliminated from the body by the kidneys (Swan and Bennett, 1991). In acute renal failure, significant alterations in drug dosages are often necessary in order to prevent toxic levels and adverse reactions. The following considerations should be kept in mind by the physician determining the dosage regimen for a patient with acute renal failure. Assessment of renal function by use of creatinine clearance is the first step of drug therapy. The pharmacokinetic characteristics of the drug to be given, the route of elimination, and the extent of protein binding are all considered.

Peak and trough drug levels are also monitored in order to gauge the effectiveness of the dosage selection. A peak level is usually drawn 1 to 2 hours after the drugs are administered and reflects the highest level achieved after the drug has been rapidly distributed and before any substantial elimination has occurred. A trough level is drawn just before the next dose is given and is an indicator of how the body has cleared the drug. Nurses are responsible for scheduling and obtaining the peak and trough blood levels at the appropriate times in order to ensure accurate results.

Many drugs are removed by dialysis, and extra doses are often required in order to avoid suboptimal drug levels. In general, drugs that are primarily water soluble, such as vitamins, cimetidine, and phenobarbital, are removed by dialysis and should be administered after dialysis. Drugs that are protein bound, lipid bound, or metabolized by the liver, such as phenytoin, lidocaine, and vancomycin, are not removed by dialysis and can be given at any time (Dunetz, 1992; Swan and Bennett, 1991). Table 12–14 lists drugs that are removed by dialysis.

DIETARY MANAGEMENT

Dietary management in patients with acute renal failure continues to be a major component of the therapeutic regimen. The average metabolic rates in acute renal failure are about 20% greater than normal, causing increased catabolism (Oldrizzi et al., 1994). Dialysis also contributes to protein catabolism. The loss of amino acids and water-soluble vitamins in the dialysate constitutes another drain on the patient's nutritional stores.

The overall goal of dietary management for acute renal failure is the maintenance of homeostasis. Nutritional recommendations include (Hirschberg and Kopple, 1991)

- Caloric intake of 30 to 35 kcal/kg of ideal body weight per day.
- Protein intake of 0.5 to 0.8 g/kg of ideal body weight per day, 75 to 80% of which contains all of the required essential amino acids.
- Sodium intake of 0.5 to 1.0 g/day.
- Potassium intake of 20 to 50 mEq/day.
- Calcium intake of 800 to 1200 mg/day.
- Fluid intake equal to the volume of the patient's urine output plus an additional 600 to 1000 ml/day.

In addition, patients undergoing dialysis usually receive multivitamins, folic acid, and occasionally an iron supplement to replace the water-soluble vitamins and other essential elements lost during dialysis.

If the patient is unable to ingest or tolerate an adequate oral nutritional intake, total parenteral nutrition is prescribed. Total parenteral nutrition therapy supplies the patient with sufficient nonprotein glucose calories, essential amino acids, fluids, electrolytes, and essential vitamins in order to create a more stable internal environment. Such an internal environment not only prevents further catabolism, negative nitrogen balance, muscle wasting, and other uremic complications, but it also enhances the patient's tubular regenerating capacity, resistance to infection, and ability to combat other multisystem dysfunctions. In order to facilitate the use of total parenteral nutrition, the physician must also prescribe early dialysis therapy.

MANAGEMENT OF FLUID, ELECTROLYTE, AND ACID-BASE IMBALANCES

Fluid Imbalance

Volume overload is generally managed by dietary restriction of salt and water and administration of diuretics and low-dose dopamine. In addition, dialysis or other renal replacement therapies may be indicated for fluid control. These modalities are discussed later in this chapter.

Table 12–14. COMMON DRUGS REMOVED BY HEMODIALYSIS*

Aminoglycosides (gentamycin, tobramycin)
Cephalosporins (cefoxitin, ceftazidime, and many others)
Penicillins (piperacillin, penicillin G, and others)
Erythromycin
Isoniazid
Sulfonamides (sulfamethoxazole, sulfisoxazole)
Trimethoprim-sulfamethoxazole (Septra)
Acetaminophen
Procainamide
Quinidine
Nitroprusside
Lithium carbonate
Water-soluble vitamins
Folic acid
Phenobarbital
Cimetidine
Ranitidine

*If possible, hold daily doses until after dialysis; supplemental doses may be required for many of these agents.

Electrolyte Imbalance

The most commonly seen electrolyte imbalances in acute renal failure are listed in Table 12–12. In general, three primary approaches are used for the treatment of hyperkalemia: reducing the body potassium content, shifting the potassium intracellularly, and antagonizing the membrane effect of the hyperkalemia. These approaches, which may be used simultaneously or separately, are summarized in Table 12–15. Only two methods are effective in reducing plasma potassium and total body potassium content in a patient with acute renal failure: (1) dialysis and (2) the use of cation exchange resins (Kayexalate) with sorbitol. The other methods listed "protect" the patient for a short time until dialysis or cation exchange resins are instituted and have had sufficient time to produce therapeutic results.

A commonly prescribed regimen for hyperkalemia consists of the following orders (Innerarity, 1992):

- Calcium gluconate, 10 ml of a 10% solution given intravenously over 5 minutes.
- Glucose (50 ml of 50% dextrose) given intravenously.
- Regular insulin, 10 U given intravenously.
- Sodium bicarbonate, 50 to 100 mEq/L given intravenously.
- Sodium polystyrene sulfonate (Kayexalate), 15 to 30 g every 3 to 4 hours with 50 to 100/ml of a 20% sorbital solution given by mouth or as a retention enema.

Hyponatremia is generally the result of water overload and is treated with fluid restriction, specifically, restriction of free water intake. Intravenous solutions of dextrose and water are avoided. Oral intake is restricted, usually to 1 L a day or less. Hypocalcemia is not routinely treated unless the patient is symptomatic. The low serum calcium levels increase when the hyperphosphatemia is corrected because calcium and phosphorus have a reciprocal relationship in the body (Felver, 1995). If treatment is required for the hypocalcemia, calcium carbonate is generally administered. Hyperphosphatemia is usually treated by restriction of dietary intake of phosphorus and administration of phosphate-binding agents (aluminum hydroxide gels and calcium carbonate). Protein-rich and calcium-rich foods are also high in phosphorus; therefore, intake of such foods should be restricted. If hypermagnesemia is present, administration of magnesium-containing antacids should be discontinued.

Acid-Base Imbalance

Metabolic acidosis is the primary acid-base imbalance seen in acute renal failure. Table 12–16 summarizes the etiology and the signs and symptoms of metabolic acidosis in acute renal failure. Treatment for metabolic acidosis depends on its severity. In mild metabolic acidosis, the lungs are able to compensate

Table 12–15. TREATMENT APPROACHES FOR HYPERKALEMIA

Approach	Methods	Efficacy
Reduce the body potassium content	Decrease potassium intake	May decrease plasma and total body potassium content over time
	Increase the fecal excretion of potassium by using cation-exchange resins such as sodium polystyrene sulfonate (Kayexalate)	Takes hours to be effective but eventually decreases both plasma and total body potassium content
	Increase the renal excretion of potassium by using mineralocorticoid agents, increasing salt intake, or using diuretic agents	Any of these would be effective in decreasing both plasma and total body potassium content if the individual has normal renal function
		Decreases both plasma and total body potassium content within a 4- to 6-h time frame
Shift the potassium intracellularly	Administer glucose and insulin intravenously	Decreases plasma potassium level for about 2 h but has no effect on total body potassium content
	Administer an alkali, e.g., sodium bicarbonate	Decreases plasma potassium level for a short time but has no effect on total body potassium content
Antagonize the cellular membrane effect	Administer calcium salts	Has no effect on either plasma or total body potassium content
	Administer hypertonic sodium salts	Has no effect on either plasma or total body potassium content

Table 12–16. METABOLIC ACIDOSIS IN ACUTE RENAL FAILURE

Etiology

Inability of kidney to excrete hydrogen ions produced by body; decreased production of ammonia by the kidney (normally assists with hydrogen ion excretion) Retention of acid end-products of metabolism, which use available buffers in the body; inability of kidney to synthesize bicarbonate

Signs and Symptoms

Increased rate and depth of respirations to excrete carbon dioxide (CO_2) from the lungs (CO_2 acts like an acid); known as Kussmaul's respiration
Lethargy and coma if severe
Low serum bicarbonate, CO_2 combining power, $PaCO_2$
Low pH of arterial blood (pH <7.35)

by excreting excess carbon dioxide (Felver, 1995). Patients with a serum bicarbonate level of less than 15 mEq/L (normal, 24 to 28 mEq/L) and a pH of less than 7.20 are usually treated with intravenous sodium bicarbonate. The goal of treatment is to raise the pH to a value greater than 7.20 in order to avoid the adverse effects of acidosis, such as decreased cardiac contractility. Rapid correction of the acidosis should be avoided, however, because tetany may occur as a result of hypocalcemia. The pH determines how much ionized calcium is present in the serum: the more acid the serum, the more ionized calcium present. If the metabolic acidosis is rapidly corrected, the serum ionized calcium level decreases as the calcium binds with albumin and other substances, such as phosphate and sulfate. For this reason, intravenous calcium gluconate may be prescribed (Lancaster, 1992). Dialysis also corrects the metabolic acidosis because it removes excess hydrogen ions and because bicarbonate is added to the dialysate cleansing solution.

DIALYSIS THERAPY

Dialysis therapy is the primary treatment for the patient with acute renal failure. Without some form of dialysis, the patient is unable to sustain life during the acute renal failure episode. Therapy may include hemodialysis, CRRT, or peritoneal dialysis.

Definition

Dialysis is defined as the separation of solutes by differential diffusion through a porous or semipermeable membrane that is placed between two solutions. This general definition permits the clinician to distin-

guish among the various types of dialyses merely by identifying the semipermeable membrane and describing the two solutions that are involved.

Indications for Dialysis

Dialysis is used for acute renal failure for many reasons. Typically, fluid overload with pulmonary edema, hypertension, heart failure, or electrolyte imbalances, such as hyperkalemia and hyponatremia, are the most common reasons for instituting dialysis. Other indications include acid-base disturbances, such as metabolic acidosis, and complications due to the uremic state, such as nausea and vomiting, pericarditis, and hematological abnormalities. Dialysis therapy is usually initiated early in the course of the renal failure in order to maintain the patient's serum creatinine level at less than 10 mg/100 ml and the BUN level at less than 100 mg/dl (Lazarus et al., 1996). Maintaining these values helps prevent infection and the complications of uremia. In addition, dialysis is often started for fluid control when total parenteral nutrition is administered.

Principles and Mechanisms Involved

Dialysis therapy is based on two physical principles that operate simultaneously: diffusion and ultrafiltration (Ismail and Hakim, 1991). *Diffusion* (or clearance) is the movement of solutes, such as urea from the patient's blood to the dialysate cleansing fluid, across a semipermeable membrane (the artificial kidney). Substances such as bicarbonate may also cross in the opposite direction, from the dialysate across the semipermeable membrane into the patient's blood. Movement of solutes across the semipermeable membrane is dependent on

- The amount of solutes on each side of the semipermeable membrane; typically, the patient's blood has larger amounts of solutes, such as urea, creatinine, and potassium.
- The surface area of the semipermeable membrane, in other words, the size of the artificial kidney.
- The permeability of the semipermeable membrane.
- The size and charge of the solutes.
- The rate of blood flowing through the artificial kidney.
- The rate of dialysate cleansing fluid flowing through the artificial kidney.

Ultrafiltration is the removal of plasma water and some low-molecular-weight particles by use of a pressure or osmotic gradient. Ultrafiltration is primarily aimed at controlling fluid volume, whereas dialysis is aimed at decreasing waste products and treating fluid and electrolyte imbalances.

Vascular Access

An essential component for all of the renal replacement therapies is an adequate, easy access to the patient's bloodstream, where blood flow is high. Four types of vascular access are used for renal replacement therapy: percutaneous venous catheters, arteriovenous fistulas, arteriovenous grafts, and external arteriovenous shunts. Temporary percutaneous catheters are most commonly used in patients with acute renal failure because they can be used immediately. They are usually inserted into the subclavian, jugular, or femoral vein (Fan, 1994). The typical catheter has a single or double lumen and is designed to be used only for short-term renal replacement therapy during acute situations. One example of such a device is the Vas-Cath catheter.

An arteriovenous fistula is an internal surgically created communication between an artery and a vein. The most frequently created fistula is the Brescio-Cimino fistula, which involves anastomosing the radial artery and cephalic vein in a side-to-side or end-to-side manner. The anastomosis permits blood to bypass the capillaries and flow directly from the artery into the vein. As a result, the vein is forced to dilate in order to accommodate the increased pressure that accompanies the arterial blood. This method produces a vessel that is easy to cannulate for the renal replacement therapies.

Arteriovenous grafts are created by use of different types of prosthetic material, most commonly polytetrafluoroethylene (PTFE), Gore-Tex, or Impra grafts (Harland, 1994). Anastomoses are made with the graft ends connected to an artery and a vein.

An external arteriovenous shunt (Quinton-Scribner) consists of a surgically implanted extracorporeal apparatus that is used to connect an artery and a vein. This type of device has become less popular since the advent of percutaneous catheters but may occasionally be used in the critical care unit. The external shunt poses a risk for infection and clotting problems.

Nursing Care of Arteriovenous Fistula or Graft

The nurse is always protective of the vascular access site. An arteriovenous fistula or graft should be auscultated for a bruit and palpated for the presence of a thrill or buzz every 4 to 8 hours. The extremity that has a fistula or graft must never be used for drawing blood specimens or obtaining blood pressure measurements. Such activities could produce pressure changes within the altered vessels that could result in clotting or rupture. The nurse can alert other health care personnel of the presence of the fistula or graft by posting a large sign near patient's head that indicates which arm should be used. Constrictive clothing and jewelry must be avoided on the affected arm. Patients should be cautioned against sleeping on the affected arm. All of these situations may decrease blood flow through the fistula or graft and cause clotting. The presence and strength of the distal pulse past the fistula or graft is evaluated. Inadequate collateral circulation past the fistula or graft may result in loss of this pulse. The physician is notified immediately if no bruit is auscultated, no thrill is palpated, or the distal pulse is absent.

Nursing Care of Percutaneous Catheters

Strict aseptic technique must be applied to any percutaneous catheter placed for dialysis. Exit sites should be inspected daily for signs of infection, such as redness, drainage, and swelling. Dressing changes should be performed by use of sterile technique. There is minimal manipulation of the catheter in order to avoid accidental dislodging. The catheter is not used for the administration of fluids or medications or for the sampling of blood unless a specific order is obtained to do so. Heparin is placed in the catheter by dialysis personnel in order to maintain patency, and the catheter is clamped.

Hemodialysis

Hemodialysis is the most frequently used renal replacement therapy used to treat acute renal failure. Hemodialysis consists of simply cleansing the patient's blood through an artificial kidney or dialyzer by use of diffusion and ultrafiltration. Water and waste products of metabolism are easily removed. Hemodialysis is efficient and corrects biochemical disturbances quickly. Treatments are typically 3 to 4 hours long. Hemodialysis has several disadvantages. Hemodialysis requires special staff education training, equipment is expensive, machine availability may be a problem at any specific time, and complications are numerous.

Complications of Hemodialysis

An assortment of complications may occur in the patient undergoing hemodialysis. Hypotension occurs in approximately 10 to 50% of patients (Lazarus et al., 1996) and is usually the result of preexisting hypovolemia, excessive amount of fluid removal, or too-rapid removal of fluid. Other factors that may contribute to hypotension during hemodialysis include left ventricular dysfunction from preexisting heart disease or medications, autonomic dysfunction resulting from medication or diabetes, and inappropriate vasodilation resulting from sepsis or antihypertensive drug therapy. Dialyzer membrane incompatibility may also cause hypotension.

Dysrhythmias may occur during dialysis and are often caused by a rapid shift in the serum potassium level, clearance of antiarrhythmic medications, preexisting coronary artery disease, hypoxemia, or hypercalcemia resulting from rapid influx of calcium from the dialysate solution.

Muscle cramps may occur during dialysis, but they occur more commonly in chronic renal failure. Cramping is thought to be caused by ischemia of the skeletal muscles that results from aggressive fluid removal. The cramps typically involve the legs, feet, and hands and occur most often during the last half of the dialysis treatment.

A decrease in the arterial oxygen content of the blood occurs in about 90% of patients undergoing hemodialysis (Lazarus et al., 1996). Usually, the decrease ranges from 5 to 35 mm Hg (mean, 15 mm Hg) and is not clinically significant except in the critically ill patient. Several theories have been offered to explain the hypoxemia, including leukocyte interactions with the artificial kidney and a decrease in carbon dioxide levels, either resulting from an acetate dialysate solution or a loss of carbon dioxide across the semipermeable membrane (Lazarus et al., 1996).

Dialysis disequilibrium syndrome is most likely to occur after the first or second dialysis treatment or in patients who have had sudden large decreases in BUN and creatinine levels as a result of the hemodialysis. Because of the blood-brain barrier, dialysis does not deplete the concentrations of BUN, creatinine, and other uremic toxins in the brain as rapidly as it does those substances in the extracellular fluid. An osmotic concentration gradient established in the brain allows fluid to enter until the concentration levels equal that of the extracellular fluid. The extra fluid in the brain tissue creates a state of cerebral edema for the patient, resulting in severe headaches, nausea and vomiting, twitching, mental confusion, and occasionally seizures. The incidence of dialysis disequilibrium syndrome may be decreased by the use of shorter, more frequent, dialysis treatments (Peschman, 1992). Mannitol, an osmotic diuretic, may help prevent the fluid shifts into the brain. Phenytoin (Dilantin) may be used in the new hemodialysis patient in order to decrease the central nervous system symptoms.

Infectious complications associated with hemodialysis include vascular access infections and hepatitis C. Vascular access infections are usually caused by a break in sterile technique, whereas hepatitis C is usually transfusion acquired.

Hemolysis, air embolism, and hyperthermia are rare complications of hemodialysis. Hemolysis can occur when the patient's blood is exposed to incorrectly mixed dialysate solution or hypotonic chemicals (formaldehyde and bleach). An air embolism can occur when air is introduced into the bloodstream through a break in the dialysis circuit. Hyperthermia may occur if the temperature control devices on the dialysis machine malfunction. Complications of hemodialysis are summarized in Table 12–17.

Nursing Care of the Hemodialysis Patient

The critical care nurse is responsible for the following tasks in regard to hemodialysis:

- Monitor laboratory values as ordered and report abnormal results to nephrologist and dialysis staff.
- Weigh patient daily; 1 kg of body weight gain is equal to 1000 ml of retained fluid.
- On the day of dialysis, withhold any dialyzable (water-soluble) medications until after treatment; check with dialysis nurse or pharmacist if you are unsure of which medications to withhold; administer supplemental doses as ordered after treatment.
- Avoid administering antihypertensive agents for 4 to 6 hours before treatment, if possible. Reduce as much as possible other medications that lower blood pressure (narcotics, sedatives).
- Assess percutaneous catheter, fistula, or graft

Table 12–17. DIALYSIS COMPLICATIONS

Hypotension
Cramps
Bleeding/clotting
Anaphylaxis
Hemolysis
Leukopenia
Arrhythmias
Infections
Hypoxemia
Pyrogen reactions
Dialysis disequilibrium syndrome
Angioaccess dysfunction
Technical mishaps—incorrect dialysate mixture, contaminated dialysate, air embolism, spallation, incorrect replacement solution

Adapted from Brenner B. (Ed.) (1996). *Brenner and Rector's the kidney* (5th ed., Vol. II) (p. 2472). Philadelphia: W. B. Saunders Co.

frequently; report any unusual findings, such as loss of bruit, redness, or drainage at site.
- Assess patient frequently after treatment for signs of bleeding, hypovolemia, and dialysis disequilibrium syndrome.

Continuous Renal Replacement Therapy (Hemofiltration)

Continuous renal replacement therapy provides continuous ultrafiltration of fluids and clearance of uremic toxins. It uses the process of hemofiltration, a convective mode of blood cleansing in which solutes cross the semipermeable membrane as a result of differences in pressures on each side of the membrane. Several techniques or approaches to performing CRRT exist; continuous arteriovenous hemofiltration (CAVH) and continuous arteriovenous hemodialysis (CAVHD) are two methods.

Indications for Continuous Renal Replacement Therapy

The clinical indications for CRRT include many of the same indications as for dialysis, such as treatment for hypervolemia, cardiac failure, electrolyte imbalances, and acid-base imbalances and facilitation of aggressive hyperalimentation therapy. However, CRRT has several advantages over hemodialysis:

- CRRT has more gradual solute removal than hemodialysis.
- The risk of hemodynamic instability is less with CRRT than with hemodialysis.
- CRRT allows increased flexibility in fluid administration.
- CRRT requires only minimal heparinization.
- CRRT is relatively inexpensive.
- CRRT requires minimal staff education for implementation of the therapy.
- CRRT is ideal for physiologically unstable patients.

Continuous renal replacement therapy is generally prescribed for patients who are too hemodynamically unstable to tolerate hemodialysis. Disadvantages of CRRT include the following:

- The patient must remain in bed during the entire therapy.
- Vascular access and mild anticoagulation are necessary with CRRT.
- One-to-one nursing must be available for the patient undergoing CRRT.

Principles of Continuous Renal Replacement Therapy

Basically, CRRT is extracorporeal circulation of blood through a filter for the removal of fluid and small solutes, which are then collected in an attached drainage bag. Vascular access is necessary for the performance of CRRT. Because both arterial and venous accesses are required, the femoral artery and vein are usually cannulated so that adequate blood flow can be obtained. Several different types of hemofilters are available, but all have highly porous membranes that permit the clearance of molecules less than 50,000 daltons (Ronco et al., 1995). Some drugs are removed with hemofiltration, requiring supplemental dosing.

Blood flows from the patient's arterial access through the hemofilter and returns through the patient's venous access (Fig. 12–6). The patient's own blood pressure pumps the blood through the system. Fluid removal or ultrafiltration is controlled by the total pressure applied to the filter's porous membrane, known as the total transmembrane pressure. The total transmembrane pressure is influenced by the patient's hydrostatic and oncotic pressures as well as the negative pressure supplied by gravity on the drainage collection bag. A constant heparin infusion is usually necessary to keep the filter from clotting.

Several factors influence blood flow through the hemofilter. First, the diameter of the arterial access and that of the venous access need to be the same so that obstruction is avoided. Second, the patient's mean arterial blood pressure should be at least 60 mm Hg so that blood flows through the filter at 20 ml/min. Last, because blood viscosity influences flow through the system, the patient's hematocrit value needs to be less than 45% (Baldwin and Elderkin, 1995).

Methods of Continuous Renal Replacement Therapy

Continuous arteriovenous hemofiltration is often the therapy of choice when moderate fluid and solute removal is needed. The average fluid lost with CAVH is 500 to 800 ml/h; therefore, replacement fluid is necessary for the prevention of dehydration and electrolyte imbalance (Price, 1992). Replacement fluid is usually 0.9% sodium chloride or lactated Ringer's solution with electrolytes added based on the patient's laboratory values.

Continuous arteriovenous hemodialysis is used if aggressive management of uremia is required and the patient is experiencing extreme volume overload. With CAVHD, either a standard peritoneal dialysate solution or a custom-made dialysate solution is infused in the direction opposite that of the patient's blood flow

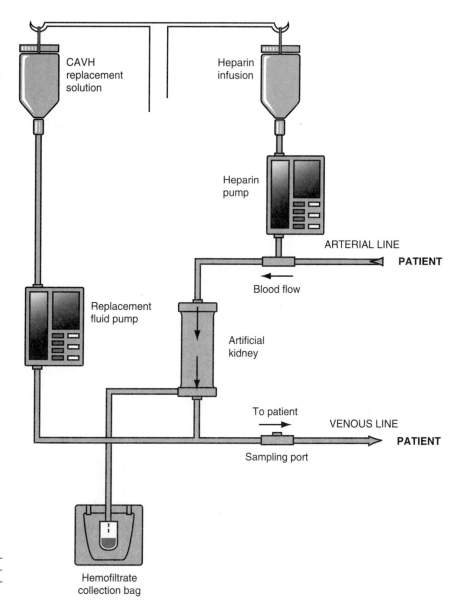

Figure 12–6. Schematic of continuous arteriovenous hemodialysis. CAVH = continuous arteriovenous hemofiltration.

through the hemofilter. The typical flow rate of the dialysate solution is 1000 ml/h. As with hemodialysis, solutes are removed based on their concentration gradient. Small solutes, such as urea and creatinine, are easily cleared across the semipermeable membrane of the hemofilter. The aggressive fluid removal seen in CAVHD is facilitated by the dextrose in the dialysate solution. Because large amounts of fluid are removed with CAVHD, replacement fluid is also necessary.

Complications of Continuous Renal Replacement Therapy

Numerous complications are associated with CAVH and CAVHD:

- Depletion of vitamins, amino acids, and other substances.
- Acid-base imbalances.
- Fluid and electrolyte imbalances.
- Hemorrhage resulting from anticoagulation or disruption of the filter or tubing.
- Infection.
- Rupture or leakage of the filter.
- Clotting of the filter.
- Loss of the vascular access site.

Responsibilities of the Critical Care Nurse

The critical care nurse is responsible for the following tasks in regard to CRRT:

Article Reference

Van Bommel, E. F., Bouvy, N. D., So, K. L., Zietse, R., Vincent, H. H., Bruining, H. A., et al. (1995). Acute dialytic support for the critically ill: Intermittent hemodialysis versus continuous arteriovenous hemodiafiltration. *American Journal of Nephrology, 15*(6), 192-200.

Review of Study Methods and Findings

The purpose of this study was to determine whether continuous renal replacement therapy (continuous arteriovenous hemodialysis (CAVHD)) is more effective than hemodialysis in the treatment of critically ill patients with acute renal failure. The researchers reviewed medical records of 94 patients in a surgical intensive care unit (SICU) who developed acute renal failure that required renal replacement therapy.

The causes of the acute renal failure were varied and often multifactorial. The mean age of patients was 61 years (range, 17 to 85 years); 46 of the 94 patients were aged 65 years or older. Indications for dialysis in the study group were azotemia, severe hyperkalemia, refractory acidosis, and/or severe volume overload. The patients received either acute intermittent hemodialysis treatments (34 patients) or CAVHD (60 patients). For assessment of the severity of illness and establishment of whether the groups were comparable, the Acute Physiology and Chronic Health Evaluation (Apache) II score was used at the start of the treatment. In addition, the number of organ system failures was also calculated. For each patient, the probability of death was then calculated according to the Apache II equation.

Significant differences existed between the 34 patients treated with hemodialysis and the 60 patients treated with CAVHD. First of all, significant variation existed in the severity of illness between the groups. The patients in the CAVHD group had higher Apache II scores, lower mean arterial blood pressures, and more additional organ system failures and required greater ventilator and vasopressor support. The patients in the CAVHD group tolerated the treatment better hemodynamically. Severe hypotension occurred in 25 of the 130 (19%) hemodialysis treatments. In addition, 13 of the 130 hemodialysis procedures were complicated by cardiac dysrhythmias (supraventricular tachycardia and ventricular fibrillation). In the CAVHD group,

no significant change in heart rate or blood pressure was observed. Superior metabolic control was also demonstrated in the CAVHD group, as evidenced by a significant decrease in serum urea levels within 72 hours. The duration of treatment time was approximately the same for both groups: 8.9 days for the CAVHD group versus 8.1 days for the hemodialysis group. Regarding patient outcomes, 26 (43%) of the 60 patients in the CAVHD group survived to leave the SICU, and 23 (38%) of the 60 were later discharged from the hospital. In the hemodialysis group, 20 (59%) of the 34 patients left the SICU, and 19 (55%) of the 34 were discharged. These differences were not statistically significant. Interestingly, the mean Apache II score of patients in the CAVHD group who survived was similar to that of the patients in the hemodialysis who died. Forty-seven percent of the patients in the CAVHD group regained renal function, compared with 53% of the patients receiving hemodialysis; however, this finding was not statistically significant.

Study Strengths and Weaknesses

One strength of the study is its relatively large sample size, especially of CAVHD group. There has been a general lack of research comparing the two methods of renal replacement therapy; therefore, the researchers should be commended for undertaking this project. The results of this study support physicians who believe that continuous renal replacement therapies are superior to intermittent hemodialysis in the critically ill patient with acute renal failure.

One weakness of this study is that the design was retrospective. In addition, the patient population was nonrandomized. Treatment selection bias became evident to the researchers as the study progressed. It was believed, however, that careful assessment of the disease severity with the Apache II score and other clinical and laboratory data allowed a meaningful comparison between the two groups.

Implications for Nursing Practice

Nurses who care for these patients in the critical care unit need to be aware of each mode of therapy because either one may be used in their particular setting. Understanding the benefits of each mode of therapy and the patients who are the best candidates for each is beneficial for the critical care nurse collaborating with the physician in the treatment of the acute renal failure patient.

- Monitor hemodynamic status hourly.
- Assess ultrafiltration rate hourly and administer appropriate replacement fluid.
- Assess hemofilter every 2 to 4 hours for clotting (as evidenced by dark fibers, rapid decrease in amount of ultrafiltration without a change in patient's hemodynamic status). If clotting is suspected, flush system with 50 ml of normal saline and observe for dark streaks or clots; system may need to be changed (Pinson, 1992).
- Monitor results of serum chemistries, clotting studies, and other tests as ordered.
- Frequently assess CRRT system: keep filter and lines visible at all times, avoid kinks, and keep tubing warm to the touch.
- Assess ultrafiltrate for blood (pink-tinged to frank blood), which is indicative of membrane rupture.
- Maintain heparin infusion per hospital protocol.
- Collaborate with the nephrologist and dialysis nurse for system or patient problems.
- Maintain sterile technique: swab ports with povidone-iodine (Betadine) before any blood is removed for samples, during dressings changes, or when the system is changed.

Peritoneal Dialysis

Peritoneal dialysis is the removal of solutes and fluid by diffusion through an individual's own semipermeable membrane (the peritoneal membrane) with the use of a dialysate solution that has been instilled into the peritoneal cavity. The peritoneal membrane surrounds the abdominal cavity and lines the organs inside the abdominal cavity. This renal replacement therapy is not as frequently used for the treatment of acute renal failure because of its comparatively slow ability to alter the biochemical imbalances.

Indications for Peritoneal Dialysis

Clinical indications for peritoneal dialysis include acute and chronic renal failure, severe water intoxication, electrolyte disorders, and drug overdose. It offers several advantages:

- The equipment is easily and rapidly assembled and relatively inexpensive.
- Minimal physical preparation of the patient is required.
- The danger of acute electrolyte imbalances or hemorrhage is minimal.
- The dialysate solution can be easily individualized.
- The process can be implemented in either general care or specialty care areas.

Peritoneal dialysis also has several disadvantages:

- It is time-intensive, usually requiring at least 36 hours for a therapeutic effect to be achieved.
- Biochemical disturbances are corrected slowly.
- Protein loss is about 30 g per a 36-hour dialysis session.
- Access to the peritoneal cavity is sometimes difficult.

Complications of Peritoneal Dialysis

Although rare, many complications can result from peritoneal dialysis. The complications can be divided into three categories: mechanical problems, metabolic difficulties, and inflammatory reactions.

The potential complications resulting from mechanical problems include the following:

- The abdominal viscera may be perforated during insertion of the catheter.
- Hemorrhage may result from the catheter insertion.
- The catheter may be improperly placed.
- Poor drainage may occur as a result of catheter blockage.
- Fluid may leak around the catheter.
- The patient may experience pain during the catheter insertion.
- The patient may experience discomfort as a result of the pressure of the fluid within the peritoneal cavity.
- Pulmonary complications may occur as a result of the pressure of the fluid in the peritoneal cavity.

Complications that may result from metabolic difficulties are as follows:

- Hypovolemia and hypernatremia may result from too rapid a removal of fluid.
- Hypervolemia may result from impaired drainage of fluid.
- Hypokalemia may result from the use of potassium-free dialysate.
- Alkalosis may result from the use of an alkaline dialysate.
- Disequilibrium syndrome may result from too rapid a removal of fluid and waste products.
- Hyperglycemia may result from the high glucose concentration of the dialysate.

The complications that may result from inflammatory reactions are

- Peritoneal irritation produced by the catheter.
- Peritonitis resulting from bacterial infection.

NURSING CARE PLAN FOR THE PATIENT WITH ACUTE RENAL FAILURE

Nursing Diagnosis	Patient Outcomes	Nursing Interventions
Fluid volume excess related to sodium and water retention, and excess intake.	Intake and output will be balanced. Body weight will be within 2 lb of dry weight. Vital signs will be stable. Central venous pressure will be 0–8 mm Hg Skin turgor, moisture and elasticity will be normal. Oral mucosa will be normal, hydrated. Serum laboratory values will be within normal limits.	Monitor intake and output every 4 h. Obtain daily weights. Monitor laboratory values daily (blood urea nitrogen, creatinine, potassium) Assess vital signs every 2 h head-to-toe assessment every 8 h. Monitor urine (color, odor, pH, specific gravity, protein level, and glucose level). Administer all fluids and medications precisely. Administer blood before or during dialysis. Prepare patient for dialysis or continuous arteriovenous hemofiltration and continuous arteriovenous hemodialysis.
Risk for infection related to depressed immune response secondary to uremia and impaired skin integrity.	Infection will be absent. Patient will be afebrile. Skin temperature will be normal. Breath sounds, chest x-ray study will be normal. Urination pattern will be normal for patient. Culture will be negative for all body fluids and wound areas. White blood cell count and differential will be normal.	Monitor environment, visitors, and personnel caring for patient for possible contamination. Assess all abrasions, cuts, incisions every 8 h. Inspect all intravenous sites every 2–4 h. Monitor temperature every 4 h. Avoid invasive equipment whenever possible. Monitor laboratory values and diagnostic tests daily (white blood cell count, cultures). Perform pulmonary preventive program (turn, cough, deep breathing).
Altered nutrition (less than body requirements) related to uremia, altered oral mucous membrane, and dietary restrictions.	Nutritional intake will be adequate. Body weight will be consistent with individual. Caloric intake will be appropriate. Energy level will be appropriate. Serum laboratory values will be consistent with patient's condition. Patient will verbalize comfort of oral cavity. Patient will verbalize ability to taste food appropriately.	Monitor body weight and caloric intake daily. Monitor serum laboratory values daily. Provide diet with essential nutrients but within restrictions. Provide food and fluids at comfortable temperature. Provide small frequent feedings. Remove noxious stimuli from patient's environment. Promote dietary goals with patient. Administer vitamins, medications, and nutritional supplements as prescribed. Administer hyperalimentation precisely as ordered. Assess oral cavity every 4 h. Assist with oral care every 2 h, before meals, and at bedtime.
Risk for anxiety related to diagnosis, treatment plan, prognosis, and unfamiliar environment.	Patient will have relaxed facial expression and body posture. Patient will demonstrate reduced anxiety level. Patient will demonstrate effective coping mechanisms. Patient will participate in treatment plan.	Monitor for signs of anxiety: tachycardia, hypertension, muscle tension, inappropriate behaviors. Use calm, trusting approach with patient and family. Explain all procedures to patient. Provide calm, relaxed environment; attempt to decrease stimulation. Allow patient to make decisions as appropriate. Administer sedatives as ordered.
Knowledge deficit related to disease process and therapeutic regimen.	Patient will have sufficient, accurate information to be an informed participant in own care. Patient will verbalize information known and ask questions about disease process and health care regimen. Patient will cooperate and participate in own care.	Assess content of patient's verbalizations and questions daily. Provide specific and factual information about the disease process, its impact on the patient, and its effect on care. Reinforce information and update daily. Include family in process.

Peritonitis is the most common complication encountered in peritoneal dialysis therapy and is usually caused by contamination in the system. It is manifested by abdominal pain, cloudy peritoneal fluid, fever and chills, nausea and vomiting, and difficulty draining fluid from the peritoneal cavity. Appropriate antibiotic treatment is indicated for peritonitis.

Contraindications to Peritoneal Dialysis

Although conflicting opinions exist regarding contraindications for peritoneal dialysis, the following conditions are considered contraindications (Smith, 1992):

- Acute active peritonitis.
- Recent or extensive abdominal surgery.
- Known peritoneal adhesions.
- Severe abdominal trauma or burns.
- Massive intraperitoneal hematoma.
- Any major abdominally located vascular anastomosis.

Any or all of these renal replacement therapies are likely to be prescribed by physicians attempting to formulate the best intervention plan for the patient with acute renal failure. Table 12–18 summarizes the major types of renal replacement therapy used in acute renal failure. The following guidelines (Brady et al., 1996) are often used by the physician deciding what form of renal replacement therapy to use:

- If the patient is extremely volume-overloaded but hemodynamically stable, perform hemodialysis; if hemodynamically unstable, perform CRRT.

- If the patient is extremely hypercatabolic, use either hemodialysis or CRRT.
- If the patient has a severe cardiac history and does not require large amounts of fluid removal, peritoneal dialysis may be the best choice.
- If vascular access is not available, such as with severe peripheral vascular disease, peritoneal dialysis may be an option.
- If rapid removal of drugs is needed because of an overdose or error, hemodialysis is the best option.
- If the patient needs frequent moving or transport to procedures, CRRT should not be used.

Outcomes

With appropriate interventions, expected patient outcomes for the patient with acute renal failure include the following:

- Fluid balance and hemodynamic status are stable.
- Body weight is within 2 pounds of dry weight.
- Vital signs are stable and are consistent with baseline.

Table 12–18. RENAL REPLACEMENT THERAPIES

Mode	Indications	Complications
Hemodialysis	Emergent catabolic fluid overloaded states Hyperkalemia Overdoses	Hemodynamic instability (hypotension, dysrhythmias, ischemia) Hypoxemia Fluid and electrolyte shifts Access complications (clotting, bleeding, infection) Systemic bleeding from anticoagulation Disequilibrium syndrome
Peritoneal dialysis	Hemodynamically unstable or bleeding patient Vascular access is unavailable or difficult Hemodialysis unavailable	Peritonitis Exit site and tunnel infections Fluid retention Peritoneal fluid drainage failure Reduced diaphragmatic compliance (decreased ventilation) Hyperglycemia, hyperosmolarity (hypertonic glucose)
Continuous arteriovenous hemofiltration (CAVH)	Hemodynamically unstable, fluid-overloaded patient	Access complications (bleeding, clotting, infection) Loss of limb from distal arterial ischemia Excessive fluid removal
Continuous arteriovenous hemodialysis (CAVHD)	Hemodynamically unstable patients with azotemia Catabolic acute renal failure Electrolyte imbalances	Access complications (clotting, bleeding, infection) Loss of limb from distal arterial ischemia Fluid and electrolyte shifts

Data from Brenner, B. (Ed.) (1996). *Brenner and Rector's the kidney* (5th ed.) (p. 2472). Philadelphia: W. B. Saunders Co.

- Skin turgor is normal, and oral mucosa is intact and well hydrated.
- Serum laboratory values and arterial blood gas results are within normal limits.
- Infection is absent.
- Nutritional intake is adequate for the maintenance of the desired weight.
- Patient and family are able to participate in patient's care and are able to make informed decisions.

Summary

The patient with acute renal failure poses an immense clinical challenge for all health care personnel. Many of these patients have multisystem failure and require intensive and aggressive care. In addition, the development of acute renal failure is an event that often catches the patient and family unprepared. Nurses can play a pivotal role in promoting positive patient outcomes through prevention, sharp assessment skills, and supportive nursing care.

CRITICAL THINKING QUESTIONS

1. What laboratory criteria are commonly used to differentiate between prerenal azotemia and intrinsic azotemia?
2. Why is the administration of diuretics often stopped in the patient with acute renal failure?
3. How can the critical care nurse help prevent acute renal failure?
4. A patient has muscle weakness, tented T waves, prolonged PR interval, and abdominal cramps. What electrolyte imbalance do you suspect? What treatment do you anticipate? Explain how each treatment works to correct this imbalance.
5. Why is low-dose dopamine occasionally ordered in acute renal failure?

REFERENCES

Anderson, R. (1993). Prevention and management of acute renal failure. *Hospital Practice, 28*(8), 61–75.

Baer, C., & Lancaster, L. (1992). Acute renal failure. *Critical Care Nursing Quarterly, 14*(4), 1–21.

Baldwin, I., & Elderkin, T. (1995). Continuous hemofiltration: Nursing perspectives in critical care. *New Horizons: The Science and Practice of Acute Medicine, 3*(4), 738–747.

Brady, H., Brenner, B., & Lieberthal, W. (1996). Acute renal failure. In B. Brenner (Ed.), *The kidney* (5th ed., Vol. II) (pp. 1200–1252). Philadelphia: W. B. Saunders Co.

Chernecky, C., Krech, R., & Berger, B. (1993). *Laboratory Tests and diagnostic procedures.* Philadelphia: W. B. Saunders Co.

Chmielewski, C. (1992). Renal anatomy and overview of nephron function. *American Nephrology Nurses Association Journal, 19*(1), 34–40.

Dolleris, P. (1992) Diuretic and vasopressor usage in acute renal failure: A synopsis. *Critical Care Nursing Quarterly, 14*(4), 28–31.

Dunetz, P. (1992). If your med/surg patient is on dialysis. *RN, 55*(9), 46–53.

Fan, P. (1994). Acute vascular access: New advances. *Advances in Renal Replacement Therapy, 1*(2), 90–98.

Feest, T., Round, A., & Hamad, S. (1993). Incidence of severe acute renal failure in adults: Results of a community-based study. *British Medical Journal, 306*, 481–483.

Felver, L. (1995). Fluid and electrolyte homeostasis and imbalances. In L. Copstead (Ed.), *Perspectives on pathophysiology* (pp. 524–537). Philadelphia: W. B. Saunders Co.

Felver, L. (1995). Acid-base homeostasis and imbalances. In L. Copstead (Ed.), *Perspectives on pathophysiology* (pp. 538–545). Philadelphia: W. B. Saunders Co.

Finn, W. (1993). Recovery from acute renal failure. In J. Lazarus, & B. Brenner (Eds.), *Acute renal failure* (3rd ed.) (p. 553). New York: Churchill Livingstone.

Harland, R. (1994). Placement of permanent vascular access devices: Surgical considerations. *Advances in Renal Replacement Therapy, 1*(2), 99–106.

Hirschberg, R., & Kopple, J. (1991). Nutritional therapy in patients with renal failure. In D. Levine (Ed.), *Care of the renal patient* (2nd ed.) (pp. 169–180). Philadelphia: W. B. Saunders Co.

Holechek, M. (1992). Glomerular filtration and renal hemodynamics. *American Nephrology Nurses Association Journal, 19*(3), 237–248.

Innerarity, S. (1992). Hyperkalemic emergencies. *Critical Care Nursing Quarterly, 14*(4), 32–39.

Ismail, N., & Hakim, R. (1991). Hemodialysis. In D. Levine (Ed.), *Care of the renal patient* (2nd ed.) (pp. 220–246). Philadelphia: W. B. Saunders Co.

Lancaster, L. (1992). *Core curriculum for nephrology nursing* (2nd ed.). Pitman, NJ: Anthony Jannetti.

Lazarus, J., Denker, B., & Owen, W. (1996). Hemodialysis. In B. Brenner (Ed.), *The kidney* (5th ed., Vol. II) (pp. 2424–2506). Philadelphia: W. B. Saunders Co.

Llach, F. (1993). *Clinical nephrology* (3rd ed.). Boston: Little, Brown & Co.

Oldrizzi, L., Rugiu, C., & Maschio, G. (1994). Nutrition and the kidney: How to manage patients with renal failure. *Nutrition in Clinical Practice, 9*(1), 3–10.

Peschman, P. (1992). Acute hemodialysis: Issues in the critically ill. *AACN Clinical Issues, 3*(3), 545–557.

Pinson, J. (1992). Preventing complications in the CAVH patient. *Dimensions of Critical Care Nursing, 11*(5), 242–248.

Price, C. (1992). An update on continuous renal replacement therapies. *AACN Clinical Issues, 3*(3), 597–604.

Ronco, C., Barbacini, S., Digito, A., & Zoccali, G. (1995). Advances and new directions in continuous renal replacement therapies. *New Horizons: The Science and Practice of Acute Medicine, 3*(4), 708–716.

Shuler, C., Golper, T., & Bennett, W. (1996). Prescribing drugs in renal disease. In B. Brenner (Ed.), *The kidney* (5th ed., Vol. II) (pp. 2653–2702). Philadelphia: W. B. Saunders Co.

Smith, L. (1992). Peritoneal dialysis in the critically ill patient. *AACN Clinical Issues, 3*(3), 558–569.

Stark, J. (1994). Interpreting BUN/creatinine levels: It's not as simple as you think. *Nursing, 24*(9), 58–61.

Stark, J. (1992). Acute tubular necrosis: Differences between oliguria and nonoliguria. *Critical Care Nursing Quarterly, 14*(4), 22–27.

Swan, S., & Bennett, W. (1991). Drug use in renal patients and the extracorporeal treatment of poisoning. In D. Levine (Ed.), *Care of the renal patient* (2nd ed.) (pp. 130–138). Philadelphia: W. B. Saunders Co.

Swan, S., & Bennett, W. (1993). Nephrotoxic acute renal failure. In B. Brenner & J. Lazarus (Eds.), *Acute renal failure* (3rd ed.) (p. 357). New York: Churchill Livingstone.

Tische, C., Madsen, K. (1996). Anatomy of the kidney. In B. Brenner (Ed.), *The kidney* (5th ed., Vol. I) (pp. 3–71). Philadelphia: W. B. Saunders Co.

Wagener, O., Lieske, J., & Toback, G. (1995). Molecular and cell biology of acute renal failure: New therapeutic strategies. *New Horizons: The Science and Practice of Acute Medicine, 3*(4), 634–639.

RECOMMENDED READINGS

Aragon, D., & Goshorn, J. (1994). How to recognize and treat rhabdomyolysis. *American Journal of Nursing, 94*(11), 56I–56P.

Butler, B. (1991). Nutritional management of catabolic acute renal failure requiring renal replacement therapy. *American Nephrology Nurses Association Journal, 18*(3), 247–259.

Byers, J., & Goshorn, J. (1995). How to manage diuretic therapy. *American Journal of Nursing, 95*(2), 38–44.

Carlson, K. (1995). Renal failure. In L. Copstead (Ed.), *Perspectives on pathophysiology* (pp. 587–600). Philadelphia: W. B. Saunders Co.

Douglas, S. (1992). Acute tubular necrosis: Diagnosis, treatment, and nursing implications. *AACN Clinical Issues, 3*(3), 688–697.

Dunn, S. (1993). How to care for the dialysis patient. *American Journal of Nursing, 93*(6), 26–34.

Hodgson, B., Kizior, R., & Kingson, R. (1995). *Nurses drug handbook 1995.* Philadelphia: W. B. Saunders Co.

Hulman, P., & Wolfson, M. (1993). The patient with acute renal failure. *Hospital Medicine, 29*(7), 82–89.

Kelleher, R. (1992). Dialysis in the surgical intensive care patient: A case study. *Critical Care Nursing Quarterly, 14*(4), 72–77.

Kierdorf, H. (1995). The nutritional management of acute renal failure in the intensive care unit. *New Horizons: The Science and Practice of Acute Medicine, 3*(4), 699–707.

King, B. (1994). Detecting acute renal failure. *RN, 57*(3), 34–40.

Kroh, U. (1995). Drug administration in critically ill patients with acute renal failure. *New Horizons: The Science and Practice of Acute Medicine, 3*(4), 748–759.

Price, C. (1991). Continuous renal replacement therapy: The treatment of choice for acute renal failure. *American Nephrology Nurses Association Journal, 18*(3), 239–244.

Richard, C. (1995). Renal function. In L. Copstead (Ed.), *Perspectives on pathophysiology* (pp. 548–569). Philadelphia: W. B. Saunders Co.

Stark, J. (1994). Acute renal failure in trauma: Current perspectives. *Critical Care Nursing Quarterly, 16*(4), 49–60.

Toto, K. (1992). Acute renal failure: A question of location. *American Journal of Nursing, 92*(11), 44–57.

Varella, L., & Utermohlen, V. (1993). Nutritional support for the patient with renal failure. *Critical Care Nursing Clinics of North America, 5*(1), 79–96.

Wood, J., & Bosley, C. (1995). Acute postrenal failure: Reversing the problem. *Nursing, 25*(3), 48–50.

13

Hematological and Immune Disorders

Anne-Marie Jones, M.S.N., R.N., CCRN

OBJECTIVES

- Explain the basic anatomy and physiology and the normal functioning of the hematological and immune systems.
- Describe the pathophysiological processes that affect the hematological and immune systems.
- Discuss the clinical manifestations, the nursing care, and the medical management of anemias, leukemia, disseminated intravascular coagulation, and thrombocytopenia.

- Discuss the concepts of immunity, host defenses, and immune responses.
- Discuss the various disorders of, and the treatments for, the immunocompromised patient, including human immunodeficiency virus infection and acquired immunodeficiency syndrome.
- Develop plans of care for the patient with a bleeding disorder and for the immunocompromised host.

Introduction

Whenever a patient is critically ill, the hematological and immune systems become involved. Proper functioning of these systems is necessary for basic processes, such as gas exchange, tissue perfusion, nutrition, acid-base balance, hemostasis, and protection against infection. Problems affecting these systems have been increasingly seen in critical care patients. Life-threatening disorders, such as disseminated intravascular coagulation (DIC) and acquired immunodeficiency syndrome (AIDS), are two examples of such problems. The increased use of invasive monitoring and invasive procedures has placed patients at risk

for iatrogenic infections. Additionally, progress in the treatment of malignancies and immunotherapy related to organ transplantation has introduced new problems for critical care patients and their caregivers.

Because critical care nurses are frequently challenged by hematological and immune system disorders, a basic understanding of the anatomy and physiology and the normal functioning of these two systems is necessary for comprehensive patient assessment and treatment. Knowledge of the pathological processes that affect these systems and subsequent medical and nursing interventions are necessary in order for the critical care nurse to provide the standard of care. In this chapter, hematological and immune anatomy and physiology are reviewed. Pathophysiology, medical treatment, and nursing management of selected disorders are then discussed.

Review of Hematological Anatomy and Physiology

The hematological system, through its various components, is involved in many cellular processes. In addition to transporting oxygen, carbon dioxide, nutrients, and waste, the blood is vital in hemostasis, temperature regulation, acid-base balance, and defense against infection.

HEMATOPOIESIS AND THE HEMATOLOGICAL FUNCTION OF ORGANS

Hematopoiesis is the formation and development of blood cells. Theoretically, all blood cells are derived from hematopoietic stem cells, and these cells differentiate into erythrocytes (red blood cells [RBCs]), leukocytes (white blood cells [WBCs]), or thrombocytes (platelets) (Fig. 13–1). The hormone erythropoietin stimulates the formation and differentiation of RBCs, whereas a substance known as thrombopoietin regulates the production and maturation of platelets. The bone marrow is the site of blood cell production. In young children, most bones are filled with blood-forming red marrow; in adults, productive bone marrow is found in the vertebrae, skull, chest cage, ilium, and proximal long bones (Guyton, 1991).

The spleen is a highly vascular organ that is involved in the production of lymphocytes; the filtering and destruction of erythrocytes; the filtering and trapping of foreign matter, including bacteria and viruses; and the storage of blood. Although it is not necessary for survival, the spleen plays an important role in hemostasis and protection against infection.

The liver produces clotting factors, produces bile from RBC breakdown, and detoxifies many substances in the blood; its proper functioning is essential for normal hemostasis and metabolism. The liver filters and stores blood in addition to its many other metabolic functions (Guyton, 1991).

The thymus gland and lymph nodes are also part of the hematopoietic system; they are primarily involved in immunological functions.

CHARACTERISTICS OF BLOOD

Blood volume varies depending on such physiological factors as weight, sex, pregnancy, body position, age, and nutritional status, and on such environmental factors as temperature and altitude. It represents approximately 8% of body weight. In the adult male, about 5 L of blood is generally present; in the adult female, about 3.5 to 4.5 L. In an adult with a blood volume of 5 L, 4500 ml is in the systemic circuit. Of this, about 76% is in the veins and venules, 18% is in the arteries, and 6% is in the capillaries. The pulmonary circulation contains the remaining 500 ml of blood: 24% is in the arteries, 50% is in the capillaries, and 30% is in the veins and venules (Jackson and Jones, 1988b).

The specific gravity of blood normally ranges from 1.048 to 1.066 and depends to a large extent on the number of circulating RBCs. The higher the specific gravity, the more viscous the blood. The degree of viscosity affects the blood flow: the higher the viscosity, the slower the flow. Problems, such as abnormal clotting, are more likely to occur in the presence of sluggish blood flow.

In a normal state, arterial blood is bright red, and venous blood is darker. The depth of color reflects the degree of hemoglobin oxygenation. The osmotic pressure of blood, which is determined by the amount of salts, glucose, waste, dissolved crystalloids, and plasma proteins present, is maintained within normal limits by the kidneys. It averages 300 mOsm/kg of water.

The pH, or the hydrogen ion concentration, must remain within a narrow range in order for homeostasis to be maintained. The normal range is 7.35 to 7.45, which is slightly alkaline. Various buffering mechanisms in the body are involved in maintaining the pH within a normal range.

COMPONENTS OF BLOOD

Plasma

The blood contains both circulating cells and plasma (Fig. 13–2). Plasma, a pale yellow liquid, makes up about 55% of total blood volume and is composed of serum and fibrinogen, which is a blood protein. Plasma contains a large number of substances, the highest percentage of weight being made up of the plasma proteins: albumin, serum globulins, fibrinogen, prothrombin, and plasminogen. These proteins participate in various functions, including coagulation, blood clot dissolution, wound healing, transport of various substances, and maintenance of intravascular blood volume through osmotic pressure (Jackson and Jones, 1988b).

Cells

Cells constitute the remaining 45% of blood volume and include erythrocytes, leukocytes, and platelets (Table 13–1).

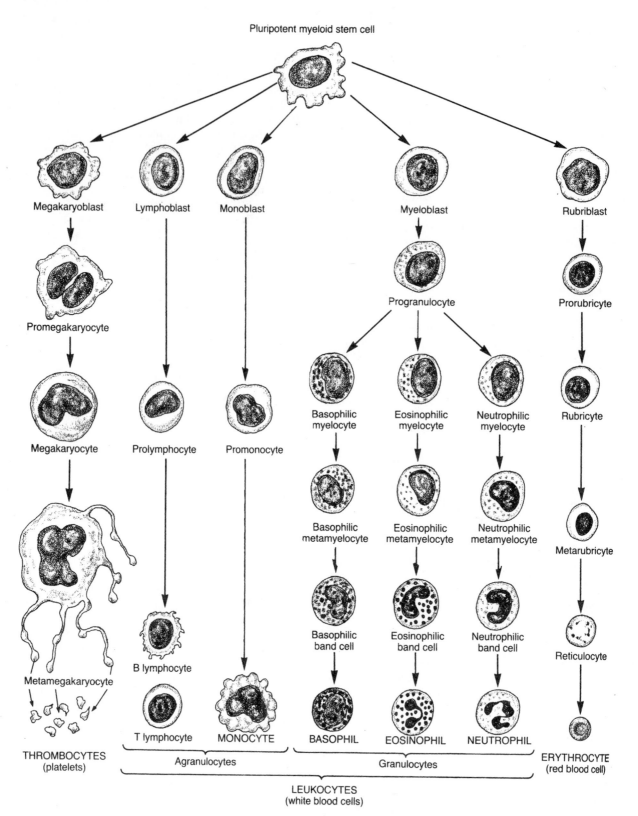

Pluripotent myeloid stem cell

Megakaryoblast

Lymphoblast

Monoblast

Myeloblast

Rubriblast

Promegakaryocyte

Progranulocyte

Prorubricyte

Megakaryocyte

Prolymphocyte

Promonocyte

Basophilic
myelocyte

Eosinophilic
myelocyte

Neutrophilic
myelocyte

Rubricyte

Basophilic
metamyelocyte

Eosinophilic
metamyelocyte

Neutrophilic
metamyelocyte

Metarubricyte

B lymphocyte

Basophilic
band cell

Eosinophilic
band cell

Neutrophilic
band cell

Reticulocyte

Metamegakaryocyte

T lymphocyte

MONOCYTE

BASOPHIL

EOSINOPHIL

NEUTROPHIL

THROMBOCYTES
(platelets)

Agranulocytes

Granulocytes

ERYTHROCYTE
(red blood cell)

LEUKOCYTES
(white blood cells)

Figure 13–1. Origin, development, and structure of thrombocytes, leukocytes, and erythrocytes from the pluripotent stem cell. (From Pavel, J., Plunkett, A., & Sink, B. (1993). Basic concepts of hematology. In J. M. Black, & E. Matassarin-Jacobs (Eds.), *Luckmann and Sorensen's medical-surgical nursing* (4th ed.) (p. 1320). Philadelphia: W. B. Saunders Co.)

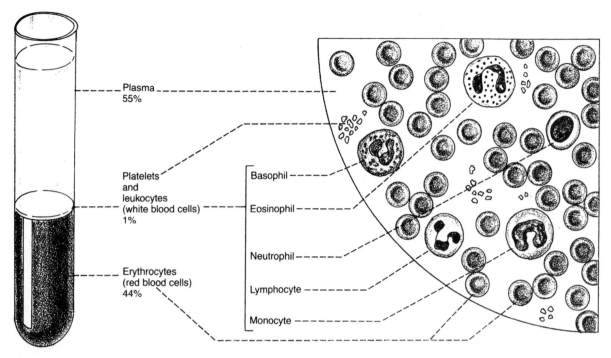

Figure 13–2. Composition of blood. (Adapted from Pavel, J., Plunkett, A., & Sink, B. (1993). Basic concepts of hematology. In J. M. Black, & E. Matassarin-Jacobs (Eds.), *Luckmann and Sorensen's medical-surgical nursing* (4th ed.) (p. 1319). Philadelphia: W. B. Saunders Co.)

Erythrocytes

Erythrocytes (RBCs) are flexible biconcave discs without nuclei whose primary component is hemoglobin. Because of their unique configuration, RBCs can travel at high speeds and can bend, twist, and elongate in order to facilitate passage through small areas and to expose more surface area for gas exchange. For each milliliter of blood, approximately 5 million RBCs exist; they have a life span of about 120 days (Jackson, 1988a).

Red blood cells are generated from precursor stem cells under the influence of growth factors and erythropoietin. Erythropoietin is secreted by the kidney in response to hypoxia and anemia (Jackson and Jones, 1988b).

Oxygen transport is the main function of erythrocytes. Hemoglobin binds with oxygen in the lungs and transports it to the tissues. The affinity of hemoglobin for oxygen depends on several factors, including blood pH, temperature, and concentration of 2,3-diphosphoglycerate (2,3-DPG). Erythrocytes are also vital in the maintenance of acid-base balance in the body (Jackson and Jones, 1988b).

Reticulocytes are immature RBCs. Maturation of RBCs takes 4 to 5 days. When the demand for RBCs is great, as in hemorrhage or hemolysis, many of the cells released from the marrow are not mature, and an increase in reticulocytes is seen. Reticulocytes circulate about 24 hours before maturing (Guyton, 1991). If the demand for RBCs continues or increases, an increase in normoblasts may be seen; these cells are even more immature (Jackson and Jones, 1988b).

The hematocrit value is an expression of the ratio of RBCs to plasma. In males, a normal hematocrit value is approximately 45%; in females, 40%. The normal hematocrit value, however, has a wide range and is affected by many factors, such as the level of hydration and the altitude at which the patient lives. Hemoglobin values range between 14 and 18 g/dl in the male and 12 to 16 g/dl in the female. In laboratory studies, the RBC count, hematocrit value, and hemoglobin value usually follow the same trends. For example, increased values in all three parameters occur in dehydration, hemoconcentration resulting from blood loss, and polycythemia. Values are decreased in anemia, fluid overload, and recent hemorrhage.

Leukocytes

Leukocytes (WBCs) are mobile cells that are larger and less numerous than RBCs and have nuclei. Various leukocytes exist; they are specialized for dif-

Table 13–1. FUNCTIONS AND NORMAL VALUES OF BLOOD CELLS

Cell	Functions	Normal Value	Alterations
Erythrocyte (red blood cell (RBC))	Respiration Oxygen transport Acid-base balance	5 million/μl	Increased: polycythemia, dehydration Decreased: anemia, fluid overload, hemorrhage
Leukocyte (white blood cell (WBC))	Immmune response Defend against infection, foreign tissue	4500–11,000/μl	Increased: inflammation, tissue necrosis, leukemia Decreased: bone marrow depression (radiation, immune disorders)
Granular leukocytes Neutrophils	Polymorphonuclear neutrophils Phagocytosis of invading organisms	50–70% of WBCs	Increased: inflammation, infection, surgery, myocardial infarction Decreased: aplastic anemia, hepatitis, some pharmacological agents
Eosinophils	Defend against parasites; detoxification of foreign proteins Phagocytosis	1–5% of WBCs	Increased: allergic attacks, autoimmune diseases, parasitic infections Decreased: stress reactions
Basophils	Release heparin, serotonin, and histamine in allergic reactions; inflammatory response	0–1% of WBCs	Increased: postsplenectomy, hemolytic anemia, radiation
Nongranular leukocytes Monocytes	Mature into macrophages; phagocytosis of necrotic tissue, debris, foreign particles	1–8% of WBCs	Increased: bacterial, parasitic, and some viral infections
Lymphocytes	Defend against microorganisms	20–40% of WBCs	Increased: bacterial and viral infections, lymphocytic leukemia Decreased: chemotherapy, immunodeficiencies
B lymphocytes	Humoral immunity and production of antibodies		
T lymphocytes	Cell-mediated immunity		
Thrombocytes (platelets)	Blood clotting; hemostasis	150,000–400,000/μl	Increased: polycythemia vera, postsplenectomy Decreased: leukemia, bone marrow failure, DIC, hemorrhage, hypersplenism

DIC = disseminated intravascular coagulation.

ferent functions and are classified by their structure and their affinity for certain dyes. The normal amount of WBCs ranges from 4500 to 11,000/μl of blood in the adult. Although WBCs are transported in the blood, many reside in the tissues. An increase in the total WBC count may be seen in inflammation, tissue necrosis, and leukemia. A decreased total WBC count reflects bone marrow depression, as may result from radiation, viral infections, and immune disorders.

Primarily involved in the body's immune response, WBCs play a key role in the defense against infectious organisms and foreign antigens. They produce and transport factors such as antibodies that are vital in maintaining immunity. Although varied and possessing specialized functions, WBCs work in an integrated fashion to protect the body.

White blood cells are classified into two categories: granulocytes (polymorphonuclear leukocytes, polymorphonuclear neutrophils) and nongranular leukocytes. The polymorphonuclear neutrophils include

neutrophils, eosinophils, and basophils. Nongranular leukocytes include monocytes and lymphocytes (see Fig. 13–1 and Table 13–1).

Granulocytes

Neutrophils. Neutrophils, the most numerous of the granulocytes, constitute 50 to 70% of the total white cell count. They are further broken down into segmented neutrophils, in which filaments in the cell give the nuclei an appearance of having lobes, and band neutrophils, which are immature and have a thicker or U-shaped nucleus. Normally, segmented neutrophils make up approximately 56% of WBCs, whereas band neutrophils constitute only about 3% (Jackson and Jones, 1988b). The phrase "a shift to the left" refers to an increased number of "bands," or band neutrophils, as compared with mature neutrophils on a complete blood count report. This finding generally indicates an acute infectious process that draws on the WBC reserves in the bone marrow, causing less mature forms to be released. Likewise, a "shift to the right" indicates an increased number of circulating mature neutrophils (Gawlikowski, 1992). Infection, surgical procedures, myocardial infarction, or any inflammatory process may cause an increase in neutrophils. An unusually high proportion of mature neutrophils may be seen in such disorders as liver disease, cancer of the gastrointestinal tract, pernicious anemia, and chronic morphine addiction, as well as after tissue breakdown. A decrease in neutrophils occurs with certain disorders, such as hepatitis, aplastic anemia, and various viral infections, as well as after the administration of pharmacological agents, such as sulfonamides and antihistamines (Chernecky et al., 1993).

The survival time of neutrophils and the other granulocytes is short—once released from the bone marrow, they circulate in the blood 4 to 8 hours before migrating to the tissues, where they live another 4 to 5 days (Guyton, 1991). When serious infection is present, neutrophils may live only a few hours while they phagocytize infectious organisms. Because of this short life span, drugs that affect rapidly multiplying cells (e.g., chemotherapeutic agents) quickly decrease the neutrophil count and thus alter the patient's ability to fight infection.

Neutrophils are attracted to and migrate to areas of inflammation or bacterial invasion by the process of *chemotaxis,* which is mediated by substances released at the site of injury. There they ingest and kill invading microorganisms by *phagocytosis* (Fig. 13–3).

Phagocytosis is the process by which antigens and damaged cells are removed from the tissues; this process is carried out by granulocytes (especially neutrophils) and macrophages (matured monocytes). These phagocytes operate on a "search and destroy" principle. Once they have been attracted to an area by chemotaxis, a process called *opsonization* occurs, in which antibody and complement attach to the phagocytic cells in order to enhance phagocytosis of bacteria. Once the bacteria have been engulfed, they are killed and digested within the cell by lysosomal enzymes. By the process of phagocytosis, pus formation, or *suppuration*, occurs. Phagocytosis is a rapid process that is initiated within minutes of cellular injury (Fidler, 1988).

Phagocytosis also occurs in the lymphoreticular organs, which include the lymph nodes, thymus, spleen, and liver. When infectious organisms escape the local immune response, they enter the bloodstream and lymphatic channels. In the bloodstream, they are engulfed and destroyed by macrophages in the liver and spleen; in the lymph system, pathogenic substances are filtered by the lymph nodes and are phagocytized by tissue macrophages. Here, they may also stimulate the immune response by the lymphoid cells (Guyton, 1991).

Eosinophils. Eosinophils are larger than neutrophils and make up 1 to 5% of the normal WBC count. They are important in the defense against parasites and are thought to be involved in the detoxification of foreign proteins (Jackson and Jones, 1988b). Eosino-

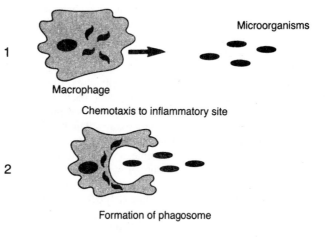

1 — Macrophage / Microorganisms — Chemotaxis to inflammatory site

2 — Formation of phagosome

3 — Release of lysosomal enzymes

Figure 13–3. Chemotaxis and phagocytosis. (Adapted from Janusek, L. (1993). Structure and function of the immune system. In J. M. Black, & E. Matassarin-Jacobs (Eds.), *Luckmann and Sorensen's medical-surgical nursing* (4th ed.) (p. 533). Philadelphia: W. B. Saunders Co.)

phils are found largely in the tissues of the intestinal tract and lungs; their numbers increase during an allergic reaction. Like neutrophils, eosinophils migrate to areas of infection and inflammation through chemotaxis; in these areas, they participate in phagocytosis. Eosinophils contain bactericidal substances and lysosomal enzymes that aid in the destruction of invading organisms. An increase in circulating eosinophils is seen during allergic attacks, autoimmune diseases, and parasitic infections (Jackson, 1988a). A decrease in circulating eosinophils may occur in severe stress reactions because of the high levels of epinephrine and adrenocorticotropic hormone (Chernecky et al., 1993).

Basophils. The third type of granulocyte is the basophil, which has large granules that contain heparin, serotonin, and histamine. Basophils participate in the body's inflammatory and allergic responses by releasing these substances. Basophils, which constitute zero to 1% of the total WBC count, are not phagocytes but play an important role in acute systemic allergic reactions as well as in the inflammatory response. They, like the other granulocytes, have a short life span. An increase in basophils may occur after splenectomy, with radiation therapy, and in hemolytic anemia (Chernecky et al., 1993).

Nongranular Leukocytes

Monocytes. Monocytes are the largest of the leukocytes, although they constitute only 1 to 8% of the total WBC count. Once they migrate from the bloodstream into the tissues, monocytes mature into tissue macrophages, which are phagocytes that function as "seek and destroy" scavengers. In the lung, these tissue macrophages are known as alveolar macrophages; in the liver, they are Kupffer's cells; in connective tissue, they are histiocytes (Guyton, 1991). In addition to "eating" large foreign particles and cell fragments, macrophages are vital in the phagocytosis of necrotic tissue and debris. Like eosinophils, macrophages contain lysosomal enzymes and bactericidal substances. When activated by antigens, macrophages also secrete substances called monokines, which act as chemical communicators between the cells involved in the immune response. For example, a monokine known as interleukin-1 influences the growth and division of lymphocytes, a process that enhances immunity. Although monocytes may circulate only 36 hours, they can survive for months or even years as tissue macrophages (Guyton, 1991). Monocyte values are increased in bacterial, parasitic, and some viral infections, as well as in collagen diseases and some malignancies (Jackson, 1988a).

Lymphocytes. Approximately 20 to 40% of the total WBC count is made up of lymphocytes in the adult. Lymphocytes are vital in the body's defense against bacteria, viruses, and other microorganisms;

they also play a major role in tumor immunity (surveillance for abnormal cells), delayed hypersensitivity reactions, autoimmune diseases, and foreign tissue rejection. Lymphocytes are primarily concerned with the specific immune responses and participate in two types of immunity: humoral immunity, which is mediated by B lymphocytes, and cellular immunity, which is mediated by T lymphocytes. B lymphocytes, or B cells, originate in the bone marrow and are thought to mature there also. Their name is derived from the bursa of Fabricius, the site of B-cell maturation in birds. T lymphocytes, or T cells, compose most of the circulating lymphocytes; they also live longer than B cells and participate in long-term immunity. T cells are produced in the bone marrow but migrate to the thymus for maturation (Fig. 13–4). After maturation, T cells migrate to other lymphoid tissue or to the bloodstream, where they "patrol" for antigens. A third type of lymphocyte, the natural killer cell, is responsible for surveillance and destruction of virus-infected and malignant cells. The life span of lymphocytes may be close to a year or more, while they circulate in and out of tissues (Guyton, 1991). Lymphocytes are increased in bacterial and viral infections, multiple myeloma, and lymphocytic leukemia. A decrease is seen in patients taking chemotherapeutic drugs, in those in immunodeficiency states, such as AIDS, and in those experiencing some forms of sepsis (Jackson, 1988a). The immune response and the function of lymphocytes are covered in depth in the immune anatomy and physiology section.

Platelets (Thrombocytes)

Platelets, or thrombocytes, are the smallest of the formed elements of the blood. A normal platelet count ranges from 150,000 to 400,000/μl of blood. Platelets are necessary for blood clotting and hemostasis. They adhere to injured blood vessel walls and other surfaces, where they occlude rents and tears, thereby preventing blood loss. Platelets also release mediators necessary for the clotting process. These substances include epinephrine and serotonin, which contribute to vasospasm; adenosine diphosphate, which is necessary for platelet adhesion and aggregation; and calcium and phospholipids, which are necessary in various steps of the clotting process.

Adhesion refers to the attachment of platelets to nonplatelet surfaces; *aggregation* is the adherence of platelets to each other for the formation of plugs. Platelets have a life span of 7 to 14 days and are continually being used in the repair of small vascular injuries that occur normally. Most are circulating throughout the blood, although the spleen normally stores up to 20% of platelets.

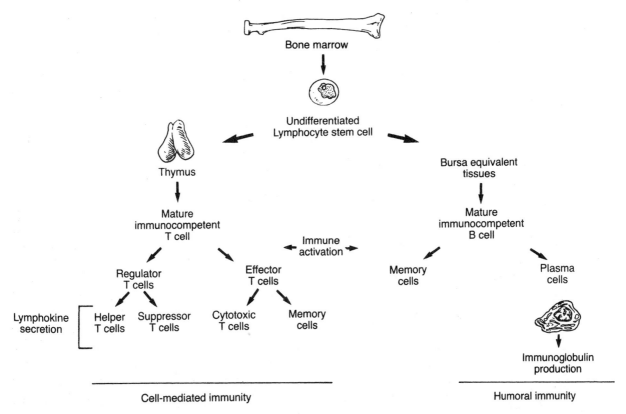

Figure 13–4. The pathway of lymphocyte maturation. (Adapted from Janusek, L. (1993). Structure and function of the immune system. In J. M. Black, & E. Matassarin-Jacobs (Eds.), *Luckmann and Sorensen's medical-surgical nursing* (4th ed.) (p. 533). Philadelphia: W. B. Saunders Co.)

Thrombocytopenia is a deficiency of platelets; *relative thrombocytopenia* refers to a functional abnormality of platelets, although the count may be normal. Platelets are increased in polycythemia vera, in leukemia, after splenectomy, in some malignant diseases, and as a compensatory mechanism after hemorrhage. A decrease in platelets is seen in bone marrow failure, hypersplenism, DIC, hemorrhage, and certain autoimmune diseases associated with increased destruction of platelets (Jackson, 1988a).

HEMOSTASIS

Hemostasis is the prevention of blood loss, or the process by which the body arrests bleeding. It involves several events and processes that are interrelated and occur both simultaneously and sequentially.

When injury occurs to a blood vessel that results in the escape of blood, the following physical events take place: (1) vascular spasm or vasoconstriction occur, (2) exposure of endothelial surfaces causes platelets to become sticky in order to enhance adhesion, (3) platelets aggregate to form plugs and release sub-

stances that facilitate the coagulation process, (4) a blood clot is formed through the activation of plasma coagulation factors, (5) clot retraction occurs in order to stabilize the clot, (6) fibrous repair of damaged tissue is initiated, and (7) the clot is eventually lysed (Jackson and Jones, 1988b) (Fig. 13–5).

COAGULATION

The function of the body's blood coagulation system is the formation of a fibrin clot on the surface of the platelet plug. It involves a series of biochemical reactions that ultimately convert fibrinogen to fibrin, thereby forming the fibrin clot. Fibrin threads trap platelets, RBCs, and plasma as the clot forms. The clot occludes the vessel lumen, then retracts, pulling the vessel edges together.

Coagulation occurs by two distinct pathways, the intrinsic and the extrinsic, which share a common "final" pathway, where the blood clot is formed (Fig. 13–6). These separate pathways are basically alternate modes of activating a critical clotting factor, factor X. Both pathways begin with an initiating event and have

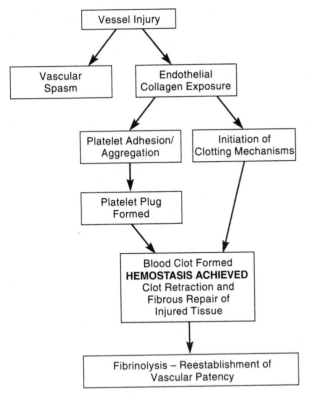

Figure 13–5. Hemostasis.

a cascade sequence of factor activation. Each factor is activated by a preceding reaction.

The coagulation factors are mostly plasma proteins that circulate as inactive enzymes (Table 13–2). With the exception of factors VIII and XIII, synthesis of these factors takes place in the liver. Hence, liver disease or injury can lead to problems with blood coagulation and bleeding. Several of the factors are vitamin K dependent, and thus a vitamin K deficiency can also lead to bleeding problems. Coagulation factors are designated by roman numerals according to their order of discovery, not their position in the clotting cascade.

Intrinsic Pathway

All factors needed for clot formation are contained in circulating blood. When blood is exposed to subendothelial collagen or is "injured," factor XII is activated to XIIa, which initiates coagulation via the intrinsic pathway. Factor XI is then converted to XIa, which, in the presence of calcium, activates factor IX. The sequence continues as factors IXa, VIII, calcium, and platelet phospholipids participate to activate factor X. The common pathway is thus triggered.

Extrinsic Pathway

When tissue injury occurs, a substance known as tissue factor, or thromboplastin (factor III), and phospholipids are released. The presence of calcium activates factor VII, which converts factor X to Xa; thus, the final common pathway for coagulation is entered.

Common Pathway

In the common pathway, activated factor X (Xa) converts prothrombin (factor II) to thrombin in the presence of calcium and other cofactors. Thrombin, a powerful procoagulant, then converts fibrinogen (factor I) to fibrin, which forms a fibrin mesh and blood clot.

Thrombin also stimulates platelet aggregation, activates and enhances the activity of other clotting factors, and initiates the fibrinolytic system by converting plasminogen to plasmin.

Coagulation Antagonists and Clot Lysis

A system of checks and balances exists in order to maintain a balance between clot formation and bleeding. Of the procoagulant forces, thrombin is the most powerful. Enough prothrombin is present in 10 ml of blood to clot 2500 ml of plasma in only 15 seconds (Jackson and Jones, 1988b). Thus, anticoagulant forces must be effective in preventing abnormal clotting.

Normal vascular endothelium is smooth and intact, thereby preventing the collagen exposure that initiates the intrinsic clotting pathway. In addition, negatively charged proteins are present on the endothelium that repel positively charged clotting factors. Rapid blood flow serves to dilute and disperse clotting factors. Clotting factors that are not contained within a formed clot are filtered and removed from the circulation by the liver. Several plasma proteins are present that localize clotting to the site of injury; they include antiplasmin and antithrombin III. However, the most potent anticoagulant forces are the fibrin threads, which absorb 85 to 90% of thrombin during clot formation, and antithrombin III, which inactivates thrombin that is not contained within the clot (Guyton, 1991). Heparin, which is produced in small quantities by basophils and tissue mast cells, acts as a potent anticoagulant. Heparin combines with antithrombin III to greatly increase the effectiveness of the latter; this complex removes several of the activated coagulation factors from the blood (Guyton, 1991).

Once hemostasis has been accomplished and blood vessel integrity has been restored, blood flow

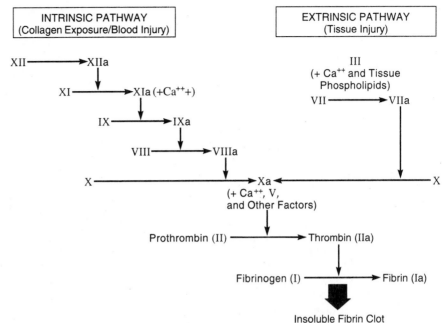

Figure 13–6. Coagulation pathways—intrinsic, extrinsic, and common.

must be reestablished. This goal is accomplished by the fibrinolytic system, by which clots are broken down (lysed) and removed. Fibrinolysis is mediated by plasmin, an enzyme that digests fibrinogen and fibrin (Fig. 13–7). A plasma protein, plasminogen, is the inactive form of plasmin; it is incorporated into the blood clot as it forms and cannot initiate clot lysis until it is activated. Many substances found in the body are capable of activating plasminogen, including thrombin and other activated clotting factors, lysosomal enzymes, urokinase (which is found in the urine), and streptokinase (which is released from streptococcal bacteria).

Fibrinolysis is active within the microcirculation,

Table 13–2. BLOOD COAGULATION FACTORS

Factor	Common Names	Comments
I	Fibrinogen	Synthesized in liver
II	Prothrombin	Synthesized in liver; vitamin K dependent
III	Tissue thromboplastin Tissue factor	Extrinsic pathway's first factor
IV	Calcium	Necessary in several steps of coagulation
V	Labile factor	Synthesized in liver
VI	Not assigned	
VII	Proconvertin Stable factor	Synthesized in liver; extrinsic pathway
VIII	Antihemophilic factor A	Required in intrinsic pathway
IX	Plasma thromboplastin component (PTC) Christmas factor Antihemophilic factor B	Synthesized in liver; vitamin K dependent
X	Stuart-Prower factor	Synthesized in liver; vitamin K dependent; intrinsic and extrinsic pathways
XI	Plasma thromboplastin antecedent (PTA) Antihemophilic factor C	Required in intrinsic pathway
XII	Hageman factor	Intrinsic pathway's first factor
XIII	Fibrin-stabilizing factor	Stabilizes clot formation

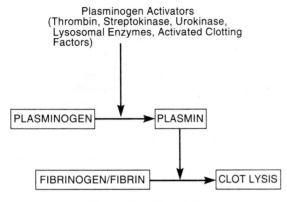

Figure 13–7. Fibrinolysis.

where it maintains the patency of the capillary beds. Larger vessels contain less plasminogen activator; this characteristic may predispose them to clot formation (Jackson and Jones, 1988b).

When plasmin digests fibrinogen, fragments are produced that function as potent anticoagulants. These fragments are known as fibrin split products or fibrin degradation products. In cases of excessive clotting and clot lysis, these fibrin split products contribute to the coagulopathy. The fibrin split products are not normally present in the circulation but are seen in some hematological disorders as well as with thrombolytic therapy (e.g., the administration of streptokinase or tissue plasminogen activator).

Laboratory studies that evaluate coagulation are listed in Table 13–3.

Assessment of the Hematological System

Any hematological alteration can affect such vital body functions as tissue perfusion, respiration, and hemostasis. A thorough hematological assessment is performed in order to determine the existence of, or the risk for, hematological problems.

Table 13–3. COAGULATION PROFILE STUDIES

Test	Normal Value	Comments
Lee-White clotting time	6–12 min	Nonspecific for clotting abnormalities
Partial thromboplastin time	60–80 sec	General indicator of blood's clotting ability—evaluates intrinsic pathway
Activated partial thromboplastin time	30–45 sec	Used to monitor heparin therapy and detect bleeding tendencies, hemorrhagic disorders Increased in anticoagulation therapy, liver disease, vitamin K deficiency, DIC
Prothrombin time	11–16 sec	Evaluates extrinsic pathway; used to monitor oral anticoagulant therapy Increased in warfarin sodium therapy, liver disease, vitamin K deficiency, obstructive jaundice
Thrombin time	10–15 sec	Used to detect fibrinogen abnormalities, monitor heparin therapy Increased in fibrinogen abnormalities, multiple myeloma, cirrhosis of liver, heparin therapy
Fibrinogen level	200–400 mg/dl	Decreased in DIC and fibrinogen disorders
Fibrin degradation products	<10 μg/ml	Evaluates hematologic disorders Increased in DIC, fibrinolysis, thrombolytic therapy
Platelet count	150,000–400,000/μl	Measures number of circulating platelets Decreased in thrombocytopenia
Platelet aggregation test	3–5 min	Measures platelet adherence ability Decreased in von Willebrand's disease, acute leukemia, idiopathic thrombocytopenic purpura, liver cirrhosis, aspirin use
Bleeding time	1–4 min	Evaluates platelet function Increased in thrombocytopenia and aspirin therapy
Calcium	9–11 mg/dl	Decreased with massive transfusions of stored blood

A complete health history is obtained, including allergies, past illnesses (specifically, hematological problems), hospitalizations, surgeries, and relevant family history. The nurse is alert for a history of anemia, excessive bleeding, blood clots, delayed wound healing, recurrent infections, alcoholism, or renal or liver disease. Surgical procedures, such as splenectomy, tumor removal, valve replacement, and gastrointestinal resection, can alter normal hematological function. If the patient has received transfusions of blood or blood products, the nurse determines why the procedures were performed and whether any reaction occurred. The nurse determines what medications (prescription and over-the-counter drugs) the patient is taking, including anticoagulants, drugs containing aspirin, nonsteroidal anti-inflammatory drugs, and bone marrow suppressants (e.g., chemotherapeutic agents). Lifestyle factors that can alter hematological function include nutrition, history of alcohol or substance abuse, and occupational exposure to chemicals or radiation (Shannon-Bodnar, 1993).

During the physical examination, the nurse notes the patient's general appearance and assesses for signs of fatigue, acute illness, or chronic disease. The patient's neurological status is assessed for changes in level of consciousness and cognition; such changes might indicate hypoxia. The patient is questioned about syncope, and his or her reflexes are evaluated. Skin color is assessed for jaundice, cyanosis, or pallor. In addition, the color of the nail beds and the presence of clubbing of fingers are assessed. Skin integrity is assessed, and signs of infection or poor healing are noted. The nurse checks for petechiae or ecchymoses, especially in pressure areas, and assesses venipuncture sites for signs of infection or bleeding. Cardiovascular assessment includes heart rate and rhythm, heart sounds, blood pressure, peripheral pulses, and presence of edema or jugular venous distention. Respiratory rate and effort are noted, as are breath sounds. The nurse assesses for abdominal pain and for liver and spleen enlargement or tenderness. The nurse also checks for any signs of bleeding from the respiratory, gastrointestinal, and urinary systems, as evidenced by frank or occult blood in respiratory or nasogastric secretions, stool, and urine. The nurse is alert to any assessment findings that indicate hypoxia, alteration in tissue perfusion, infection, or bleeding.

Diagnostic tests for hematological function include a complete blood count with differential and coagulation studies. A bone marrow aspiration and biopsy may be performed for the assessment of blood cell production and morphology of cells. The peripheral blood smear also evaluates the morphology of blood cells and can assist in the diagnosis of various anemias and blood dyscrasias (Shannon-Bodnar, 1993).

Selected Hematological Disorders

Many pathological conditions affect the hematological system, ranging from mild anemias to life-threatening bleeding disorders. In critical care, nurses see many of these disease states. The purpose of this section is to review those disorders that are most frequently seen in critical care and pose the greatest risk to the patient.

RED BLOOD CELL DISORDERS

Anemias

Pathophysiology

The term *anemia* refers to a reduction in the number of circulating RBCs or hemoglobin. Simply put, too few RBCs and/or too little hemoglobin exists for full oxygenation of the tissues. When the blood's hemoglobin content is less than that needed to meet the body's demands, tissue hypoxia results. Although symptoms may vary depending on the type, cause, or severity of anemia, the basic clinical findings are the same.

As tissues become hypoxic, 2,3-DPG increases to cause hemoglobin to release oxygen. Blood flow is redistributed to areas where oxygenation is most vital, that is, the brain and the heart.

Anemia has many causes that are frequently seen in critical care. Posthemorrhagic anemia is caused by acute or chronic blood loss, such as from gastrointestinal bleeding or severe trauma. In aplastic anemia, bone marrow failure results in the inadequate production of all blood cells, including RBCs. Hemolytic anemia is an increase in the rate of destruction of RBCs. Causes of hemolytic anemia include autoimmune diseases; hereditary states, such as sickle cell disease; trauma to cells, resulting from malfunctioning prosthetic heart valves or extracorporeal circulation; drug therapy; and certain infectious organisms (Jackson, 1988b).

Sickle cell disease, which is a form of hereditary hemolytic anemia, is occasionally seen in critical care when the patient is in crisis. Because of an abnormal amount of hemoglobin S in relation to hemoglobin A, RBCs assume a sickle or crescent shape when a decrease in the oxygen concentration, a decrease in pH, or an increase in 2,3-DPG level occurs. This sickling alters the blood viscosity, impairing flow and leading to occlusion of the microvasculature. Although the sickling is reversible with the administration of supplemental oxygen, patients carry a varying number of irreversibly sickled cells that, when removed by the body, are hemolyzed and result in anemia. Sickle cell crisis is potentially life threatening because occlusion of the microvasculature leads to hypoxia, exacerbation of sickling, anoxia, infarction, and thrombosis in tissues and organs, such as the brain, kidneys, spleen, and lungs (Belcher, 1989).

Assessment/Clinical Manifestations

Symptoms of the various anemias are related to the tissue hypoxia and the body's resulting compensatory activities; the body shunts blood away from nonvital organs (e.g., the skin and kidneys) to perfuse the vital organs. General signs and symptoms include pallor, fatigue, weakness, and lethargy. More specific assessment findings, caused by the body's attempt to compensate for the lack of oxygen in the tissues, are tachycardia, palpitations, angina, systolic murmurs, dyspnea, and tachypnea.

Posthemorrhagic anemia results in symptoms of hypovolemia, such as thirst, hypotension, and decreased urine output. Additionally, because of the altered perfusion and oxygenation of the brain, the patient may be restless and disoriented.

In addition to the aforementioned symptoms, the patient with aplastic anemia may also present with bruising, nosebleeds, petechiae, and decreased ability to fight infections. These result from thrombocytopenia and decreased WBC counts, which occur when the bone marrow fails to produce blood cells.

Assessment of the patient with hemolytic anemia may reveal jaundice, abdominal pain, and enlargement of the spleen or liver; these findings result from the increased destruction of RBCs, their sequestration (abnormal distribution in the spleen and liver), and the accumulation of breakdown products.

Patients with sickle cell anemia may also have joint swelling or pain and delayed physical and sexual development. In crisis, the sickle cell patient often has decreased urine output and peripheral edema and signs of uremia because the renal tissue perfusion is impaired as a result of sluggish blood flow.

Laboratory findings in anemia include decreased RBC count and decreased hemoglobin and hematocrit levels. The reticulocyte count is usually increased, indicating increased RBC production. Hemolytic anemia patients also have an increased bilirubin level. In aplastic anemia, the reticulocyte, platelet, and WBC counts are decreased because the marrow fails to produce any cells. In sickle cell disease, a stained blood smear reveals sickled cells.

Nursing Diagnoses

Nursing diagnoses of the anemic patient may include:

- Decreased cardiac output related to decreased circulating blood volume.
- Altered tissue perfusion related to decreased or dysfunctional RBCs and/or hemoglobin.
- Impaired gas exchange related to decreased or dysfunctional RBCs and/or hemoglobin.
- Risk for fluid volume excess/deficit related to fluid replacement and/or hemorrhage.
- Impaired skin integrity related to inadequate perfusion and tissue hypoxia.
- Pain related to tissue ischemia and microvascular occlusions.
- Risk for infection related to bone marrow failure and low WBC count.
- Risk for injury related to transfusions.
- Activity intolerance related to tissue hypoxia.

Medical Interventions

Medical treatment of anemia includes identification and removal of any causative agents or conditions, improvement of tissue oxygenation with supplemental oxygen and blood component therapy, and cardiovascular system support as needed. For certain types of anemia, other interventions may be needed, such as splenectomy for hemolytic anemia or bone marrow transplantation for aplastic anemia. In sickle cell disease, oxygenation and correction of dehydration are important for the reversal or prevention of sickling of the erythrocytes. Synthetic erythropoietin may also be used for stimulation of RBC production. Other promising therapies being researched include the use of thrombopoietin and gene therapy for congenital deficiencies.

Nursing Interventions

Nursing management of anemia is based on a continuous, thorough nursing assessment and the prescribed medical treatment.

Physical assessment in anemia is vital; monitoring of vital signs, the electrocardiogram, hemodynamics, heart and lung sounds, and peripheral pulses assists the nurse in the assessment of tissue perfusion and gas exchange. Tachycardia and orthostatic hypotension are particularly important signs that indicate that the patient is not tolerating the anemia. Additionally, mental status, urine output, and skin color and temperature are important indicators of adequate perfusion. Pain management and comfort measures are instituted as needed. Scrupulous skin care is given in order to prevent tissue breakdown, and signs of infection are monitored closely. For patients at risk for further blood loss, bleeding precautions are instituted. Interventions for patients at risk for bleeding or infection are listed later in this chapter.

Laboratory results, such as the complete blood

count, are carefully monitored. Other vital nursing interventions include promotion of rest; skin care; careful administration of blood components, drug therapy, and intravenous (IV) fluids; and monitoring of patient response to the therapy.

Patient Outcomes

The following are the goals of care for the patient with anemia:

- Optimal tissue perfusion, oxygenation, and gas exchange will be maintained, as evidenced by the patient's response to treatment, e.g., normal vital signs, hemodynamics, mental status and organ function, and ability to tolerate activity.
- The complete blood count will reflect an adequate RBC and hemoglobin count.
- The patient will have adequate hydration and absence of transfusion reaction, pain, and infection.

WHITE BLOOD CELL DISORDERS

Many pathological conditions exist that can be classified as WBC disorders. Depending on the cells or tissues affected, the conditions include neutropenia, various types of leukemias, lymphomas, and malignant myeloma. Leukemia is briefly addressed here. Lymphomas and malignant myeloma are not discussed in this text; for this information, the reader is referred to a more comprehensive reference on oncological disorders.

Neutropenia

Pathophysiology

Neutropenia occurs when the absolute neutrophil count is less than 1000 cells/μl of blood, resulting from the suppression of the bone marrow and its failure to produce adequate neutrophils (Jassak et al., 1993). Patients with such low counts are predisposed to infections because of the body's reduced phagocytic ability. Neutropenia may be caused by acute or overwhelming infections, radiation, exposure to chemicals and drugs (benzenes, vinblastine, phenytoin, chloramphenicol), or other disease states (aplastic anemia, multiple myeloma, uremia).

Assessment/Clinical Manifestations

Fever may be the only sign of infection in the patient with neutropenia. Without phagocytosis, inflammation, heat, redness, and pain may be absent. Other clinical signs may include fatigue and weakness,

chills, oral ulcers, sore throat, diarrhea, and tachycardia. Areas of heavy bacterial colonization (e.g., oral mucosa, perineal area, and venipuncture and catheter sites) have a high risk of infection. The complications of neutropenia are most commonly septicemia and pneumonia, which result from the body's inability to defend itself adequately against infection.

Nursing Diagnoses

Two important nursing diagnoses in neutropenia are

- Risk for infection.
- Altered oral mucous membranes.

Medical Interventions

Medical treatment of neutropenia has primarily been aimed at preventing and treating infection. Anti-infective agents and reverse isolation may be ordered; granulocyte transfusions may be necessary for the replacement of deficient cells. New therapies are being developed and researched in order to enhance and hasten bone marrow recovery—for example, the use of granulocyte-macrophage colony-stimulating factor and other naturally occurring substances (Dudjak and Fleck, 1991).

Nursing Interventions

Interventions for protecting the patient from infection include close observation for signs of infection, alertness to the presence of fever, maintenance of skin integrity, promotion of adequate fluid and nutritional intake, assurance of perineal hygiene, use of reverse isolation as needed, and administration of antibiotics (see Nursing Care Plan for the Immunocompromised Patient). The patient's diet should not include raw fruits and vegetables, because these are potential sources of infection. Scrupulous oral hygiene is necessary in order to promote the integrity of mucous membranes and to prevent infection. *The most crucial intervention in the prevention of infection is consistent proper hand washing.*

Patient Outcomes

The following are the goals of care for the patient with neutropenia:

- Patient will remain free from infection, as evidenced by absence of fever, redness, swelling, pain, and heat.
- Laboratory study results (WBCs, differential,

urinalysis, cultures) will remain within normal limits.
- Adventitious breath sounds will be absent.
- Chest x-ray study will show no infiltrates.

Leukemia

Pathophysiology

Leukemia is a malignant disease that involves the blood-forming tissues and is characterized by a proliferation of abnormal or immature leukocytes. These cells accumulate in the lymphoid tissue and eventually infiltrate tissues throughout the body, involving all organs. The leukemias are classified by the type of cell and tissue involved as well as the course and duration of the disease. For instance, acute lymphocytic leukemia causes hyperplasia of lymphoid tissue and has a rapid onset and progression. Leukemia results in a loss of normal WBCs, thereby predisposing the patient to infection, as well as anemia and coagulation disorders because the bone marrow is unable to produce normal cells.

Assessment/Clinical Manifestations

Clinically, the patient with leukemia may present with signs of recurrent infection or bleeding. The abnormal or immature WBCs are not able to protect the body from infectious microorganisms, and the marrow fails to produce sufficient numbers of platelets. Mouth ulcers, pneumonia, gum bleeding, and epistaxis may be noted. Fatigue, lethargy, weakness, and pallor may result from anemia; the patient may also experience tachycardia and shortness of breath. Anorexia and weight loss may also be present. Other symptoms vary depending on the organ involved and include decreased urine output, neurological changes, and enlargement of the liver, spleen, and lymph nodes.

Laboratory studies reveal an increased WBC count ($\geq$15,000 to 500,000/μl) and a decreased number of RBCs and platelets. Massive numbers of WBCs are present on bone marrow biopsy (Belcher, 1989).

Nursing Diagnoses

Nursing diagnoses in leukemia include

- Risk for infection.
- Altered tissue perfusion related to anemia.
- Risk for injury (bleeding).
- Ineffective individual or family coping.
- Anxiety related to fear of dying, procedures, and the unknown.
- Anticipatory grieving.

Medical Interventions

Medical treatment of leukemia is aimed at stopping the proliferation of abnormal leukocytes and their infiltration into tissues. Medications depend on the classification of leukemia but may include antineoplastics, such as methotrexate and corticosteroids. Radiation may be used to kill leukemic cells in the bone marrow. When blood flow is severely compromised as a result of leukocytosis, high blood viscosity, and abnormal coagulation, leukopheresis may be performed in order to quickly lower the WBC count, although the WBC count is preferably lowered with the use of chemotherapeutic agents (Schiffer, 1991). Bone marrow transplantation is performed in order to provide normal productive tissue. Transfusions may be necessary for the correction of anemia or coagulation disorders. Infection is treated with antibiotics; reverse isolation techniques are instituted in order to protect the patient from infection. Additionally, IV hydration is maintained, and analgesics may be prescribed in order to relieve pain.

Nursing Interventions

Infection in this population must be prevented whenever possible. The nurse must continually assess for the presence of infection. Methods for the prevention and assessment of infection are the same as those listed for neutropenia. (Also see the Nursing Care Plan for the Immunocompromised Patient.) Interventions for the bleeding patient are covered in depth under bleeding disorders. Psychosocial support of patients with leukemia and their families is ongoing and includes allowing the expression of feelings and fostering communication. Other members of the health care team, such as social workers and clergy, are available to offer emotional support. Significant others are included in patient teaching and in patient care if possible.

Patient Outcomes

The following are the goals of care for the patient with leukemia:

- Patient will remain free of infection and bleeding, maintain optimal tissue perfusion, remain comfortable and free of pain, and be adequately hydrated and nourished.
- Health care providers will promptly recognize and treat any signs of infection, bleeding, pain, or dehydration.
- The patient and family will be able to cope effectively and receive adequate emotional support and education.

BLEEDING DISORDERS

Patients with difficulty maintaining hemostasis are frequently seen in critical care. These bleeding disorders, referred to as coagulopathies, may be caused by problems involving platelets, coagulation factors, or other pathological states. They may be inherited, such as hemophilia or von Willebrand's disease, or acquired, such as DIC and vitamin K deficiency.

Disseminated Intravascular Coagulation

Pathophysiology

Disseminated intravascular coagulation is a serious bleeding disorder that is characterized by an exaggeration of normal coagulation and profuse bleeding. Because clotting factors are used up in the abnormal coagulation process, this disorder is also known as consumption coagulopathy. It is always secondary to another process and can be triggered by many disease states (Table 13–4). It is a complication commonly seen in the treatment of the critically ill. Mortality in those with DIC is high, although the severity of the illness depends on the extent of the underlying disease process.

Disseminated intravascular coagulation can exist in chronic, acute, and subacute forms. The chronic form is most often caused by malignancy but may result from renal, liver, or metabolic disease. Acute DIC, the variety most often seen in the intensive care unit, develops rapidly and is the most serious form of acquired coagulopathy. With subacute DIC, the patient has no clinical signs or symptoms, but laboratory findings may indicate coagulation abnormalities (Pavel et al., 1993).

Whatever the initiating event in DIC, procoagulants are released that cause diffuse uncontrolled clotting. The intrinsic and/or extrinsic pathways can be activated. Large amounts of thrombin are produced, which results in the deposition of fibrin in the microvasculature, the consumption of available clotting factors, and the stimulation of fibrinolysis.

Clotting in the microvasculature of the patient with DIC causes organ ischemia and necrosis. The skin, lungs, and kidneys are most often damaged. Thrombophlebitis, pulmonary embolism, cerebrovascular accident, gastrointestinal bleeding, and renal failure may result from thrombosis. Additionally, microvasculature thrombosis may result in acral cyanosis, purpura fulminans, or infarction and gangrene of the digits or tip of the nose.

The fibrinolysis that follows results in the release of fibrin degradation products, which are potent anticoagulants that interfere with thrombin, fibrin, and platelet activity. RBCs are damaged as they try to pass through the blocked capillary beds; the damage to RBCs causes excess hemolysis. The lack of available clotting factors coupled with the anticoagulant forces results in an inability to form clots as needed and predisposes the patient with DIC to hemorrhage (Fig. 13–8). The patient bleeds from venipuncture sites, catheters, incisions, body orifices, and into the skin.

Assessment/Clinical Manifestations

Clinically, the patient with DIC presents with bleeding ranging from mild oozing from venipuncture sites to massive hemorrhage from all body orifices (Table 13–5). Petechiae, ecchymosis, and purpura may be present in the skin, and gingival bleeding and epistaxis may be noted. Blood in the stool, emesis, and urine are common (see Table 13–6 for bleeding terminology). Signs of organ ischemia and necrosis that result from microvasculature clotting include angina, decreased urine output, gastrointestinal bleeding, dyspnea, and alterations in mental status. Acral cyanosis and infarction of digits and the tip of the nose may occur if the DIC is severe. Occult bleeding into body cavities, such as the peritoneal and retroperitoneal spaces, may be detected by vital sign changes or other classic signs of blood loss. Earlier signs of DIC may include more subtle changes, including mental status

Table 13–4. CAUSES OF DISSEMINATED INTRAVASCULAR COAGULATION

Cause	Examples
Infections	Bacterial (especially gram-negative), fungal, viral, mycobacterial, protozoan, rickettsial
Trauma	Burns, head, crush, or multiple injuries, snakebite
Obstetrical	Abruptio placentae, placenta previa, amniotic fluid embolism, retained dead fetus, missed abortion, eclampsia, hydatidiform mole
Hematological/ immunological disorders	Transfusion reaction, transplant rejections, anaphylaxis, autoimmune disorders, sickle cell crisis
Oncological disorders	Carcinomas, leukemias
Miscellaneous	Extracorporeal circulation, pulmonary or fat embolism, anoxia, acidosis, hyperthermia or hypothermia, hypovolemic or hemorrhagic shock, ARDS, sustained hypotension

ARDS = adult respiratory distress syndrome.

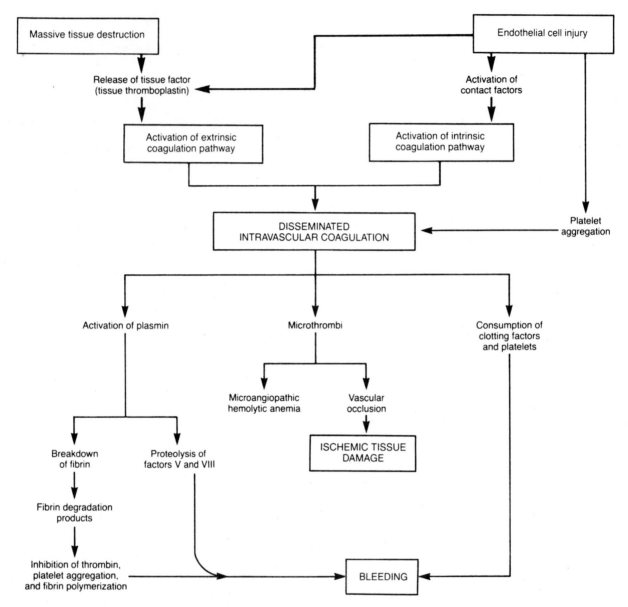

Figure 13–8. Pathophysiology of disseminated intravascular coagulation. (Adapted from Cotran, R. S., Kumar, V., & Robbins, S. L. (1989). *Robbins pathological basis of disease* (4th ed.) (p. 700). Philadelphia: W. B. Saunders Co.)

changes, restlessness, confusion, dyspnea, and hypotension (Ruggiero and Barie, 1993).

Diagnosis of DIC may be difficult but is made on the basis of a combination of clinical symptoms, patient history, and results of laboratory studies. Laboratory findings in DIC are listed in Table 13–7.

Nursing Diagnoses

The patient with DIC may have the following nursing diagnoses:

- Altered tissue perfusion related to abnormal clotting and thrombosis (cerebral, peripheral, renal, cardiopulmonary, and gastrointestinal), decreased cardiac output (secondary to hemorrhage or cardiac ischemia), or anemia.
- Fluid volume deficit related to hemorrhage.
- Impaired gas exchange related to pulmonary ischemia (e.g., pulmonary embolism).
- Altered pattern of urinary elimination related to decreased renal blood flow.

Table 13–5. SYMPTOMS OF DISSEMINATED INTRAVASCULAR COAGULATION

Oozing or bleeding from venipuncture sites, incisions, wounds

Bleeding around tubes: endotracheal, nasotracheal or nasogastric, urethral catheters

Bleeding from mucosal surfaces/body orifices: epistaxis, hematemesis, hemoptysis, melena, hematochezia, hematuria; gingival, scleral bleeding

Skin: ecchymoses, petechiae, pallor, mottling

Neurological: headache, altered level of consciousness, vertigo, lethargy, irritability, confusion, restlessness, focal deficits, seizures, coma

Cardiovascular: hypotension, tachycardia, ST-T wave changes

Renal: oliguria, hematuria

Gastrointestinal: abdominal pain, distention, hyperactive or absent bowel sounds

Other: anxiety, dyspnea, muscle weakness, fatigue, acral cyanosis, acidosis, hematomas, signs of thrombophlebitis

---

- Impaired skin integrity related to immobility, trauma, and invasive procedures.
- Anxiety related to the fear of dying, the procedures being performed, and the unknown.
- Pain related to tissue ischemia, bleeding into tissues, and therapeutic/diagnostic interventions.

Medical Interventions

Medical treatment of DIC is aimed at identifying and treating the underlying cause, stopping the abnormal coagulation, and controlling the bleeding (Table

Table 13–6. BLEEDING TERMINOLOGY

Term	Refers to
Ecchymosis	Blue or purplish hemorrhagic spot on skin or mucous membrane, round or irregular, nonelevated
Epistaxis	Bleeding from the nose
Hemarthrosis	Blood in a joint cavity
Hematochezia	Blood in stool; bright red
Hematoma	Collection of blood in tissue, space or organ; usually clotted
Hematemesis	Blood in emesis
Hematuria	Blood in urine
Hemoglobinuria	Hemoglobin in urine
Hemoptysis	Coughing of blood
Melena	Blood pigments in stool; dark or black
Menorrhagia	Excessive bleeding during menstruation
Petechia	Purplish red hemorrhagic spot, nonelevated, pinpoint, round

Table 13–7. LABORATORY FINDINGS IN DISSEMINATED INTRAVASCULAR COAGULATION

Test	Normal Value	Alteration
Platelet count	150,000–400,000/μl	Decreased
Prothrombin time	11–16 sec	Prolonged
Activated partial thromboplastin time	30–45 sec	Prolonged
Thrombin time	10–15 sec	Prolonged
Fibrinogen	200–400 mg/dl	Decreased
Fibrin degradation products	<10 μg/ml	Increased
Antithrombin III	>50% of control (plasma)	Decreased
D-Dimer assay	<100 μg/L	Increased

13–8). Correction of hypotension, hypoxemia, and acidosis is vital, as is treatment of infection. If the cause is obstetrical, evacuation of the uterus for retained fetal or other tissue must be performed. Blood volume expanders and crystalloid IV fluids, such as lactated Ringer's solution or normal saline, are given in order to counteract hypovolemia caused by blood loss.

Blood component therapy is used in DIC in order to replace deficient platelets and clotting factors and to treat hemorrhage; packed RBCs, whole blood, fresh frozen plasma, platelets, and cryoprecipitate may be given (Table 13–9). Transfusions of whole blood and

Table 13–8. MEDICAL TREATMENT OF DISSEMINATED INTRAVASCULAR COAGULATION

Correct underlying problem
1. Intravenous fluids, pharmacological therapy, respiratory and cardiovascular support to correct hypotension, infection, hypoxemia, acidosis, shock, electrolyte disturbances

Stop abnormal coagulation
1. Heparin to interfere with thrombin—bolus followed by continuous or intermittent infusion (controversial)
2. Antithrombin III to inhibit thrombin

Control bleeding/restore hemostasis
1. Blood component therapy (platelets, fresh frozen plasma, cryoprecipitate) to replace platelets, clotting factors
2. Stabilize formed clots—aminocaproic acid used with caution to inhibit fibrinolysis

Treat/prevent complications
1. Blood components to correct anemia from hemorrhage
2. Cardiovascular and respiratory support to maintain cardiac output, optimal gas exchange, and tissue perfusion

Table 13-9. SUMMARY OF BLOOD PRODUCTS AND ADMINISTRATION

Blood Component	Description	Actions	Indications	Administration	Complications
Whole blood	RBCs, plasma, and stable clotting factors	Restores oxygen-carrying capacity and intravascular volume	Symptomatic anemia with major circulating volume deficit Massive hemorrhaging with shock	Donor and recipient must be ABO compatible and Rh compatible Use microaggregate filter Rate of infusion: usually 2 to 4 h but more rapid in cases of shock	Hemolytic reaction Allergic reaction Hypothermia Electrolyte disturbances Citrate intoxication Infectious diseases
Red blood cells (RBCs)	RBCs centrifuged from whole blood	Restores oxygen-carrying capacity and intravascular volume	Symptomatic anemia when patient is at risk for fluid overload Acute hemorrhaging	Donor and recipient must be ABO compatible and Rh compatible Use microaggregate filter Rate of infusion: 2 to 4 h but more rapid in cases of shock	Infectious diseases Hemolytic reaction Allergic reaction Hypothermia Electrolyte disturbances Citrate intoxication
Leukocyte-poor cells or washed red blood cells	RBCs from which leukocytes and plasma proteins have been reduced	Restores oxygen-carrying capacity and intravascular volume	Symptomatic anemia when patient has history of repeated febrile nonhemolytic transfusion reactions Acute hemorrhaging	Donor and recipient must be ABO compatible and Rh compatible Use microaggregate filter Rate of infusion: 2–4 h but more rapid in cases of shock	Allergic reaction Hemolytic reaction Hypothermia Electrolyte disturbances Citrate intoxication Infectious diseases
Fresh frozen plasma	Plasma rich in clotting factors with platelets removed	Replaces clotting factors	Deficit of coagulation factors as in disseminated intravascular coagulopathy, liver disease, and coagulopathies from massive transfusions Major trauma victims with signs/symptoms of hemorrhage	Donor and recipient must be ABO compatible and Rh compatible Rate of infusion: 10 ml/min	Allergic reaction Febrile reactions Circulatory overload Infectious diseases

Component	Preparation	Action	Indications	Special considerations	Complications
Platelets	Removed from whole blood	Increases platelet count and improves hemostasis	Thrombocytopenia Platelet dysfunction (prophylactically for platelet counts <10,000–20,000/μl or evidence of bleeding with platelet count <50,000/μl)	Do not use microaggregate filter; component filter obtained from blood bank ABO testing not necessary unless contaminated with RBCs but is usually done: usually give 6 units at one time	Infectious diseases Allergic reactions Febrile reactons
Cryoprecipitate antihemophilic factor (AHF)	Primarily coagulation factor VIII with 250 mg of fibrinogen and 20–30% of factor XIII	Used primarily with classic hemophilia A patients and patients with von Willebrand's disease, factor XIII, and fibrinogen deficiencies	Hemophilia A, von Willebrand's disease Hypofibrinogenemia Factor XIII deficiency	Repeat doses may be necessary to attain satisfactory serum level Rate of infusion: approximately 10 ml of diluted component per minute	Allergic reactions Hepatitis
Albumin	Prepared from plasma	Intravascular volume expander by increasing osmotic pressure	Hypovolemic shock Liver failure	Special administration set with vial Rate of infusion over 30–60 min	Circulatory overload Febrile reaction
Granulocytes	Prepared by centrifugation or filtration leukopheresis, which removes granulocytes from whole blood	Increase the leukocyte level	Decreased WBCs usually from chemotherapy or radiation	Must be ABO compatible and Rh compatible Rate of infusion: one unit over 2–4 h; closely observe for reaction	Rash Febrile reaction Hepatitis
Plasma protein	Pooled from human plasma	Intravascular volume expander by increasing osmotic pressure	Hypovolemic shock	ABO compatibility not necessary Rate of infusion: over 30–60 min	Circulatory overload Febrile reaction

From Orsi, A. J. (1993). The hematologic system. In R. L. Boggs, & M. Wooldridge-King (Eds.), AACN procedure manual for critical care (3rd ed.) (pp. 692–693). Philadelphia: W. B. Saunders Co.

WBC = white blood cell.

packed RBCs are given in order to replace cells lost in hemorrhage. Fresh frozen plasma is administered judiciously to patients who have factor depletion; it contains clotting factors V, VIII, XIII, and antithrombin III. Platelet infusions are often necessary because these patients almost always have thrombocytopenia. Cryoprecipitate replaces fibrinogen and factor VIII.

Heparin is sometimes given in DIC in order to interfere with the effects of thrombin, although its use is controversial, and studies have failed to show consistent benefit from its use in DIC (Ruggiero and Barie, 1993). The use of heparin is aimed at preventing further clotting and thrombosis that may lead to organ ischemia and necrosis. Although heparin's antithrombin activity prevents further clotting, it may increase the risk of bleeding, causing further problems.

Other pharmacological therapy in DIC includes the administration of synthetic antithrombin III, which, like heparin, inhibits thrombin, and the administration of aminocaproic acid (Amicar), which inhibits fibrinolysis by interfering with plasmin activity. Antithrombin III concentrates may shorten the course of the disease and may increase survival rate (Vinazzer, 1989). Aminocaproic acid is given in combination with heparin to prevent the lysis of existing clots, thereby preventing the release of fibrin degradation products and contributing to the rapid cessation of hemorrhage. Many other treatments are being investigated for use in DIC, including administration of other thrombin inhibitors and monoclonal antibodies, whose products may neutralize endotoxins released in sepsis that trigger DIC (Levi et al., 1993.)

Nursing Interventions

Nursing care of the patient with DIC is aimed primarily at the prevention and recognition of thrombotic and hemorrhagic events. Continuous assessment for complications and aggressive interventions by the nurse determine patient outcome. Psychosocial support of the patient and family, as in any critical illness, is of great importance (see nursing care plan, p. 399).

The patient is assessed for signs of altered perfusion and cardiac output. These parameters can be assessed through monitoring of vital signs, the electrocardiogram, hemodynamic parameters, arterial blood gases, mental status, bowel sounds, and urine output. Cardiovascular signs include chest pain, dysrhythmias, hypotension, murmurs, and tachycardia. The patient is monitored for dyspnea, tachypnea, abnormal breath sounds, cyanosis, and hemoptysis, which indicate inadequate pulmonary perfusion. Gastrointestinal involvement might cause abdominal pain, distension, nausea and vomiting, altered bowel sounds, and blood in the stool or gastrointestinal secretions. Altered cerebral perfusion can cause mental status changes, such as restlessness, confusion, irritability, or changes in reflexes. Peripheral pulses, capillary refill, and skin temperature and color are evaluated. In addition, the skin is assessed for petechiae, ecchymoses, mottling, and edema. Medical treatment is administered per orders, and patient response is monitored, including the response to vasoactive and antiarrhythmic drugs, respiratory support and oxygen, anticoagulants, IV fluids, and blood component therapy. Good skin and oral care is provided in order to enhance circulation and promote skin integrity.

The fluid volume deficit in patients with DIC is assessed thoroughly and is corrected by careful administration of fluids and blood components. Accurate intake and output measurements are performed hourly and include measurement of blood loss. Further bleeding is prevented or is promptly detected and controlled. For the prevention of further bleeding, skin integrity is protected. Laboratory coagulation studies are carefully followed. Signs and symptoms of bleeding are carefully monitored, including any oozing from venipunctures, catheters, incisions, mucous membranes, or body orifices. The nurse assesses urine, emesis, and stool for the presence of blood. Gastrointestinal function may be determined through bowel sounds and by the presence of nausea, vomiting, abdominal distention, or cramps. Skin is assessed thoroughly for bruising or pressure areas. Careful cleaning and lubrication of the skin, frequent turning, and protection of pressure areas are necessary in order to keep skin intact. If possible, a flotation or air-fluidized mattress is used. Suctioning is performed only when necessary because even minimal pressure can cause trauma. Cuff blood pressures, including the use of noninvasive blood pressure machines, are used as infrequently as possible. Use of rectal thermometers, suppositories, enemas, and douches is avoided. Venipunctures and other needle sticks are also avoided if possible; when such measures are necessary, only small-gauged needles are used, and pressure is held on sites for 10 minutes afterward. Blood samples can be obtained through central lines, although placement of lines may also result in hemorrhage. Frequent oral hygiene with sponge-tipped or cotton swabs and normal saline rinses helps protect oral mucosa; toothbrushes and alcohol-containing solutions are not used. An electric razor can be used if the patient must be shaved. Only paper tape is used in order to avoid tissue trauma and bleeding on removal.

Pulmonary function is monitored in order to assess for impaired gas exchange. The patient's respiratory rate, depth, and pattern are observed, and breath sounds are auscultated so that rales or rhonchi can be detected. Arterial blood gases are monitored, and the patient is assessed for restlessness, chest pain, or sputum production. Supplemental oxygen or ventilatory assistance is administered as ordered, and the patient is encouraged to turn, cough, and deep breathe and/or perform incentive spirometry as able.

The patient with DIC and his or her family are assessed for the level of anxiety and coping mechanisms available. Communication is encouraged, and feelings are acknowledged. Involvement in the planning and implementation of care may return a sense of control to the patient and family. The nurse is available to listen to, reassure, and support both the patient and the family. The information given is accurate, and false assurance is avoided. Maintenance of an open, honest, and supportive environment, may enable stress and anxiety to be lessened.

Pain relief and promotion of comfort may also diminish anxiety in the patient with DIC. The location, intensity, and quality of the patient's pain are assessed, along with the patient's response to discomfort. Pain medication is offered as ordered, with attention given to response to analgesics. The patient is medicated before painful procedures, when possible. Positioning, with support and proper body alignment and frequent changes, also enhances the patient's level of comfort.

Patient Outcomes

The following are the goals of care for the patient with DIC:

- Adequate tissue perfusion will be maintained as abnormal clotting and thrombosis are controlled and as hypotension and anemia are corrected.
- Cardiac output and gas exchange will be sufficient to provide adequate tissue oxygenation; the patient will be normovolemic and will have adequate coronary blood flow.
- Bleeding or thrombotic events will be prevented or promptly recognized and treated; care will be provided in such a manner as to prevent any injury to tissues that might cause bleeding.
- Skin integrity will be maintained and healing promoted.
- The patient will be able to verbalize fears and will have sufficient emotional support. Effective coping patterns will be fostered.
- The patient will remain as comfortable as possible.

Thrombocytopenia

Pathophysiology

A quantitative deficiency of platelets is termed *thrombocytopenia*; this condition is a common cause of severe hemorrhage if it is not corrected. The pathophysiology may be related to decreased production of platelets by the bone marrow, increased destruction of platelets, or sequestration of platelets (abnormal distribution). Decreased production may result from bone marrow depression by toxic or chemotherapeutic agents, radiation, infection, or such disorders as aplastic anemia. Destruction of platelets is caused by their overconsumption, as occurs in DIC, or by autoimmune disorders. Prosthetic heart valves, extracorporeal circulation, and balloon counterpulsation may also damage platelets. Many drugs used frequently in critical care have been implicated as contributors to thrombocytopenia, although the mechanism is not understood (Ruggiero and Barie, 1993) These agents include quinidine, phenytoin, diazepam, and digitoxin.

Assessment/Clinical Manifestations

Clinically, the patient with thrombocytopenia presents with petechiae, purpura, and ecchymosis, with oozing from mucous membranes. Laboratory findings reveal a platelet count of less than 150,000/μl, predisposing the patient to an increased risk of bleeding. When the count drops to less than 40,000/μl, spontaneous bleeding may occur. Fatal hemorrhage is a great risk when the count is less than 10,000/μl (Jackson and Jones, 1988a).

Nursing Diagnoses

In addition to many of the nursing diagnoses listed in DIC, the thrombocytopenic patient may have the following:

- Risk for injury related to bleeding.
- Altered tissue perfusion related to bleeding.
- Impaired skin integrity and pain related to bleeding into tissues (Pavel et al., 1993).

Medical Interventions

Medical treatment of thrombocytopenia includes infusions of platelets in order to maintain hemostasis, steroids or plasmapheresis if the cause is an autoimmune disease, and splenectomy if the condition is refractory.

Nursing Interventions

Nursing interventions for the patient with thrombocytopenia are similar to those listed for DIC.

Patient Outcomes

The following are the goals of care for the patient with thrombocytopenia:

- Patient will maintain adequate tissue perfusion, as evidenced by stable vital signs, hemodynamics, absence of dysrhythmias, adequate urine output, and normal mental status.
- Tissue integrity will be maintained, and any bleeding will be promptly recognized and treated.
- Pain will be managed so that the patient will be as comfortable as possible.

White Clot Syndrome. This phenomenon is also known as heparin-induced or heparin-associated thrombocytopenia. Although it is a rare complication of heparin therapy, the seriousness of the syndrome warrants suspicion when a patient receiving antiembolic drug therapy presents with multiple emboli. The disorder gets its name from the "white clot" aggregates of platelets and fibrin. It is thought to be an immune-mediated response that results in the destruction of platelets, and it is not dose related. Clinical signs of this disorder, which appear 2 or more days after the initiation of heparin therapy, include symptoms of thrombosis or emboli (e.g., changes in extremity pulse, color, or temperature; respiratory difficulty; and chest pain), a platelet count of less than 100,000/µl, and a positive platelet aggregation test result. An increasing resistance to the anticoagulation effects of heparin is also seen.

Treatment is immediate cessation of heparin therapy. Other anticoagulants, such as warfarin sodium (Coumadin), aspirin, dipyridamole (Persantine), and dextran, may be substituted if necessary (Kuhar and Hill, 1991). IV fluids and volume expanders may be administered in order to correct fluid deficit and maintain hydration. Bleeding precautions are carefully observed. The patient must not receive *any* subsequent heparin. Arterial, central, and peripheral IV lines are flushed with saline or some other solution, such as sodium citrate 1.4% (Waldrop et al., 1991). Warning signs are placed at the bedside, and allergy alerts are placed on the chart and sent to the pharmacy.

Other Coagulation Disorders

In addition to DIC and thrombocytopenia, several other disorders are seen in critical care areas that predispose patients to bleeding. These disorders include vitamin K deficiency, liver disease, hemophilia, and von Willebrand's disease. Patients who receive massive transfusions of stored blood or packed cells also are at risk for coagulation problems.

Vitamin K Deficiency

Vitamin K is fat-soluble and is not stored in the body; thus, its presence in the body depends on dietary intake and gastric absorption. It is essential in the formation of several of the clotting factors. Vitamin K deficiency may result from malabsorption, lack of intake, or liver disease. Laboratory studies reveal prolonged prothrombin time and partial thromboplastin time, although administration of vitamin K corrects the abnormalities in 12 to 48 hours (Jackson and Jones, 1988a). The underlying cause of the deficiency is treated, and supplements are administered as necessary.

Liver Disease

One of the most common causes of bleeding disorders is liver disease (Jackson and Jones, 1988a). The patient with liver disease has an impaired ability to synthesize clotting factors, especially those that are vitamin K dependent. Portal hypertension may lead to enlargement of the spleen and sequestration of platelets, further contributing to bleeding tendency. A prolonged prothrombin time is found in laboratory studies; partial thromboplastin time may also be prolonged, and most clotting factors are reduced. Treatment includes administration of fresh frozen plasma in order to replace clotting factors; platelets replacement may also be necessary. Vitamin K may be given parenterally because malabsorption is common.

Massive Transfusions, Hemophilia, and von Willebrand's Disease

Hemorrhaging patients who receive only packed cells, stored whole blood, and crystalloid and/or colloid fluids lack replacement of clotting factors and platelets (Rick, 1991). Fresh frozen plasma and platelet infusions must also be given for the maintenance of hemostasis (see Table 13–9).

Hemophilia and von Willebrand's disease are hereditary disorders in which factor VIII is deficient. Treatment consists of local measures for the control of bleeding, cryoprecipitate infusion, and factor VIII or IX replacement. Desmopressin has been found to be an effective new treatment for many patients with mild-to-moderate disease (Ruggiero and Barie, 1993). Administration of this agent causes the release of endogenous factor VIII from plasma storage sites.

Nursing diagnoses, interventions, and patient outcomes are similar to those for any bleeding or coagulation disorder (see Nursing Care of the Patient with a Bleeding Disorder*).

Review of Immunological Anatomy and Physiology

The body's ability to resist and fight infection is termed *immunity*. Our bodies are constantly exposed

NURSING CARE PLAN FOR THE PATIENT WITH A BLEEDING DISORDER

Nursing Diagnosis	Patient Outcomes	Nursing Interventions
Altered tissue perfusion related to abnormal clotting, hypotension, and/or anemia.	Adequate perfusion will be maintained and damage to vital organs will be prevented, as evidenced by: Vital signs and hemodynamics stable and within normal limits. Normal mental status. Arterial blood gas (ABG) results within normal limits. Urine output > 30 ml/h. Absence of cardiac dysrhythmias. Adequate peripheral pulses, skin warm with normal color.	Monitor hemodynamics, vital signs, electrocardiogram, ABGs, intake and output, and laboratory results. Provide good skin and oral care in order to promote circulation. Assess for and report signs of altered perfusion: Cardiovascular: dysrhythmias, angina, hypotension, murmurs, tachycardia, dyspnea. Cerebral: decreased level of consciousness, restlessness, confusion, irritability, pupillary changes, reflexes. Pulmonary: dyspnea, tachypnea, rales/rhonchi, cyanosis, hemoptysis. Renal: decreased urine output, hematuria. Gastrointestinal: abdominal pain, distention, nausea/vomiting, hyperactive or absent bowel sounds, hematemesis, hematochezia/melena. Peripheral: pallor, acral cyanosis, mottling, ecchymoses, petechiae, absence of or diminished pulses, edema. Administer medical treatment per orders and observe response: Vasoactive, antiarrhythmic drugs. Respiratory support; oxygen. Antibiotics. Heparin, aminocaproic acid. Blood component therapy.
Fluid volume deficit related to hemorrhage.	Patient will be free of bleeding and will be normovolemic, as evidenced by: Absence of oozing/bleeding. Laboratory study results within normal limits. Vital signs and hemodynamics stable and within normal limits.	Monitor hemodynamics, vital signs, intake and output, and laboratory study results. Weigh dressings/linens to estimate blood loss. Check body fluids for occult blood. Assess for, note presence and degree, and report signs of bleeding. General: oozing or bleeding from venipunctures, intravenous access sites, incisions, wounds, mucous membranes and body orifices. Cardiovascular: dysrhythmias, hypotension, murmurs, tachycardia, dyspnea. Cerebral: decreased level of consciousness, restlessness, confusion, irritability, pupillary changes, reflexes abnormal. Pulmonary: dyspnea, tachypnea, crackles/rhonchi, cyanosis, hemoptysis. Renal: decreased urine output, hematuria. Gastrointestinal: abdominal pain, distention, nausea/vomiting, hyperactive or absent bowel sounds, hematemesis, hematochezia/melena. Peripheral: hematomas, pallor, cyanosis, mottling, ecchymoses, petechiae, edema, bone and joint pain. Control bleeding: Use ice packs, pressure dressings or direct pressure over bleeding sites. Leave existing clots undisturbed. Administer topical hemostatic agents as ordered.

Continued on following page

NURSING CARE PLAN FOR THE PATIENT WITH A BLEEDING DISORDER *Continued*		
Nursing Diagnosis	Patient Outcomes	Nursing Interventions

		Prevent trauma:
		  Provide frequent, gentle skin and oral care.
		  Avoid venipunctures, injections, cuff blood pressures, rectal/vaginal examinations, or intramuscular medications.
		  Frequent position changes; air or flotation mattress; sheepskins.
		  Use electric razor only.
		  Administer stool softeners, soft diet.
		Administer medical treatment per orders and observe response:
		  Aminocaproic acid.
		  Blood component therapy.

Anxiety related to fear of death, procedures, the unknown.	Behavior will reflect diminished level of anxiety. Patient and family will be able to state verbal understanding of disease process and treatments; verbalize questions, fears, anxieties. Patient and family will participate in the planning and implementation of care.	Provide emotional support; develop rapport with patient and family; be available to patient and family; maintain open lines of communication; be honest, avoid false reassurance. Assess level of anxiety, knowledge of disease process, and treatments. Educate patient and family about disease process, treatments. Explain procedures. Involve patient and family in the planning and implementation of care. Use relaxation/imagery techniques; keep stressors to minimum. Support positive coping mechanisms.
Pain related to bleeding, altered tissue perfusion, procedures.	Optimal comfort will be maintained, pain will be relieved, as evidenced by verbal statements and behavioral clues of relief of pain.	Assess location, intensity, duration, and quality of pain. Administer analgesics as ordered or needed; observe response. Position patient for comfort using proper body alignment, pillows for support, and padding pressure areas. Use heat/cold treatments as warranted. Provide quiet, calm, reassuring environment. Remain with patient during procedures; allow family visitation as appropriate.

to bacteria, viruses, fungi, and parasites (some of which are normally present on the skin and many mucous membranes) that are capable of causing disease. In the healthy individual, an intact and responsive immune system provides adequate protection. However, the person whose immune system is not functioning properly is at risk for overwhelming, life-threatening infection. Such factors as disease, age, stress, and medical therapy can compromise an individual's immune system, resulting in an inadequate defense.

In critical care, patients' immune systems are often compromised by disease, procedures, and medications. Infectious disease processes can overwhelm the body's ability to "fight back." Diagnostic and therapeutic interventions, such as invasive and surgical procedures, put the patient at risk for infection. Additionally, many of the drugs and treatments administered can depress patients' immune systems. In the case of organ transplantation, this immunosuppression is intentional, but it can result in the patient's inability to fight infection.

Critical care nurses' understanding of the normal immune system and its proper response to an assault is paramount to good assessment skills and use of therapeutic interventions.

NURSING CARE PLAN FOR THE IMMUNOCOMPROMISED PATIENT

Nursing Diagnosis	Patient Outcomes	Nursing Interventions

Risk for infection related to immunocompromise or immunosuppression, invasive procedures, presence of opportunistic pathogens.	Patient will remain free of infection, as evidenced by absence of fever, redness, swelling, pain, and heat; laboratory studies (white blood cell (WBC) and differential, urinalysis, cultures) within normal limits; chest x-ray study without infiltrates, absence of adventitious breath sounds.	Establish baseline assessment with documented history, physical examination, and laboratory study results.
		Assess patient for signs/symptoms of infection.
		  Monitor vital signs with temperature at least every 4 h—any elevation in temperature is reported and investigated.
		  Monitor laboratory results: white blood cell (WBC) and differential, blood, urine, sputum, wound, and throat cultures; report abnormal results.
		  Note presence of chills, tachycardia, dysuria.
		  Pulmonary: observe for cough, sputum production, dyspnea; monitor arterial blood gas (ABG) results for hypoxemia; assess breath sounds at least every 4 h; monitor chest x-ray study for infiltrates, changes; obtain sputum cultures as indicated.
		  Skin/mucous membranes/wound: observe mouth, skin, perineum, axillae, areas of pressure, breakdown, or excoriation, presence of lesions; note any pain, redness, swelling, pus formation, or heat at venipuncture, intravenous (IV) site, wound, or incision sites; culture areas as indicated.
		Use strict hand washing before, during, and after any patient contact.
		Promote optimal nutrition and hydration.
		Encourage incentive spirometry every 1 h; position changes and pulmonary toilet every 2 h; perform chest physiotherapy and postural drainage; use strict aseptic technique for suctioning.
		Avoid breaks in skin/mucous membrane integrity; provide meticulous skin care, keeping all areas clean, dry, and lubricated as appropriate; position changes every 2 h.
		Use meticulous oral hygiene with nonirritating solutions and soft bristled brush.
		Change dressing as ordered to wound, incision, and invasive line sites, using strict aseptic technique.
		Limit number of invasive devices/procedures as able (e.g., IV, central, Foley catheters); use strict aseptic technique when devices necessary.
		Use private room and reverse isolation as necessary; limit number of visitors; restrict visitors/caregivers to those without infection; use gown, masks, gloves as needed.
		Provide diet of well-cooked foods; avoid fresh fruits or vegetables if patient is neutropenic.
		Keep room uncluttered and well cleaned; no standing water sources; discard any open containers or unused fluid solutions.
		Continued on following page

Continued on following page

Nursing Diagnosis	Patient Outcomes	Nursing Interventions
Risk for impaired skin integrity and altered oral mucous membranes related to immobility, invasive devices and procedures, dehydration, malnutrition, immunosuppression.	Patient's skin and mucous membranes will remain intact; will be absent of signs of pressure areas, breakdown, lesions, excoriation; skin turgor and moisture of mucous membranes will remain adequate; patient will remain free of signs of infection.	Assess skin and mucous membranes every shift for signs of pressure, breakdown, lesions, and excoriation. Monitor incisions, IV and venipuncture sites, axillae, perineal areas, and so forth, for redness, swelling, pain, heat. Provide meticulous skin care; keep skin clean, dry, and lubricated. Provide frequent mouth care with nonirritating solutions and soft-bristled brush; maintain moisture of mucous membranes. Turn/reposition the patient at least every 2 h and as needed. Use air-fluidized/alternating pressure mattresses, or eggcrate mattresses/pad bony prominences and pressure points. Treat any pressure ulcers or areas of breakdown promptly; provide protection from further damage. Maintain adequate hydration and optimal nutritional status. Assist with mobility as able.
Altered nutrition (less than body requirements) related to fasting (NPO) status (endotracheal or nasogastric tubes, surgery), anorexia, nausea/vomiting, painful oral mucosa.	Patient will maintain optimal nutritional status, as evidenced by adequate caloric and protein intake; ideal/stable body weight; laboratory values will remain within normal limits (total protein, serum albumin, electrolytes, hemoglobin, and hematocrit).	Assess baseline nutritional status. Height and weight. Laboratory values. Presence of weakness, fatigue, infection, or other signs of malnutrition, food preferences, and deterrents to adequate intake of protein and calories. Obtain dietary consult to determine nutrients/intake required. Establish food preferences. Determine deterrents to adequate intake: fasting (NPO) status, presence of, e.g., anorexia, nausea, vomiting, stomatitis. Monitor daily weight, laboratory values, protein and caloric intake, intake and output. Encourage small, frequent, high-calorie and high-protein meals. Provide meticulous mouth care before and after meals. Encourage meals from home/significant others and relaxed atmosphere/socialization during meals. Administer antiemetics as needed, 30 min before meals. Assess need for enteral/parenteral nutritional therapy; administer as ordered and observe response.
Knowledge deficit related to disease process; critical routines, procedures or treatments; immunosuppressive therapy.	Patient verbalizes understanding of disease process, treatments, medication regimens.	Assess patient's level of understanding and ability to comprehend information, readiness to learn. Orient patient to critical care unit, routines, procedures. Instruct patient/significant others about diagnosis, treatments, medications, need for optimal nutrition and adherence to medication regimen. Answer questions promptly and honestly; maintain atmosphere of mutual respect and approachability; be available to patient and family to answer questions. Reinforce patient education and compliance with plan of care.

CONCEPTS IN IMMUNOLOGY

To understand immune physiology, the critical care nurse should have a working knowledge of a few key concepts, including *antigen, self versus nonself, tolerance, autoimmunity, and specificity.*

An *antigen* is any substance that is capable of stimulating an immune response in the host. Microorganisms (e.g., bacteria, viruses, fungi, and parasites), abnormal or mutated cells, foreign or transplanted cells, and foreign molecules (e.g., penicillin) can act as antigens (Miller and Habicht, 1991). An antigen is seen by the body as being foreign, or *nonself.* The body normally protects cells or molecules that it senses as being *self* and attempts to destroy those that are nonself. Self can be recognized as nonself if it undergoes mutation, is in an abnormal location, or changes structure (Fidler, 1988).

The body's response to an antigen is determined by many factors, such as genetics, amount of antigen, and route of exposure (Miller and Habicht, 1991). Once a substance is recognized as an antigen, the body puts its natural and acquired defenses into action to destroy the invader and prevent disease.

Tolerance is the body's ability to recognize self as self and therefore protect itself. In *autoimmunity*, the body for some reason attacks self as nonself (i.e., it has no tolerance), and an immune response is activated against body tissues. Autoimmunity can result from injury to tissues, infection, or malignancy, although in many cases, the cause is not known. An example of an autoimmune disease is systemic lupus erythematosus.

Specificity refers to the fact that an immune response stimulates cells to develop immunity for a specific antigen (Fidler, 1988). B lymphocytes are sensitized and produce antibodies that recognize, react with, and destroy specific antigens.

Whereas a *specific* immune response refers to the sensitization of lymphocytes and the production of antibodies, *nonspecific* defenses include the processes of phagocytosis and inflammation. In *active* immunity, the body actively produces cells and mediators that result in the destruction of the antigen. *Passive* immunity is that which is transferred from another person (e.g., maternal antibodies transferred to the newborn through the placenta and breast milk).

ORGANS INVOLVED IN IMMUNOLOGICAL FUNCTION

The immune system is diffuse—it functions throughout the body and involves several different cells and organs. The lymphoreticular system consists of lymphoid tissue, lymphatic cells, and phagocytic cells in the body that engulf and process foreign materials in order to protect the body from invasion. The organs included in the lymphoreticular system are the bone marrow, thymus, lymph nodes, spleen, and liver (Fidler, 1988) (Fig. 13–9).

All bloosd cells are produced in the bone marrow, including those involved in immune defenses. The bone marrow is thought to be the site of maturation of B lymphocytes, which provide humoral immunity through antibody formation. The thymus has two main functions: the maturation of T lymphocytes, which are involved in cellular immunity, and the production of hormones critical in the maturation of the immune system. It is located in the anterior mediastinum just beneath the sternum. The thymus is the central organ of the lymphatic system and is largest during puberty, after which it begins to involute. Lymph nodes are small, bean-shaped structures located in the head, neck, axillae, groin, and abdomen; they are connected by lymphatic vessels. Their function is the filtering and cleansing of interstitial fluid and the circulation of lymphocytes.

The blood is filtered in the spleen; foreign material, dead or abnormal cells, and debris are removed

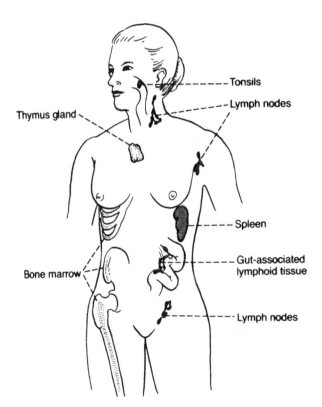

Figure 13–9. Organs of the immune system. (Adapted from Janusek, L. (1993). Structure and function of the immune system. In J. M. Black, & E. Matassarin-Jacobs (Eds.), *Luckmann and Sorensen's medical-surgical nursing* (4th ed.) (p. 535). Philadelphia: W. B. Saunders Co.)

by phagocytes. The spleen also stimulates B-lympho-cyte and T-lymphocyte proliferation, differentiation, and production of antibodies in response to antigenic material that has been trapped, recognized, and processed. The liver also acts as a filter through phagocytosis—blood is cleansed of bacteria, and foreign material absorbed from the gut (Fidler, 1988).

CELLS INVOLVED IN IMMUNOLOGICAL FUNCTION

Leukocytes are essential to the body's defense against invasion by foreign organisms. Both granulocytes and nongranulocytes are vital to immunity. The characteristics and functions of granulocytes (neutrophils, eosinophils, and basophils) and nongranulocytes (monocytes and lymphocytes) are discussed in the hematological anatomy and physiology review section.

IMMUNE MECHANISMS

An intact and healthy immune system consists of both natural, or nonspecific, defenses and acquired, or specific, defenses. The nonspecific defenses are the first line of protection; when they fail to protect the body from invasion, the specific defenses are put into action.

Nonspecific Defenses

The body's nonspecific defenses consist of the physical and chemical barriers to invasion, the protective and repairing processes of inflammation and phagocytosis, and other substances that stimulate the body to fight back.

Epithelial Surfaces

The body's first line of defense against infection consists of physical and chemical barriers. The epithelial surfaces are those that are exposed to the environment and are already colonized by a "normal" bacterial flora. These normal flora help to protect the body from pathogens; because they are attached to the epithelial surfaces, they prevent pathogens from doing so and gaining access to the body.

Intact skin and mucous membranes provide a protective covering; they also secrete substances that have antimicrobial effects. For instance, sweat glands produce lysozyme, an antimicrobial enzyme, and sebaceous glands secrete sebum, which has antimicrobial and antifungal properties. The skin is also constantly exfoliating, a process that sloughs off bacterial and chemical hazards.

The pH of the skin and mucosa of the gastrointes-tinal and urinary tracts inhibits the growth of many pathogens. Secretory immunoglobulin A (IgA), an antibody, and phagocytic cells are present in respiratory and gastrointestinal secretions. In the respiratory tract, mucus and cilia work together to trap and remove harmful substances. Macrophages present in the alveoli engulf and destroy pathogens. The motility of the intestines maintains an even distribution of bacterial flora, thereby preventing overgrowth and invasion and promoting evacuation of pathogens (Fidler, 1988).

Inflammation and Phagocytosis

The second line of defense involves the processes of inflammation and phagocytosis. Inflammation is initiated by cellular injury and is necessary for tissue repair, but it can be harmful if it is uncontrolled. When cellular injury occurs, specific substances are released that act as mediators; they include histamine, serotonin, kinins, lysosomal enzymes, prostaglandin, clotting factors, and complement, which is a series of proteins that act in a cascade fashion to enhance the immune and inflammatory responses. These mediators increase blood flow, capillary permeability, and vasodilation, and they promote chemotaxis and phagocytosis by neutrophils. The signs of inflammation, heat, pain, redness, and swelling are caused by these responses (Fidler, 1988). Antibody activity, phagocytosis, and inflammation are enhanced by complement components (Fidler and Keen, 1988).

Other Nonspecific Defenses

Another defense involves the release of *cytokines* from WBCs. Cytokines secreted by monocytes and macrophages are known as monokines, whereas those secreted by lymphocytes are known as lymphokines. These substances, which include interleukins, tumor necrosis factor, colony-stimulating factors, and interferons, mediate various interactions between immune system cells (Janusek, 1993) (Table 13–10). Interleukin-1, originally called endogenous pyrogen, is a monokine that increases body temperature in infection, thereby inhibiting the growth of pathogens. Interferons act to inhibit viral replication; they also have been found to have antitumor effects. Through recombinant DNA technology, interferons and these other naturally occurring substances are now being produced for the research and treatment of many disorders. Interferon is currently approved by the United States Food and Drug Administration (FDA) for the treatment of certain malignant disorders (Dudjak and Fleck, 1991).

Table 13–10. MAJOR CYTOKINES

Cytokine	Principal Effects
Interleukin-1 (IL-1)	Lymphocyte activation Macrophage and neutrophil stimulation Stimulation of acute phase proteins Fever and sleep Pituitary hormone regulation
Interleukin-2 (IL-2)	Enhances T-cell growth and function
Interleukin-3 (IL-3)	Stimulates differentiation of hematopoietic cells (colony-stimulating factor)
Interleukin-4 (IL-4)	B-cell growth factor
Interleukin-5 (IL-5)	B-cell growth and differentiation
Interleukin-6 (IL-6)	B-cell growth and differentiation Stimulates the acute phase response
Tumor necrosis factor (TNF)	Activates macrophages, granulocytes, and cytotoxic cells Cachexia Mediates septic shock Increases leukocyte adhesion Enhances antigen presentation
Colony-stimulating factor (CSF)	Stimulates division and differentiation of bone marrow stem cells
Interferon	Antiviral factor

From Janusek, L. (1993) Structure and function of the immune system. In J. M. Black & E. Matassarin-Jacobs (Eds.) *Luckmann and Sorensen's medical-surgical nursing* (4th ed.) (p. 540). Philadelphia: W. B. Saunders Co.

Specific (Acquired) Defenses: The Immune Response

The immune response protects the body from disease by recognizing, processing, and destroying foreign invaders. It also aids in the removal of damaged body tissues and cells and defends the body against the proliferation of abnormal or malignant cells. It involves the interaction of macrophages and B and T lymphocytes.

Two "arms" to the immune response exist—humoral immunity and cell-mediated immunity. These two forms are not mutually exclusive; they act together to provide immunity.

Humoral Immunity

Humoral immunity is mediated by B lymphocytes and involves the formation of antibodies in response to specific antigens. Antigens bind to receptors on B lymphocytes. This binding activates B lymphocytes and causes the proliferation and differentiation of plasma cells and the production of antibodies in response to specific antigens (Fig. 13–10). Once antibodies have been synthesized and released, they bind to their target antigen and form an antigen-antibody complex (Fig. 13–11). This complex is targeted for phagocytosis by neutrophils and macrophages. The antigen-antibody complex also activates complement. The humoral response and proliferation of B lymphocytes is regulated by the activity of T lymphocytes. Helper T cells promote B-lymphocyte activity and the production of antibodies, whereas suppressor T cells downgrade the humoral response (Fig. 13–12).

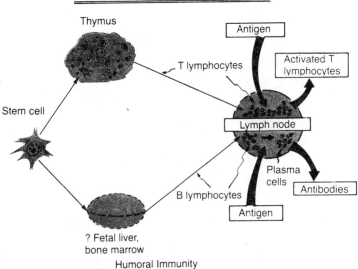

Figure 13–10. Formation of antibodies and sensitized lymphocytes in response to antigens. (From Guyton, A. C. (1991). *Textbook of medical physiology* (8th ed.) (p. 375). Philadelphia: W. B. Saunders Co.)

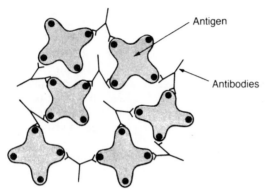

Figure 13–11. Binding of antigens and antibodies. (From Guyton, A. C. (1991). *Textbook of medical physiology* (8th ed.) (p. 378). Philadelphia: W. B. Saunders Co.)

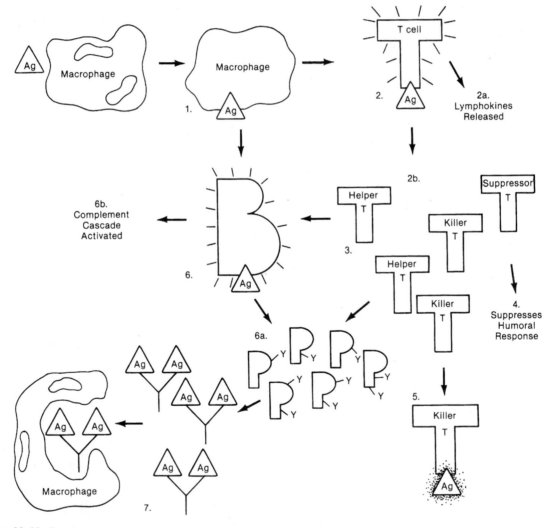

Figure 13–12. The immune response. (*1*), Macrophages process antigen (Ag) and present to T lymphocytes. (*2*), T lymphocytes (T cells) recognize antigen—in response (*2a*) they release lymphokines (e.g., interleukin 2) and (*2b*) differentiate into helper T cells, suppressor T cells, and killer T cells. (*3*), Helper T cells promote B-cell activity and antibody production. (*4*), Suppressor T cells downgrade the humoral response. (*5*), Killer T cells bind with and destroy antigens. (*6*), B lymphocytes (B cells) become activated after contact with antigen. (*6a*), They proliferate and differentiate into antibody-producing plasma cells (P = plasma cells; Y = antibodies). (*6b*), Activated B cells also activate complement. (*7*), Antibodies bind with antigen, enhancing their phagocytosis and destruction by macrophages and neutrophils.

There are two responses in humoral immunity: the primary immune response and the secondary response. In the primary response, antigens that have evaded the nonspecific defenses are engulfed and processed by macrophages. The macrophages then present the processed antigens to the lymphocytes, which proliferate, differentiate, and produce antibodies. In this first exposure, antibodies appear in the serum after 7 to 10 days. Immunoglobulin M (IgM) is the first antibody to appear, then immunoglobulin G (IgG). The total antibody titer peaks at about 21 days. In this primary response, the cells develop an immunological memory for antigens; this memory provides the basis for the secondary response on subsequent exposure (Fidler, 1988).

When a second or subsequent exposure to the antigen occurs, even if it occurs after many years, the secondary response occurs, which is much quicker, stronger, and longer lasting than the first. An overwhelming IgG response occurs; antibodies peak within 7 to 10 days and may be detectable in serum for years (Miller and Habicht, 1991).

Humoral immunity and antibodies can be passively transferred through serum. When an individual is deficient in B lymphocytes (e.g., in X-linked agammaglobulinemia and common variable immunodeficiency), sufficient antibodies cannot be produced, and the individual is at risk, especially for bacterial infections.

Immunoglobulins. Antibodies, also known as immunoglobulins, are produced in specific response to certain antigens. Five classes of immunoglobulins exist: IgG, IgM, IgA, immunoglobulin E (IgE), and immunoglobulin D (IgD) (Table 13–11).

The most abundant of the immunoglobulins is IgG, which is found in most body fluids. It is unique in that it crosses the placenta and provides passive immunity to the newborn through a variety of antibodies. Immunoglobulin G also activates and fixes complement; complement, in turn, enhances the effects of antibodies.

Immunoglobulin M is the first immunoglobulin synthesized in an immune response. It is the largest antibody, and it is present mostly in the bloodstream. It causes agglutination, or the clumping together of antigenic particles; it causes cell lysis; and it activates the complement cascade.

Immunoglobulin A, also called secretory IgA, is an important part of the body's nonspecific first line of defense and prevention of disease. It is present in many secretions, such as saliva, sweat, tears, mucus, and breast milk. The breast-feeding infant receives protection from intestinal pathogens through the ingestion of colostrum and breast milk. Immunoglobulin A inhibits the adherence of pathogens to epithelial cells.

Table 13–11. IMMUNOGLOBULINS

Immunoglobulin (Ig)	Comments
IgG	Most abundant immunoglobulin Present in intravascular and extravascular spaces Crosses placenta Coats microorganisms in order to enhance phagocytosis Activates complement
IgM	First Ig produced in response to antigen Present mostly in intravascular space Activates complement
IgA	Present in many body secretions: saliva, tears, sweat, mucus Protects epithelial surfaces Passes to newborn through colostrum and breast milk Activates complement
IgE	Important in allergic and inflammatory responses, parasitic infections
IgD	Function not well understood; ? role in lymphocyte differentiation

Immunoglobulin E is normally present in very low concentrations in the serum, but it is important in allergic reactions. It binds with mast cells and basophils in epithelial surfaces, thereby effecting the release of histamine and vasoactive substances, resulting in allergic symptoms. Immunoglobulin E also plays an important role in the defense against parasitic infections.

The function of IgD is not understood, but it is thought to play a role in the differentiation of lymphocytes (Janusek, 1993).

Cell-Mediated Immunity

Cellular, or cell-mediated, immunity is mediated by the T lymphocyte. When macrophages recognize foreign materials as being nonself, they trap, process, and present such materials to T lymphocytes. T lymphocytes recognize these antigens processed by macrophages; the T lymphocytes then proliferate, differentiate, and migrate to the site of the antigen, which is neutralized or destroyed. Differences between B and T lymphocytes are displayed in Table 13–12.

Once contact is made with a specific antigen, the T lymphocyte differentiates into helper/inducer T cells; suppressor T cells; and cytotoxic, or killer, cells. Although these T cells are microscopically identical, they can be distinguished by molecules present on the cell surface called *cluster designations* (CDs) (Fig. 13–13) (Janusek, 1993). Helper T cells (also known as T_4 cells

Table 13–12. COMPARISON OF B AND T LYMPHOCYTES

	B Lymphocyte	T Lymphocyte
Mediates:	Humoral immunity	Cell-mediated immunity
Origin:	Bone marrow	Bone marrow
Differentiation/ maturation:	Bursa equivalent in bone marrow/peripheral lymph tissue	Thymus
Function:	Immunoglobulin (Ig) synthesis	
	IgG	Defense against viral, protozoan, and fungal infections
	IgM	Stimulates macrophages
	IgA	Regulates humoral response
	IgE	Transplant rejection
	IgD	Immunosurveillance for mutant or malignant cells
Transfer:	By serum	Only through injection of cells

because they carry a CD4 marker) enhance the humoral immune response by stimulating B cells to differentiate and produce antibodies. Suppressor T cells downgrade and suppress the humoral and cell-mediated responses. In autoimmune diseases, the activity of these suppressor cells is decreased, and an overactive immune response results in the attack on body tissues. The ratio of helper to suppressor T cells is normally 2:1; a normal immune response is dependent on the relationship between these two cells. An alteration in this ratio may cause disease. For instance, a depressed ratio (a decrease of helper T cells in relation to suppressor T cells) is found in AIDS, whereas a higher ratio (a decrease in suppressor T cells in relation to helper T cells) is a feature of an autoimmune disease (Miller and Habicht, 1991). Cytotoxic, or killer, T cells, participate directly in the destruction of antigens by binding to and altering the membrane surface and

disrupting the intracellular environment, which ultimately destroys the cell. Killer cells also release cytotoxic substances into the antigen cell that causes cell lysis.

Additionally, T cells provide the body with immunosurveillance, in which they monitor blood, body fluids, and tissue for abnormal cells or tissue. This mechanism is responsible for the rejection of transplanted tissue, which is recognized by T cells as nonself.

Cell-mediated immunity cannot be transferred through serum; transfer takes place only through injection of sensitized T cells. Whereas humoral immunity is an immediate response, cell-mediated immunity is a more delayed reaction. It is important in viral, fungal, and intracellular infections and is the mechanism involved in transplant rejection. Cell-mediated immunity is also important in the fight against neoplastic cells.

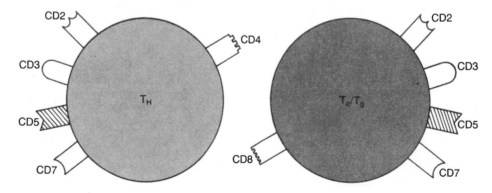

Figure 13–13. T lymphocyte markers. (Adapted from Janusek, L. (1993). Structure and function of the immune system. In J. M. Black, & E. Matassarin-Jacobs (Eds.), *Luckmann and Sorensen's medical-surgical nursing* (4th ed.) (p. 534). Philadelphia: W. B. Saunders Co.)

Assessment of Immune Function

If any component of the immune system is altered, the body is at risk for disease, specifically overwhelming infection, autoimmune disorders, or malignancies. A thorough assessment is performed in order to determine the existence of, or risk for, an immune system alteration.

A complete health history is obtained, including chronic diseases, past illnesses, hospitalizations, surgeries, and relevant family history. Any history of allergies, infections, or neoplastic disorders is well documented. The nurse determines whether the patient has suffered from delayed wound healing, persistent cough, lymphadenopathy, anorexia, nausea and vomiting, diarrhea, fever, or night sweats. Joint pain, limited range of motion, and bone tenderness are noted because they might indicate the presence of an autoimmune or malignant disorder. Any medications the patient is taking are noted; many drugs suppress bone marrow function, resulting in altered immune function. Any treatment with antibiotics, radiation, chemotherapeutic agents, steroids, or other immunosuppressants is emphasized.

Dietary practices are assessed because inadequate protein or caloric intake alters immune functions, such as antibody formation and phagocytosis. Any history of IV drug use is documented. The patient is questioned about possible occupational exposure to chemicals or radiation that may cause depressed bone marrow function or place the patient at risk for certain types of cancer. The patient's use of alcohol, tobacco, or illicit drugs is assessed. The nurse determines sexual behaviors that might place the patient at risk for infectious diseases, such as infection with human immunodeficiency virus (HIV), that can be detrimental to immune function (Shannon-Bodnar, 1993).

During the physical examination, the patient's general appearance, signs of fatigue, acute illness, and chronic disease are noted. The patient's neurological status is assessed for changes in level of consciousness and cognition, which might indicate central nervous system infection (e.g., HIV, toxoplasmosis, and cryptococcal meningitis). The head and neck are examined for swollen lymph nodes, presence of pain, tenderness, or meningeal irritation (e.g., as indicated by headache, stiff neck). Skin integrity is evaluated, and any impairment, sign of infection, or poor healing is noted. The nurse checks for rashes or lesions, such as the characteristic purplish-brown lesions of Kaposi's sarcoma. Respiratory rate and effort are noted, as are breath sounds and the presence of shortness of breath, dyspnea, or cough. In addition, the abdomen is assessed for distention or tenderness, and the liver and spleen are assessed for enlargement or tenderness, as may be found in many immune disorders.

Diagnostic tests for immune function include WBC count with differential in order to determine the presence of infection. Total B-cell counts and absolute lymphocyte counts may be performed in order to assess for specific cell abnormalities, and complement assessments can be performed. Skin testing is helpful in assessing cell-mediated immunity and in determining allergens. A bone marrow aspiration and biopsy may be performed in order to assess for WBC disorders. Lymph node or liver biopsy may also be used for diagnosis. Noninvasive tests include nuclear scans, computed tomography, and magnetic resonance imaging in order to determine abnormal enlargement or tumors of the bone marrow, spleen, liver, or lymph nodes. Two tests are commonly used for diagnosing HIV infection: the enzyme-linked immunosorbent assay (ELISA) and the Western blot, both of which test for the presence of antibodies to HIV. T-cell counts may be performed in order to determine how susceptible the patient is to infection. This count is obtained by measuring the cell-surface markers present on the cell membranes of lymphocytes, most frequently, CD4 and CD8 cell markers (basically, the numbers of helper/inducer and cytotoxic T cells). The CD4 count is used in the clinical staging of patients infected with HIV (Saag, 1995).

Selected Immunological Disorders

Many pathological states can alter the body's ability to fight disease. The immune system can fail to develop properly, lose its previous ability to react to invasion by pathogens, overreact to otherwise harmless antigens, or turn immune functions against self. Included in the long list of disorders of the immune system are hypersensitivity and anaphylaxis, autoimmune diseases, congenital immune disorders, acquired immune disorders, and malignant or neoplastic diseases of the lymphoid organs or tissues. However, in the intensive care unit, the predominant immune system problem seen is that of immunocompromise. This section focuses on the recognition and treatment of the immunocompromised patient.

A nursing diagnosis seen frequently in critical care is "risk for infection" (see Nursing Care Plan for the Immunocompromised Patient). Immunocompromise in the critically ill is caused by many factors. In addition to existing immunodeficiency diseases and life-threatening illness, immune defenses are altered by invasive monitoring, procedures, and presence of opportunistic pathogens. These factors can worsen the patient's preexisting state or can contribute to the development of new problems.

Immune disorders can affect any or all of the various components of the immune system. Cell-mediated or humoral immune responses may be affected. The defect may be in the ability to phagocytize pathogens or in the complement cascade. Any defect in the immune system, whatever the component, puts the body at risk for disease.

PRIMARY IMMUNODEFICIENCY

Primary immune disorders or immunodeficiencies are those in which the primary dysfunction exists in the immune system. Most primary immunodeficiencies are congenital; some part of the immune system fails to develop (Fidler and Keen, 1988). Many disorders fall into this category (Table 13–13).

Table 13–13. PRIMARY AND SECONDARY IMMUNODEFICIENCIES

Immunodeficiency	Examples
Primary	
B cell defects	Bruton's agammaglobulinemia (X-linked)
	Common variable immunodeficiency
	IgA deficiency
T cell defects	DiGeorge's syndrome
	Nezelof's syndrome
Combined defects	Severe combined immunodeficiency disease
	Ataxia-telangiectasia
Phagocytic defects	
Complement defects	
Secondary	
Infections	Measles, tuberculosis, acute viral, cytomegalovirus, human immunodeficiency virus (acquired immunodeficiency syndrome)
Malignancies	Hodgkin's disease, acute and chronic leukemias, multiple myeloma
Autoimmune states	Systemic lupus erythematosus, rheumatoid arthritis
Chronic disease	Diabetes mellitus, renal disease, alcoholic cirrhosis
Drugs	Cytotoxic agents (chemotherapeutics, immunosuppressants), antibiotics, phenytoin, anesthetic agents
Other	Aging, stress, malnutrition, radiation, burn injuries, trauma

When the deficiency is in the stem cell, both humoral and cell-mediated immunity is diminished or absent, as occurs in severe combined immunodeficiency disease. A congenital humoral disorder results in a deficient production of immunoglobulin and manifests through recurrent, severe, or unusual infections with extracellular bacteria (Fidler and Keen, 1988). X-linked agammaglobulinemia and common variable immunodeficiency are examples of congenital humoral defects. When the defect is in cell-mediated immunity or the T cell, the patient has an impaired defense against fungi and intracellular microorganisms, as occurs in DiGeorge's syndrome. Other primary disorders affect the function of complement or phagocytosis. Complement defects diminish the activity of antibodies, of phagocytes, and of the process of inflammation. Phagocytic defects can result in an inadequate number or dysfunction of phagocytic cells (Fidler and Keen, 1988).

SECONDARY IMMUNODEFICIENCY

In a secondary immunodeficiency, the immune disorder is the result of factors outside the immune system and involves the loss of a previously functional immune defense. Also known as acquired immunodeficiency, secondary immunodeficiency causes may include stress, aging, malnutrition, malignancies, chronic disease, pharmacological agents (e.g., chemotherapeutic agents, immunosuppressants), and infectious diseases (e.g., HIV infection) (see Table 13–13).

Stress

Although stress has not been definitively shown to *cause* disease, it does affect the body's ability to protect itself against disease. When the body is stressed, physically or emotionally, an increased release of adrenal hormones and, subsequently, cortisol, occurs. These substances cause a decrease in the numbers of circulating eosinophils and lymphocytes (Guyton, 1991). A history of burns or trauma, serious illness, noise, lights, constant activity, procedures, and equipment are patient stressors in critical care units. Social factors, such as bereavement, job loss, or divorce, are stressors, as are pathological conditions, such as tuberculosis, myocardial infarction, diabetes, and malignancy (Fidler and Keen, 1988). Surgery also causes stress, and many anesthetics used in surgery further depress the immune response.

Age

The very young and the very old are immunocompromised. The newborn is protected by maternal antibodies up to several weeks or months after birth but then becomes susceptible to infection until it develops a competent immune system of its own. Elderly patients have diminished immunity. With age, thymus involution results in a decreased cell-mediated immunity. Antibody production and response diminish, and immune memory is also affected. The incidence of autoimmune and malignant diseases also increases (Gurka, 1989).

Malnutrition

Malnutrition affects the ability to fight disease. Especially in protein and caloric deficiencies, a decrease in immunocompetent WBCs occurs. Cell-mediated immunity and complement activity are particularly diminished. The thymus gland and lymph nodes atrophy, particularly in the presence of iron deficiency (Gurka, 1989). The malnourished patient is more susceptible to infection, especially by fungi, viruses, and intracellular bacteria (Fidler and Keen, 1988). In critical care patients, malnutrition is common. Inadequate intake caused by endotracheal tubes, nasogastric suction, or surgical status as well as anorexia, nausea, and vomiting caused by drugs, treatment, or illness contribute to malnutrition in the critically ill.

Malignancy

Malignancies, or neoplastic diseases, that cause secondary immunodeficiency include Burkitt's lymphoma, chronic lymphocytic leukemia, acute leukemia, multiple myeloma, and Hodgkin's disease. In these and other malignancies, therapeutic treatment, such as chemotherapy and radiation, also severely compromise immunity. Radiation destroys both B and T lymphocytes and causes shrinkage of lymphoid tissue. The resulting decreased resistance to infection may last a year or longer (Fidler and Keen, 1988). Chemotherapy also causes a decrease in lymphocytes. Most chemotherapeutic drugs alter the proliferation and differentiation of stem cells, resulting in decreased WBCs.

Chronic Disease

Most patients with chronic disease are in a debilitated state, which places them at risk for infection. In renal disease or renal failure, a decrease in circulating lymphocytes occurs. This, in conjunction with the presence of uremic toxins, acidosis, and malnutrition, depresses the immune response (Gurka, 1989). Diabetes also results in an increased susceptibility to infection. High blood glucose level, neuropathy, and vascular insufficiency contribute to this increased risk.

Pharmacological Agents

Drugs other than chemotherapeutic agents can cause immune system depression. The chronic abuse of alcohol results in a decrease in granulocytes and diminished cell-mediated immunity. Antibiotics can alter the normal bacterial flora of the gastrointestinal and respiratory tracts, a situation that allows pathogenic organisms to attach and invade more easily. Steroids cause an increase in neutrophils while decreasing lymphocyte activity and the numbers of monocytes and eosinophils. They also may diminish production of IgG. When used on a long-term basis, cell-mediated immunity is impaired. Interleukin-2 is decreased, and the migration of T lymphocytes and macrophages is affected (Dattwyler, 1991).

Therapeutic Immunosuppression

In transplantation, immunosuppression is the ultimate goal; it prevents the body from recognizing the transplanted tissue as nonself, or foreign. Advances in immunosuppressive drug therapy have improved the survival and quality of life for transplant recipients. Although the drugs used in immunosuppressive therapy vary depending on the tissue or organ transplanted, kidney, bone marrow, heart, lung, liver, and pancreas transplants all require some degree of immunosuppression. Drugs used for immunosuppression include corticosteroids, antimetabolites, monoclonal and polyclonal antibodies, and others, such as cyclosporine. Corticosteroids affect lymphocytes, especially T cells. Thus, their long-term use impairs cell-mediated immunity. An antimetabolite used in transplants is azathioprine (Imuran), which seems to primarily affect T cells. Antibodies used in therapeutic immunosuppression are those that have been synthesized in animals injected with human blood cells. Antilymphocyte serum suppresses humoral and cell-mediated immunity; antithymocyte globulin depresses primarily T cells. OKT3, a monoclonal antibody, is also used to depress T-cell function. Cyclosporine is another immunosuppressant; it inhibits T-lymphocyte function but leaves humoral immunity and phagocytosis intact (Dattwyler, 1991).

Besides placing the patient at greater risk for infection, immunosuppressants have other deleterious side effects and require close nursing supervision during their administration. Monitoring for patient response and side effects is very important.

Infectious Diseases

Many infectious diseases, such as measles, tuberculosis, acute viral infections, and cytomegalovirus (CMV), result in immunocompromise. AIDS is currently one of the nation's greatest health problems.

Acquired Immunodeficiency Syndrome

Having reached epidemic proportions worldwide, AIDS is seen in all settings of health care, including critical care. AIDS also exists as a "hidden" disease because many individuals may have been infected with HIV, the disease-causing virus, unknowingly. Although the incidence of AIDS continues to increase, these patients are living longer and have a better quality of life because of advances in treatment. In critical care, the AIDS patient typically presents with life-threatening opportunistic infections.

Acquired immunodeficiency syndrome was first recognized as a syndrome in 1981, when the Centers for Disease Control and Prevention (CDC, formerly the Centers for Disease Control) reported an increased incidence of a rare pneumonia and cancer in homosex-

ual males. By 1982, the syndrome was defined by the CDC as AIDS and was noted to affect individuals other than homosexuals; patients with hemophilia A were also infected. In 1984, the causative virus was isolated by physicians in the United States and France at approximately the same time and was given two different names: the human T-cell leukemia/lymphoma virus (HTLV-3) and lymphadenopathy-associated virus (LAV). The virus was renamed human immunodeficiency virus in 1987 (Coletti et al., 1989).

Acquired immunodeficiency syndrome in the United States is most common in males, in those living in urban areas, and in blacks and Hispanics. Whereas homosexuals constitute the majority of those infected, the incidence in that population is decreasing, whereas heterosexual transmission in women and adolescents is increasing dramatically. The incidence of AIDS in

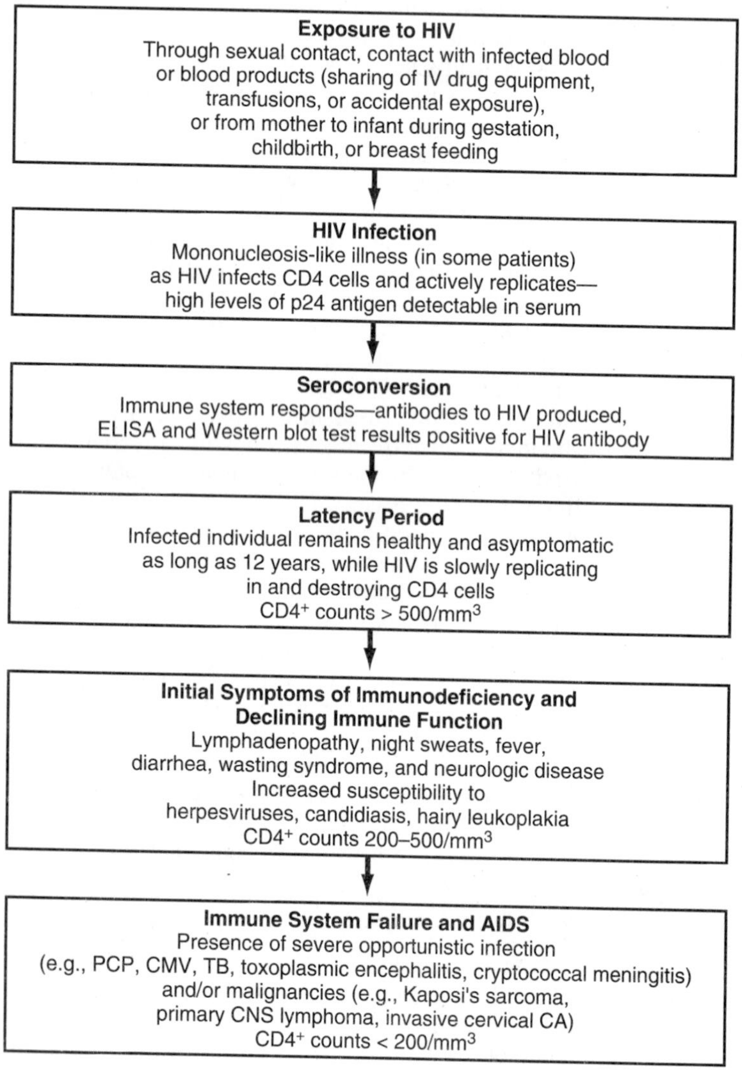

Exposure to HIV
Through sexual contact, contact with infected blood or blood products (sharing of IV drug equipment, transfusions, or accidental exposure), or from mother to infant during gestation, childbirth, or breast feeding

HIV Infection
Mononucleosis-like illness (in some patients) as HIV infects CD4 cells and actively replicates— high levels of p24 antigen detectable in serum

Seroconversion
Immune system responds—antibodies to HIV produced, ELISA and Western blot test results positive for HIV antibody

Latency Period
Infected individual remains healthy and asymptomatic as long as 12 years, while HIV is slowly replicating in and destroying CD4 cells
$CD4^+$ counts > 500/mm^3

Initial Symptoms of Immunodeficiency and Declining Immune Function
Lymphadenopathy, night sweats, fever, diarrhea, wasting syndrome, and neurologic disease Increased susceptibility to herpesviruses, candidiasis, hairy leukoplakia
$CD4^+$ counts 200–500/mm^3

Immune System Failure and AIDS
Presence of severe opportunistic infection (e.g., PCP, CMV, TB, toxoplasmic encephalitis, cryptococcal meningitis) and/or malignancies (e.g., Kaposi's sarcoma, primary CNS lymphoma, invasive cervical CA)
$CD4^+$ counts < 200/mm^3

Figure 13–14. Pathophysiology of human immunodeficiency virus (HIV) infection. ELISA = enzyme-linked immunosorbent assay; IV = intravenous; PCP = *Pneumocystis carinii* pneumonia; CMV = cytomegalovirus; TB = tuberculosis; CA = cancer; CNS = central nervous system.

male and female heterosexuals who inject drugs is increasing, as are cases in rural areas (Klimek, 1992). The percentage of AIDS cases in children is also rising dramatically as infants are born to infected mothers (Durham, 1994).

Pathophysiology. Human immunodeficiency virus causes AIDS by disrupting the body's immune response; it is manifested by recurrent opportunistic infections and/or rare malignancies that are seldom seen in immunocompetent individuals. AIDS is primarily a dysfunction of cell-mediated immunity: the HIV virus causes a deficiency in helper T cells.

Human immunodeficiency virus infects primarily helper T cells and macrophages; it then reproduces and kills the cells. HIV is a retrovirus, which transcribes its genetic material, RNA, into DNA in the host cell nucleus by using an enzyme called reverse transcriptase. Once an individual is infected with HIV, a burst of viral activity occurs as HIV replicates in CD4 cells. Seroconversion, which usually occurs within 2 to 12 weeks of exposure, takes place as antibodies to HIV are developed; the patient may experience "acute seroconversion syndrome" with symptoms similar to those of mononucleosis. This immune response is followed by a decrease in the HIV titer as infected cells are sequestered in the lymph nodes (Cohn, 1993; Fan et al., 1994). During this period, which may last 10 years or more, the patient may remain totally asymptomatic, although viral particles are being actively produced. The immune system is slowly destroyed as HIV continues to replicate; this phenomenon is evident through the decreasing CD4 cell counts as the disease progresses. As the CD4 count decreases, the patient becomes more susceptible to various opportunistic infections and malignancies; AIDS is the final stage of HIV infection (Fig. 13–14).

The virus is transmitted through exposure to infected body fluids, blood, or blood products. This transmission can occur through rectal or vaginal intercourse with an infected person, IV drug use with contaminated equipment, transfusion with contaminated blood or blood products, accidental exposure through needle sticks or breaks in the skin, or gestation or childbirth (from mother to fetus) (Table 13–14). Transmission via breast feeding has also occurred. Transmission appears to be dose related, and the disease is not known to be spread by casual contact. Risk of transmission apparently is more likely when the infected individual has advanced disease (Greenberg, 1993), *although transmission of HIV can occur at any time or stage of infection.* The risk to those requiring transfusions has been greatly decreased through the screening of all blood products, which began in April 1985 (Cohn, 1993). The risk of transmission to health care workers, although small, does exist; through con-

sistent observance of protective guidelines, such as universal precautions, this risk can be minimized. Universal precautions recommended by the Centers for Disease Control and Prevention are displayed in Table 13–15.

Table 13–14. RISK FACTORS/TRANSMISSION OF HUMAN IMMUNODEFICIENCY VIRUS

Rectal or vaginal intercourse with frequent, multiple partners
Intravenous drug abuse/sharing needles
Transfusion with contaminated blood or blood products
Transmission from mother to fetus during gestation or childbirth or to newborn through breast feeding
Occupational exposure to infected blood or body fluids through needle sticks, sharp instruments, or nonintact skin

---

Table 13–15. UNIVERSAL PRECAUTIONS TO PREVENT TRANSMISSION OF HUMAN IMMUNODEFICIENCY VIRUS IN HEALTH CARE SETTINGS*

1. *Gloves* should be worn whenever blood or body fluids, mucous membranes, or nonintact skin is touched, whenever any items or surfaces soiled with blood or body fluids are handled, whenever venipuncture or other vascular access procedures are performed. Gloves should be changed after contact with each patient.
2. *Masks, protective eyewear, or face shields* should be worn for any procedure in which droplets of blood or body fluids might be generated or when splattering might occur.
3. *Gowns or aprons* should be worn for any patient care or procedure in which splattering of blood or body fluids might occur.
4. *Hands and skin surfaces* should be washed immediately and thoroughly after any contact with blood or body fluids, and after removal of gloves.
5. *Needles, scalpels, and other sharp instruments* should be handled with extreme care during procedures, cleaning, and disposal in order to prevent accidental injuries. Needles should *not* be recapped, broken, removed, or otherwise manipulated; they should be placed in a puncture-resistant container for disposal. Puncture-resistant containers should be placed in patient care areas for ready access and should be changed before becoming overfull.
6. *Mouthpieces, resuscitation bags, or ventilation devices* should be readily accessible for emergency use.

Adapted from Centers for Disease Control. (1987). Recommendations for prevention of HIV transmission in health-care settings. *Morbidity and Mortality Weekly Report, 36*(2S), 3–18.
*Universal blood and body fluid precautions should be used consistently for *all* patients.
Blood and body fluids to which universal precautions apply include blood and other body fluids containing visible blood; semen and vaginal secretions; and cerebrospinal, synovial, pleural, peritoneal, pericardial, and amniotic fluids.

Table 13–16. SYMPTOMS OF HUMAN IMMUNODEFICIENCY VIRUS INFECTION

Fever
Night sweats
Fatigue, weakness
Generalized lymphadenopathy
Malaise
Anorexia
Weight loss
Diarrhea
Dementia
Peripheral neuropathy
Malignancies: Kaposi's sarcoma, lymphoma, cervical cancer
Opportunistic infections (see Table 13–17)

Assessment/Clinical Manifestations. The signs and symptoms of AIDS vary greatly, depending on the particular opportunistic infections or malignancies and the degree of patient immunosuppression present (Ta-

ble 13–16). AIDS is indicated by a CD4 count of less that 200/μl and clinical signs of opportunistic infections (Table 13–17), malignancies, wasting syndrome, or dementia (Fan et al., 1994; Barrick, 1988). The diagnosis is confirmed by the presence of HIV antibodies, detected by enzyme-linked immunosorbent assay and confirmed by the Western blot test. In addition to decreasing CD4 counts and HIV antibody tests, laboratory findings in AIDS may include an abnormal helper to suppressor ratio (<1.0), leukopenia, and thrombocytopenia. The p24 test, which detects HIV directly through the presence of the core antigen (p24), may also be performed. A positive test result indicates the presence of HIV infection, although a negative p24 test result does not rule out the presence of HIV infection (Cohn, 1993).

Acute illness can be gradual or sudden and includes complaints of fatigue, malaise, fever, night sweats, lymphadenopathy, anorexia, persistent diarrhea, weight loss, cough, and shortness of breath (Barrick, 1988). Although patients with AIDS experience many opportunistic infections, pneumonia caused by

Table 13–17. OPPORTUNISTIC INFECTIONS IN ACQUIRED IMMUNODEFICIENCY SYNDROME

Pathogen	Effect	Treatment
Pulmonary		
Pneumocystis carinii	Pneumonia	First line: trimethoprim-sulfamethoxazole (TMP/SMX); second line: intravenous pentamidine, trimetrexate, atovaquone
Mycobacterium tuberculosis	Tuberculosis; disseminated illness	Combination: isoniazid, rifampin, pyrazinamide, and ethambutol or streptomycin
Central Nervous System		
Toxoplasma gondii	Encephalitis	Pyrimethamine and sulfadiazine
Cryptococcus neoformans	Cryptococcal meningitis; disseminated illness	Amphotericin B followed by fluconazole
Cytomegalovirus	Retinitis, encephalitis, and disseminated illness	Ganciclovir, foscarnet
JC virus	Progressive multifocal encephalopathy	None effective at present
Gastrointestinal		
Candida albicans	Oral, pharyngeal, gastrointestinal candidiasis; vaginitis	Fluconazole, clotrimazole, ketoconazole, nystatin
Cryptosporidium parvum	Gastroenteritis	No standard—possibly azithromycin; intravenous fluids
Isospora belli, human immunodeficiency virus	Gastroenteritis	TMP/SMX
Salmonellae	Diarrhea, bacteremia	Ciprofloxacin, ampicillin, chloramphenicol, TMP/SMX
General/Other		
Mycobacterium avium, Mycobacterium intracellulare	Disseminated illness: fever, night sweats, diarrhea, weight loss, abdominal pain	Clarithromycin or azithromycin, with ethambutol
Herpes simplex virus, types 1 and 2	Painful oral, genital, or perirectal lesions	Acyclovir; foscarnet if resistant
Herpes zoster virus	Painful cutaneous lesions	Acyclovir; foscarnet if resistant

Data from American Foundation for AIDS Research. (1995). *AIDS/HIV Treatment Directory.* 7(4). Rockville, MD: Author.

the protozoan *Pneumocystis carinii* is most frequently seen in critical care.

Pneumocystis carinii pneumonia (PCP) is the predominant pulmonary infection in AIDS; this organism causes tremendous morbidity and mortality in the HIV-infected population. Acutely ill patients present with tachypnea, fever, hypoxemia, and diffuse infiltrates on chest x-ray study; they may report a recent history of nonproductive cough, dyspnea, fever, and fatigue (Timby, 1992). Without intervention, respiratory failure and death occur. Diagnosis is made by arterial blood gas results, chest x-ray study, gallium lung scan, and sputum induction; the more risky procedures of bronchoscopy with bronchoalveolar lavage, transbronchial biopsy, or open lung biopsy of tissue for the identification of the organism may be required (Timby, 1992).

Another cause of pulmonary disease in AIDS is CMV. Patients present similarly to those with PCP: diffuse infiltrates on chest x-ray study and hypoxemia. CMV may be isolated from bronchoscopy specimens or blood cultures; antibodies to CMV may be present in serum as well. Mortality in patients with CMV infection is high, especially if the patient also has PCP (Singer et al., 1990). CMV more frequently affects the eyes, causing retinitis; this is a major cause of blindness in AIDS patients. It is also known to cause symptoms in the hepatic as well as the gastrointestinal and central nervous systems.

Kaposi's sarcoma is a malignant tumor of the endothelium. On the skin, it appears as a purplish brown lesion, usually on the extremities. Kaposi's sarcoma may also affect tissue in the lymph nodes, lung, gastrointestinal tract, liver, or bone. Diagnosis is made by tissue biopsy. Other malignancies frequently seen in AIDS are non-Hodgkin's lymphomas, leukemias, and squamous cell carcinoma of the mouth and rectum (Coletti et al., 1989). Cervical cancer is increasing as the incidence of AIDS in women increases (Cohn, 1993).

Neurological manifestations of AIDS can be caused by opportunistic infections of the brain and spinal cord, malignancies, pharmacological therapies, or direct infection of the central nervous system with HIV. AIDS dementia complex, also known as HIV encephalopathy, is caused by direct infection with HIV; it is the most common cause of neurological symptoms in patients with AIDS (Loder, 1993). Symptoms include personality changes, apathy, social withdrawal, loss of fine motor coordination, weakness, tremor, ataxia, and problems with memory and cognition. AIDS dementia progresses over months. In the advanced stages, patients suffer from severe dementia, incontinence, and paraplegia.

Toxoplasmic encephalitis is another major cause of neurological problems in the AIDS population. A protozoan parasite, *Toxoplasma gondii* causes inflammation that destroys brain cells. Transmission of this organism can occur through handling infected cat feces or ingesting uncooked or undercooked meat. Symptoms include fever, headache, subtle mental status changes, and focal neurological abnormalities, such as hemiparesis. Diagnosis of toxoplasmic encephalitis is made by imaging studies and cerebrospinal fluid examinations; definitive diagnosis is made by brain tissue biopsy (Mocsny, 1992).

Other common opportunistic disorders in AIDS include bacterial infections caused by *Mycobacterium avium* complex, streptococci, *Shigella* species, and *Campylobacter* species; cryptococcal meningitis; candidiasis infection of the mouth, esophagus, or vagina; other fungal infections, such as histoplasmosis, blastomycosis, and coccidioidomycosis; diarrhea caused by *Cryptosporidium;* and herpes simplex or herpes zoster infections. Drug-resistant tuberculosis has increasingly become a problem in the AIDS population.

Nursing Diagnoses. Nursing care of the patient with AIDS is complex, especially in critical care. The list of nursing diagnoses, actual and potential, is long and depends on the particular manifestations seen.

- Risk for infection related to immunosuppression, disease process, malnutrition, chemotherapy, and opportunistic pathogens.
- Impaired gas exchange related to pulmonary infection.
- Impaired tissue integrity related to invasive lines and/or procedures, diarrhea, malnutrition, malignant lesions (Kaposi's sarcoma), chemotherapy, or immobility.
- Hyperthermia related to infectious process.
- Risk for fluid volume deficit related to nausea and vomiting, diarrhea, or malabsorption.
- Altered oral mucous membranes related to oral infections or lesions, malignancy, or treatment side effects.
- Altered nutrition (less than body requirements) related to diarrhea, malabsorption, anorexia, painful oral lesions, or fasting (NPO) status.
- Diarrhea related to gastrointestinal infection, antibiotics, cytotoxic drugs, or enteral feedings.
- Risk for injury (seizures) related central nervous system infection or malignancy.
- Activity intolerance related to weakness, fatigue, malnutrition, neurological involvement, respiratory problems, or infectious processes.
- Altered thought processes related to central nervous system infection, malignancy, or pharmacological interventions.

- Pain related to infections, neuropathy, lesions, chemotherapy, procedures, immobility, and/or treatments.
- Knowledge deficit regarding disease transmission, course of disease, opportunistic infections, treatments, or medications.
- Anxiety related to diagnosis, uncertain outcome of disease, fear of death or procedures, or reaction of significant others to diagnosis.

Medical Interventions. Medical treatment of AIDS consists of primary treatment of HIV as well as prevention, early detection, and treatment of opportunistic infections (see Table 13–17) and malignancies. This regimen includes management of symptoms and prevention of complications. In addition to specific medications (Table 13-18), treatment may include chest physiotherapy, respiratory support, oxygen, nutritional support, administration of blood products and/or IV fluids, administration of analgesics, and physical therapy.

Primary therapy for HIV includes the use of antiretroviral agents. By inhibiting replication of HIV, these drugs are given in order to prevent or delay the progression of disease. Zidovudine (AZT) was the first antiretroviral to be approved for use by the FDA; it remains the drug of choice because it decreases the frequency and severity of opportunistic infections and prolongs the survival of patients with AIDS (Hoth et al., 1993). AZT therapy is recommended when the patient's CD4 count decreases to less than 500/µl. AZT toxicity is common and may require lowering of the dosage or discontinuation of the drug. The major adverse reactions include anemia and leukopenia; these may be treated with epoetin alfa (Epogen, Procrit), which increases RBC counts, or granulocyte colony-stimulating factor, which increases WBC counts (Cohn, 1993). Other FDA-approved antiretrovirals are didanosine (ddI, Videx), zalcitabine (ddC, Hivid), and stavudine (d4T, Zerit). Although didanosine is used when AZT toxicity or resistance has developed, zalcitabine is most effective when used in conjunction with AZT (Cohn, 1993). The most recently approved of these drugs is stavudine. Didanosine, zalcitabine, and stavudine have similar adverse reactions; pancreatitis or painful peripheral neuropathy are the most common dose-limiting reactions. Another antiretroviral drug currently in investigational trials is lamivudine (3TC); it is being used especially in combination with other antiretrovirals. Other primary HIV therapy being researched involves the enhancement of immune function through the administration of cytokines, such as interleukin-2 (Kovacs et al., 1995).

The first-line medical treatment of PCP in critical care is administration of trimethoprim-sulfamethoxazole. Alternative choices are IV pentamidine, clindamycin with primaquine, trimetrexate, and atovaquone. Although these drugs have improved the prognosis and survival in PCP, they have deleterious side effects, such as leukopenia, thrombocytopenia, anemia, severe rashes, and hepatotoxicity (Hopewell and Masur, 1995). Corticosteroids may be used for the prevention of respiratory failure; these agents should be administered carefully because they may result in further immunosuppression (Bartlett et al., 1993). Oxygen is administered, and the patient may also require mechanical ventilation.

Malignancies, such as Kaposi's sarcoma, lymphomas, and cervical cancer, are typically treated with chemotherapeutic agents and radiation. Research evaluating the use of monoclonal antibodies and cytokines in the treatment of malignancies is encouraging.

In direct HIV infection, such as occurs in AIDS dementia complex, AZT is the drug used in treatment; it is known to cross the blood-brain barrier (Scherer, 1990).

Preferred medical treatment of toxoplasmosis infection is pyrimethamine and sulfadiazine, although toxicity is a problem with many patients. Other drugs used include clindamycin with pyrimethamine, azithromycin, and atovaquone. Folic acid may be given in order to counteract the side effects of pyrimethamine (Bartlett et al., 1993). Corticosteroids may also be administered for the control of cerebral edema.

Other pharmacological treatments for opportunistic disorders include ganciclovir and foscarnet in CMV infections; azithromycin or clarithromycin with ethambutol for *Mycobacterium avium* complex, amphotericin B followed by fluconazole for cryptococcal meningitis; fluconazole, clotrimazole, ketoconazole, or nystatin for candidiasis; and acyclovir for herpes simplex or zoster. Tuberculosis is initially treated with isoniazid, rifampin, or pyrazinamide, in combination with ethambutol or streptomycin, drug sensitivities must be performed to guide clinical decisions. Second-line drugs are available for most infections if the patient cannot tolerate or is resistant to the preferred treatment. Many drugs are being investigated or are currently in trials for the treatment of these disorders; hence, advances and changes in recommended treatment occur rapidly.

Drug prophylaxis has become the routine treatment for HIV-infected individuals. Based on the CD4 lymphocyte count, drugs are administered in order to prevent the development or recurrence of certain opportunistic infections, such as PCP and *M. avium* complex disease (Anastasi and Rivera, 1994).

Research. The pathogenesis and treatment of HIV and AIDS continue to be vigorously researched, and many areas are open to investigation. These areas include the use of antiviral agents, the use of immune

Table 13–18. DRUGS USED IN HUMAN IMMUNODEFICIENCY VIRUS / ACQUIRED IMMUNODEFICIENCY SYNDROME

Drug	Actions/Uses Used Primarily In	Dosage/Route	Common Side Effects	Nursing Implications
Zidovudine (AZT, Retrovir)	Antiretroviral: inhibits HIV replication HIV infection	200 mg q 4 h po 1–2 mg/kg IV q 4 h over 1 h	Anemia, thrombocytopenia, leukopenia, rash, myalgias, nausea, headache, weakness, diarrhea, abdominal pain	Monitor CBC; give with light food in order to avoid nausea Administer po when possible
Didanosine (ddl, Videx)	Antiretroviral HIV infection; AZT resistance or intolerance	Based on weight—125–300 mg bid po	Peripheral neuropathy, pancreatitis, nausea, vomiting, diarrhea, anorexia, liver failure	Administer 30 min ac or 2 h pc; pills must be chewed, crushed, or dissolved Monitor LFT results, CBC
Zalcitabine (ddC, Hivid)	Antiretroviral HIV infection; given in combination with AZT	0.75 mg + 200 mg AZT q 8 h po	Peripheral neuropathy, pancreatitis, oral ulcers	Do not give with food. Monitor amylase level; increased risk of pancreatitis with pentamidine
Stavudine (d4T, Zerit)	Antiretroviral HIV infection; AZT resistance or intolerance	>60 kg: 40 mg po bid <60 kg: 30 mg po bid	Peripheral neuropathy, anemia, headache, rash, diarrhea, myalgia	Monitor aminotransferase levels; may be of most use in combination therapy (research ongoing)
Trimethoprim sulfamethoxazole (TMP/SMX)	Antibacterial *Pneumocystis carinii* pneumonia—acute	15–20 mg/kg/d + 75–100 mg/kg/d in 4 divided doses	Rash, fever, nausea, vomiting, leukopenia, thrombocytopenia	Dilute drug in 125–250 ml 5% DW; infuse over 60–90 min; monitor CBC for dyscrasias
Pentamidine (Pentam)	Antiprotozoal *P. carinii* pneumonia—acute	4 mg/kg/d IV over 1–2 h	Hypotension, metallic taste, hypoglycemia, renal toxicity, anxiety, chills, headache	Monitor BP closely during administration; check CBC, glucose, LFT results, BUN, Cr (creatinine)
Trimetrexate (Neu Trexin)	*P. carinii* pneumonia—moderate to severe	30–45 mg/m²/d IV	Hepatic, renal toxicity; bone marrow suppression	Monitor LFT results, Cr, BUN, CBC for dyscrasias
Atovaquone (Mepron)	*P. carinii* pneumonia—mild to moderate	750 mg po tid	Rash, fever, headache, nausea, vomiting, diarrhea, anemia, leukopenia	Administer with food Monitor CBC, LFT results
Pyrimethamine (Daraprim) (given with sulfadiazine)	Folic acid antagonist, toxoplasmic encephalitis	100 mg × 1 day; then 50–75 mg/d po	Anemia, leukopenia, thrombocytopenia, anorexia, vomiting	Monitor CBC for dyscrasias; give with milk or food
Sulfadiazine	Toxoplasmic encephalitis	200 mg/kg (4–8 g) po or IV in divided doses qd	Rash, fever, leukopenia, crystalluria	Monitor CBC for dyscrasias Encourage fluid intake *Table continued on following page*

417

Table 13–18. DRUGS USED IN HUMAN IMMUNODEFICIENCY VIRUS/ACQUIRED IMMUNODEFICIENCY SYNDROME *Continued*

Drug	Actions/Uses Used Primarily In	Dosage/Route	Common Side Effects	Nursing Implications
Amphotericin B (Fungizone)	Antifungal Cryptococcal meningitis	0.3–0.8 mg/kg/d IV	Anemia; renal, hepatic toxicity, electrolyte disturbances; hypotension, headache, fever, chills, nausea, vomiting, diarrhea	Administer under close supervision; monitor renal function, LFT results, serum electrolyte levels May require premedication with acetaminophen, diphenhydramine
Ganciclovir (Cytovene)	Antiviral Cytomegalovirus (CMV) retinitis	5 mg/kg IV q 8–12 h	Neutropenia, thrombocytopenia, anemia, fever, rash	Monitor CBC for dyscrasias; BUN, Cr Discontinue if neutrophil count drops below 25,000/mm³; monitor LFT results, blood glucose level
Foscarnet (Foscavir)	Antiviral Cytomegalovirus	60 mg/kg IV q 8 h	Renal toxicity, anemia, electrolyte disturbances, nausea, vomiting, diarrhea, seizures, fever, myalgias	Central line preferred for administration; flush with NS after administration Monitor for CBC, electrolyte abnormalities, renal function (BUN, Cr), LFT results
Acyclovir (Zovirax)	Antiviral Herpes viruses (herpes simplex viruses I and II, varicella-zoster virus)	200–800 mg po five × d; 5–12 mg/kg IV q 8 h	Local reaction at IV site; renal dysfunction, bone marrow suppression; nausea, vomiting, diarrhea	Monitor renal function (BUN, Cr), CBC for dyscrasias Maintain adequate hydration
Azithromycin (Zithromax)	Antibiotic *Mycobacterium avium* complex, *M. intracellulare*	500 mg po × 1 d, then 250 mg qd × 4 d	Diarrhea, nausea, abdominal pain, rash	Administer 1 h ac or 2 h pc Given in combination with ethambutol
Clarithromycin (Biaxin)	Antibiotic *M. avium* complex, *M. intracellulare*	500–1000 mg po bid	Diarrhea, nausea, altered taste, headache, abdominal pain, rash	Given in combination with ethambutol
Fluconazole (Diflucan)	Antifungal Cryptococcal meningitis; oral, pharyngeal, vaginal candidiasis	400 mg/d po or IV 100–200 mg po qd	Nausea, vomiting, abdominal pain, headache, rash, diarrhea, abnormal LFT results	Monitor LFT results
Clotrimazole	Antifungal Candidiasis	10 mg po five × d	Abnormal LFT results	Monitor LFT results
Ketoconazole (Nizoral)	Antifungal Candidiasis	200–400 po qd	Hepatotoxicity, nausea, vomiting, anorexia	Monitor LFT results Administer on empty stomach

Adapted from Deglin, J. H., & Vallerand, A. H. (1995). *Davis's drug guide for nurses* (4th ed.). Philadelphia: F. A. Davis Co.
5% D/W = 5% dextrose in water; po = orally; q = every; bid = twice a day; tid = three times a day; CBC = complete blood count; ac = before meals; LFT = liver function test; BP = blood pressure; BUN = blood urea nitrogen; Cr = creatinine; NS = normal saline.

modulators, and the possible development of a vaccine. Examples of drugs being researched or in clinical trials include lamivudine, soluble CD4, protease inhibitors, and other immunological therapy (Cohn, 1993). Thalidomide, which is well-known for its teratogenic effects in the 1950s, is being researched in the treatment of oral and esophageal ulceration in HIV disease. In one study, 19 of 20 patients showed significant improvement in the healing of ulcers; some experienced desired weight gain (Paterson et al., 1995). Immune modulators being investigated include interferon alfa and interferon gamma and interleukin-2. Use of these drugs is aimed at boosting the depressed immune system by increasing the number of T cells or enhancing their function.

One area of interest of study pertains to a small percentage of HIV-positive patients who have failed to develop AIDS even after 7 or more years after seroconversion. These patients, termed "long-term nonprogressors," have been able to maintain healthy, intact immune function with CD4$^+$ cell counts of greater than 600/μl, although the mechanism for this phenomenon is not understood (Pantaleo et al., 1995). Some are possibly infected with a strain of HIV that lacks part of a gene needed to cause significant immune system damage. Others apparently have a stronger immune response to HIV infection and are able to keep the virus from destroying T cells. Whatever the reason or mechanism, researchers may be able to learn how to bolster the immune response and control HIV disease in others, perhaps even develop an effective vaccine.

Vaccination is an important and controversial area of HIV research and is considered a priority. Goals of development are the production of a successful preventive vaccine to inhibit transmission as well as a therapeutic vaccine to slow the progression of HIV disease in infected individuals. Vaccine development, still a long way off, is impeded for several reasons. First, many different strains of HIV exist; because HIV mutates quickly, it exists in many antigenic forms. Also, the specific immune response that inhibits HIV infection has not yet been identified (Cohn, 1993). The lack of suitable animal models is an additional problem. Ethical, social, liability, and logistical issues concerning vaccine trials in humans abound. However, trials are being conducted that test various therapeutic vaccines in HIV infection (Zurlinden and Verheggen, 1994; Haynes, 1993).

Nursing Interventions. Thorough hand washing is carried out before, during, and after any patient contact. Vital signs and hemodynamic parameters are monitored at least every 4 hours and as needed; any temperature increase is immediately investigated. Usual signs of infection may be absent in any immunocom-promised patient, and fever often is the only indicator; thorough baseline documentation and frequent assessment are necessary for the detection of subtle changes that may indicate the presence of a dangerous infection.

Breath sounds are auscultated for adventitious sounds, and the rate, depth, and rhythm of respirations are noted. The nurse observes for dyspnea, cough, sputum production, or use of accessory muscles for respiration. The nurse monitors arterial blood gas results for signs of hypoxemia, acidosis, or hyperventilation (respiratory alkalosis), or changes from baseline values. The patient is assessed for cyanosis and tachycardia. Oxygen therapy and/or respiratory support is administered as ordered, and the patient's response is monitored. The patient is positioned in a semi- to high-Fowler's position in order to ease respiratory effort. Pulmonary toilet, including spirometry, chest physiotherapy, and postural drainage, is performed at least every 2 hours while the patient is awake. Sputum cultures are obtained if infection is suspected. Antibiotics and other antimicrobials are administered as ordered, and the patient is closely observed for side effects.

Strict aseptic technique is used for any invasive procedures, suctioning, or dressing changes. Skin, axillae, groin areas, and mucous membranes are assessed for signs of infection or breakdown; any signs of opportunistic infections, such as thrush, herpes, diarrhea, and mental changes, are reported. Intravenous sites, incisions, and wounds are frequently assessed for redness, swelling, heat, or tenderness, although these signs may be masked. Meticulous body hygiene is provided in order to prevent breakdown and infection, and the skin is kept clean and dry, although moisturized. Frequent oral care is performed with nonirritating, nondrying solutions and soft bristled brushes. Trauma to the skin is avoided; the patient is turned at least every 2 hours, and padding is provided for bony prominences. If possible, an air-fluidized or alternating-pressure mattress is used for the prevention of pressure ulcers. Mobility is encouraged as appropriate.

Wound, urine, sputum, and throat cultures are obtained as indicated and as ordered. Results of laboratory studies (complete blood count, urinalysis, cultures) are monitored for increases or decreases in WBC and differential counts or presence of bacteria. Adequate fluid balance and optimal nutritional status are maintained. Other signs to assess for are chills, dyspnea, and diaphoresis.

The patient's baseline height and desired weight are assessed. Caloric and protein intake, intake and output, and daily weights are recorded. Dietary consultation is provided if needed, and significant others are encouraged to bring preferred foods to the hospital.

Results of laboratory studies, especially total protein, serum albumin, hematocrit, and hemoglobin determinations, are monitored. Vitamin, mineral, and caloric supplements are administered as ordered. The patient is encouraged to eat small, frequent, high-protein and high-calorie meals and snacks. Antiemetics are administered 30 minutes before meals as needed. Meticulous oral hygiene and relief measures are provided for painful oral lesions. The nurse also determines the need for supplements or diet changes. Enteral feedings or hyperalimentation is administered as ordered, and the patient is closely observed for a response.

The patient is observed for diarrhea, and the frequency, amount, consistency, and presence of blood, fat, mucus, or undigested particles are noted. Bowel sounds are monitored at least every shift. Anti-infectives and antidiarrheals are administered as ordered, and the patient's response is noted. Adequate hydration status is maintained through fluid replacement as necessary. The nurse also assesses for electrolyte disturbances (e.g., the laboratory results are monitored, and the patient is assessed for dysrhythmias, weakness, or cramps). Stool cultures are obtained and evaluated for microbial growth. The rate and strength of enteral feedings are adjusted if necessary. The perineum is kept clean and dry; the patient is assessed and treated for excoriation and breakdown.

The patient's baseline mental, emotional, and neurological status is assessed. Seizure precautions, such as padded side rails, are implemented as indicated, and antiepileptics are administered as ordered. The patient is monitored for neurological changes, such as headache, confusion, dizziness, and visual disturbances. Mood alterations and problems with memory or cognition are noted. The patient is reoriented as necessary and is protected from injury. A calm environment is promoted, and information is provided in simple terms that are easy to understand; the information is reinforced as needed. Emotional support and reassurance are provided to the patient and significant others.

Pain is assessed for location, duration, intensity, precipitating factors, and character. Analgesics and anti-inflammatory drugs are administered as needed and ordered; the nurse anticipates the patient's need when possible and monitors for response. The patient is positioned for comfort, and support is provided with pillows or padding. The patient's position is changed every 2 hours and as needed. Massage and hot and cold applications are administered as effective. Diversional activities, relaxation, and imagery techniques are encouraged.

The patient, family, and significant others' level of anxiety is anticipated when possible, and positive coping mechanisms are determined. Rapport and an atmosphere of mutual acceptance are established. Open, honest communication and expression of feelings are encouraged. The critical care nurse is available to the patient and significant others; he or she provides reassurance without false hope. The nurse provides information regarding the disease process, transmission, treatments, medications, and procedures. The patient and significant others are oriented to the critical care environment, and the patient and significant others are encouraged to participate in the planning and implementation of care. The nurse remains with the patient during procedures or periods of anxiety.

Patient Outcomes. The following are the goals of care for the patient with AIDS:

- Infection will be prevented or promptly recognized and treated.
- Gas exchange will be optimized, as evidenced by lack of air hunger or respiratory distress, absence of cyanosis, and arterial blood gas results within normal limits.
- Adequate hydration and optimal nutritional status will be maintained, as evidenced by adequate urine output and skin turgor, stable body weight, and laboratory values within normal limits.
- Skin and mucous membrane integrity will be maintained, as evidenced by absence of infection, breakdown, or lesions.
- Pain relief, comfort, and rest will be promoted, as evidenced by absence of discomfort and patient's ability to sleep.
- Anxiety will be minimized, and patient will be alert and oriented.
- Diarrhea will be controlled through medication; dehydration will be prevented through adequate fluid intake.
- Patient will be free of injury related to seizures; seizures will be controlled when possible through medication.
- Patient will have a thorough understanding of disease transmission, course of disease, symptoms of opportunistic infections, treatments, and medications.

Nursing concerns regarding AIDS are many and are relevant to the nurse as well as to the patient. The prevention of transmission of HIV in the clinical setting is of vast importance. Universal precautions are practiced at all times with all patients, by all members of the health care team (see Table 13–18). Hand washing continues to be the single most important action taken. As discussed earlier, protecting the immunosuppressed AIDS patient from infection is of primary importance. Assessments must be continuous and thorough. Staff must have access to ongoing support because caring for AIDS patients is demanding as well as challenging and poses quite an emotional strain. The risk of exposure also places a constant emotional stressor on nurses. Continuing education must be available that addresses prevention of transmission, current research, and treatments. Staff support, education, and research will continue to improve AIDS patient outcomes.

TREATMENT OF THE IMMUNOCOMPROMISED PATIENT

Whatever the cause of the immunodeficiency, the patient has the potential to develop infection, which is the leading cause of death in immunocompromised patients. Immunosuppressed patients do not respond to infection in a typical fashion; the signs and symptoms of infection vary greatly and may be absent or masked. Close monitoring consisting of thorough assessment,

early detection and treatment, and prevention of complications is paramount in the treatment of the immunocompromised patient.

Medical and surgical treatments are aimed at the cause of symptoms and the prevention of complications. In primary immunodeficiencies, B-cell and T-cell defects are treated with specific replacement therapy or bone marrow transplants (Fidler and Keen, 1988). In the future, many types of inherited immune disorders may be treated with somatic gene therapy; research and clinical trials are progressing in these areas (Cournoyer and Caskey, 1993). In secondary immunodeficiencies, the underlying condition is treated. Malnutrition is corrected, administration of immunosuppressants is stopped if possible, and medications are given for the treatment of infections or other disease states.

RESEARCH APPLICATION

Article Reference

El-Sadr, W., & Gettler, J. (1995). Unrecognized human immunodeficiency virus infection in the elderly. *Archives of Internal Medicine, 155*, 184-186.

Review of Study Methods and Findings:

Excess serum samples were collected from patients older than 60 years with no history of human immunodeficiency virus (HIV) infection who died during a 1-year period at the researchers' institution. The serum samples were tested for the presence of HIV antibodies by use of the enzyme-linked immunosorbent assay and the Western blot analysis; charts of those patients found to be HIV positive were then reviewed. Of a total of 257 serum samples tested, 13 (5.05%) tested positive for HIV antibodies. Of those 13, six (6.2%) of the 92 men and seven (8.9%) of the 78 women were infected. There were no HIV-positive patients older than 79 years. None of the 13 deaths were attributable to HIV infection, according to chart reviews. Four of the 13 infected patients had a history of injection drug use, and one had a history of blood transfusion; the remaining eight patients had no documented identifiable risk for HIV infection.

Critique of Study Strengths/Weaknesses:

The population studied was limited—hospitalized patients who died at an inner city institu-

tion. Thus, the findings should not be generalized to a larger pool of elderly persons. In order to determine the true incidence of HIV infection in the elderly, further studies using more random populations should be conducted.

Implications of the Study for Nursing Practice

HIV infection has typically been seen as affecting patients younger than the age of 60, with identifiable risk behaviors. This study suggests that HIV infection in certain populations of the elderly may be a significant problem. Additionally, most HIV-infected individuals may have no identifiable risk for acquisition of the disease. This study also suggests a higher prevalence of infection in elderly women than had been previously thought.

Public health education campaigns have primarily been aimed at a younger population. Nurses should be aware that HIV affects all age groups and that the elderly are also in need of HIV education, testing, and counseling. Nursing assessments of the elderly should include questions about risk behaviors. Further studies concerning the prevalence of HIV infection in the elderly, as well as the impact of unrecognized infection on the clinical outcome of these patients, should be conducted. Additionally, nurses should practice universal precautions at all times with all patients; age is not an indicator of HIV status or risk.

A detailed, documented database containing the patient's history, physical examination, and laboratory studies is paramount. Other nursing goals, as in AIDS, are aimed at prevention of infection; nutritional support; maintenance of skin and mucous membrane integrity, fluid and electrolyte balance, and renal function; emotional support; alleviation of discomfort; and promotion of rest (Dattwyler, 1991) (see Nursing Care Plan for the Immunocompromised Patient, p. 401.)

Summary

All patients in critical care have the potential for alterations in function of the hematological and immune systems. A thorough understanding of normal anatomy and physiology provides the critical care nurse with a basis on which a comprehensive assessment and treatment approach can be built. Because nurses play a key role in the outcome of patients with serious alterations in the hematological and immune systems, such as those with DIC or AIDS, this knowledge is critical and has great impact on the well-being of their patients.

CRITICAL THINKING QUESTIONS

1. What disorders do you see in critical care that are associated with anemia?
2. Why does the treatment of DIC (blood products, heparin) often exacerbate the problem?
3. What factors lead to risky behaviors for HIV transmission and why are these behaviors so difficult to eliminate or modify?
4. What accounts for the variability between individuals regarding the time required to progress from HIV infection to frank AIDS?
5. Why is the critical care unit often a dangerous place for the immunosuppressed patient to be in?

REFERENCES

American Foundation for AIDS Research. (1995). *AIDS/HIV treatment directory 7*(4).
Anastasi, J. K., & Rivera, J. (1994). Understanding prophylactic therapy for HIV infections. *American Journal of Nursing, 94*(2), 37–42.
Barrick, B. (1988). Caring for AIDS patients: A challenge you can meet. *Nursing '88, 18*(11), 50–59.
Bartlett, J. A., Gallis, H. A., Shipp, K. W., & Nabors, K. L. (1993). Diagnosis and treatment of the patient with HIV infection. In J. A. Bartlett (Ed.), *Care and management of patients with HIV infection* (pp. 103–135). Durham, NC: Glaxo.
Belcher, A. E. (1989). Hematolymphatic system. In J. M. Thompson,

G. K. Mcfarland, J. E. Hirsch, S. M. Tucker, & A. C. Bowers (Eds.), *Mosby's manual of clinical nursing* (2nd ed.) (pp. 1400–1445). St. Louis: C. V. Mosby Co.
Chernecky, C. C., Krech, R. L., & Berger, B. J. (1993). *Laboratory tests and diagnostic procedures.* Philadelphia: W. B. Saunders Co.
Cohn, J. A. (1993). Human immunodeficiency virus and AIDS: 1993 update. *Journal of Nurse Midwifery, 38*(2), 65–85.
Coletti, M., German, M., Zeller, J. M., & Balkstra, R. (1989). Immunologic system. In J. M. Thompson, G. K. Mcfarland, J. E. Hirsch, S. M. Tucker, & A. C. Bowers (Eds.), *Mosby's manual of clinical nursing* (2nd ed.) (pp. 1302–1399). St. Louis: C. V. Mosby Co.
Cotran, R. S., Kumar, V., & Robbins, S. L. (1989). *Robbins pathological basis of disease* (4th ed.). Philadelphia: W. B. Saunders Co.
Cournoyer, D., & Caskey, C. T. (1993). Gene therapy of the immune system. *Annual Review of Immunology, 11,* 297–329.
Dattwyler, R. J. (1991). Immunomodulation: Therapeutic manipulation of the immune system. In J. T. Dolan (Ed.), *Critical care nursing: Clinical management through the nursing process* (pp. 1181–1203). Philadelphia: F. A. Davis Co.
Dudjak, L. A., & Fleck, A. E. (1991). BRMs: New drug therapy comes of age. *RN, 54*(10), 42–48.
Durham, J. D. (1994). The changing HIV/AIDS epidemic: Emerging psychosocial challenges for nurses. *Nursing Clinics of North America, 29*(1), 9–18.
Fan, H., Conner, R. F., & Villareal, L. P. (1994). *The biology of AIDS.* Boston: Jones & Bartlett Publishers.
Fidler, M. R. (1988). Immunologic anatomy and physiology. In M. R. Kinney, D. R. Packa, & S. B. Dunbar (Eds.), *AACN's clinical reference for critical-care nursing* (2nd ed.) (pp. 1171–1201). New York: McGraw-Hill Book Co.
Fidler, M. R., & Keen, M. F. (1988). The immunocompromised patient. In M. R. Kinney, D. R. Packa, & S. B. Dunbar (Eds.). *AACN's clinical reference for critical-care nursing.* (2nd ed.) (pp. 1249–1269). New York: McGraw-Hill Book Co.
Gawlikowski, J. (1992). White cells at war. *American Journal of Nursing, 92*(3), 44–51.
Greenberg, P. (1993). Immunopathogenesis of HIV infection. In L. Corey (Ed.), *AIDS: Problems and prospects* (pp. 17–29). New York: W. W. Norton & Co.
Gurka, A. M. (1989). The immune system: Implications for critical care nursing. *Critical Care Nurse, 9*(7), 24–35.
Guyton, A. C. (1991). *Textbook of medical physiology* (8th ed.). Philadelphia: W. B. Saunders Co.
Haynes, B. F. (1993). Scientific and social issues of human immunodeficiency virus vaccine development. *Science, 260,* 1279–1286.
Hopewell, P. C., & Masur, H. (1995). *Pneumocystis carinii* pneumonia: Current concepts. In M. A. Sande, & P. A. Volberding (Eds.), *The medical management of AIDS* (pp. 367–401). Philadelphia: W. B. Saunders Co.
Hoth, D. F., Jr., Myers, M. W., & Stein, D. S. (1993). Current status of HIV therapy: I. Antiretroviral agents. In L. Corey (Ed.), *AIDS: Problems and prospects* (pp. 51–70). New York: W. W. Norton & Co.
Jackson, B. S. (1988a). Hematopoietic data acquisition. In M. R. Kinney, D. R. Packa, & S. B. Dunbar (Eds.), *AACN's clinical reference for critical-care nursing* (2nd ed.) (pp. 1136–1142). New York: McGraw-Hill Book Co.
Jackson, B. S. (1988b). Hyperviscosity and anemias. In M. R. Kinney, D. R. Packa, & S. B. Dunbar (Eds.), *AACN's clinical reference for critical-care nursing* (2nd ed.) (pp. 1143–1155). New York: McGraw-Hill Book Co.
Jackson, B. S., & Jones, M. B. (1988a). Coagulopathies. In M. R. Kinney, D. R. Packa, & S. B. Dunbar (Eds.), *AACN's clinical reference for critical-care nursing* (2nd ed.) (pp. 1156–1167). New York: McGraw-Hill Book Co.

Jackson, B. S., & Jones, M. B. (1988b). Hematologic anatomy and physiology. In M. R. Kinney, D. R. Packa, & S. B. Dunbar (Eds.), *AACN's clinical reference for critical-care nursing* (2nd ed.) (pp. 1113–1135). New York: McGraw-Hill Book Co.

Janusek, L. (1993). Structure and function of the immune system. In J. M. Black, & E. Matassarin-Jacobs (Eds.), *Luckmann and Sorensen's medical-surgical nursing* (4th ed.) (pp. 529–547). Philadelphia: W. B. Saunders Co.

Jassak, P. F., Petty, J., & Krol, M. A. (1993). Treatment modalities for neoplastic disorders. In J. M. Black, & E. Matassarin-Jacobs (Eds.), *Luckmann and Sorensen's medical-surgical nursing* (4th ed.) (pp. 501–525). Philadelphia: W. B. Saunders Co.

Klimek, J. J. (1992). Notes from the VIII International Conference on AIDS. *Asepsis, 14*(2), 16–20.

Kovacs, J. A., Baseler, M., Dewar, R. J., Vogel, S., Davey, R. T., Falloon, J., et al. (1995). Increases in CD4 T lymphocytes with intermittent courses of interleukin-2 in patients with human immunodeficiency virus infection: A preliminary study. *New England Journal of Medicine, 332*(9), 567–575.

Kuhar, P. A., & Hill, K. M. (1991). White clot syndrome: When heparin goes haywire. *American Journal of Nursing, 91*(3), 59–60.

Levi, M., ten Cate, H., van der Poll, T., & van Deventer, S. J. H. (1993). Pathogenesis of disseminated intravascular coagulation in sepsis. *JAMA, 270*(8), 975–979.

Loder, P. A. W. (1993). HIV infections of the central nervous system: What are the nursing implications? *Nursing Clinics of North America, 28*(4), 839–847.

Miller, F., & Habicht, G. (1991). Immune system: Underlying principles. In J. T. Dolan (Ed.), *Critical care nursing: Clinical management through the nursing process* (pp. 1155–1175). Philadelphia: F. A. Davis Co.

Mocsny, N. (1992). Toxoplasmic encephalitis in the AIDS patient. *Journal of Neuroscience Nursing, 24* (1), 30–33.

Orsi, A. J. (1993). The hematologic system. In R. L. Boggs, & M. Wooldridge-King (Eds.), *AACN procedure manual for critical care* (3rd ed.) (pp. 691–717). Philadelphia: W. B. Saunders Co.

Pantaleo, G. P., Menzo, S., Vaccarezza, M., Graziosi, C., Cohen, O. J., Demarest, J. F., et al. (1995). Studies in subjects with long-term nonprogressive human immunodeficiency virus infection. *New England Journal of Medicine, 332*(4), 209–216.

Paterson, D. L. (1995). Thalidomide as treatment of refractory aphthous ulceration related to human immunodeficiency virus infection. *Clinical Infectious Disease, 20*(2), 250–254.

Pavel, J., Plunkett, A., & Sink, B. (1993). Nursing care of clients with hematologic disorders. In J. M. Black, & E. Matassarin-Jacobs (Eds.), *Luckmann and Sorensen's medical-surgical nursing* (4th ed.) (pp. 1335–1401). Philadelphia: W. B. Saunders Co.

Rick, M. E. (1991). Hemorrhagic and thrombotic disorders. In J. E. Parrillo (Ed.), *Current therapy in critical care medicine* (pp. 288–292). Philadelphia: B. C. Decker.

Ruggiero, J. T., & Barie, P. S. (1993). Hematologic disease and surgical hemostasis. In P. S. Barie, & G. T. Shires (Eds.), *Surgical intensive care* (pp. 667–680). Boston: Little, Brown, & Co.

Saag, M. S. (1995). AIDS testing now and in the future. In M. A. Sande, & P. A. Volberding (Eds.), *The medical management of AIDS* (pp. 65–88). Philadelphia: W. B. Saunders Co.

Scherer, P. (1990). How AIDS attacks the brain. *American Journal of Nursing, 90*(1), 44–52.

Schiffer, C. A. (1991). Therapeutic cytapheresis. In P. H. Wiernik, G. P. Canellos, R. A. Kyle, & C. A. Schiffer (Eds.), *Neoplastic diseases of the blood* (pp. 853–862). New York: Churchill Livingstone.

Shannon-Bodnar, R. (1993). Immune system and blood. In P. G. Morton (Ed.), *Health assessment in nursing* (2nd ed.) (pp. 547–585). Springhouse, PA: Springhouse Corp.

Singer, P., Askanazi, J., Akiva, L., Bursztein, S., & Kvetan, V. (1990). Reassessing intensive care for patients with the acquired immunodeficiency syndrome. *Heart and Lung, 19*(4), 387–394.

Timby, B. K. (1992). Pneumocystis in patients with acquired immunodeficiency syndrome. *Critical Care Nurse, 12*(7), 64–71.

Vinazzer, H. (1989). Therapeutic use of antithrombin III in shock and disseminated intravascular coagulation. *Seminars in Thrombosis and Hemostasis, 15*(3), 347.

Waldrop, G. B., Cervenka, B. S., Moffett, S. A., Bedenbaugh, J. C., Bishop, L. B., & Crouch, M. A. (1991). Heparin-induced thrombocytopenia and thrombosis. *Dimensions of Critical Care Nursing, 10*(6), 330–343.

Zurlinden, J., & Verheggen, R. (1994). HIV vaccines: A report from the front. *RN, 57*(1), 36–40.

RECOMMENDED READINGS

Alspach, J. G.(1991). *Core curriculum for critical care nursing* (4th ed.). Philadelphia: W. B. Saunders Co.

Bailes, B. K. (1992). Disseminated intravascular coagulation: Principles, treatment, nursing management. *AORN Journal, 55*(2), 517–529.

Birnbaum, D. (1993). Universal precautions: An off-target response. *Critical Care Nurse, 13*(3), 160.

Cohen, F. L. (1991). The pharmacologic treatment of HIV infection and AIDS in adults. *Nursing Clinics of North America, 26*(2), 315–329.

Cordisco, M. E. C. (1994). Fighting DIC. *RN, 57*(8), 36–40.

Crow, S. (1983). Nursing care of the immunosuppressed patient. *Infection Control, 4*(6), 465–467.

Davey, R. J. (1991). Blood product therapy. In J. E. Parrillo (Ed.). *Current therapy in critical care medicine* (pp. 292–296). Philadelphia: B. C. Decker.

Epstein, C., & Bakanauskas, A. (1991). Clinical management of DIC: Early nursing interventions. *Critical Care Nurse, 11*(10), 42–53.

Esparaz, B., & Green, D. (1990). Disseminated intravascular coagulation. *Critical Care Nursing Quarterly, 13*(2), 7–13.

Fidler, M. R., & Morgan, M. S. (1988). Immunologic data acquisition. In M. R. Kinney, D. R. Packa, & S. B. Dunbar (Eds.), *AACN's clinical reference for critical-care nursing* (2nd ed.) (pp. 1202–1234). New York: McGraw-Hill Book Co.

Golightly, M. G. (1991). Clinical application: Immunodeficiency disorders. In J. T. Dolan (Ed.), *Critical care nursing: Clinical management through the nursing process* (pp. 1213–1226). Philadelphia: F. A. Davis Co.

Golightly, M. G., & Dolan, J. T. (1991). Assessment of immunologic function. In J. T. Dolan (Ed.), *Critical care nursing: clinical management through the nursing process* (pp. 1176–1180). Philadelphia: F. A. Davis Co.

Gurevich, I. (1985). The competent internal immune system. *Nursing Clinics of North America, 20*(1), 151–161.

Harrington, L., & Hufnagel, J. M. (1990). Heparin-induced thrombocytopenia and thrombosis syndrome: A case study. *Heart and Lung, 19*(1), 93–98.

Henry, S. B., & Holzemer, W. L. (1992). Critical care management of the patient with HIV infection who has *Pneumocystis carinii* pneumonia. *Heart and Lung, 21*(3), 243–249.

Jennings, B. M. (1991). The hematologic system. In J. G. Alspach (Ed.), *Core curriculum for critical care nursing* (pp. 675–747). Philadelphia: W. B. Saunders Co.

Mocsny, N. (1992). Cryptococcal meningitis in patients with AIDS. *Journal of Neuroscience Nursing, 24*(5), 265–268.

Mocsny, N. (1993). Toxoplasmic encephalitis in the AIDS patient. *Rehabilitation Nursing, 18*(1), 20–22, 25.

Moran, T. A. (1989). AIDS: Current implications and impact on nursing. *Journal of Intravenous Nursing, 12*(4), 220–226.

Taber, J. (1989). Nutrition and HIV infection. *American Journal of Nursing, 89*(11), 1446–1451.

Talan, D. A., Johnson, G. A., & Sepkowitz, K. A. (1993). When the AIDS patient crashes. *Patient Care, 27*(1), 140–158.

Ungvarski, P. J., & Schmidt, J. (1992). AIDS patients under attack. *RN, 55*(11), 36–45.

Waltzer, W. C. (1991). Clinical application: Clinical organ transplant. In J. T. Dolan (Ed.), *Critical care nursing: Clinical management through the nursing process* (pp. 1204–1212). Philadelphia: F. A. Davis Co.

Young, L. M. (1990). DIC: The insidious killer. *Critical Care Nurse, 10*(10), 26–33.

14

Gastrointestinal Alterations

Joanne M. Krumberger, M.S.N., R.N., CCRN
Beth Hammer, B.S.N., R.N.

OBJECTIVES

- Review the anatomy and physiology of the gastrointestinal system.
- Describe general assessment of the gastrointestinal system.
- Discuss nutritional assessment and therapies used for providing optimal nutrition.

- Compare the pathophysiology, assessment, nursing diagnoses, outcomes, and interventions for acute upper gastrointestinal bleeding, acute pancreatitis, and hepatic failure.
- Formulate a plan of care for the patient with acute upper gastrointestinal bleeding, acute pancreatitis, and hepatic failure.

Introduction

Body cells require water, electrolytes, and nutrients (carbohydrates, fats, and proteins) in order to obtain the energy necessary to fuel body functions. The primary function of the alimentary tract (oropharyngeal cavity, esophagus, stomach, small and large intestines) and accessory organs (pancreas, liver, and gallbladder) is to provide the body with a continual supply of nutrients. Additionally, food must move through the system at a slow enough rate for digestive and absorptive functions to occur but must also be fast enough to meet body needs. Meeting these goals requires the appropriate and timely movement of nutrients through the gastrointestinal (GI) tract (motility), the presence of specific enzymes to break down nutrients (digestion), and the existence of transport mechanisms to move the nutrients into the bloodstream (ab-

sorption). Each part is adapted for specific functions, including food passage, storage, digestion, and absorption. This chapter provides a brief physiological review of each section of the GI system and a general assessment of the GI system, which provide the foundation for the discussion of the GI disorders most commonly encountered in the critical care setting: acute upper GI bleeding, acute pancreatitis, and liver failure. The remainder of the chapter reviews the pathophysiology of each disorder, nursing and medical assessments, nursing diagnoses, nursing and medical interventions, and patient outcomes. Complete nursing plans of care for select nursing diagnoses are provided; these serve as valuable summaries of the most common patient care problems and collaborative interventions. Nutritional assessment and nutritional support therapies are also presented because altered nutrition is a common nursing diagnosis in patients with GI disorders.

Review of Anatomy and Physiology

GASTROINTESTINAL TRACT

The anatomical structure of the GI system is shown in Figure 14–1. It comprises the alimentary canal (beginning at the oropharynx and ending at the anus) and the accessory organs (liver, pancreas, and gallbladder) that empty their products into the canal at certain points. A review of the anatomy of the gut wall is provided as an introduction to this section because it provides the foundation for the understanding of absorption of nutrients and GI protective mechanisms.

Gut Wall

The GI tract begins in the esophagus and extends to the rectum; it is composed of multiple tissue layers.

Mucosa. The innermost layer, the mucosa, is the most important physiologically. This layer is exposed to food substances, and it therefore plays a role in nutrient metabolism. The mucosa is also protective. The cells in this layer are connected by tight junctions that produce an effective barrier against large molecules and bacteria and protect the GI tract from bacterial colonization. The goblet cells in the mucosa secrete mucus, which provides lubrication for food substances and protects the mucosa from excoriation.

Gastric Mucosal Barrier. In the stomach, the special architecture of cells of the mucosa and the mucus that is secreted are known as the gastric mucosal barrier. This physiological barrier is impermeable to hydrochloric acid, which is normally secreted in the stomach, but it can be permeable to other substances, such as salicylates, alcohol, steroids, and bile salts. The disruption of this barrier by these types of substances is thought to play a role in ulcer development. Additionally, these cells have a special feature—they regenerate rapidly—which explains how disruptions in the mucosa can be quickly healed.

Submucosa. The second layer of the gut wall, the submucosa, is composed of connective tissue, blood vessels, and nerve fibers. The muscular layer is the major muscular layer of the wall. The serosa is the outermost layer.

Beneath the mucosa, submucosa, and muscular layer are various nerve plexuses that are innervated by the autonomic nervous system. Disturbances in these neurons in a given segment of the GI tract cause a lack of motility.

Oropharyngeal Cavity

Mouth. Food substances are ingested into the oral cavity primarily according to the intrinsic desire for food called hunger. Food in the mouth is initially subject to mechanical breakdown by the act of chewing (mastication). Chewing of food is important for digestion of all foods, but particularly for digestion of fruits and raw vegetables, because they require the cellulose membranes around their nutrients to be broken down. The muscles of chewing are innervated by the motor branch of the fifth cranial nerve.

Saliva is the major secretion of the oropharynx and is produced by three pairs of salivary glands: submaxillary, sublingual, and parotid. Saliva is rich in mucus, which provides lubrication of food. Salivary amylase, a starch-digesting enzyme, is also secreted. Stimuli such as sight, smell, thoughts, and taste of food stimulate salivary gland secretion. Parasympathetic stimulation promotes a copious secretion of watery saliva. Conversely, sympathetic stimulation produces a scanty output of thick saliva. The normal daily secretion of saliva is 1200 ml.

Pharynx. Swallowing is a complex mechanism involving oral (voluntary), pharyngeal, and esophageal stages. It is made more complex because the pharynx serves several other functions, the most important of

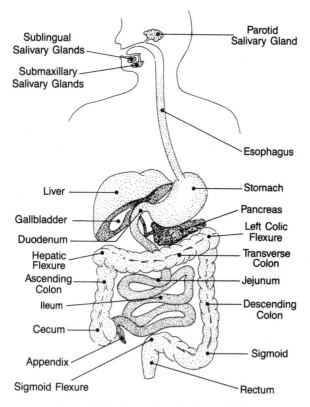

Figure 14–1. The gastrointestinal system.

which is respiration. The pharynx participates in the function of swallowing for only a few seconds at a time in order to aid in the propulsion of food, which is triggered by the presence of fluid or food in the pharynx. Table 14–1 outlines the three broad stages of swallowing.

Esophagus

Once fluid or food enters the esophagus, it is propelled through the lumen by the process of peristalsis, which involves the relaxation and contraction of esophageal muscles that are stimulated by the bolus of food. This process occurs repeatedly until the food reaches the lower esophageal sphincter, which is the last centimeter of the esophagus. This area is normally contracted and thus prevents reflux of gastric contents into the esophagus, a phenomenon that would damage the lining by gastric acid and enzymes. Waves of peristalsis cause this sphincter to relax and allow food to enter the stomach. Mucosal layers in the esophagus secrete mucus, which protects the lining from damage by gastric secretions or food and also serves as a lubricant.

Stomach

The stomach is located at the distal end of the esophagus. It is divided into four regions: the cardia, the fundus, the body, and the antrum (Fig. 14–2). The muscular walls form multiple folds that allow for greater expansion of the stomach. The opening at the distal end of the stomach opens into the small intestine and is surrounded by the pyloric sphincter. The motor functions of the stomach include storage of food until it can be accommodated by the lower GI tract, mixing of food with gastric secretions until it forms a semi-fluid mixture called chyme, and slow emptying of the chyme into the small intestine at a rate that allows for proper digestion and absorption. Motility is accomplished through peristalsis. The pyloric sphincter at the distal end of the stomach prevents duodenal reflux.

Gastric secretions are produced by mucus-se-

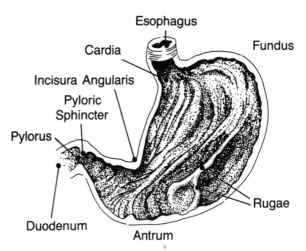

Figure 14–2. The stomach.

creting cells that line the inner surface of the stomach and by two types of tubular glands:

- Oxyntic (gastric) glands
- Pyloric glands

Table 14–2 summarizes the major gastric secretions.

An oxyntic gland is composed of three types of cells: mucous neck cells, which secrete mostly mucus; peptic, or chief, cells, which secrete pepsinogen; and oxyntic, or parietal cells, which secrete hydrochloric acid. Mucous cells secrete a viscid and alkaline mucus that coats the stomach mucosa, thereby providing protection and lubrication for food transport. Parietal cells secrete hydrochloric acid solution, which begins the digestion of food in the stomach. Hydrochloric acid is very acidic (pH, 0.8), and the rate of its secretion is normally 2 to 3 mEq/h. Stimulants of hydrochloric acid secretion exist, including vagal stimulation, gastrin, and the chemical properties of chyme, that increase its secretion rate 10-fold. Histamine, which stimulates the release of gastrin, also stimulates the

Table 14–1. SWALLOWING STAGES

Oral: Voluntary
  Initiates swallowing process; usually stimulated by bolus of food in the mouth near the pharynx
Pharyngeal: Involuntary
  Passage of food through pharynx to esophagus
Esophageal: Involuntary
  Promotes passage of food from pharynx to stomach

Table 14–2. GASTRIC SECRETIONS

Gland / Cells	Secretion
Cardiac gland	Mucus
Pyloric gland	Mucus
Fundic (gastric) gland	
Mucous neck cells	Mucus
Parietal cells	Water
	Hydrochloric acid
	Intrinsic factor
Chief cells	Pepsinogen
	Mucus

Table 14–3. ELECTROLYTE/ACID-BASE DISTURBANCES ASSOCIATED WITH THE GASTROINTESTINAL TRACT

Fluid Loss	Imbalances
Gastric juice	Metabolic alkalosis Potassium deficit Sodium deficit Fluid volume deficit
Small intestine juice	Metabolic acidosis Potassium deficit Sodium deficit Fluid volume deficit
Large intestine juice (recent ileostomy)	Metabolic acidosis Potassium deficit Sodium deficit Fluid volume deficit
Biliary or pancreatic fistula	Metabolic acidosis Sodium deficit Fluid volume deficit

secretion of hydrochloric acid. Current drug therapies for ulcer disease use H_2 histamine receptor blockers that block the effects of histamine and therefore hydrochloric acid stimulation. The acidic environment of the stomach promotes the conversion of pepsinogen, a proteolytic enzyme secreted by gastric chief cells, to pepsin. Pepsin begins the initial breakdown of proteins. Pepsin is active only in a highly acidic environment (pH <5); therefore, hydrochloric acid secretion is essential for protein digestion.

An essential protein secreted only by the stomach's parietal cells is intrinsic factor. Intrinsic factor is necessary for the absorption of vitamin B_{12} in the ileum. Vitamin B_{12} is critical for the formation of red blood cells, and a deficiency in this vitamin causes anemia.

In addition to hydrochloric acid and pepsinogen secretion, the stomach secretes fluid that is rich in sodium and potassium and other electrolytes. Therefore, losses of these fluids via vomiting or gastric suction place the patient at risk for fluid and electrolyte imbalances, as well as acid-base disturbances (Table 14–3).

Small Intestine

The segment spanning the first 10 to 12 inches of the small intestine is called the duodenum. This anatomical area is physiologically important in that pancreatic juices and bile from the liver empty into this structure. The duodenum also contains an extensive network of mucus-secreting glands called Brunner's glands. The function of this mucus is to protect the duodenal wall from digestion by gastric juice. Secretion of mucus by Brunner's glands is inhibited by sympathetic stimulation, which leaves the duodenum unprotected from gastric juice. This inhibition is thought to be one of the reasons why this area of the GI tract is the site for more than 50% of peptic ulcers.

The segment spanning the next 7 to 8 feet of the small intestine is called the jejunum, and the remaining 10 to 12 feet consists of the ileum. The opening into the first part of the large intestine is protected by the ileocecal valve, which prevents reflux of colonic contents back into the ileum.

The movements of the small intestine include mixing contractions and propulsive contractions. The chyme in the small intestine takes 3 to 5 hours to move from the pylorus to the ileocecal valve, although this activity is greatly increased after meals. Digestion and absorption of food stuffs occur primarily in the small intestine. The anatomical arrangement of villi and microvilli in the small intestine greatly increases the surface area in this part of the intestine, accounting for its highly digestive and absorptive capabilities. Located on the entire surface of the small intestine are small pits called crypts of Lieberkühn, which produce intestinal secretions at a rate of 2000 ml/d. These secretions are neutral in pH and supply the watery vehicle necessary for absorption.

In the small intestine, digestion of carbohydrates, fats, and proteins begins with degradation by pancreatic enzymes that are secreted into the duodenum. Pancreatic juice contains enzymes necessary for digesting all three major types of food: proteins, carbohydrates, and fats (Table 14–4). It also contains large quantities of bicarbonate ions, which play an important role in neutralizing acidic chyme that is emptied from the stomach into the duodenum. Pancreatic juice is primarily secreted in response to the presence of chyme in the duodenum.

The small intestine also handles water, electrolyte,

Table 14–4. PANCREATIC ENZYMES AND THEIR ACTIONS

Enzyme	Action
Trypsin*	Digests proteins
Chymotrypsin*	Digests proteins
Carboxypolypeptidase*	Digests proteins
Ribonuclease	Digests proteins
Deoxyribonuclease	Digests proteins
Pancreatic amylase	Digests carbohydrates
Pancreatic lipase	Digests fats
Cholesterol esterase	Digests fats

*Becomes activated only after it is secreted into the intestinal tract.

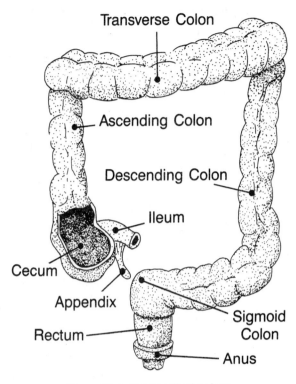

Figure 14–3. The intestinal system.

and vitamin absorption. Up to 10 L of fluid enters the GI tract daily, and fluid composition of stool is only about 200 ml. Sodium is actively reabsorbed in the small intestine. In the ileum, chloride is absorbed and sodium bicarbonate is secreted. Potassium is absorbed as well as secreted in the GI tract. Vitamins, with the exception of B_{12}, and iron are absorbed in the upper part of the small bowel. As mentioned earlier, vitamin B_{12} is absorbed in the terminal ileum in the presence of intrinsic factor.

Large Intestine

The large intestine, or colon, is anatomically divided into the ascending colon, the transverse colon, the descending colon, and the rectum (Fig. 14–3). The functions of the colon are absorption of the water and electrolytes from the chyme and storage of fecal material until it can be expelled. The proximal half of the colon performs primarily absorptive activities, whereas the distal half performs storage activities. The characteristic contractile activity in the colon is called "haustration," which propels fecal material through the tract. A mass movement moves feces into the rectal vault, and then the urge to defecate is elicited. The mucosa of the large intestine is lined with crypts of

Lieberkühn, but the cells contain very few enzymes. Rather, mucus is secreted, which protects the colon wall against excoriation and serves as a medium for holding fecal matter together.

ACCESSORY ORGANS

Pancreas

The pancreas is located in both upper quadrants of the abdomen, with the head in the upper right quadrant and the tail in the upper left quadrant. The head and tail are separated by a midsection called the body of the pancreas (Fig. 14–4). Because the pancreas lies retroperitoneally, it cannot be palpated, and this characteristic explains why diseases of the pancreas can cause pain that radiates to the back. Additionally, a well-developed pancreatic capsule does not exist, and this may explain why inflammatory processes of the pancreas can freely spread and affect the surrounding organs (stomach and duodenum).

The pancreas has both exocrine (production of digestive enzymes) and endocrine (production of insulin and glucagon) functions. The cells of the pancreas, called acini, secrete the major pancreatic enzymes essential for normal digestion (see Table 14–4). Trypsinogen and chymotrypsinogen are secreted in an inactive form so that autodigestion of the gland does not occur. Bicarbonate is also secreted by the pancreas and plays an important role in enabling the pancreatic enzymes to work to break down food stuffs. After breakdown by pancreatic enzymes, food is further digested by enzymes in the small intestine and is absorbed into the bloodstream. The presence of acid in the stomach stimulates the duodenum to produce the hormone secretin, which stimulates pancreatic secretions. Protein substances in the duodenum stimulate the production of cholecystokinin.

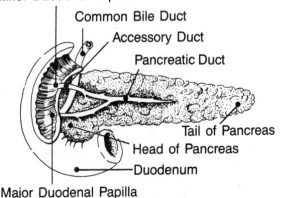

Figure 14–4. The pancreas.

The endocrine functions of the pancreas are accomplished by groups of alpha and beta cells that compose the islets of Langerhans. Beta cells secrete insulin, and alpha cells secrete glucagon. Both are essential to carbohydrate metabolism. When beta cells are affected by disease, blood glucose levels can increase.

The exocrine and endocrine functions of the pancreas are essential to digestion and carbohydrate metabolism, respectively. Therefore, pancreatic dysfunction can predispose the patient to malnutrition and accounts for many clinical problems.

The pancreatic response to low-flow states (decreased cardiac output), or hypotension, is often ischemia of the pancreatic cells. This ischemia is thought to play a role in the release of cardiotoxic factors (myocardial depressant factor), which are known to decrease cardiac output. Pancreatic ischemia can also result in acute pancreatitis, which is discussed later in the chapter.

Liver

The liver is the largest internal organ of the body; it is located in the right upper abdominal quadrant. The basic functional unit of the liver is the liver lobule (Fig. 14–5). Hepatic cells are arranged in cords that radiate from the central vein into the periphery. Blood from portal arterioles and venules empties into channels called sinusoids. Lining the walls of the sinusoids are specialized phagocytic cells called *Kupffer's cells*. These cells remove bacteria and other foreign material from the blood.

The liver has a rich blood supply—it receives blood from both the hepatic artery and the portal vein, which drains structures of the GI tract. The blood supplied to the liver by these two vessels accounts for approximately 25% of the cardiac output.

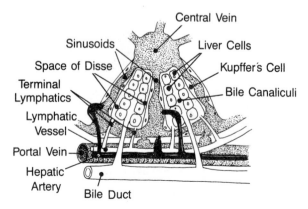

Figure 14–5. The normal liver lobule.

Table 14–5. FUNCTIONS OF THE LIVER

Vascular Functions

Blood storage
Blood filtration

Secretory Functions

Production of bile salts
Secretion of bilirubin
Conjugation of bilirubin

Metabolic Functions

Carbohydrate metabolism
Fat metabolism
Protein metabolism
Synthesis of blood clotting components (factors II, VI, VII, VIII, IX, X)
Removal of activated clotting factors
Detoxification of drugs, hormones, and other substances

Storage Functions

Blood
Glucose
Vitamins (A, B_{12}, D, E, K)
Fat

The liver performs more than 400 functions. The following discussion of hepatic functions is based on the classification by Guyton (1991) and includes vascular, secretory, and metabolic functions. These actions are summarized in Table 14–5.

Vascular Functions

Blood Storage. Resistance to blood flow (hepatic vascular resistance) in the liver is normally low. Any increase in pressure in the veins that drain the liver causes blood to accumulate in the sinusoids and causes the sinusoids to distend in order to handle the increased blood volume. The liver sinusoids can store up to 400 ml of blood. This blood volume can serve as a compensatory mechanism in cases of hypovolemic shock; in this mechanism, blood from the liver can be shunted into the circulation in order to increase blood volume.

Filtration. As mentioned earlier, Kupffer's cells that line the sinusoids cleanse the blood of bacteria and foreign material that has been absorbed through the GI tract. These cells are extremely phagocytic and thus normally prevent almost all bacteria from reaching the systemic circulation.

Secretory Functions

Bile Production. The secretion of bile is a major function of the liver. Bile is composed of water, electrolytes, bile salts, phospholipids, cholesterol, and bilirubin. Approximately 500 to 1000 ml of bile is produced daily. Bile salts emulsify fats and foster their absorption. The bile salts are reabsorbed in the terminal portion of the ileum and are then transported back to the liver, where they can be used again. Bile travels to the gallbladder via the common bile duct, where it is stored and concentrated.

Bilirubin Metabolism. Bilirubin, a physiologically inactive pigment, is a metabolic end-product of the degradation of hemoglobin. Bilirubin enters the circulation bound to albumin in the plasma and is "free," or unconjugated, in this state. This portion of the bilirubin is reflected in the "indirect" serum bilirubin level. Accumulation of unconjugated bilirubin is toxic to cells. Conjugation of bilirubin by the liver, which results in the binding of bilirubin to albumin, prevents toxic effects of unconjugated bilirubin from occurring. Approximately 80% of bilirubin transported to the liver is conjugated in hepatic cells, and the rest is conjugated with other substances. Some conjugated bilirubin does return to the blood and is reflected in the "direct" serum bilirubin level. Almost all bilirubin is secreted into bile. Excess bilirubin accumulation in the blood results in jaundice. Jaundice has several causes, including hepatocellular, hemolytic, and obstructive. Hemolytic jaundice results from increased red blood cell destruction, such as that resulting from blood incompatibilities and sickle cell disease. Viral hepatitis is the most common cause of hepatocellular jaundice (jaundice caused by hepatic cell damage). Cirrhosis and liver cancer can also decrease the liver's ability to conjugate bilirubin. Obstructive jaundice is usually caused by gallbladder disease, such as gallstones.

Metabolic Functions

Carbohydrate Metabolism. The liver plays an important role in the maintenance of normal blood glucose concentration. When the concentration of glucose increases to greater than normal levels, it is stored as glycogen (glycogenesis). When blood glucose levels decrease, glycogen stored in the liver is split to form glucose (glycogenolysis). If blood glucose levels decrease to less than normal and glycogen stores are depleted, the liver can make glucose from proteins and fats (gluconeogenesis).

Protein Metabolism. All nonessential amino acids are produced in the liver. All amino acids must be deaminated (removal of ammonia) to be used for energy by cells or converted into carbohydrates or fats. Ammonia is released and then removed from the blood by conversion to urea in the liver. The urea that is secreted by the liver into the bloodstream is excreted by the kidneys.

With the exception of gamma globulins, the liver also produces all plasma proteins in the blood. The major types of plasma proteins are albumins, globulins, and fibrinogen. Albumin maintains blood osmotic pressure and prevents plasma loss from the capillaries. Globulins are essential for cellular enzymatic reactions. Fibrinogen helps form blood clots.

Fat Metabolism. Almost all cells in the body are capable of lipid metabolism; however, the liver metabolizes fats so rapidly that it is the primary site for these functions. The liver is also the primary site for the conversion of excess carbohydrates and proteins to triglycerides.

Production and Removal of Blood Clotting Factors. In addition to fibrinogen, the liver is the site of synthesis of prothrombin (factor II); accelerator globulin (factor V); and factors VII, VIII, IX, and X. Factors II, VII, IX, and X are vitamin K dependent. The liver also removes active clotting factors from the circulation, and therefore prevents clotting in the macrovasculature and microvasculature.

Detoxification. Drugs, hormones, and other toxic substances are metabolized by the liver to inactive forms for excretion. This process is usually accomplished by conversion of the fat-soluble compounds to water-soluble compounds. They can then be excreted via the bile or the urine.

Vitamin and Mineral Storage. Excess amounts of vitamins A, B_{12}, D, E, and K are stored in the liver. The liver also contains up to 30% of the total body iron supply. Magnesium is also stored in the liver.

Gallbladder

The gallbladder is a saclike structure that lies beneath the right lobe of the liver. Its primary function is the storage and concentration of bile. The gallbladder can hold approximately 70 ml of bile. Bile salts are secreted into the duodenum when nutrients are ingested. The gallbladder is connected to the duodenum via the common bile duct. Bile flow is controlled by contraction of the gallbladder and relaxation of the sphincter of Oddi, which is located at the junction of the common bile duct and the duodenum. Contraction of the gallbladder is controlled by hormonal (cholecystokinin) and central nervous system signals and is initiated by the presence of food in the duodenum. Bile salts emulsify fats and also assist in the absorption of fatty acids.

NEURAL INNERVATION OF THE GASTROINTESTINAL SYSTEM

Functions of the GI system are influenced by neural and hormonal factors. The autonomic nervous system exerts multiple effects. In general, parasympathetic cholinergic fibers or drugs that mimic parasympathetic effects are stimulatory to GI secretion and motility, whereas sympathetic stimulation or drugs with adrenergic effects tend to be inhibitory. Parasympathetic and sympathetic fibers also innervate the gallbladder and the pancreas. Other neural regulators of gastric secretions are stimulated by sight, smell, and thoughts of food, as well as by the presence of food in the mouth. In this phase (cephalic), the brain centers reflexively cause parasympathetic stimulation of gastric secretions by chief and parietal cells.

HORMONAL CONTROL OF THE GASTROINTESTINAL SYSTEM

The GI tract is considered to be the largest endocrine organ in the body. Hormones that influence GI function include those produced by specialized cells in the GI tract as well as these produced by other endocrine organs (pancreas and gallbladder). Gastrointestinal hormones modulate such activities as motility, secretion, absorption, and maturation of GI tissues. Table 14–6 summarizes the common GI hormones and their actions.

BLOOD SUPPLY OF THE GASTROINTESTINAL SYSTEM

Blood supply to organs within the abdomen is referred to as the splanchnic circulation. The GI system receives the largest single percentage of the cardiac output. Approximately one third of the cardiac output supplies these tissues. The superior and inferior mesenteric and celiac arteries supply the stomach, small and large intestines, pancreas, and gallbladder. The liver has a dual blood supply and receives part of its blood supply from the hepatic artery. Circulation to the GI system is unique in that venous blood draining the system empties into the portal vein, which then perfuses the liver. The portal vein supplies approximately 70 to 75% of liver blood flow.

Because of the large percentage of cardiac output that perfuses the GI tract, the GI tract is a major source of blood flow during times of increased need, such as during exercise or as a compensatory mechanism in hemorrhage. Conversely, prolonged occlusion or hypoperfusion of a major artery supplying the GI tract can lead to mucosal ischemia and eventually necrosis. Necrosis of intestinal villi can destroy the GI tract's barrier to harmful toxins and bacteria. It is thought that these bacteria can then enter the blood supply and cause septic shock.

General Assessment of the Gastrointestinal System

A comprehensive assessment of the abdomen includes a history, inspection, auscultation, percussion, and palpation. Of utmost importance is the timing of auscultation; this assessment is performed before the abdomen is manipulated so that the frequency of bowel sounds is not altered. Optimal positioning of the patient in order to relax the abdomen is performed before auscultation is begun. A supine position with the patient's arms at the sides or folded at the chest is usually the recommended position. Placing a pillow under the knees also helps relax the abdominal wall.

Mapping of the abdomen for descriptive purposes is usually performed by use of the four-quadrant method by drawing imaginary lines crossing at the umbilicus: right upper, right lower, left upper, and left lower. Symptoms such as pain may also be described by use of these landmarks.

HISTORY

An assessment of the GI system begins with a history unless an emergency situation exists that re-

Table 14–6. ACTIONS OF GASTROINTESTINAL HORMONES

Action	Gastrin	Cholecystokinin	Secretin	Gastric Inhibitory Peptide
Acid secretion	Stimulates	Stimulates	Inhibits	Inhibits
Gastric motility	Stimulates	Stimulates	Inhibits	—
Gastric emptying	Inhibits	Inhibits	Inhibits	Inhibits
Intestinal motility	Stimulates	Stimulates	Inhibits	—
Mucosal growth	Stimulates	Stimulates	Inhibits	—
Pancreatic HCO_3 secretion	Stimulates	Stimulates	Stimulates	0
Pancreatic enzyme secretion	Stimulates	Stimulates	Stimulates	0
Pancreatic growth	Stimulates	Stimulates	Stimulates	—
Bile HCO_3 secretion	Stimulates	Stimulates	Stimulates	0
Gallbladder contraction	Stimulates	Stimulates	Stimulates	—

0 = no effect; dash = not yet tested; HCO_3 = bicarbonate.

quires immediate physiological assessment and intervention. The patient is questioned about any past problems with indigestion, difficulty swallowing (dysphagia), pain on swallowing, nausea and vomiting, heartburn, belching, abdominal distention or bloating, diarrhea, constipation, or bleeding. All symptoms should be explored in terms of when the symptoms became apparent, any precipitating factors, what treatment was sought, factors that relieved or made the symptoms worse, and whether the symptom is current.

A careful pain assessment should also be performed and is a challenging aspect of the history. Pain receptors in the abdomen are less likely to be localized and are mediated by common sensory structures projected to the skin. Therefore, distinguishing the pain of a peptic ulcer or cholecystitis from that of a myocardial infarction is often difficult. Abdominal pain is most often caused by engorged mucosa, pressure in the mucosa, distention, or spasm. Visceral pain is more likely to cause pallor, perspiration, bradycardia, nausea and vomiting, weakness, and hypotension and should also be assessed. Increasing intensity of pain, especially after a therapeutic regimen, is always significant and usually signifies complicating factors, such as increasing inflammation, gastric distension, hemorrhage into tissue or the peritoneal space, or peritonitis from perforation or anastomosis leakage. If possible, the nurse obtains a description of the location and the type of pain in the patient's own words.

A history of any GI surgeries, including the specific type and dates, should also be discussed. A current list of medications is also important, especially because many drugs have gastrointestinal side effects.

INSPECTION

General inspection of the abdomen should focus on the following characteristics: skin color and texture, symmetry and contour of the abdomen, masses and pulsations, and peristalsis and movement.

Skin Color and Texture

The nurse observes for pigmentation of skin (jaundice), lesions, discolorations, old or new scars, and vascular and hair patterns. General nutrition and hydration status may also be discerned.

Symmetry and Contour of Abdomen

The nurse notes the size and shape of the abdomen and visible protrusions and adipose distribution. Abdominal distention, particularly in the presence of pain, should always be investigated because it usually

indicates trapped air or fluid within the abdominal cavity.

Masses and Pulsations

The nurse looks for any obvious abdominal masses, which are best seen on deep inspiration. Pulsations, if they are seen, usually originate from the aorta.

Peristalsis and Movement

Motility of the stomach may be reflected in movement of the abdomen in lean individuals and therefore is a normal sign. However, strong contractions are abnormal and indicate the presence of disease.

AUSCULTATION

Bowel sounds are high-pitched gurgling sounds caused by air and fluid as they move through the GI tract. They are best heard with the diaphragm of the stethoscope and are systematically assessed in all four quadrants of the abdomen. The frequency and character of the sounds are noted. The frequency of bowel sounds has been estimated at 4 to 34 per minute, and the sounds are usually irregular. Therefore, the abdomen must be auscultated at least 5 minutes before an assessment of complete absence of bowel sounds can be made. Table 14–7 reviews common causes of increased and decreased bowel sounds as they relate to acute illness.

Vascular sounds, such as bruits, may also be heard and indicate dilated, tortuous, or constricted vessels. Venous hums are also normally heard from the inferior vena cava. A hum in the periumbilical region in a patient with cirrhosis indicates an obstructed portal circulation. Peritoneal friction rubs may also be heard and may indicate infection, abscess, or tumor in the abdomen.

Table 14–7. CAUSES OF INCREASED AND DECREASED BOWEL SOUNDS

Causes of Decreased Bowel Sounds	Causes of Increased Bowel Sounds
Peritonitis	Early pyloric or intestinal obstruction
Gangrene	Bleeding ulcers or electrolyte disturbances
Reflux ileus	
Surgical manipulation of bowel	Varices
Late bowel obstruction	Diarrhea
	Subsiding ileus

PERCUSSION

Percussion is aimed at detecting fluid, gaseous distention, or masses in the abdomen. Because of the presence of gas within the GI tract, percussed tympany predominates. Solid masses percuss as dull. Organ borders of the liver, spleen, and stomach may also be ascertained. Abnormal findings are typically diagnosed by radiological tests in the critical care setting.

PALPATION

Palpation is used for evaluating the major organs with respect to shape, size, position, mobility, consistency, and tension. Palpation is performed last because it often elicits pain and/or muscle spasm. Deep abdominal tenderness and rebound tenderness need to be differentiated. Rebound tenderness occurs when pain is elicited after the examiner's hand is quickly released after deep palpation. Rigidity or guarding of the abdomen is also noted. Masses in the liver, spleen, kidneys, gallbladder, and descending colon can also be felt through palpation.

Nutritional Assessment and Therapy

ASSESSMENT

Adequate nutritional support of the critically ill patient is an aspect of nursing care that needs to be considered early in the patient's illness. Increased morbidity and mortality rates, delayed wound healing, and altered normal immune responses are all associated with malnutrition. Early feeding via any method is recommended in all acutely ill patients.

Body homeostasis requires that a balance exist between energy supply and energy expenditure. The basal metabolic rate is the energy that a person requires for the performance of physiological processes at rest. Logically, stressors such as fever, trauma, and sepsis negatively affect energy balance (increase the basal metabolic rate) and need to be considered in the care of the critically ill patient. Nitrogen balance is also important and reflects whether the body is building protein. Anabolism reflects a positive nitrogen balance, or the fact that the body is building protein. Catabolism, or a negative nitrogen balance, represents body breakdown of protein. Most critically ill patients, by virtue of their injury or disease process, are in a catabolic state, and this characteristic needs to be considered in the assessment and in the application of nutritional therapies.

Complete nutritional assessment consists of history taking, including usual and current weight, and biochemical measurements and allows for the quanti-

fication of nutritional health (Dudek, 1993). The parameters the nurse most commonly uses to assess nutritional balance in a critically ill patient are albumin and nitrogen balance. Normal serum albumin level is 3.5 to 5.2 values. Nitrogen balance is calculated according to the following equation:

$$\text{Nitrogen Balance} = \frac{\text{Protein Intake}/6.25}{\text{Urinary Urea Nitrogen} + 4}$$

If the number calculated is zero, nitrogen balance is present. If the number is positive, protein synthesis is occurring. If the number is negative, protein catabolism exists, and the patient is malnourished. A diet history may also help to determine the patient's nutritional state before illness.

The final step in performing a nutritional assessment is determination of the patient's caloric needs. This value is normally calculated by use of a basal energy requirement calculation (Harris-Benedict equation) (Table 14–8).

THERAPY

Total Parenteral Nutrition

Total parenteral nutrition (TPN) is a successful way to provide nutrients to patients who are unable to maintain adequate nutritional status by oral intake. Formulas for TPN contain all known essential nutrients, including water, protein, carbohydrate, fat, electrolytes, vitamins, and trace elements. The proportion of these elements as well as the total calories given are calculated according to the patient's needs. The mixture usually comprises 20 to 30% glucose and 3.5 to 5.0% amino acids. The ratio of glucose, which supplies calories, to nitrogen or amino acids is about 200:1, which maintains nitrogen balance and promotes weight gain, wound healing, and anabolism. Electrolytes are also added to the solution, including sodium, potassium, and chloride. Fats are either supplied by intravenous supplement or mixed in the TPN bag.

Table 14–8. BASAL ENERGY REQUIREMENT FORMULAS*

Women
  BEE = 655 + (9.6 × Wt) + (1.8 × Ht) − (4.7 × Age)
Men
  BEE = 66 + (13.7 × Wt) + (5 × Ht) − (6.8 × Age)

---

*Used to determine caloric requirements; weight in kilograms; height in centimeters; age in years.
  Ht = height; Wt = weight; BEE = basal energy expenditure.

Medications such as insulin and histamine blockers may also be added. Adjustments in the formula are made as the patient's energy expenditure changes during the course of the illness.

Nurses are responsible for the administration of TPN. Major complications of TPN include sepsis and fluid and electrolyte imbalance. Maintaining the sterility of the TPN set-up is essential. All tubing is changed at least every 24 to 48 hours. No intravenous push or piggyback medications are given in the same line. Intravenous site care is meticulous. Because TPN solution is hyperosmolar, it is usually administered through either a peripherally inserted central catheter or a central line, which can become infected in the absence of meticulous care by nurses and physicians. Monitoring for fluid and electrolyte balance and monitoring for early signs of infection are important aspects of nursing care related to this therapeutic modality. Glucose overfeeding and other electrolyte imbalances are also complications of TPN therapy. Therefore, serum glucose and other electrolyte levels also need to be monitored. Patients receiving TPN undergo blood glucose monitoring by fingerstick every 6 hours until glucose tolerance is assessed. When the blood glucose level stabilizes, blood glucose level can be monitored less frequently. Occasionally, insulin needs to be administered with TPN therapy, especially in patients in whom insulin secretion and regulation is impaired. It is also important to remember that patients receiving TPN need to be weaned from it slowly in order to prevent hypoglycemic reactions.

Enteral Nutrition

Enteral nutrition refers to the delivery of nutrients into the GI tract. It is most commonly selected for patients with neuromuscular impairment; patients who cannot meet their nutritional needs by oral intake alone; patients who are hypercatabolic; or patients who are unable to eat as a result of their underlying illness, such as those on ventilators or with hypoperfusion states. The use of enteral feedings, even if the gut cannot handle a full enteral feeding schedule, is thought to be advantageous because it prevents bacterial overgrowth and potential bacterial entry into the bloodstream. These benefits are crucial in critically ill patients. TPN is used in combination with enteral nutrition in order to meet the nutritional needs of the patient.

To accommodate diverse patient needs, many types of enteral formulas have been developed. All contain protein, carbohydrates, and fat, but the proportion of each differs depending on the formula used. The osmolality or ionic concentration is important to consider in the selection of a formula for enteral feedings. Two major types of formulas exist: intact and hydrolyzed. Complete proteins, protein isolates, and blenderized formulas are considered to be intact protein formulas. These formulas are lower in osmolality and require normal digestion for absorption. Hydrolyzed formulas can be used as a transition between TPN and standard feedings because they consist of partially or totally "predigested" proteins, carbohydrates, and fats. These formulas have a higher osmolality. Patients receiving feedings with higher osmolality must be assessed for severe diarrhea, electrolyte depletion, and dehydration. Enteral feeding formulas have been introduced as a means of providing for the immunological and metabolic needs of critically ill patients. Formulas containing glutamine, arginine, lipids, nucleotides, and aurine provide necessary fuel and enhance immune function (Table 14–9) (Alexander, 1993; Keithley and Eisenberg, 1993).

Enteral nutrition depends on an intact bowel that is able to absorb nutrients. The mouth is the ideal method of enteral nutrition, but for patients who are unable to consume food orally, various routes are available for the administration of enteral nutrition. The most common route is nasogastric. Nasogastric tube length is dependent on placement of the tube in the GI tract. A 36-inch tube is standard and reaches the stomach if it is inserted via the nose.

Feeding schedules may be either intermittent or continuous. The stomach is normally a reservoir for intermittent receipt of food. Therefore, an intermittent schedule is recommended by most authorities. Feedings delivered in this manner are delivered by gravity and are regulated with a roller clamp to infuse over the course of 40 to 60 minutes. Delivery of tube feeding by use of a syringe is not recommended because of the risk of pulmonary aspiration (Metheny, 1993). Feedings delivered into the small intestine are delivered by constant infusion because the intestinal mucosa normally receives nutrients from the stomach in peristaltic waves. Enteral feeding pumps are recommended for delivery.

Complications of enteral feedings include

- Mechanical complications resulting from tube obstruction.
- Pulmonary complications caused by improper tube placement or aspiration.

Table 14–9. ENTERAL FEEDING PRODUCTS AVAILABLE FOR IMMUNONUTRITION

Impact	Perative
Immun-Aid	Alitraq
Vivonex T.E.N.	

- Gastrointestinal complications, such as diarrhea and dumping syndrome (abdominal distention, delayed gastric emptying, cramping, and constipation).
- Metabolic complications, such as hyperglycemia, hypercapnia, and electrolyte imbalance.

Table 14–10 reviews common enteral feeding complications and nursing interventions. The most common complication of tube feedings is diarrhea. It can be caused by many factors, including concomitant drug therapy; lactose, lipid, or fiber content of the formula; osmolality of the feeding; bacterial contamination; and rate of infusion. Pulmonary complications are potentially the most serious and can result from improper tube placement or aspiration. Tube placement should be checked after initial placement. Gastric residuals should be checked every 4 hours. Measurement of pH can also be used to verify tube placement (see Research Application).

In summary, enteral feedings are a safe form of nutritional therapy. The most common complications are gastrointestinal. The nurse is responsible for the prevention of these complications; prevention can be accomplished through careful monitoring. On the basis of the current research, we recommend the following:

- All patients undergoing tube feedings should have standing orders or protocols that provide guidelines for confirming correct tube placement, handling formulas, administering formulas, and managing complications.
- Fine-bore tubes need to be carefully assessed because they are easily dislodged. Food coloring can be added to all feedings in order to help detect aspiration or tube displacement. The nurse checks for gastric residual every 4 hours.
- Good hand washing technique is used in the preparation of delivery sets or in the reconstitution of formulas (e.g., half strength). The delivery set is rinsed with water before new formula is added. Hanging time of formulas at room temperature is limited to 8 to 12 hours. Delivery sets are changed every 24 hours.
- Blood glucose levels are monitored by fingerstick every 6 hours until blood glucose levels are stable. Daily weights, daily electrolyte panels, blood urea nitrogen (BUN) level, and glucose level are assessed until they are stabilized. Trace elements are monitored every week.
- A controller pump is used to administer feedings at a constant rate. Feeding tubes are flushed every 4 hours during continuous feedings, after intermittent feedings are given, and after medications are given.
- Ongoing nutritional assessments are provided.

Acute Upper Gastrointestinal Bleeding

PATHOPHYSIOLOGY

Many causes of acute upper GI bleeding necessitate admission of a patient to the critical care unit. Table 14–11 reviews the most common causes of this GI emergency.

Peptic Ulcer Disease

Duodenal and gastric ulcers are the most common cause of upper GI bleeding. Duodenal and gastric ulcers are characterized by a break in the mucosa that extends through the muscularis mucosae. The ulcer crater is usually surrounded by either acutely or chronically inflamed cells. Over time, the inflamed tissue is replaced by necrotic tissue, then granulation tissue, and finally scar tissue.

The role of gastrin, which stimulates excess secretion of acid, is important in the pathogenesis of duodenal ulcer disease. Research indicates that parietal cell mass in this patient population is 1.5 to 2.0 times greater than in persons with no ulcer disease. In patients with normal acid secretion, impaired mucosal resistance to acids is being studied as a cause of duodenal ulcer disease. Duodenal ulcer disease is also associated with several chronic diseases, including chronic pulmonary disease, cirrhosis, renal failure and transplantation, renal stones, and coronary artery disease.

Risk factors for the development of this disease have also been widely studied. Although certain foods, beverages, and spices may cause dyspepsia (Table 14–12), no supportive data indicate that diet causes or reactivates duodenal ulcers. Furthermore, a cause and effect relationship between a bland diet or milk consumption in duodenal ulcer disease has not been substantiated.

Known risk factors for duodenal ulcer disease are listed in Table 14–13. Alcoholic beverages are acid-secretion stimulants and in high concentrations cause damage to the gastric mucosal barrier. Intake of alcoholic beverages is associated with duodenal lesions and upper gastrointestinal bleeding.

Aspirin and other nonsteroidal anti-inflammatory drugs may cause acute gastric mucosal damage and chronic ulcers and may precipitate upper gastrointestinal bleeding.

Cigarette smoking has been causally linked to duodenal ulcer disease. Smoking is thought to impair ulcer healing, is associated with recurrences, and increases patient risk for complications. It has been proposed that smoking induces bile reflux, stimulates acid

Table 14–10. TUBE FEEDING COMPLICATIONS AND NURSING INTERVENTIONS

Complication	Nursing Interventions
Mechanical	
Tube obstruction	Flush feeding tube with at least 30 ml of water every 4 h during continuous feedings, after medications, after intermittent feedings, and before and after gastric residuals are checked. Use polyurethane tube. Use medications in elixir form whenever possible. If the tube becomes obstructed, irrigate it with either water or cola.
Pulmonary	
Improper tube placement	Verify the position of all small-bore feeding tubes by x-ray study. Identify patients at risk for malposition: e.g., those with impaired gag/cough reflex, those who are obtunded, those who are heavily sedated, or those receiving neuromuscular blocking agents. Note: Air insertion into tube with auscultation can be misleading. Attempting to aspirate gastric contents may also be difficult because small-bore tubes collapse easily.
Aspiration	Monitor residuals every 4 h and temporarily discontinue feedings if volume is greater than 100–150 ml/h for 2 consecutive h. Monitor for abdominal distention with abdominal girth measurements. Assess bowel sounds. Monitor for tube position every 4 h by aspirating fluid. Note the appearance of the aspirate and check pH (should be acidic unless patient is taking histamine blockers or antacids). (See Research Application, pp 470–471.) Mark feeding tube at exit site. To prevent reflux, keep head of bed elevated 30–40° during feedings. Discontinue feedings for 10–15 min before patient's head is rolled for therapies. Color tube feedings with dye. Monitor pulmonary secretions.
Gastrointestinal	
Diarrhea	Review medications the patient is receiving. Administer fiber-enriched formulas or bulking agents in order to normalize stool consistency (e.g., Metamucil). Prevent bacterial contamination: • When possible, use full-strenth, ready-to-use formula. • Use meticulous hand washing techniques in the handling of all formulas and supplies. • Avoid touching inside of delivery sets. • Wash delivery sets with soapy water and rinse after intermittent feedings. Change delivery set every 24 h. • Limit hanging time of formulas at room temperature to 8 h. (Exception: prefilled sets; read manufacturer recommendations.)
Dumping syndrome	Limit bolus feedings to <300 ml. Slow the rate and frequency of bolus if abdominal distention or cramping persists.
Metabolic	
Hyperglycemia	Monitor urine glucose and acetone levels every 3–6 h until stable. Monitor blood glucose level every 24 h. Observe for signs and symptoms of hyperglycemia. Administer insulin as ordered, usually per sliding scale. Use delivery methods that ensure administration of feeding at a constant rate.
Hypercapnia	Use formulas with lower carbohydrate and higher fat content for respiratory-compromised and ventilator-dependent patients. Monitor partial pressure of arterial carbon dioxide.
Electrolyte imbalance	Monitor fluid status closely. Monitor serum sodium, potassium, and phosphate levels.

Table 14–11. CAUSES OF UPPER GASTROINTESTINAL BLEEDING

Duodenal ulcer	Mallory-Weiss tear
Gastric ulcer	Gastritis
Cushing's ulcer	Esophagitis
Curling's ulcer	Esophageal or
Stress ulcer	gastric varices

secretion, decreases prostaglandin synthesis, and alters gastric blood flow.

Strong evidence also supports a genetic basis for duodenal ulcer disease. Twenty to 50% of duodenal ulcer patients report a positive family history (Soll, 1990).

Emotional factors also influence gastric function; however, the specific role of personality types and responses to stressful events as mediated by the central nervous system has not been clearly linked to duodenal ulcer disease and needs further study.

The cause of gastric ulcers is poorly understood. Whether acid and pepsin damage the mucosa or whether acid and pepsin cause the ulceration once mucosal damage occurs is not known. Gastric mucosal ischemia is also believed to be an important pathogenesis of acute mucosal injury (see Stress Ulcers next). Abnormalities in mucus production and/or bicarbonate secretion have also been widely studied. Theoretically, patients with gastric ulcer might secrete lower than normal amounts of mucus or bicarbonate, or they may produce an inferior quality of mucus. Gastric ulcers tend to recur frequently, usually at the same site.

Helicobacter pylori bacteria has been associated with the pathogenesis of various gastroduodenal diseases, including peptic ulcer formation. The literature on this topic is controversial, but anti–*H. pylori* therapy has proved to be effective in several clinical trials in the long-term prevention of *H. pylori* infection associated with ulcer development (NIH Consensus, 1994). As a result of these findings, antibiotics have been added to the therapeutic regimen for the treatment of peptic ulcer disease. At present, *H. pylori* research is centered around establishing methods for diagnosis of

Table 14–12. DIETARY STIMULANTS OF ACID SECRETION

Unrefined wheat	Acid-neutralized coffee
Coffee	7-Up
Cola drinks	Beer
(Coca-Cola)	Tea
Diet colas	

Table 14–13. KNOWN RISK FACTORS FOR DUODENAL ULCER DISEASE

Alcohol
Drugs
    Aspirin
    Nonsteroidal anti-inflammatory drugs
    ?Corticosteroids (>30 days; >1 g)
Smoking
Genetic predisposition
    Acid hypersecretion
    Altered mucosa
Defense mechanism
?Stress

the infection and the cost, benefits, and risks of anti–*H. pylori* therapy in the clinical setting.

Stress Ulcers

A stress ulcer is an acute gastric mucosal erosion that commonly occurs in patients in intensive care units. The lesions are associated with severe trauma, long-term sepsis, severe burns (Curling's ulcer), cranial or central nervous system disease (Cushing's ulcer), and long-term ingestion of drugs that have known adverse effects on the gastric mucosa. Abnormalities range from small surface hemorrhages to deep ulcerations with massive gastrointestinal hemorrhage and occasionally perforation. Massive upper gastrointestinal bleeding usually occurs 3 to 7 days after the initial insult and significantly increases the mortality rate for the critically ill patient.

Factors associated with stress ulcers are reviewed in Table 14–14. Acid hypersecretion is not associated with all causes of stress ulcers, but some amount of acid is necessary for the formation of an ulcer. Cardiogenic shock directly impairs oxygen supply to the stomach and therefore may impair vascular perfusion of the stomach, causing mucosal anoxia. Stress may reduce both the quality and the quantity of mucus in the stomach. Mucus, a natural defense mechanism in the stomach, delays the diffusion of hydrogen ions into the mucosa. Lowered mucosal pH (<3.5) and decreased regeneration of mucosal cells also have been implicated in the development of stress ulcers.

Table 14–14. PATHOGENESIS OF STRESS ULCERS

Acid hypersecretion
Gastric anoxia (hypotension)
Altered mucosal defense mechanisms
Decreased mucosal pH

Mallory-Weiss Tear

A Mallory-Weiss tear is an arterial bleed from an acute longitudinal tear in the gastroesophageal mucosa and accounts for 10 to 15% of upper GI bleeding episodes. It is associated with long-term nonsteroidal anti-inflammatory drug or aspirin ingestion and with excessive alcohol intake. The upper GI bleed usually occurs after episodes of forceful retching. Bleeding usually spontaneously resolves; however, lacerations of the esophagogastric junction may cause a massive GI bleed, which requires surgical repair.

Esophageal Varices

In chronic cirrhotic liver failure, liver cell structure and function are impaired, resulting in increased portal venous pressure, which is called portal hypertension (see Liver Failure section). As a result, part of the venous blood in the splanchnic system may be diverted from the liver to the systemic circulation by the development of connections to neighboring low-pressure veins. This phenomenon is termed *collateral circulation*. The most common sites for the development of these collateral channels are the submucosa of the esophagus and rectum, the anterior abdominal wall, and the parietal peritoneum. Figure 14–6 shows a liver with collateral circulation. The normal portal venous pressure is 2 to 6 mm Hg. As pressure increases in these veins, they become distended with blood, the vessels enlarge, and varices develop. Formation of varices requires that this pressure increase to more than 10 mm Hg. The most common sites for the development of these varices are the esophagus and the upper portion of the stomach. In summary, esophageal and gastric varices represent massively dilated submucosal veins that divert splanchnic venous blood from the high-pressure portal system. These varices tend to have a low tolerance for pressure and thus tend to bleed. Studies indicate that a portal venous pressure of at least 12 mm Hg is needed for varices to bleed (Goff, 1993).

ASSESSMENT

Clinical Presentation

Patients manifest blood loss from the gastrointestinal tract in several ways. *Hematemesis* is bloody vomitus that is either bright red, which indicates fresh blood, or "coffee-ground," that is older blood that has been in the stomach long enough for the gastric juices to act on it. Blood may also be passed via the colon. *Melena* is shiny, black, foul-smelling stool and results from the degradation of blood by stomach acids or intestinal bacteria. Bright red or maroon blood, *hema-*

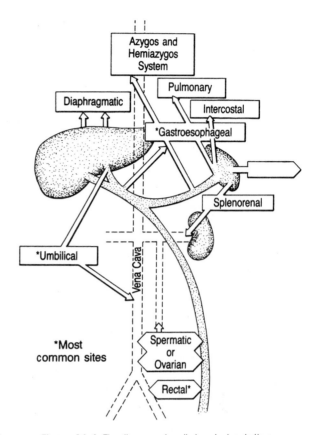

Figure 14–6. The liver and collateral circulation.

tochezia, can also be passed from the rectum. Gastrointestinal blood loss can also be occult, or detected only by testing of the stool with a chemical reagent (guaiac). However, stool and nasogastric drainage can test guaiac positive for up to 10 days after a bleed and are associated with chronic bleeds. Hematemesis, melena, or hematochezia indicates an episode of acute upper GI bleeding. Hematemesis results from the collection of large amounts of blood in the stomach, accompanied by nausea. Hematochezia is usually a sign of lower GI bleeding. When hematochezia is from an upper GI source, it is associated with a massive bleed (greater than 1000 ml). Upper GI bleeding may also be accompanied by mild epigastric pain or abdominal distress, although it is not very common. Pain is thought to arise from the acid's bathing the ulcer crater.

Finally, patients may present with clinical signs and symptoms of blood loss, such as hypotension, tachycardia, dizziness, dyspnea, restlessness and anxiety, decreased level of consciousness, decreased urine output, and shock. Table 14–15 summarizes the common presenting manifestations of an acute upper GI bleed. Rapid assessment of the patient is undertaken

Table 14–15. CLINICAL SIGNS AND SYMPTOMS OF UPPER GASTROINTESTINAL BLEEDING

Hematemesis
Melena
Hematochezia
Abdominal discomfort
Signs and symptoms of hypovolemic shock
   Hypotension
   Tachycardia
   Cool, clammy skin
   Changes in level of consciousness
   Decreased urine output
   Decreased gastric motility

to determine the seriousness of the bleeding, that is, whether it is acute or chronic, and to determine whether the patient is hemodynamically stable or unstable. Patients with acute upper GI bleeding commonly have signs or symptoms of hypovolemic shock (see Chapter 8). Figure 14–7 describes the pathophysiology of acute upper GI bleeding.

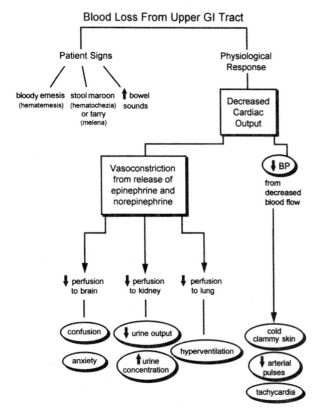

Figure 14–7. Pathophysiology flow diagram of acute upper gastrointestinal (GI) bleeding. BP = blood pressure.

Nursing Assessment

Assessment of the severity of blood loss is the first priority and includes the frequent monitoring of vital signs and assessments of body systems for signs of shock. Blood pressure and heart rate depend on the amount of blood loss, the suddenness of the blood loss, and the degree of cardiac and vascular compensation (Lieberman, 1993). Vital signs should be monitored at least every 15 minutes. As blood loss exceeds 1000 ml, the shock syndrome progresses, causing decreased blood flow to the skin, lungs, liver, and kidneys. As a result of decreased blood flow to the skin, the patient's skin is cool and clammy. Decreased blood flow to the lungs causes hyperventilation in order to maintain adequate oxygenation. As blood flow decreases to the kidney, waste products accumulate in the blood, as reflected in an increasing BUN level. Urine output is a sensitive measure of systemic tissue perfusion and blood flow, and therefore output must be measured at least every hour. Abdominal assessment may reveal a soft or distended abdomen. Bowel sounds most often are hyperactive as a result of the sensitivity of the bowel to blood. Hypotension is an advanced sign of shock. As a rule, a systolic pressure of less than 100 mm Hg or a postural decrease in blood pressure of greater than 10 mm Hg and/or a heart rate of greater than 120 beats/min reflect a blood loss of at least 1000 ml—25% of the total blood volume. As blood pressure decreases, it can be assumed that more blood has been lost. Rarely, a central venous pressure or pulmonary artery catheter is inserted in order to evaluate the patient's hemodynamic response to the blood loss. The central venous pressure and/or the pulmonary capillary wedge pressure (PCWP) is decreased in the patient with hemorrhagic shock. The electrocardiogram (ECG) may also show ST-segment depression or flattening of the T waves, both of which indicate decreased coronary blood flow.

In addition to the physical examination, a history is taken in order to ascertain if there have been previous episodes of bleeding or surgery for bleeding; a family history of bleeding; or a current illness that may lead to bleeding, such as coagulopathies, cancer, and liver disease. Concurrent diseases also affect the patient's response to the hemorrhage and to the treatment modalities. Patterns of drug or alcohol ingestion and other risk factors need to be assessed and may also help ascertain the cause.

Medical Assessment

Laboratory Studies

The common laboratory studies ordered for a patient with acute upper GI bleeding are listed in Table

14–16. A complete blood count is always ordered. However, the hematocrit (Hct) value does not change substantially during the first few hours after an acute GI bleed. During this time, the severity of the bleed must not be underestimated; this severity is best evaluated with the vital signs mentioned earlier. Only when extravascular fluid enters the vascular space in order to restore volume does the Hct value decrease. This effect is further complicated by fluids and blood that are administered during the resuscitation period. Platelet and white blood cell counts may also be increased, reflecting the body's attempt to restore homeostasis. An electrolyte profile is also ordered. Decreases in potassium and sodium levels are common as a result of the accompanying vomiting. Later, serum sodium levels may increase as a result of the loss of vascular volume. Glucose level is often increased on account of the stress response. Increases in the BUN level and creatinine level reflect decreased perfusion to the liver and kidneys, respectively. Liver functions tests, clotting profile, and serum ammonia level are usually ordered in order to rule out preexisting liver disease. An arterial blood gas analysis is also ordered in order to evaluate the patient's acid-base and oxygenation status. Respiratory alkalosis is common with GI bleeding as a result of the effects of the sympathetic nervous system on the lungs and patient anxiety. As shock progresses, the patient may present with metabolic acidosis as a result of anaerobic metabolism. Hypoxemia may also be present as a result of decreased circulating hemoglobin levels.

Barium Study and Endoscopy

The history and physical examination are not definitive diagnostic examinations, because they do not define the bleeding lesion that is necessary before definitive treatment can be initiated. In a patient who is admitted to the critical care unit, endoscopy is the procedure of choice. Endoscopy allows for direct mucosal inspection with the use of a fiberoptic scope. Flexible scopes allow this test to be performed at the patient's bedside, which is preferable in an unstable critically ill patient. Endoscopic evaluation of the source of the bleed is not undertaken until the patient has been hemodynamically stabilized with conventional medical therapies (see Intervention section). Barium studies can be performed in order to help define the presence of peptic ulcers, the sites of bleeding, the presence of tumors, and the presence of inflammatory processes.

NURSING DIAGNOSES

The actual and potential nursing diagnoses most commonly seen in patients with acute GI bleeding include

- Fluid volume deficit related to decreased circulating blood volume.
- Anxiety related to hemorrhage, pain or discomfort, hospitalization, or fear of the unknown.
- Altered systemic tissue perfusion related to decreased circulating blood volume.
- Knowledge deficit related to disease process and therapeutic interventions.
- Impaired gas exchange related to loss of oxygen-carrying capacity.
- Risk for fluid volume excess related to fluid overload from treatment regimen.
- Risk for aspiration of blood related to vomiting of gastric contents.

Additionally, patient problems that can result from the disease process or treatment regimen include

- Altered electrolyte balance related to loss of blood and gastric contents and administration of fluids and blood products.
- Hepatic encephalopathy related to altered cerebral metabolism from increased circulating ammonia.

(See the Nursing Care Plan for the Patient with Acute Upper Gastrointestinal Bleeding.)

Table 14–16. LABORATORY TESTS FOR UPPER GASTROINTESTINAL BLEEDING

Complete blood count
  Hemoglobin—normal, then decreases
  Hematocrit—normal, then decreases
  White blood cell count—elevated
  Platelet count—initially elevated, then decreased

Electrolyte panel
  Serum potassium level—decreases, then increases
  Serum sodium level—elevated
  Serum calcium level—normal or decreased
  Serum blood urea nitrogen, creatinine
    level—elevated
  Serum ammonia level—possibly elevated
  Serum glucose level—hyperglycemia common
  Serum lactate level—elevated

Hematology profile
  Prothrombin time, partial thromboplastin
    time—usually decreased

Serum enzyme levels—elevated

Arterial blood gases—respiratory alkalosis
  Respiratory alkalosis/metabolic acidosis

Gastric aspirate for pH and guaiac—
  Possibly acidotic pH; guaiac +

NURSING CARE PLAN FOR THE PATIENT WITH ACUTE GASTROINTESTINAL BLEEDING

Nursing Diagnosis	Patient Outcomes	Nursing Interventions
Fluid volume deficit related to decreased circulating blood volume.	Circulating body fluid volume will be normal. Hemorrhage will be controlled or resolved. Preload indicators will be within normal limits. Hematocrit (Hct) and hemoglobin (Hgb) levels will be stable. Weight will be stable. Intake and output will be balanced.	Monitor vital signs for hemodynamic instability; orthostatic changes. Measure preload indicators: central venous pressure (CVP), pulmonary capillary wedge pressure (PCWP). Monitor electrocardiogram, skin, urine output, daily weights, amount, and characteristics of gastrointestinal secretions. Monitor response to fluid replacement. Monitor laboratory values: serial Hct, Hgb, blood urea nitrogen, potassium, sodium. Monitor nature of bowel sounds. Monitor for clinical manifestations of perforation: severe persistent abdominal pain; board-like abdomen. Lavage as ordered until clear. Administer medications, parenteral fluids. Prepare for endoscopy, assist as necessary, monitor for complications.
Altered tissue perfusion related to decreased circulating blood volume.	Signs and symptoms of decreased perfusion will be absent. Decreased sensorium, chest pain, renal failure will be absent. Hemodynamics will be stable. Urine output will be > 30 ml/h. Skin will be warm and dry. Bowel sounds will be within normal limits.	Monitor for hypoperfusion and hemodynamic instability. Monitor vital signs every 15 min until stable. Measure CVP, PCWP, cardiac output every hour until stable. Monitor for presence of tachycardia, chest pain, ST-segment elevation, diaphoresis, cool/clammy extremities. Measure urine output every 4 h. Monitor for alterations in level of consciousness. Assess bowel sounds. Monitor for increased bilirubin. Notify physician of changes, abnormalities.
Anxiety related to hospitalization, hospital regimen.	Patient and family will demonstrate decreased anxiety with nursing intervention, e.g., explanations of environment. Patient and family will verbalize understanding of disease, medical and nursing interventions used.	Assess level of anxiety. Explain intensive care unit (ICU) environment and all procedures. Provide reassurance to patient and family. Approach patient and family in a calm, concerned manner. Structure ICU environment to provide rest; limit stimuli as possible. Describe disease process and all therapeutics instituted. Anticipate treatments and procedures and provide explanations and reassurance. Provide for patient comfort. Liberalize or restrict family visitation as necessary. Involve patient and family in planning care. Encourage patient and family to verbalize fears and concerns.

NURSING CARE PLAN FOR THE PATIENT WITH ACUTE GASTROINTESTINAL BLEEDING *Continued*

Nursing Diagnosis	Patient Outcomes	Nursing Interventions
Risk for fluid volume excess related to fluid overload from treatment regimen.	Respiratory pattern will be normal. Lung congestion or pulmonary edema will be absent.	Carefully monitor hemodynamic response to all fluids given. Monitor breath sounds at least every hour during fluid administration. Monitor for sudden restlessness or anxiety, dyspnea, tachycardia, coughing, coarse crackles throughout all lung fields, productive white or pink-tinged frothy sputum, dysrhythmias, abnormal arterial blood gas results, acute changes in blood pressure, increased CVP, jugular vein distention. Record accurate intake and output. Obtain daily weights. Document and report any abnormalities.
Risk for infection related to contaminated surgical wound or translocation to blood (postoperative surgical).	Patient will be free of infection. Patient will be afebrile. The wound will be clean and dry and without redness, swelling, erythema, pain, or purulent drainage.	Use aseptic technique for all dressing changes. Monitor appearance of incision and surrounding tissue; note any redness, warmth, swelling, or complaints of pain or tenderness. Document and report all wound drainage, color, amount, odor. Culture any suspicious drainage. Monitor white blood cell count, temperature trends. Monitor nutritional status, nitrogen balance, albumin levels. Teach patient and family signs and symptoms of wound infection for discharge planning.
Risk for ineffective breathing pattern related to obstruction of the airway by the Sengstaken-Blakemore tube.	Airway obstruction will be prevented or detected early.	Maintain prescribed pressures in all balloon ports. Deflate balloon ports as ordered (*always* deflate the esophageal balloon before the gastric balloon). Maintain traction on ports as ordered. Keep patient on bed rest with head of bed elevated. Sedate patient as necessary; provide for safety. Irrigate nasogastric tube every 2 h and as needed to maintain patency; note gastric contents. Suction nasopharynx frequently. Keep scissors at bedside and cut entire tube and remove if there is an episode of sudden respiratory distress or if gastric balloon deflates before esophageal balloon. Cleanse and lubricate all skin in contact with tube or traction device.

COLLABORATIVE MANAGEMENT: NURSING AND MEDICAL CONSIDERATIONS

The management of acute GI bleeding initially consists of hemodynamically stabilizing the patient and then consists of diagnosing the cause of bleeding and initiating specific and supportive therapies (Table 14–17). The nurse's role during the initial management of acute GI bleeding includes assessing the patient carrying out prescribed medical therapy, monitoring the patient's physiological and psychosocial responses to the interventions, monitoring for complications of the disease process or treatment regimen, and providing supportive care. Patient and family support during the acute phase is a nursing priority. Explanations of the diagnostic tests, the medical therapies, and the intensive care environment are extremely important to patients, who are often anxious about their diagnosis and the outcome.

Hemodynamic Stabilization

Patients who are hemodynamically unstable need to have immediate venous access (using large-bore intravenous tubes) and administration of fluid must be started. For the restoration of vascular volume, fluids must be infused as rapidly as the patient's cardiovascular status allows and until the patient's vital signs return to baseline. The physician may order colloids, crystalloids, or albumin initially in order to achieve this purpose. The nurse's role is to gain venous access and to initiate prompt fluid resuscitation. Because the blood pressure is the most sensitive measure of adequacy of vascular volume, frequent monitoring of vital signs, at least every 5 to 15 minutes, is a priority. Often, intra-arterial lines are inserted for continuous blood pressure monitoring. The nurse can use reversal

---

Table 14–17. MANAGEMENT OF UPPER GASTROINTESTINAL BLEEDING

Hemodynamic stabilization
  Colloids
  Crystalloids
  Blood/blood products
Definitive and supportive therapies
  Gastric lavage
  Pharmacological therapies
    Antacids
    H_2 histamine blockers
  Endoscopic therapies
    Sclerotherapy
    Heater probe
    Laser
  Surgical therapies

---

of the signs of hemorrhagic shock as a means of assessing the adequacy of fluid administration. These signs include normal skin color and temperature, absence of tachycardia, and adequate urine output. The goal of fluid therapy is improvement of the circulation of red blood cells. Oxygen administration may also be started, which assists in tissue oxygenation.

Patients who continue to bleed or who have an excessively low Hct value (<25%) and clinical symptoms may be resuscitated with blood and blood products. The physician's decision to use blood products is based on laboratory data and clinical examination. Blood is transfused in order to improve oxygenation by increasing the number of red blood cells and/or to improve coagulation (by replacing platelets and plasma). An Hct value may not initially reflect actual blood volume during the first 24 to 72 hours after a bleed and until vascular volume is restored. A reasonable goal for the management of blood transfusions is an Hct value of 30%, but this goal is individually determined for the patient based on clinical assessments. One unit of packed red blood cells can be expected to increase the hemoglobin (Hgb) value by 1 g/dL and the Hct value by 2 to 3%, but this effect is influenced by the patient's intravascular volume status and by whether the patient is actively bleeding.

Maintenance of bed rest with the head of the bed elevated is important supportive care geared to prevent further bleeding and to decrease the risk of aspiration. Exertion increases intra-abdominal pressure, which predisposes the patient to more bleeding. Keeping the head of the bed elevated also may help prevent reflux of gastric contents into the esophagus. Clearing the nasopharynx of secretions is a nursing priority for the prevention of aspiration, particularly in patients who have an altered level of consciousness and impaired swallowing reflexes. Suction and intubation equipment needs to be readily accessible.

In addition to monitoring the effects of fluid resuscitation and blood product administration, the nurse also monitors for complications of the therapy. In patients with preexisting cardiovascular, pulmonary, or renal disease, central venous or pulmonary artery pressure monitoring may be instituted in order to prevent fluid administration overload. Frequent assessments of breath sounds by the nurse during fluid administration are an important aspect of care. Careful monitoring for complications of blood transfusion therapy is also important. These complications include hypercalcemia, hyperkalemia, infection, increased ammonia levels, hypothermia, and anaphylactic reactions.

Gastric Lavage

Gastric lavage may be ordered, but this is a controversial therapy in the treatment of an upper GI

445

bleed. Physicians in favor of gastric lavage claim that it helps indicate the rapidity of the bleed, helps ascertain whether there is active bleeding in the GI tract, and serves to cleanse the stomach in preparation for endoscopy. If lavage is ordered, 1000 to 2000 ml of room-temperature normal saline is usually instilled via nasogastric tube and is then gently removed by manual or intermittent suction until the secretions are clear. The use of ice lavage is used in some centers, although this regimen is controversial. After lavage, the nasogastric tube may be left in or removed. Some research indicates that nasogastric tubes left in place may increase hydrochloric acid secretion in the stomach and may cause increased bleeding (Lieberman, 1993). Eighty to 90% of upper GI bleeds are self-limiting and stop with lavage therapy alone or on their own. The nurse must carefully document the nature of the nasogastric secretions or vomitus, such as the color, amount, and pH.

Pharmacological Therapy

Pharmacological agents are used to decrease gastric acid secretion or to reduce acid effects on gastric mucosa. The most common agents used include antacids, histamine antagonists (H_2 histamine blockers), and mucosal barrier enhancers. Table 14–18 summarizes these major drugs, including actions, dosage and route, side effects, and nursing implications.

Antacids. These agents act as a direct alkaline buffer to control the pH of the gastric mucosa. Administration of antacids is usually ordered every 1 to 2 hours initially. If a nasogastric tube is left in place, antacids may be ordered in order to maintain the gastric pH at greater than 5. The nurse is responsible for obtaining the gastric pH, for administering the antacid, and for monitoring for side effects of the therapy. The major side effects of antacids include diarrhea, electrolyte disturbances (increased magnesium and sodium ion content), and metabolic alkalosis.

Histamine Blockers. These agents act to block all factors that stimulate the parietal cells in the stomach to secrete hydrochloric acid. The most common H_2 histamine blockers are cimetidine, ranitidine, and famotidine. A more recent complication associated with all drugs that increase gastric pH is microbial colonization of the stomach, which may predispose intubated patients to tracheal colonization. This effect may increase the risk for nosocomial pneumonia in these patients.

Mucosal Barrier Enhancers. These agents act on the gastric mucosa to reduce the effects of acid secretion. Prostaglandins are known to improve the mucosal barrier. Sucralfate is a drug used in the treatment of duodenal ulcers and acts to form a protective barrier over the ulcer site. Colloidal bismuth binds to the ulcer base and also stimulates mucus secretion, which prevents further mucosal damage.

Antibiotics. *Helicobacter pylori* has been associated with the development of ulcers in peptic ulcer disease. A combination of tetracycline, metronidazole, and bismuth subsalicylate has been shown in some studies to be effective in eradicating *H. pylori*. Amoxicillin may be substituted for tetracycline. This combination may be ordered in the prophylactic treatment of bleeding gastric ulcers, particularly in patients who have recurrent bleeding (NIH Consensus, 1994).

Endoscopic Therapy

Several endoscopic therapies have been developed for the control of peptic ulcer bleeding. The advantage of these therapies is that they can be applied at the time of diagnosis. Sclerotherapy involves injecting the bleeding ulcer with a necrotizing agent. The most common agents used are morrhuate sodium, ethanolamine, and tetradecyl sulfate. These agents work by traumatizing the endothelium, causing necrosis and eventual sclerosis of the bleeding vessel. Thermal methods of endoscopic therapy include use of the heater probe, laser photocoagulation, and electrocoagulation. All of these therapies act to tamponade the vessel in order to stop active bleeding. Because they are performed at the patient's bedside, the nurse assists with the procedures and monitors for untoward effects.

Maintenance of airway and breathing during endoscopic procedures is of major concern. Placement of the patient in a left lateral reverse Trendelenburg's position can help prevent respiratory complications. Other common complications of sclerotherapy include fever and oozing from the bleeding site. A more serious complication that can occur when morrhuate sodium is used is the development of adult respiratory disease syndrome (ARDS), which is thought to result from the exposure of lung tissue to fatty substances liberated from the necrotizing agent that is used to sclerose the bleeding vessel (see Chapter 11).

Surgical Therapy

Surgery may be considered in patients who have a massive GI bleed that is immediately life-threatening, in patients who continue to bleed despite medical therapies, and in patients with perforation or unremitting pyloric obstruction.

The purpose of emergency surgery in patients with a massive upper GI bleed is the prevention of death from exsanguination. The patient is usually admitted to an intensive care unit for initial management, such as fluid and cardiorespiratory resuscitation, to

Table 14–18. PHARMACOLOGICAL INTERVENTIONS FOR UPPER GASTROINTESTINAL BLEEDING

Drug	Action/Uses	Dosage/Route	Common Side Effects	Nursing Implications
Antacids	Acid neutralizer.	30–60 ml po/NG every 1–2 h	Depends on antacid used. See medication formulary for specific drug side effects; most common include diarrhea and constipation.	Monitor patients with renal failure closely. Avoid antacids containing aluminum if the patient has renal failure (see Chapter 12).
Histamine (H₂) blockers Cimetidine (Tagamet)	Competitive inhibitor of the action of histamine at the H₂ receptors of the parietal cells.	300 mg IV every 6 h	Confusional states, decreased WBC count, nephrotoxicity, pancreatitis, somnolence, rash, diarrhea, thrombocytopenia, arthralgias, drug interactions.	Monitor closely in patients with renal failure; monitor for complications with other drugs. Monitor platelet counts.
Ranitidine (Zantac)	H₂ receptor antagonist.	50 mg IV every 6–8 h	Leukopenia, thrombocytopenia, malaise, dizziness, depression, tachycardia, diarrhea, constipation, hepatitis, arthralgias.	Monitor closely in patients with hepatic and renal failure. Monitor platelet count.
Famotidine (Pepcid)	H₂ receptor antagonist.	200 mg/dl 5% D/W IV every 6 h	CNS (headache, dizziness, hallucinations), GI disturbances, increased BUN and creatinine levels, thrombocytopenia (rare), rash, irritation around IV site.	No incompatibilities with IV fluids. Solution is stable for 48 h after diluting. Oral doses are most effective if administered at bedtime.
Omeprazole (Prilosec)	Hydrogen/ potassium adenosine triphosphatase inhibitor. More research is needed regarding its effectiveness during the acute GI bleed phase.	20 mg po daily; may be increased to as much as 40 mg daily for patients with poor response to H₂ blockers	CNS (headache, dizziness), GI disturbances, cough, rash, back pain.	Sustained release must be swallowed intact, not opened, chewed, or crushed. Now available in elixir. If daily dosage is >80 mg, administer in divided doses. Documented interactions with ampicillin, iron derivatives, ketoconazole (omeprazole decreases absorption of these drugs). Increased serum levels noted with diazepam, phenytoin, and warfarin.

po = oral; IV = intravenous; NG = nasogastric; 5% D/W = 5% dextrose in water; CNS = central nervous system; GI = gastrointestinal; BUN = blood urea nitrogen.

stabilize the patient as much as possible in preparation for the emergent surgery. The most common reason for emergency surgery is massive rebleeding that occurs within 8 hours of admission to the hospital.

Patients may also become surgical candidates if they continue to bleed despite aggressive medical intervention. Criteria for delayed surgery varies from institution to institution, but it is usually considered in patients who require more than 8 units of blood within a 24-hour period.

Impaired emptying of solids or liquids from the stomach into the small intestine (gastric outlet obstruction) may also necessitate surgical intervention. The major symptoms of obstruction include vomiting and continued ulcer pain that is localized in the epigastrium.

Surgical therapies for peptic ulcer disease include gastric resections (antrectomy, gastrectomy, gastroenterostomy, vagotomy) or combined surgeries to restore GI continuity (Billroth I, Billroth II) or to prevent GI complications of the surgery (vagotomy and pyloroplasty). An antrectomy may be performed for duodenal

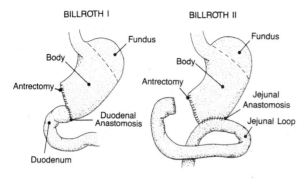

Figure 14–8. Billroth I and II procedures.

ulcers in order to decrease the acidity of the duodenum by removing the antrum, which secretes gastric acid. A vagotomy decreases acid secretion in the stomach by dividing the vagus nerve along the esophagus. A pyloroplasty may be performed in conjunction with a vagotomy in order to prevent stomach atony, a common complication of the vagotomy procedure. A Billroth I procedure involves vagotomy, antrectomy, and anastomosis of the stomach to the duodenum. A Billroth II procedure involves vagotomy, resection of the antrum, and anastomosis of the stomach to the jejunum (Fig. 14–8). A perforation can be treated by simple closure by use of a patch to cover the gastric mucosal hole (omental patch), or by excision of the ulcer and suturing of the surrounding tissue.

Postoperative nursing care is focused on prevention and monitoring of potential complications. Fluid and electrolyte imbalances are commonly related to loss of fluids during the surgical procedure and the drains that are left in place to either decompress the stomach (nasogastric tube) or drain the surgical site. Additionally, the GI system may not function normally for a period of time after surgery, resulting in nausea, vomiting, ileus, or diarrhea. The provision of adequate nutrition, which is essential for proper wound healing, is necessary. In cases of prolonged ileus after surgery, TPN may be considered. Monitoring for proper wound healing is also a nursing responsibility. Signs and symptoms of wound infection (erythema, swelling, tenderness, drainage, fever, increased white blood cell count) need to be documented and reported accordingly. A systemic infection may result from peritonitis in the case of perforation in which stomach or intestinal contents spill into the peritoneum. Postoperative rupture of the anastomosis may also lead to this complication.

Pain is also an important postoperative nursing concern. Abdominal incisions are associated with more postoperative discomfort because of their anatomical location. In addition, postoperative lung infections are more common in patients with abdominal incisions because the patient tends to splint respirations because of incisional pain. Deep breathing and coughing exercises are also more painful in this patient population.

Specific nursing diagnoses associated with the postoperative care of the patient with upper GI bleeding include

- Risk for infection (wound).
- Risk for infection related to inflammation of the peritoneum.
- Risk for altered nutrition (less than body requirements) related to dysfunctional bowel.
- Acute pain related to incision.
- Impaired gas exchange and ineffective airway clearance related to anesthesia, surgery, decreased activity, pain, splinting, and use of nasogastric tube.

Recognition of Potential Complications

Perforation of the gastric mucosa is the major GI complication of peptic ulcer disease. The nurse needs to be familiar with the signs and symptoms of acute perforation, which are reviewed in Table 14–19. The most common signs of this complication are an abrupt onset of abdominal pain, followed rapidly by signs of peritonitis. The goal for the treatment of this patient is preparation for emergent surgery. Fluid and electrolyte resuscitation and treatment of any immediate complications are priorities. These patients almost always have nasogastric tubes placed for gastric decompression. Broad-spectrum antibiotics are also usually prescribed before surgery. Antacids and histamine blockers may or may not be indicated, depending on the cause of the upper GI bleeding. Mortality rates for patients with perforations range from 10 to 40%, depending on the age and condition of the patient at the time of surgery.

TREATMENT OF VARICEAL BLEEDS

Hemorrhaging esophageal or gastric varices are usually a medical emergency because they usually

Table 14–19. SIGNS OF ACUTE GASTRIC PERFORATION
Abrupt onset of severe abdominal pain
Abdominal tenderness
Board-like abdomen
Usually absent bowel sounds
Leukocytosis
Presence of free air on x-ray study

cause massive upper GI bleeding. The patient typically presents with hemodynamic instability and signs and symptoms of shock. Often, the cause of the bleeding is unknown unless the patient has a known history of cirrhosis or has previously bled from varices. Initial treatment of patients with esophageal or gastric varices is therefore the same. Top priorities include hemodynamic stabilization and establishment of a patent airway. Gastric lavage may be used in order to clear the stomach and to document the amount of blood loss. Diagnosis of the cause of the bleeding through endoscopy is the next priority before definitive treatment for the varices can be started.

Vasopressin

Vasopressin (Pitressin) (Table 14–20) is a synthetic antidiuretic hormone. Introduction of this hormone into the bloodstream reduces bleeding in 35 to 60% of patients bleeding from varices. It acts directly on gastrointestinal smooth muscle as a vasoconstrictor. Vasopressin lowers portal venous pressure by vasoconstriction and decreases venous blood flow. Ultimately, it decreases pressure and flow in liver collateral circulation channels in order to decrease bleeding. Vasopressin is administered in a dose of 0.2 to 0.4 U/min via an infusion pump. Because it is a vasoconstrictor, vasopressin should be infused via a central line. Vasopressin may be administered for up to 36 hours, and then it is usually slowly weaned if no signs of rebleeding exist (Henderson et al., 1993).

Table 14–20. VASOPRESSIN (PITRESSIN) THERAPY

Mechanism of Action
Vasoconstrictor: constricts splanchnic vascular bed, contracts intestinal smooth muscle, and lowers portal vein pressure.

Dose
Most commonly given by IV route, although may be given intra-arterially. IV infusion is started at 0.2 U/min initially. May be increased to 0.4 U/min. Maximum recommended dose is 0.9 U/min. Vasopressin should be continued for at least 24 h after bleeding is controlled.

Side Effects
Gastrointestinal: nausea and vomiting, cramping.
Cardiovascular: hypertension, cardiac dysrhythmias, exacerbation of heart failure.
Neurological: tremors, headache, vertigo.
Integumentary: pallor, localized gangrene.

Nursing Considerations
Monitor for angina.
Infuse through a central line.

IV = intravenous.

The critical care nurse's assessments are important during vasopressin administration because although its major action is constriction of splanchnic blood flow, it has many harmful systemic effects. Continuous ECG and blood pressure monitoring is essential because of the vasopressin's constriction effects on the coronary arteries. Chest pain, dysrhythmias, and other symptoms of coronary ischemia are additional common side effects of vasopressin. Some studies have shown increased control of bleeding and decreased side effects of vasopressin when a nitroglycerin infusion at a rate of 40 μg/min was also used (Henderson et al., 1993). Renal vasoconstriction is another side effect that may induce renal failure and associated complications. Strict intake and output, daily weights, and serum laboratory values need to be closely monitored. Concurrent liver failure and its associated fluid imbalances further complicate the picture. Because vasopressin is an antidiuretic hormone, its mechanism of action also induces water retention. Consequently, ascites and edema associated with liver failure often worsen.

Balloon Tamponade

If bleeding continues despite vasopressin therapy, balloon tamponade with a Sengstaken-Blakemore tube may be considered (Fig. 14–9). The adult Sengstaken-Blakemore tube has three lumens: one for gastric aspiration, similar to that in a nasogastric tube; one for inflation of the esophageal balloon; and one for inflation of the gastric balloon. A variation of this tube is the Minnesota tube, which has an additional fourth lumen that allows for esophageal aspiration. Inflation of the balloon ports applies pressure to the vessels supplying the varices to decrease blood flow, thereby stopping the bleeding.

The tip of the balloon is inserted into the stomach, and the gastric balloon is inflated and clamped. The tube is then withdrawn until resistance is felt so that pressure is exerted at the gastroesophageal junction. Correct positioning and traction are maintained by use of an external traction source or a nasal cuff around the tube at the mouth or nose. External traction can be attached to a helmet or to the foot of the bed. Proper amounts of traction are essential because too little traction lets the balloon fall away from the gastric wall and thereby does not put enough pressure on the bleeding vessels. Too much traction can cause discomfort, gastric ulceration, or vomiting. If bleeding does not stop with inflation of the gastric balloon, the esophageal balloon is inflated and clamped. Normal inflation pressure is 20 to 45 mm Hg. Monitoring of inflation pressures is important for the prevention of tissue damage.

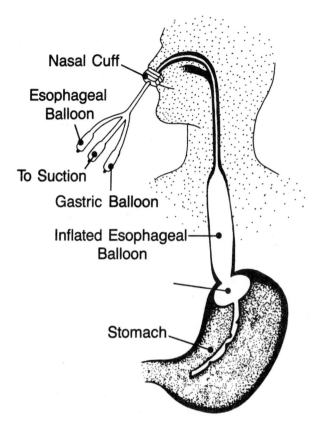

Figure 14–9. Sengstaken-Blakemore tube.

The critical care nurse is responsible for maintaining balloon lumen pressures and patency of the system. The gastric balloon port placement below the gastroesophageal junction must be confirmed by x-ray study. Ideally, the balloons should be deflated every 8 to 12 hours in order to decompress the esophagus and gastric mucosa. The status of the bleeding varices can also be assessed at this time, and the nurse must be prepared for hematemesis during this procedure. Of most importance is that the esophageal balloon be deflated before the gastric balloon is deflated or else the entire tube displaces upward and occludes the airway.

Spontaneous rupture of the gastric balloon and upward migration of the tube and occlusion of the airway are other possible complications that need to be assessed. Esophageal rupture may also occur and is characterized by the abrupt onset of severe pain. In the event of either of these two life-threatening emergencies, all three lumens are cut, and the entire tube is removed. For this reason, scissors are generally kept at the patient's beside at all times.

Other complications of the Sengstaken-Blakemore tube include ulcerations of the esophageal or gastric mucosa. Additionally, sores can develop around the mouth and nose as a result of the traction devices. Frequent cleansing and lubrication of these areas can help prevent skin breakdown. The nasopharynx also requires frequent suctioning because of an increase in secretions from the irritating tube and a decreased swallowing reflex. The nasogastric tube is also irrigated at least every 2 hours in order to ensure patency and to keep the stomach empty. This measure helps prevent aspiration. Additionally, blood that is allowed to accumulate in the stomach of a patient with liver failure is problematic because it promotes increased ammonia production that cannot be handled by the patient. Ammonia intoxication may ensue.

Sclerotherapy

Sclerotherapy is another option in the treatment of bleeding varices. After the varices are identified, the sclerosing agent is injected into the varix and the surrounding tissue. Usually, several applications of the sclerosing agent several days apart are needed in order to decompress the bleeding varix.

Transjugular Intrahepatic Portosystemic Shunt

Transjugular intrahepatic portosystemic shunting is a nonsurgical treatment for recurrent variceal bleeding after sclerotherapy. Placement of the shunt is performed by use of fluoroscopy. A stainless steel stent is used for the creation and maintenance of an opening in the intrahepatic tract, thus creating a portosystemic shunt in the liver and decreasing portal pressures (Adams and Soulen, 1993). Decreasing portal pressures decrease pressure within the varix, thereby decreasing the risk for acute hemorrhage. Long-term evaluation of the efficacy of this treatment is currently in progress.

The nurse should continuously monitor the patient's heart rhythm for bradycardia and ventricular dysrhythmias during the transjugular intrahepatic portosystemic shunting. Atropine and lidocaine should be readily available during the procedure for the treatment of these potentially life-threatening rhythms.

Surgical Interventions

Permanent decompression of portal hypertension can be achieved only through surgical procedures that divert blood around the blocked portal system. These are called portacaval shunts. In these types of surgery, a connection is made between the portal vein and the inferior vena cava, which diverts blood flow into the vena cava in order to decrease portal pressure. Several variations of this procedure exist, including the end-to-side shunt and the side-to-side shunt (Fig. 14–10). Although the end-to-side shunt is technically the easiest, it does divert all blood from the gut directly into the general circulation before detoxification can occur, thereby increasing the risk of portal encephalopathy. The side-to-side shunt attempts to prevent this complication by allowing some of the portal blood to flow back into the liver for detoxification.

Other surgical techniques for reduction of portal pressure include splenorenal and mesocaval shunting. The major complication of these procedures is a high thrombosis rate. Portal systemic shunting reduces portal hypertension and therefore decreases bleeding from esophageal varices. The nurse needs to be aware that a temporary increase in ascites occurs after all of these procedures, and careful assessments and interventions are needed in the care of this patient population (see Hepatic Failure).

PATIENT OUTCOMES

Expected patient care outcomes for each nursing diagnosis for the patient experiencing an acute GI bleed include the following:

Fluid Volume Deficit

- Circulating body fluid volume will be normal.
- Hemorrhage will be controlled or resolved.
- Preload indicators (central venous pressure and PCWP) will be within normal limits.
- Hematocrit and hemoglobin values will be stable.
- Weight will be stable, and intake and output will be balanced.

Anxiety

- Patient will demonstrate decreased level of anxiety resulting from nursing interventions, such as teaching and explanations.
- Patient will demonstrate an understanding of disease and medical and nursing interventions.

Decreased Tissue Perfusion

- Signs of decreased perfusion of body organs will be absent.
- Decreased sensorium will be absent.
- Urine output will be greater than 30 ml/h.
- Renal failure will be absent.
- Hemodynamics will be stable.
- Bowel sounds will be within normal limits.
- Skin will be warm and dry.

Impaired Gas Exchange

- Hemoglobin value will be greater than 10 mg/dl.

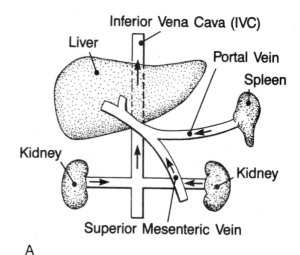

A

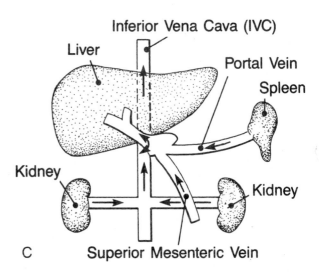

B

C

Figure 14–10. Types of portacaval shunts. (A), Normal portal circulation. (B), End-to-side shunt. (C), Side-to-side shunt.

- Partial pressure of arterial oxygen will be greater than 80 to 100 mm Hg (or returned to patient's baseline value).

Knowledge Deficit

- Patient and family will understand the patient's condition and treatment regimen.
- Patient and family will ask appropriate questions and voice concerns.

High Risk for Fluid Volume Excess

- Respiratory pattern will be normal.
- Congestion and pulmonary edema will be absent.

Altered Electrolyte Balance

- Electrolyte values will be within normal limits.

Encephalopathy

- Altered thought processes will be absent or resolved.
- Ammonia levels will be controlled.

Aspiration

- Lung fields will be clear to auscultation.

High Risk for Infection (Surgical Patient)

- Patient will be free of infection.
- Patient will be afebrile.
- Patient's wound will be clean, dry, and intact.

Acute Pain (Surgical Patient)

- Patient will be comfortable.

Risk for Ineffective Breathing Pattern (Patient with Sengstaken-Blakemore Tube)

- Respiratory pattern will be normal.
- Sengstaken-Blakemore tube will be patent.

Acute Pancreatitis

Acute pancreatitis is defined as an acute inflammatory disease of the pancreas. The intensity of the disease ranges from mild, in which the patient presents with abdominal pain and elevated blood amylase level, to extremely severe, which results in multiple organ failure. In 85 to 90% of patients, the disease is self-limiting (mild acute pancreatitis), and they generally recover rapidly. However, the disease can run a fulminant course and is associated with high mortality rates. Management of this more severe form of the disease requires intensive nursing and medical care.

PATHOPHYSIOLOGY

Acute pancreatitis is an acute inflammation of the pancreas with the potential for necrosis of pancreatic cells resulting from premature activation of pancreatic enzymes within the pancreas. Normally, pancreatic juices are secreted into the duodenum, where they are activated. These enzymes are essential to normal carbohydrate, fat, and protein metabolism. The way in which the enzymes become prematurely activated to initiate the inflammatory process has been widely studied, but the exact mechanisms remain unknown. Some theories propose that a toxic agent may alter the way in which the pancreas secretes enzymes. Another theory proposes that duodenal contents that contain activated enzymes enter the pancreatic duct, causing inflammation. Another theory implicates biliary stones that cause obstruction of the biliary ducts and therefore hypertension of the pancreas. Regardless of how the enzymes are activated, enzymatic damage to pancreatic cells (acinar cells) is the outcome of the disease process. Trypsinogen, phospholipase A, and elastase have been proposed as the primary enzymes responsible for the inflammatory process and the resulting systemic complications (Fig. 14–11).

Acute pancreatitis has been classified by the gradation of the lesions found in the pancreas. In the mild form, areas of fat necrosis are in and around pancreatic cells along with interstitial edema. Frank pancreatic necrosis is absent. This mild form may progress to a more severe form, with extensive fat necrosis in and around the pancreas, pancreatic cellular necrosis, and hemorrhage in the pancreas itself. The hemorrhagic form of this acute inflammatory disease is associated with a high mortality rate.

Endocrine and exocrine functions of the pancreas may be impaired in mild and severe manifestations of the disease. Endocrine functions include the secretion of insulin and glucagon. As mentioned earlier, exocrine functions are required for the normal metabolism of food substrates. Hyperglycemia, hypoglycemia, and nutritional depletion, therefore, are common effects of all forms of acute pancreatitis.

In most patients, acute pancreatitis resolves spontaneously within 5 to 7 days, with return of normal pancreatic endocrine and exocrine functions. Conversely, severe pancreatitis can affect every organ system in the body. Table 14–21 reviews the major systemic complications of acute fulminating pancreatitis.

It appears that as pancreatic cells are damaged, more digestive enzymes are released, which in turn causes more pancreatic damage. Local effects of pancreatitis include inflammation of the pancreas, inflammation of the peritoneum around the pancreas, and fluid accumulation in the peritoneal cavity. Acute

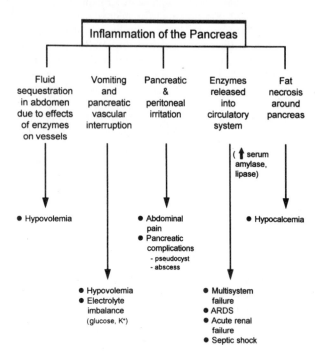

Activation of Pancreatic Exocrine Enzymes
(Trypsinogen, Phospholipase A, Elastase)

Inflammation of the Pancreas

| Fluid sequestration in abdomen due to effects of enzymes on vessels | Vomiting and pancreatic vascular interruption | Pancreatic & peritoneal irritation | Enzymes released into circulatory system | Fat necrosis around pancreas |

(↑ serum amylase, lipase)

- Hypovolemia
- Abdominal pain
- Pancreatic complications
  - pseudocyst
  - abscess
- Hypocalcemia

- Hypovolemia
- Electrolyte imbalance (glucose, K⁺)

- Multisystem failure
- ARDS
- Acute renal failure
- Septic shock

Figure 14-11. Pathophysiology flow diagram of acute pancreatitis. ARDS = adult respiratory distress syndrome; K^+ = potassium ion.

pancreatitis can also result in multisystem organ dysfunction syndrome (McFadden, 1991). The release of trypsin is known to cause abnormalities in blood coagulation and clot lysis. Disseminated intravascular coagulation and GI bleeding or infarction can be the result. The release of other enzymes (phospholipases) is thought to cause the many pulmonary complications associated with acute pancreatitis. Acute respiratory failure and ARDS are the two most common complications. Acute renal failure is thought to be a consequence of alterations in the renin-angiotensin mechanism and of hypotension. Death during the first 2 weeks of acute pancreatitis usually results from pulmonary or renal complications.

Other serious metabolic complications of acute pancreatitis include hypocalcemia and hyperlipidemia, which are thought to be related to the areas of fat necrosis resulting from acute inflammation of the pancreas. Hypocalcemia is a major complication and almost always indicates a more serious manifestation of acute pancreatitis. Various hormone imbalances, particularly parathyroid hormone imbalance, are also commonly found.

Pancreatic pseudocysts are the most common pan-

creatic complication and are a part of the necrotizing process. A pseudocyst is a collection of inflammatory debris and pancreatic secretions. The pseudocyst can rupture and hemorrhage or become infected, causing systemic sepsis (see Chapter 8).

Acute pancreatitis has numerous causes, but the most common are alcohol ingestion and gallstone disease. Table 14-22 lists many causes of this disease. Many drugs may initiate acute pancreatitis as a result of either ingestion of toxic doses or a drug reaction. Pancreatitis resulting from blunt or penetrating abdominal trauma or occurring after endoscopic exploration of the biliary tree has also been reported.

ASSESSMENT

History and Physical Examination

A diagnosis of acute pancreatitis can be made only based on careful clinical examination and the results of laboratory and radiological tests. Common

---

Table 14-21. SYSTEMIC COMPLICATIONS OF ACUTE PANCREATITIS

Pulmonary
  Arterial hypoxemia
  Atelectasis, pneumonia, pleural effusion
  Adult respiratory distress syndrome

Cardiovascular
  Hypovolemic shock
  Myocardial depression
  Cardiac dysrhythmias

Hematological
  Coagulation abnormalities
  Disseminated intravascular coagulation

Gastrointestinal
  Gastrointestinal bleeding
  Pancreatic pseudocyst
  Pancreatic abscess

Renal
  Azotemia, oliguria
  Acute renal failure

Metabolic
  Hypocalcemia
  Hyperlipidemia
  Hyperglycemia
  Metabolic acidosis

Central nervous system
  Pancreatic encephalopathy
  Retinopathy

Peripheral
  Arthritis

Adapted from Pitchumoni, C. S., Agarwal, N., & Jain, J. K. (1988). Systemic complications of acute pancreatitis. *American Journal of Gastroenterology, 83*(6), 597–603.

Table 14–22. CAUSES OF ACUTE PANCREATITIS

Alcohol
Biliary disease
    Gallstones
    Common bile duct obstruction
Drugs
    Thiazide diuretics
    Furosemide
    Estrogen
    Procainamide
    Tetracycline
    Sulfonamides
Hypertriglyceridemia
Perforation of esophagus, intestine, stomach
Opiate administration
Penetrating duodenal ulcer
Surgery
Trauma
Infectious agents
Carcinoma
Tumors
    Pancreas
    Lung
Radiation injury
Ectopic pregnancy
Ovarian cyst
Hypercalcemia
Heredity
Idiopathic

presenting signs and symptoms and laboratory and radiological findings in acute pancreatitis are listed in Table 14–23. Nurses are responsible for conducting initial and ongoing clinical assessments; monitoring, recording, reporting physical and laboratory data; and coordinating the multidisciplinary plan of care.

In most cases, patients with acute pancreatitis present with severe abdominal pain (Brown, 1991). It is most often midepigastric but may be generalized or localized in the left upper quadrant, often radiating to the back. It usually begins abruptly, commonly after a large meal or alcohol binge. The pain associated with acute pancreatitis is often steady and severe but may increase gradually for several hours. The patient may curl up with both arms over the abdomen in order to relieve the pain. On physical examination, abdominal tenderness and/or guarding may be present. Distention of the upper abdomen and tympany may also be present.

Nausea and vomiting are also common presenting symptoms. A hallmark sign of acute pancreatitis is severe abdominal pain that is unrelieved by retching or vomiting. The vomitus characteristically consists of gastric and duodenal contents. Fever is also a common symptom but is usually less than 39°C. The presence of a temperature of greater than 39°C may indicate

cholecystitis, peritonitis, or intra-abdominal abscess and is associated with more severe forms of the disease.

In severe acute hemorrhagic pancreatitis, the patient exhibits overt signs of dehydration and hypovolemic shock. Patients with more severe pancreatic disease may also have ascites, jaundice, or palpable abdominal masses. A bluish discoloration of the flanks (Grey Turner's sign) or around the umbilical area (Cullen's sign) indicates the presence of hemorrhagic pancreatitis and accumulation of blood in these areas. These signs usually do not appear for 1 to 2 weeks as more of the pancreatic gland is destroyed. Abdominal girth must be measured at least every 4 hours in order to detect internal bleeding in patients in whom hemorrhagic pancreatitis is suspected.

Diagnostic Tests

The clinical diagnosis of acute pancreatitis requires laboratory and radiological testing because the clinical history, presenting signs and symptoms, and physical findings mimic many other gastrointestinal and cardiovascular disorders. As an example, the pain associated with acute pancreatitis is like that associated with peptic ulcer disease, gallbladder disease, intestinal obstruction, and acute myocardial infarction. This similarity exists because pain receptors in the abdomen are poorly differentiated as they exit the skin surface.

Table 14–23. SIGNS AND SYMPTOMS OF ACUTE PANCREATITIS

Clinical Symptoms
Pain
Nausea and vomiting
Fever
Dehydration
Abdominal guarding, distention
Grey Turner's sign
Cullen's sign

Laboratory Diagnostics
Serum and urine amylase levels increased
Serum lipase level increased
White blood cell count increased
Hematocrit value increased with dehydration; decreased with hemorrhagic pancreatitis
Calcium level decreased
Potassium level decreased
Albumin level decreased
Glucose level increased with islet cell damage
Bilirubin, aspartate transaminase, lactate dehydrogenase levels increased
Alkaline phosphatase level increased with biliary disease

Serum lipase and amylase tests are the most specific for acute pancreatitis because as the pancreatic cells and ducts are destroyed, these enzymes are released. However, problems exist with the use of these values as pure indicators of the disease. Serum amylase and lipase levels are usually increased during the first 24 to 72 hours after the onset of symptoms. In mild pancreatitis, these levels may be close to normal, and if a few days have elapsed since the onset of symptoms, enzymes levels may be completely normal in the presence of acute pancreatitis. Further complicating the diagnosis, an increased serum amylase level is not specific to acute pancreatitis. Other conditions associated with an increased amylase level are listed in Table 14–24. Serum amylase measurement is much more specific if isoenzyme levels (i.e., isoamylase) are increased or urinary amylase level is measured. Serum amylase levels may be falsely decreased in patients with increased blood serum triglyceride levels. Serum lipase level measurement is now used in more clinical laboratories and is more specific for acute pancreatitis than serum amylase level (Panteghini and Pagani, 1991).

Advances in the diagnosis of acute pancreatitis have been in the development of improved computed tomography (CT) modalities and magnetic resonance imaging, which are used to confirm the diagnosis. These imaging techniques have proved to be superior to the previously used sonography and CT because mild edematous pancreatic changes were not usually identifiable on these scans. Gastrointestinal complications of acute pancreatitis, such as pancreatic pseudocyst, abscess or perforation, and obstruction of the biliary tree, are also distinguishable through the use of CT imaging. Additionally, radiographs of the chest and

Table 14–24. OTHER CONDITIONS ASSOCIATED WITH INCREASED SERUM AMYLASE LEVELS

Salivary gland disease
Renal insufficiency
Diabetic ketoacidosis
Intra-abdominal disease (perforations, obstructions, aortic disease, peritonitis, appendicitis)
Biliary tract disease
Pregnancy
Cerebral trauma
Pneumonia
Tumors
Chronic alcoholism
Burns
Shock
Gynecological disorders
Prostatic disease

Table 14–25. RANSON CRITERIA FOR PREDICTING SEVERITY OF ACUTE PANCREATITIS*

At admission or on diagnosis
Age >55 years (>70)
Leukocyte count >16,000/μl (>18,000)
Serum glucose level >200 mg/dl (>220)
Serum lactate dehydrogenase level >350 IU/L (>400)
Serum aspartate transaminase level >250 IU/L

During initial 48 h
Decrease in hematocrit >10%
Increase in blood urea nitrogen level >5 mg/dl (>2)
Serum calcium level <8 mg/dl
Base deficit >4 mEq/L (>5)
Estimated fluid sequestration >6 L (>4)
Partial pressure of arterial oxygen <60 mm Hg

Modified from Ranson, J. C. (1985). Risk factors in acute pancreatitis. *Hospital Practice, 20*(4), 69–73.
*When criteria values for nonalcoholic acute pancreatitis differ from those in alcohol-related disease, they are given in parentheses.

abdomen are initially obtained in patients presenting with acute abdominal pain in order to rule out intestinal ileus, perforation, pericardial effusion, and pulmonary disease. Abdominal films may also reveal intestinal gas-filled loops, which are signs of paralytic ileus.

Other common laboratory abnormalities associated with acute pancreatitis include an elevated white blood cell count resulting from the inflammatory process, and an elevated serum glucose level, resulting from beta cell damage and pancreatic necrosis. Hypokalemia may be present because of associated vomiting. Hyperkalemia may be a predominant systemic complication in the presence of acute renal failure. Hypocalcemia is common with severe disease and usually indicates pancreatic fat necrosis. Serum albumin and protein levels may be decreased as a result of the movement of fluid into the extracellular space. Increases in serum bilirubin, lactate dehydrogenase and aspartate transaminase levels, and in prothrombin time are common in the presence of concurrent liver disease. Triglycerides may be extremely increased and may be a causative factor in the development of the acute inflammatory process. Arterial blood gas analysis may show hypoxemia and retained carbon dioxide levels, which indicate the presence of associated respiratory failure, which is a common complication of the acute process.

Predicting the Severity of Acute Pancreatitis

As mentioned earlier, patients with acute pancreatitis can present with mild or fulminant disease. As a consequence, a lot of research has addressed identifying criteria for predicting the prognosis of patients with acute pancreatitis (Agarwal and Pitchumoni, 1991). The most widely used criteria in this country are those of Ranson (1985) (Table 14–25). The number of signs present within the first 48 hours of admission directly relate to the patient's chance of significant morbidity and mortality. The overall mortality rate is 10%, but it exceeds 50% in patients with hemorrhagic pancreatitis. In Ranson's (1985) research, patients with fewer than three signs have a 1% mortality rate, those with three to four signs have a 15% mortality rate, those with five to six signs have a 40% mortality rate, and those with seven or more signs have a 100% mortality rate.

NURSING DIAGNOSES

Actual or potential nursing diagnoses associated with acute pancreatitis or with systemic complications of the disease process include

- Acute pain related to the inflammatory process in the pancreas, obstruction of the pancreatic duct, and decreased blood supply.
- Fluid volume deficit related to fluid shift into the peritoneum and retroperitoneal space; serum, blood, plasma, and albumin loss into the peritoneum; or dehydration from nausea, vomiting, and fever.
- Altered nutrition (less than body requirements) related to loss of exocrine functions of the pancreas, low intake, or alcoholism.
- Impaired gas exchange related to respiratory insufficiency, atelectasis, and ARDS resulting from increased concentrations of active pancreatic enzymes.
- Risk for infection related to peritonitis resulting from leakage of pancreatic enzymes into the peritoneal cavity, formation of pancreatic pseudocyst, or abscess.
- Electrolyte imbalance related to prolonged vomiting, and fluid sequestration.

MEDICAL AND NURSING INTERVENTIONS

Nursing and medical priorities for the management of acute pancreatitis include

- Fluid resuscitation and electrolyte replacement to maintain or replenish vascular volume and electrolyte balance.
- Supportive therapies that are aimed at decreasing gastrin release from the stomach and preventing the gastric contents from entering the duodenum (resting the pancreas while maintaining the nutritional status of the patient).
- Analgesics for pain control.
- Treatment of systemic complications, the most common being respiratory.

Fluid Replacement

In patients with mild or severe acute pancreatitis, some fluid collects in the retroperitoneal space and peritoneal cavity. Initially, most patients present with some degree of dehydration and, in severe cases, hypovolemic shock. Some patients may have sequestered up to 12 L of fluid on presentation. Hypovolemia and shock are major causes of death early in the disease process. Fluid replacement then becomes a high priority in the treatment of acute pancreatitis.

The solutions ordered by the physician for fluid resuscitation are usually colloids or lactated Ringer's solution; however, fresh frozen plasma and albumin may also be used. Fluid replacement perfuses the pancreas, an effect that is thought to decrease the severity of the progression of the disease. Also, the kidneys remain perfused and may prevent the complication of acute renal failure.

Critical assessments for the evaluation of fluid replacement include accurate monitoring of intake and output and daily weights. Often, a Foley catheter is inserted in order to measure hourly urine outputs because a decrease in urine output to less than 30 ml/h is an early and sensitive measure of hypovolemia and hypoperfusion. Vital signs, including blood pressure and heart rate, are also sensitive measures of volume status. Expected patient outcomes need to be individualized, but reasonable goals would be maintenance of systolic blood pressure at greater than 100 mm Hg without an orthostatic decrease, mean arterial pressure of greater than 60 mm Hg, and a heart rate of less than 100 beats per minute. Warm extremities are an indicator of adequate peripheral circulation.

Patients with more severe manifestations of the disease may undergo pulmonary artery pressure monitoring for the evaluation of fluid status and response to treatment. The PCWP is the most sensitive measure of adequacy of volume status and left ventricular filling pressure. A PCWP between 11 and 14 mm Hg is a realistic goal for most patients.

Patients with severe disease who fail to respond to fluid therapy alone (i.e., hypotension continues) may need medications to support blood pressure (e.g., dopamine, dobutamine). Patients with acute hemorrhagic pancreatitis may also need packed red blood cells in addition to fluid therapy to restore intravascular volume.

Electrolyte Replacement

Hypocalcemia (calcium level of <8 mg/dl) is a common electrolyte imbalance. It is associated with a high mortality rate (see Ranson's prognostic signs in Table 14–25). The exact mechanism for this metabolic complication is not completely understood, but it is thought to be related to decreased binding with proteins in the plasma. Calcium is essential for catalyzing impulses for nerves and muscles, for maintaining the integrity of cell membranes and vessels, for normal clotting of blood, and for strengthening bones and teeth. Calcium is also essential for increasing contractility in the heart. An ECG sign of hypocalcemia is lengthening of the QT interval. Severe hypocalcemia (calcium level <6 mg/dl) may cause tetany, seizures, positive Chvostek's and Trousseau's signs, and respiratory distress. Patients with severe hypocalcemia should be placed on seizure precaution status, and respiratory support equipment should be available (e.g., oral airway, suction). The nurse is responsible for monitoring calcium levels, administering replacement, and monitoring the patient's response to any calcium given. Monitoring serum albumin level is also important because true serum calcium levels can be evaluated only in comparison with serum albumin levels (see Chapter 12). The patient also needs to be monitored for calcium toxicity. Symptoms include lethargy, nausea, shortening of the QT interval, and decreased excitability of nerves and muscles. Hypomagnesemia may also be present with hypocalcemia, and magnesium replacements may be needed as well.

Potassium is another electrolyte that may need to be replaced early in the treatment regimen as a result of the loss of pancreatic juices and vomiting associated with acute pancreatitis. Hypokalemia is associated with cardiac dysrhythmias, muscle weakness, hypotension, decreased bowel sounds, ileus, and irritability. Potassium should be diluted and administered slowly over 1 hour via an infusion pump.

Hyperglycemia is, surprisingly, not a common complication of acute pancreatitis, because most of the pancreatic gland must be necrosed before the insulin-secreting islet cells are affected. More commonly, hyperglycemia is a result of the normal body stress response to acute illness. Regular insulin, given according to a sliding scale, may be ordered and must be administered cautiously because glucagon levels are only transiently increased in acute pancreatitis.

Resting the Pancreas

Nasogastric suction is used in most patients with acute pancreatitis in order to suppress pancreatic exocrine secretion by preventing the release of secretin from the duodenum. Normally, secretin, which stimulates pancreatic secretion production, is stimulated when acid is in the duodenum. Nausea, vomiting, and abdominal pain may also be decreased when a nasogastric tube is placed for suctioning early in treatment. A nasogastric tube is also necessary in patients with ileus, severe gastric distention, and decreased level of consciousness in order to prevent complications resulting from pulmonary aspiration. Oral intake should not be allowed until the abdominal pain subsides and serum amylase levels have returned to normal. Starting oral intake before these goals are achieved may cause the abdominal pain to return and may induce further inflammation of the pancreas by stimulating the autodigestive disease process. Continuous stimulation of the autodigestive process increases the risk of pancreatic abscess formation. In patients with mild pancreatitis, administration of oral fluids can usually be restarted within 3 to 7 days after onset, with slow advancement of solids as tolerated.

Prolonged NPO (nothing per mouth) status is difficult for patients. Frequent mouth care and maintenance of skin integrity around the nasogastric tube through lubrication are important nursing actions to prevent injury and maximize patient comfort. Bed rest is also used in order to decrease pancreatic secretion stimulation by decreasing the patient's basal metabolic rate.

Nutritional Support

Patients with severe manifestations of the disease may be on prolonged NPO status with nasogastric suction because of paralytic ileus, persistent abdominal pain, pancreatic pseudocyst or abcesses, or other systemic complications. These patients are candidates for TPN. Because patients with acute pancreatitis often have hyperlipidemia as a part of their disease process, lipid supplementation may not be ordered.

Comfort Management

Pain control is a nursing priority in patients with acute pancreatitis not only because it produces extreme patient discomfort but also because pain increases the patient's metabolism and thus increases pancreatic secretions. The pain of pancreatitis is caused by edema and distention of the pancreatic capsule, obstruction of the biliary system, and peritoneal inflammation from pancreatic enzymes. Pain is often severe and unrelenting and is related to the degree of pancreatic inflammation.

A baseline pain assessment is performed early after the patient's admission and includes information about the onset, intensity, duration, and location (local or diffuse) of the pain. Analgesic administration is a nursing priority, and a physician's order should be obtained immediately for the treatment of the abdominal pain. It is thought that opiate analgesics (e.g., morphine) may cause spasm of the sphincter of Oddi and may exacerbate the pain associated with acute pancreatitis. Therefore, hydromorphone (Dilaudid) and meperidine (Demerol) are considered the first-line drugs of choice. Pain medications are routinely administered rather than as needed in order to prevent uncontrollable abdominal pain. Use of pain-rating scale, such as a scale of zero to 10, may also help in determining the amount of analgesia to administer and in evaluating the patient's response to medication. As mentioned earlier, insertion of a nasogastric tube connected to low intermittent suction may help ease pain considerably. Patient positioning may also be useful in relieving some of the discomfort and should be facilitated by the nurse as the patient's hemodynamic status allows.

Pharmacological Intervention

Various pharmacological therapies have been researched in the treatment of acute pancreatitis. Various drugs given in order to rest the pancreas have been studied, specifically anticholinergics, glucagon, somatostatin, cimetidine, and calcitonin, but these have not been shown to be effective. Histamine blockers and antacids are useful in preventing stress ulcers in critically ill patients, a goal that would be appropriate for this patient population.

Antibiotics have also been studied in the treatment of inflammation of the pancreas with the idea of preventing pancreatic pseudocysts or abscesses. Antibiotics have not proved to be effective and now are generally used only when a confirmed infection is present.

5-Fluorouracil and propylthiouracil decrease the metabolism of pancreatic cells and the production of enzymes and may be used during the acute phase.

Treatment of Systemic Complications

Multisystem complications of acute pancreatitis are related to the pancreas's ability to produce many vasoactive substances that affect organs throughout the body. These complications are summarized in Table 14–21.

Peritoneal lavage has been used since the 1960s for the treatment of systemic complications associated with severe acute pancreatitis. The theory behind the use of this therapy is that it removes toxic substances that are released by the damaged pancreas (e.g., trypsinogen, kinins, histamines, and prostaglandins) into the peritoneal fluid. Peritoneal lavage removes these

substances before they can be absorbed and exert their systemic effects. Presently, it is usually used when standard therapies mentioned earlier are not effective during the first few days of hospitalization.

The procedure for peritoneal lavage involves placement of a peritoneal dialysis catheter. An isotonic solution with dextrose, heparin, and potassium is added. An antibiotic may also be used in the solution. Two liters of solution is infused at a time over 15 to 20 minutes and then is drained by gravity. This cycle is repeated every 1 to 2 hours for 48 to 72 hours. If peritoneal lavage is effective, the hemodynamic response by the patient is usually immediate.

Close monitoring of respiratory status during peritoneal lavage is essential because accumulation of fluid in the peritoneum causes restricted movement of the diaphragm, a muscle used for inspiration. Hyperglycemia may be another effect of this therapy because dextrose may be absorbed from the fluid into the bloodstream.

Pulmonary complications are common in patients with both mild and severe manifestations of the disease. Arterial hypoxemia, atelectasis, pleural effusions, and pneumonia have been identified in many patients with acute pancreatitis. Arterial oxygen saturation is continuously monitored, and arterial blood gases are assessed every 8 hours for the first few days in order to monitor for hypoxemia, which is the most common pulmonary complication. Treatment of hypoxemia includes vigorous pulmonary care, such as deep breathing and coughing and frequent position changes. Oxygen therapy may also be used to improve overall oxygenation status. Pulmonary emboli have also been documented as a complication of acute pancreatitis. Careful fluid administration for the prevention of fluid overload and pulmonary congestion is also necessary.

Patients with severe disease may develop overt respiratory failure. Radiologically and clinically, this situation is indistinguishable from ARDS (see Chapter 11).

Close monitoring and management of other systemic complications of acute pancreatitis, such as coagulation abnormalities and hemorrhage, cardiovascular failure and dysrhythmias, and acute renal failure, are also important. Coagulation defects in acute pancreatitis are associated with a high mortality rate and are similar to disseminated intravascular coagulation and are treated in the same way. The cardiac depression associated with acute pancreatitis may vary, but hypovolemic shock is a grave presentation. Astute cardiovascular monitoring and volume replacement are needed in order to reverse this serious complication. Impaired renal function has been documented in many patients. Diuretics and vasodilators may be used for the treatment of this complication.

Gastrointestinal complications of acute pancreatitis include pancreatic pseudocyst and abdominal abscess. A pseudocyst should be suspected in any patient who has persistent abdominal pain and nausea and vomiting, a prolonged fever, and an elevated serum amylase level. CT can be helpful in diagnosing the location and size of the pseudocyst. Signs and symptoms of an abdominal abscess include increased white blood cell count, fever, abdominal pain, and vomiting. CT provides a definitive diagnosis. Early recognition and treatment of a pancreatic pseudocyst is important because this condition is associated with a high mortality rate.

Surgical Therapy

A pancreatic resection for acute necrotizing pancreatitis may be performed for the prevention of systemic complications of the disease process. In this procedure, dead or infected pancreatic tissue is surgically removed. In some cases, the entire pancreas is removed. Usually, the indication for surgical intervention is clinical deterioration of the patient despite the use of conventional treatments or the presence of peritonitis.

Surgery may also be indicated for pseudocysts; however, surgery is usually delayed because some pseudocysts have been known to resolve spontaneously. Surgical treatment of a pseudocyst can be performed through internal or external drainage or needle aspiration. Acute surgical intervention may be required if the pseudocyst becomes infected or perforated.

Surgery may also be performed in cases in which gallstones are thought to be the cause of the acute pancreatitis. A cholecystectomy is usually performed.

PATIENT OUTCOMES

Expected outcomes for the patient with acute pancreatitis include the following:

- Normal fluid balance will be restored, as evidenced by balanced intake and output, stable weight, normal PCWP, and urine output of greater than 30 ml/h.
- Hemodynamic stability will be restored and maintained, as evidenced by a return of blood pressure to baseline and an absence of tachycardia.
- Pain will be maintained at tolerable levels for the patient, as evidenced by subjective and objective cues that pain is diminished.
- Nutritional balance will be maintained or restored, as evidenced by a serum albumin level of greater than 4 mg/dl, positive nitrogen balance, and a stable weight.
- Pulmonary gas exchange will be maintained as evidenced by a partial pressure of arterial oxygen (PaO_2) of greater than 60 mm Hg; an arterial oxygen saturation (SaO_2) of greater than 90%; a respiratory rate of 12 to 20 breaths/min; clear lung fields; and an absence of atelectasis, pneumonia, pulmonary edema, or pleural effusion.
- Electrolyte balance will be restored, as evidenced by a serum calcium level of 8.5 to 10.5 mg/dl and a serum potassium level of 3.5 to 5.0 mEq/L.
- Systemic complications of acute pancreatitis, including hypovolemic shock, acute respiratory failure, cardiac failure, renal failure, and pancreatic complications, will be detected and reported early.

(See the Nursing Care Plan for the Patient with Acute Pancreatitis.)

Hepatic Failure

PATHOPHYSIOLOGY

Hepatic, or liver, failure results when the liver is unable to perform its many functions. These functions are reviewed in Table 14–5. Liver failure can result from necrosis or a decrease in the blood supply to liver cells. This problem is most often caused by hepatitis or inflammation of the liver. Liver failure can also result from chronic liver disease, in which healthy liver tissue is replaced by fibrotic tissue. This form of liver failure is called cirrhosis. Finally, liver cells can be replaced by fatty cells or tissue and is known as fatty liver disease.

Hepatitis

Hepatitis is an acute inflammation of liver cells, or hepatocytes. Other white blood cells in the liver may also be inflamed. This inflammation is accompanied by edema, and early in the course of the disease, no disturbance exists in the architecture of the liver. The normal liver architecture is pictured in Figure 14–5 and is characterized by a basic functional unit of the liver called a lobule. The liver lobule is uniquely made in that it has its own blood supply, which allows the liver cells to be exposed continuously to blood. As the inflammation progresses, the normal pattern of the liver is disturbed by the inflammatory process. This interrupts the normal blood supply to liver cells, causing necrosis and breakdown of healthy cells. Blood backs up in the portal system, causing increased pressure, known as portal hypertension. Liver cells do have

NURSING CARE PLAN FOR THE PATIENT WITH ACUTE PANCREATITIS

Nursing Diagnosis	Patient Outcomes	Nursing Interventions
Fluid volume deficit related to loss of fluid into peritoneal cavity, dehydration from nausea and vomiting, fever, nasogastric suction, defects in coagulation.	Heart rate will be < 100. Pulmonary capillary wedge pressure will be within normal limits. Urine output will be > 30 ml/h. Extremities will be warm, dry. Hematocrit and hemoglobin values will be stable. No bleeding will occur. Patient will be afebrile.	Monitor hemodynamic status closely, vital signs, pulmonary artery pressures, urine output, intake and output, daily weight, peripheral circulation. Administer fluid replacements, blood or blood products, and monitor patient response to treatment. Monitor for signs and symptoms of hemorrhage, hematocrit and hemoglobin values, Cullen's sign or Turner's sign; measure abdominal girth every 4 h. Monitor temperature and administer antipyretics or apply cooling blanket as needed.
Pain related to interruption of blood supply to the pancreas, edema and distention of the pancreas, and peritoneal irritation.	Pain will be within tolerable levels.	Perform a pain assessment noting onset, duration, intensity, and location. Control pain with drug of choice (meperidine). Avoid morphine, which causes spasm of the sphincter of Oddi and the ampulla of Vater, which increases pain. Schedule pain medication to prevent severe pain episodes. Differentiate pain from cardiac origin. Keep activities at a minimum. Maintain bed rest restriction. Position patient to optimize comfort. Administer sedation as needed.
Altered nutrition (less than body requirements) related to nausea and vomiting, depressed appetite, alcoholism, and impaired nutrient metabolism due to pancreatic injury and altered production of digestive enzymes.	Positive nitrogen balance will be achieved. Serum albumin level will be normal. Weight will be stable.	Assess nutritional status through clinical examination and laboratory analysis. Calculate caloric needs and compare with actual intake. Provide adequate nutritional intake as needed. Offer nutritional supplements. Administer total parenteral nutrition (TPN) as ordered. Prevent complications by attending to aseptic technique in the handling and administration of TPN and catheter care. Monitor for signs and symptoms of infection. Monitor glucose and other electrolyte levels to detect electrolyte complications of therapy.
Impaired gas exchange related to atelectasis, pleural effusions, adult respiratory distress syndrome, fluid overload during fluid administration, pulmonary emboli, and splinting from pain.	PaO_2 will be > 60 mm Hg. $PaCO_2$ will be within normal limits or at baseline. Pulmonary complications will be absent or resolved.	Monitor pulmonary status closely. Auscultate breath sounds every 4 h and as needed. Monitor respiratory rate. Administer vigorous pulmonary hygiene, coughing and deep breathing, humidification therapy. Note secretions for amount, color, consistency, and odor. Administer oxygen as prescribed. Monitor arterial blood gas results according to clinical status. Administer analgesia to prevent pain caused by splinting. Reposition patient frequently to maximize ventilation and perfusion and to prevent pooling of secretions.
Electrolyte imbalance related to prolonged nausea and vomiting, gastric suction, autodigestive process, and therapeutic regimen.	Calcium, magnesium, potassium, and glucose will be within normal limits.	Monitor electrolyte balance carefully and administer replacements according to unit protocol. Assess fluid balance by evaluating electrolyte values.

the capacity to regenerate. Over time, liver cells that become damaged can be removed from the body's immune system and are replaced with healthy liver cells. Therefore, most patients with hepatitis recover and regain normal liver function.

Hepatitis is most often caused by a viral disease. To date, five hepatitis viruses have been identified: hepatitis A, B, C, D, and E. Researchers continue to study other viruses that may be associated with acute hepatitis (Aach et al, 1992; Carey and Patel, 1992).

TYPES OF HEPATITIS

Hepatitis A. Hepatitis A is the most common type of viral hepatitis. The virus infects the liver and is eliminated by the feces. This virus is primarily spread through oral ingestion of food, water, and shellfish that have been infected by fecal contaminants. Hepatitis A was previously known as infectious hepatitis. This disease is usually mild in presentation; therefore, many individuals may have had the disease without being aware of it.

Hepatitis B. Hepatitis B usually a more serious form of hepatitis. Persons are considered infectious as long as antigens for the virus are found in the bloodstream. Hepatitis B is spread primarily by blood, blood products, and body fluids or secretions, such as semen and saliva. Hepatitis B was formerly called serum hepatitis. The virus can spread percutaneously, (e.g., via contaminated needles), through mucous membranes, or through contact with infected fluids. Modes of transmission of hepatitis B are summarized in Table 14–26. Health care providers are at risk for contracting this form of hepatitis. Of most importance, hepatitis B can result in the development of a carrier state, chronic hepatitis, cirrhosis, and liver cancer.

Hepatitis C. Hepatitis C is transmitted through blood or blood products. It also can be spread through sexual contact and is frequently seen in the male homosexual population. Hepatitis C is also the form commonly transmitted through blood transfusions. The virus is usually mild in presentation, and the patient is often asymptomatic. It rarely progresses to fulminant hepatic failure. The disease has a 50% incidence of

progression to chronic hepatitis, which may lead to cirrhosis or hepatocellular cancer (Aach et al., 1992).

Hepatitis D. Hepatitis D always occurs in the presence of hepatitis B and relies on the virus to spread. The hepatitis D virus is transmitted in the same way as the hepatitis B virus. Hepatitis D virus can result in the development of chronic liver disease.

Hepatitis E. Hepatitis E refers to an epidemic form of hepatitis that is similar in characteristics to hepatitis A. It is transmitted via the fecal-oral route and does not progress to a chronic phase. The disease is common in underdeveloped countries. Pregnant women in these countries are at the highest risk.

Assessment

Hepatitis A. Hepatitis A is diagnosed by the presence of hepatitis A antibodies in the blood. These antibodies occur within 2 to 6 weeks after exposure and remain in the blood serum indefinitely. These initial antibodies are of the immunoglobulin M class and indicate the presence of a current infection. Later, they are replaced by the immunoglobulin G class and indicate immunity to hepatitis A.

Common signs and symptoms of hepatitis A include

- Brown urine
- Depression
- Loss of appetite
- Nausea and vomiting
- Fever
- Weakness, chills
- Headache
- Right upper quadrant discomfort or pain
- Irritability
- Clay-colored feces

In addition to clinical signs and symptoms, liver function tests and coagulation test results are altered. Common liver function tests are listed in Table 14–27.

Early in hepatitis A, an incubation period exists in which the patient is asymptomatic but is contagious. Hepatitis A is most contagious before signs and symptoms occur. Because many symptoms are typical of a flulike illness, the virus may be misdiagnosed once symptoms are apparent. Some patients may become jaundiced, which causes them to come to the hospital. Generally, signs and symptoms of hepatitis A develop 2 to 7 days before the onset of jaundice. Acute symptoms can progress or disappear once jaundice is present. Usually, the patient recovers within 4 to 6 months from the onset of symptoms. Recovery is determined by a return to normal of liver function findings and the absence of clinical symptoms. Occasionally, a relapse can occur, but the symptoms are less severe.

Table 14–26. MODES OF TRANSMISSION FOR HEPATITIS

Contact with blood
Contact with blood products
Contact with semen
Contact with saliva
Percutaneously through mucous membranes
Direct contact with infected fluids/objects

Table 14–27. COMMON LIVER FUNCTION TESTS

Serum or Plasma	Alteration
Albumin	Decreased
Ammonia	Increased
Bile pigments	
Total bilirubin	Increased
Direct or conjugated bilirubin	Increased
Cholesterol	Increased
Coagulation tests	
Prothrombin time	Prolonged
Partial thromboplastin time	Prolonged
Enzymes	
Alkaline phosphatase	Increased
Aspartate transaminase	Increased
Alanine transaminase	Increased
Urine	
Bilirubin	Increased
Urobilinogen	Increased

Chronic liver disease or a carrier state usually does not follow in this type of hepatitis. After acute illness and recovery, hepatitis A is associated with lifelong immunity.

Hepatitis B. Diagnosis of hepatitis B is made through the presence of antigen-antibody systems in the blood. Hepatitis B surface antigens can be found from 1 to 10 weeks after exposure to the virus. Patients are considered infectious as long as hepatitis B surface antigens are present. Several other antigen-antibody systems can be used to diagnose hepatitis B. These include hepatitis B e antigen and hepatitis B core antigen. These antibody complexes are detectable throughout the acute stages of the illness.

The incubation period for hepatitis B can last from 6 weeks to 6 months. Clinical signs and symptoms of the acute phase are the same as for hepatitis A. Patients with hepatitis B, however, have more of a chance of developing fulminant hepatic failure, which is characterized by sudden degeneration of the liver and loss of all normal liver functions. The functional sequelae of fulminant hepatic failure are presented later in this section. The most important clinical sign is a decrease in liver size. Other signs of impending fulminant hepatic failure are listed in Table 14–28. The mortality rate for this complication is up to 5%. Patients who do survive usually do not have any residual liver failure.

Hepatitis C. Diagnosis of hepatitis C virus is made when laboratory testing for hepatitis A and hepatitis B is negative yet clinical signs and symptoms of hepatitis are present and liver function test results are abnormal. It is an important cause of transfusion-related hepatitis. This virus has an incubation period of 2 weeks to 6 months. Clinical signs and symptoms are

similar to those listed for hepatitis A. The antibody to hepatitis C virus (anti-HCV) appears 2 to 6 months after exposure to the hepatitis virus or the onset of illness.

Hepatitis D. This virus occurs only in the presence of hepatitis B. Anti-HDV is an available assay for the virus.

Hepatitis E. This virus has only been recently defined. It does not currently have an assay.

NURSING DIAGNOSES

Nursing diagnoses associated with viral hepatitis include

- Activity intolerance related to fatigue, fever, and flulike symptoms
- Altered nutrition (less than body requirements) related to loss of appetite, nausea, vomiting, and loss of liver metabolic functions
- Risk for infection related to loss of liver cell function for phagocytosis of bacteria
- Risk for altered thought processes related to medications that require liver metabolism

Medical and Nursing Interventions

No definitive treatment for acute inflammation of the liver exists. Goals for medical and nursing care include providing rest and assisting the patient in obtaining optimal nutrition.

Rest is important, particularly in the early stages of hepatitis. The patient's severe fatigue often requires frequent periods of rest. Bed rest is generally not required. Most patients can be cared for at home unless the disease becomes prolonged or fulminant failure develops. If the patient is hospitalized, the nurse can assist the individual in spacing activities in order to ensure adequate rest. Medications to help the patient rest or to decrease agitation need to be closely monitored because most of these drugs require clearance by the liver, which is impaired during the acute phase.

Maintenance of the nutritional status of the patient is a nursing priority. Loss of appetite, nausea, and vomiting may persist for weeks. A high-carbohydrate,

Table 14–28. SIGNS AND SYMPTOMS OF FULMINANT HEPATIC FAILURE

Hyperexcitability
Insomnia
Irritability
Vomiting
Decreased level of consciousness

low-protein diet is usually recommended. Patients usually avoid fatty, greasy foods. Nursing measures such as administration of antiemetics may be helpful. Small frequent meals and supplements should be offered. Evaluation of nutritional status is ongoing and includes assessments of intake, output, daily weights, serum albumin level, and nitrogen balance. Patients need to be instructed not to take any over-the-counter drugs that can cause liver damage. Table 14–29 lists common hepatotoxic drugs. Alcohol should also be avoided.

Hepatitis can lead to acute hepatic failure. The clinical manifestations of this disorder are discussed in the next section under Impaired Metabolic Processes and Impaired Bile Formation and Flow.

Special precautions must be taken to prevent spread of the virus in the care of the patient with hepatitis. These include

- Use of gloves while handling all items that are contaminated with patient's body secretions
- Use of disposable patient care items, such as thermometers, dishes, and eating utensils
- Use of a private room and bathroom for patients who are fecally incontinent
- Use of gowns when direct patient care is provided
- Double bagging and labeling of linen or any hospital equipment that is contaminated with feces or blood

Teaching the patient and family hand washing and personal hygiene techniques is important. Counseling may be needed for individuals in whom sexual transmission of the disease is suspected. Hepatitis B screening is also recommended for all pregnant women and for all patients who test positive for human immunodeficiency virus.

Prophylaxis is available for hepatitis A and hepatitis B virus in the form of a vaccine. Immune globulin can be administered to individuals both before and after exposure to the virus. Preexposure prophylaxis is recommended in persons traveling to countries where hepatitis A is prevalent. A hepatitis B vaccine was developed in the early 1980s. A series of three injections given in the deltoid muscle to produce antibodies against hepatitis B surface antigen is now used. It is also highly recommended for all health care personnel.

Table 14–29. COMMON HEPATOTOXIC DRUGS

Analgesics
  Acetaminophen (Tylenol)
  Salicylates (aspirin)

Anesthetics
  Enflurane (Ethrane)
  Halothane (Fluothane)
  Methoxyflurane (Penthrane)

Anticonvulsants
  Phenytoin (Dilantin)
  Phenobarbital (Luminal)

Antidepressants
  Monoamine oxidase inhibitors
  Amitriptyline (Elavil)
  Doxepin (Sinequan)

Antimicrobial agents
  Isoniazid
  Nitrofurantoin (Macrodantin)
  Rifampin
  Sulfonamides (sulfisoxazole acetyl (Gantrisin),
    silver sulfadiazine (Silvadene))
  Tetracycline

Antipsychotic drugs
  Haloperidol (Haldol)
  Chlorpromazine (Thorazine)
  Fluphenazine (Prolixin)
  Prochlorperazine (Compazine)
  Promethazine (Phenergan)
  Thioridazine (Mellaril)

Cardiovascular drugs
  Methyldopa (Aldomet)
  Quinidine sulfate

Hormonal agents
  Antithyroid drugs
  Oral contraceptives
  Oral hypoglycemics
    Tolbutamide (Orinase)
    Chlorpropamide (Diabinese)

Sedatives
  Chlordiazepoxide (Librium)
  Diazepam (Valium)

Others
  Cimetidine (Tagamet)

PATIENT OUTCOMES

Resolution of hepatitis can be evaluated based on the following criteria:

- Patient is able to tolerate increasing levels of activity.
- Abdominal pain is absent.
- Liver function test results return to baseline.
- Serological test results indicate the absence of active virus.
- Nutritional status is maintained.
- Infection is absent.
- Thought processes return to baseline.

Cirrhosis

Cirrhosis causes severe alterations in the structure and function of liver cells (Fig. 14–12). It is character-

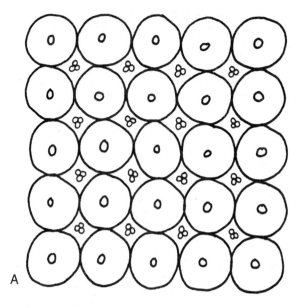

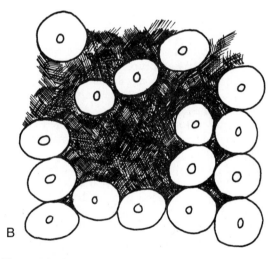

Figure 14–12. Liver architecture in cirrhosis. *(A)*, Normal liver. *(B)*, Changes occurring in cirrhosis.

ized by inflammation and liver cell necrosis that may be focal or diffuse. Fat deposits may also be present. The enlarged liver cells cause compression of the liver lobule, leading to increased resistance to blood flow and portal hypertension. Necrosis is followed by regeneration of liver tissue, but not in a normal fashion. Fibrous tissue is laid down over time, which distorts the normal architecture of the liver lobule. These fibrotic changes are usually irreversible, resulting in chronic liver dysfunction.

Four types of cirrhosis exist: (1) alcoholic

(Laënnec's) cirrhosis, (2) biliary cirrhosis, (3) cardiac cirrhosis, and (4) postnecrotic cirrhosis.

Laënnec's cirrhosis, which results from long-term alcohol abuse, is the most common type in the United States. Alcohol is known to be toxic to the liver; however, not all alcoholics develop cirrhosis. Other alcohol-induced injuries of the liver include fatty liver and alcoholic hepatitis. These may occur independently or along with the cirrhosis. Acetaldehyde, a toxic metabolite of alcohol ingestion, causes liver cell damage and death. Fibrotic tissue replaces liver cells and ultimately causes the liver to shrink. In end-stage disease, almost all liver cells are replaced by this tissue, which is unable to carry out the normal functions of the liver.

Biliary cirrhosis is caused by a decrease in bile flow, which is most commonly caused by long-term obstruction of bile ducts. It eventually leads to degeneration and fibrosis of the ducts.

Cardiac cirrhosis is most commonly caused by severe long-term right-sided congestive heart failure. Decreased oxygenation of liver cells and cellular death characterize this disease.

Postnecrotic cirrhosis can be a result of exposure to hepatotoxins, chemicals, or infection, or it can be caused by a metabolic disorder. It results in the massive death of liver cells, and it is also associated with the development of liver cancer.

Fatty Liver

Fatty liver is defined as an accumulation of excessive fats in the liver; it is morphologically distinguishable from cirrhosis. Alcohol abuse is the most common cause of this disorder. Other causes include obesity, diabetes, hepatic resection, starvation, and TPN. Damage caused by the fat deposits may result in liver dysfunction, failure, and death.

ASSESSMENT OF HEPATIC FAILURE
Presenting Clinical Signs

Initial clinical signs of hepatic failure are vague and include weakness, fatigue, loss of appetite, weight loss, abdominal discomfort, nausea and vomiting, and change in bowel habits. As destruction in the liver progresses, the systemic effects of the disease become apparent as liver function becomes impaired. This results in loss of the normal vascular, secretory, and metabolic functions of the liver (see Table 14–5). The functional sequelae of liver disease can be divided into three categories: (1) portal hypertension, (2) reduced liver metabolic processes, and (3) impaired bile formation and flow. These derangements and their clinical manifestations are summarized in Table 14–30.

Table 14–30. CLINICAL SIGNS AND SYMPTOMS OF LIVER DISEASE

Cardiac
  Hyperdynamic circulation
  Portal hypertension
  Dysrhythmias
  Activity intolerance
  Edema

Dermatological
  Jaundice
  Spider angiomas
  Pruritus

Electrolyte
  Hypokalemia
  Hyponatremia (dilutional)
  Hypernatremia

Endocrine
  Increased aldosterone
  Increased antidiuretic hormone

Fluid
  Ascites
  Water retention
  Decreased volume in vascular space

Gastrointestinal
  Abdominal discomfort
  Decreased appetite
  Diarrhea
  Gastrointestinal bleeding
  Varices
  Malnutrition
  Nausea and vomiting

Hematological
  Anemia
  Impaired coagulation
  Disseminated intravascular
    coagulation

Immune system
  Increased susceptibility to infection

Neurological
  Hepatic encephalopathy

Pulmonary
  Dyspnea
  Hyperventilation
  Hypoxemia
  Ineffective breathing patterns

Renal
  Hepatorenal syndrome

Portal Hypertension

Portal hypertension causes two main clinical problems for the patient: hyperdynamic circulation and development of esophageal and/or gastric varices. Liver cell destruction causes shunting of blood and increased cardiac output. Vasodilation is also present, which causes decreased perfusion to all body organs, even though the cardiac output is very high. This phenomenon is known as high-output failure, or hyperdynamic circulation. Clinical signs and symptoms of this disorder are identical to those of heart failure and include jugular vein distention, rales, and decreased perfusion to all organs. Initially, the patient may have hypertension, flushed skin, and bounding pulses. Blood pressure usually decreases eventually. Dysrhythmias are also common. Increased portal venous pressure causes the formation of channels that shunt blood in order to decrease pressure. These channels, or varices, are problematic because they can bleed, causing a massive upper gastrointestinal bleed (see text on upper GI bleeding). The most common sites are in the esophageal and gastric areas. Splenomegaly is also associated with portal hypertension.

Impaired Metabolic Processes

The liver is the most complex organ because of all of its metabolic processes. Liver failure causes altered carbohydrate, fat, and protein metabolism; decreased synthesis of blood clotting factors; decreased removal of activated clotting components; decreased metabolism of vitamins and iron; decreased storage functions; and decreased detoxification functions.

Altered carbohydrate metabolism may result in unstable blood glucose level. The serum glucose level is usually increased to more than 200 mg/L. This condition is termed *cirrhotic diabetes*. Altered carbohydrate metabolism may also result in malnutrition and a decreased stress response.

Altered fat metabolism may result in a fatty liver. Fat is used by all cells for energy, and altered metabolism may cause fatigue and decreased activity tolerance in many patients. Alterations in skin integrity, which are common in chronic liver disease, are also thought to be related to this metabolic dysfunction. Bile salts are also not adequately produced, which leads to an inability of fats to be metabolized by the small intestine. Malnutrition can result.

Protein metabolism is also decreased. Albumin synthesis is decreased, and serum albumin level is decreased. Albumin is necessary for colloid osmotic pressure to hold fluid in the intravascular space and for nutrition. Low albumin is also thought to be associated with the development of ascites, a complication of hepatic failure. Globulin is another protein that is essential for the transport of substances in the blood. Fibrinogen is an essential protein that is necessary for normal clotting. This, coupled with a decreased synthesis of many blood clotting factors, predisposes the patient to bleeding. Clinical signs and symptoms can range from bruising and nose and gingival bleeding to frank hemorrhage. Disseminated intravascular coagulation may also develop (see Chapter 13).

Kupffer's cells in the liver play an important role in fighting infections throughout the body. Loss of this function predisposes the patient to severe infections, particularly gram-negative sepsis (see Chapter 8).

The liver also removes activated clotting factors from the general circulation in order to prevent widespread clotting in the system. Loss of this function predisposes the patient to emboli, particularly to the lungs.

Decreased metabolism and storage of vitamins A, B_{12}, and D; iron; glucose; and fat predispose the patient to many nutritional deficiencies. The liver loses a well-known function of detoxifying drugs, ammonia, and hormones. Loss of ammonia conversion to urea in the liver is responsible for many of the altered thought processes seen in liver failure because ammonia is allowed to directly enter the central nervous system. These alterations range from minor sensory-perceptual changes, such as tremors, slurred speech, and impaired decision making, to dramatic confusion or profound coma.

Hormonal imbalances are common in liver disease. The most important physiological imbalance is the activation of aldosterone and antidiuretic hormone. Hormones are thought to contribute to some of the fluid and electrolyte disturbances commonly found in liver disease. Sodium and water retention and portal hypertension lead to a third spacing of fluid from the intravascular space into the peritoneal cavity (ascites). The resultant decrease in plasma volume causes activation of compensatory mechanisms in the body to release antidiuretic hormone and aldosterone. This situation causes further water and sodium retention. The renin-angiotensin system is also activated, which causes systemic vasoconstriction. The kidneys are most affected, and urine output decreases because of impaired perfusion. Sexual dysfunction is also common in patients with liver disease, which can lead to self-concept alterations in patients. Dermatological lesions that occur in some patients with liver failure, called "spider angioma," are thought to be related to an endocrine imbalance. These vascular lesions (Fig. 14–13) may be venous or arterial and represent the progression of liver disease.

The inability of the liver in failure to metabolize drugs is well known. Administration of all drugs metabolized by the liver needs to be restricted; the administration of such drugs could cause acute liver failure in a patient with chronic disease.

Impaired Bile Formation and Flow

The liver's inability to metabolize bile is reflected clinically in an increased serum bilirubin level and a

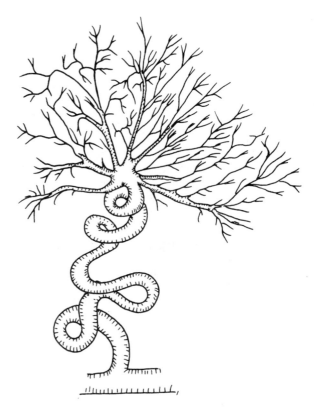

Figure 14–13. Spider angioma.

staining of tissue by bilirubin or jaundice. Jaundice is generally present in patients with a serum bilirubin level of greater than 3 mg/dl.

NURSING DIAGNOSES

The following nursing diagnoses, actual and potential, can be derived from assessment data in a patient with liver failure:

- Fluid volume deficit related to bleeding from esophageal or gastric varices, decreased production of clotting factors, and decreased effective vascular volume from ascites.
- Altered nutrition (less than body requirements) related to impaired carbohydrate, protein, and fat metabolism; decreased protein intake; and impaired absorption of fat-soluble vitamins and vitamin B_{12}.
- Activity intolerance related to impaired metabolism and decreased nutritional intake.
- Risk for ineffective breathing pattern related to elevation of the diaphragm resulting from ascites and impaired thought processes from altered ammonia detoxification.

- Altered thought processes related to impaired metabolism of ammonia and drugs, protein intake, diuretic therapy to treat ascites, GI bleeding with increased protein load, and dehydration and shock.
- Altered renal tissue perfusion related to decreased effective vascular volume from ascites and accumulation of nephrotoxic drugs from impaired liver metabolism.
- Risk for impaired skin integrity related to altered nutritional status, impaired liver metabolism of toxins and/or medications, edema, bile salt accumulation, and altered thought processes.

MEDICAL AND NURSING INTERVENTIONS

Nursing and medical management of the patient with liver failure is aimed at liver and system supportive therapies and early recognition and treatment of complications associated with the disease process (Reishtein, 1993; Young, 1993).

Diagnostic Tests

Laboratory findings in patients with liver disease (see Table 14–27) are a direct result of destruction of hepatic cells (liver enzymes) or of the effects of reduced liver metabolic processes.

In addition, parenchymal tests, such as liver biopsy, can be performed to study the liver cell architecture directly. The liver is characteristically small and has a marked decrease in functioning hepatic cell structures. This characteristic allows for a definitive diagnosis of the cause of the hepatic failure. An ultrasound study may be helpful in detecting impaired bile flow.

Supportive Therapy

Hemodynamic instability and decreased perfusion to core organs may be the end result of portal hypertension and hyperdynamic circulation. Invasive monitoring may be used in the very critically ill patient but must be weighed in terms of the potential for infection in a patient with an impaired immune response. Administration of vasoactive drugs and fluids may be ordered in order to support blood pressure and kidney perfusion, which require close monitoring by the nurse. Portal hypertension also predisposes the patient to esophageal and gastric varices, which have the potential to bleed.

The patient with liver failure is also at risk for bleeding complications because of decreased synthesis of clotting factors. Patients with a prolonged prothrom-

bin time and partial thromboplastin time and a decreased platelet count should be protected from injury through the use of padded side rails and assistance with all activity. Needlesticks should be kept to a minimum. A therapeutic touch in providing all nursing cares also reduces the risk for bleeding. Blood products may be ordered in severe cases. Gastrointestinal bleeding needs to be prevented in these patients because of the associated increase in protein load, which is not tolerated well. Antacids and H_2 histamine blockers may be ordered for the prevention of gastritis and bleeding from stress ulcers.

Treatment of Complications

Ascites

Impaired handling of salt and water by the kidneys, as well as other abnormalities in fluid homeostasis, predispose the patient to an accumulation of fluid in the peritoneum, or ascites. Ascites is problematic because as more fluid is retained, it pushes up on the diaphragm, thereby impairing the patient's breathing pattern. Nursing assessment of respiratory status through respiratory rate, breath sounds, and arterial blood gas monitoring is critical. Frequent monitoring of abdominal girths and daily weights alerts the nurse to fluid accumulation. Abdominal girths should be measured at the level of the umbilicus. Positioning the patient in a semi-Fowler's position also allows for free diaphragm movement. Frequent deep-breathing and coughing exercises and changes in position are important for the prevention of this complication. Some patients may require elective intubation until medical management of the ascites is accomplished.

Ascites is medically managed through bed rest, low-sodium diet, fluid restriction, and diuretic therapy. Diuretics must be administered cautiously, however, because if the intravascular volume is depleted too quickly, acute renal failure may be induced. Close monitoring of serum creatinine level, BUN level, and urine output is important for the early detection of this potential complication. Careful monitoring of electrolyte balance, particularly serum potassium and sodium, is also important in diuretic administration.

Paracentesis is another medical therapy for ascites, in which ascitic fluid is withdrawn through percutaneous needle aspiration. Close monitoring of vital signs during this procedure is necessary, especially as fluid is withdrawn. Major complications include sudden loss of intravascular pressure (decreased blood pressure) and tachycardia. One to two liters of fluid is generally withdrawn at one time in order to prevent these complications. The amount, color, and character of peritoneal fluid obtained should be documented.

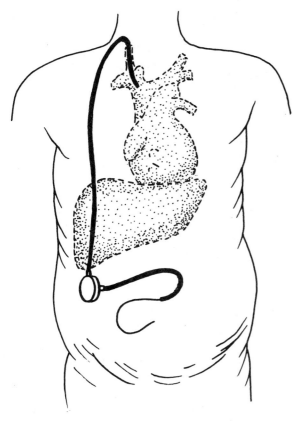

Figure 14–14. LeVeen shunt.

Often, a specimen of the fluid is sent to the laboratory for analysis. Abdominal girth should be measured before and after the procedure. Salt-poor albumin may also be administered in order to increase colloid osmotic pressure and to decrease loss of fluid into the peritoneal cavity.

Peritoneovenous shunting is a surgical procedure used to relieve ascites that is resistant to other therapies. The LeVeen shunt is inserted by placing the distal end of a tube under the peritoneum and tunneling the other end under the skin into the jugular vein or superior vena cava (Fig. 14–14). A valve that opens and closes according to pressure gradients allows ascitic fluid to flow into the superior vena cava. The patient's breathing normally triggers the valve. During inspiration, pressure increases in the peritoneum and decreases vena cava pressure, thereby allowing fluid to flow from the peritoneum into the general circulation. Major complications of this therapy include hemodilution, shunt clotting, wound infection, leakage of ascitic fluid from the incision, and bleeding problems.

A variation of this procedure is use of the Denver shunt, which involves placement of a pump in addition to the peritoneal catheter. Fluid is allowed to flow

through the pump from the peritoneum into the general circulation at a uniform rate. The pump also allows the physician or nurse to squeeze the pump percutaneously in order to increase flow or to clear the catheter of any solid matter.

Portal Systemic Encephalopathy

Portal systemic encephalopathy, commonly known as "hepatic encephalopathy," is a functional derangement of the central nervous system that causes altered levels of consciousness and cerebral manifestations ranging from confusion to coma. Impaired motor ability is also often present. Asterixis is a flapping tremor of the hand that is an early sign of hepatic encephalopathy that can be assessed by the nurse.

The exact cause of hepatic encephalopathy is unknown, but it is thought to be abnormal ammonia metabolism. Increased serum ammonia levels are thought to interfere with normal cerebral metabolism. In acute liver failure, signs and symptoms of this disorder may appear rapidly, whereas in chronic failure, they often occur over time. There are many conditions that may precipitate the development of hepatic encephalopathy, including fluid and electrolyte and acid-base disturbances, increased protein intake, portal systemic shunts, blood transfusions, GI bleeding, and many drugs, such as diuretics, analgesics, narcotics, and sedatives. Progression of hepatic encephalopathy can be divided into stages (Table 14–31).

Measures for decreasing ammonia production are necessary in the treatment of hepatic encephalopathy. Protein intake is limited to 20 to 40 g/d. Neomycin and lactulose are two drugs that can be administered in order to reduce bacterial breakdown of protein in the bowel.

Neomycin is a broad-spectrum antibiotic that de-

Table 14–31. STAGES OF PORTAL SYSTEMIC ENCEPHALOPATHY

Stage 1
  Tremors
  Slurred speech
  Impaired decision making
Stage 2
  Drowsiness
  Loss of sphincter control
  Asterixis
Stage 3
  Dramatic confusion
  Somnolent
Stage 4
  Profound coma
  Unresponsive to pain

stroys normal bacteria found in the bowel, thereby decreasing protein breakdown and ammonia production. Neomycin is given orally every 4 to 6 hours. This drug is toxic to the kidneys and therefore cannot be given to patients with renal failure. Daily renal function studies are monitored when neomycin is administered.

Lactulose creates an acidic environment in the bowel that causes the ammonia to leave the bloodstream and enter the colon. Ammonia is trapped in the bowel. Lactulose also has a laxative effect that allows for elimination of the ammonia. Lactulose is given orally or via a rectal enema.

Restriction of medications that are toxic to the liver is another important treatment. All medications that are metabolized by the liver should be reviewed for their therapeutic effect.

Nursing measures for protecting the patient with an altered mental status from harm are a priority. Many patients with hepatic encephalopathy may need to be sedated in order to prevent them from doing harm to themselves or to others. Orazepam (Serax), diazepam (Valium), or lorazepam (Ativan) may be used judiciously because they are less dependent on liver function for excretion.

Hepatorenal Syndrome

Acute renal failure that occurs with liver failure is called hepatorenal syndrome. The pathophysiology of this disorder is not well understood, but it is associated with end-stage cirrhosis and ascites, decreased albumin level, and portal hypertension. Decreased urine output and increased serum creatinine level usually occur acutely. The prognosis for the patient with hepatorenal syndrome is generally poor because therapies to improve renal function usually are ineffective. The goals of general medical therapies are to improve liver function while supporting renal function. Fluid administration and diuretic therapy are used to improve urine output. Administration of drugs that are toxic to the kidney is discontinued. Occasionally, hemodialysis may be used to support renal function if there is a chance for an improvement in liver function.

PATIENT OUTCOMES

Patient outcomes for the patient with liver failure include the following:

- Adequate fluid balance will be maintained or restored, as evidenced by
  - Absence or resolution of bleeding.
  - Hct and Hgb values returned to baseline.
  - Coagulation function test results within normal limits.

- Mean arterial pressure of greater than 60 mm Hg, heart rate of 60 to 100 beats/min, urine output greater than 30 ml/h.

- Intake of protein will be sufficient for liver regeneration, but not so much that it causes increased levels or accumulation of nitrogen waste products.
- Ascites will be absent.
- Patient's weight will be stable.
- Oxygenation and ventilation will be adequate.
- Patient's thought processes will return to baseline.
- Creatinine level and BUN level will be stable.
- Skin integrity will be maintained or restored.

(See the Nursing Care Plan for the Patient with Hepatic Failure.)

Summary

Acute upper GI bleeding, acute pancreatitis, and liver failure account for the major potentially life-threatening emergencies that require careful and astute assessments and care by the critical care nurse and medical team. Priorities for care include initial assessments and resuscitation, diagnostic testing for making a definitive diagnosis, and prompt interventions for stabilizing or reversing the pathophysiological process and preventing complications. The nurse's scope of care specifically includes ongoing assessments and monitoring, documentation and reporting of patient responses to diagnostic and treatment regimens, early detection of complications, and supportive care. Patient and family teaching of the intensive care unit routine and all therapies instituted is also a priority. As appropriate, discharge teaching of the underlying pathological process and of the dietary, medication, and activity regimens may also be initiated in the intensive care unit. Successful management of all of these patient populations requires a collaborative effort of all disciplines.

CRITICAL THINKING QUESTIONS

1. You are caring for a patient who is admitted with acute abdominal pain and vomiting. His significant admission vital signs and laboratory values include blood pressure, 94/72 mm Hg (orthostatic); heart rate, 114 beats/min; respiratory rate, 32 breaths/min; potassium level, 3.0 mEq/L; calcium level, 7.0 mg/dl; PaO_2, 58 mm Hg; SaO_2, 88%; serum amylase level, 280 IU/L; and lipase level 32 IU/dl.

NURSING CARE PLAN FOR THE PATIENT WITH HEPATIC FAILURE

Nursing Diagnosis	Patient Outcomes	Nursing Interventions
Fluid volume deficit related to variceal hemorrhage, third spacing of peritoneal fluid (ascites), and coagulation abnormalities.	Absence/resolution of bleeding. Hematocrit/hemoglobin, coagulation factors, protein, albumin values will be within normal limits (WNL). Vital signs will return to baseline.	See Nursing Care Plan for the Patient with Acute Gastrointestinal Bleeding related to varices for specific nursing interventions. Monitor blood counts and coagulation function test results. Protect patient from injury. Pad side rails and assist with activities of daily living. Monitor for petechiae and bleeding from IV site and mucous membranes. Limit punctures for blood draws, IVs. Guaiac specimens to assess occult blood. Administer fluid and blood products as ordered and monitor patient response. Administer vitamin K and other coagulation products.
Altered nutrition (less than body requirements) related to altered liver metabolism of food nutrients, insufficient intake, impaired absorption of fat-soluble vitamins, vitamin B_{12} deficiency, and anemia.	Protein intake will be sufficient for liver regeneration. No blood, accumulation of nitrogen waste products (blood urea nitrogen (BUN) level will be WNL). Liver function test results will be WNL. Serum albumin level will be WNL. Positive nitrogen balance will be achieved.	Limit protein intake. Monitor serum BUN level. Administer vitamins synthesized by the liver: A, B, D, and K. Monitor nutritional status through serum albumin level, nitrogen balance, daily weights. Consider enteral feeding or TPN if oral intake is insufficient.
Ineffective breathing pattern and impaired gas exchange related to dyspnea from ascites, increased risk of pulmonary infections from decreased activity of Kupffer's cells.	Effective lung expansion will occur. Dyspnea will be absent. Arterial blood gases (ABGs) will be WNL or returned to baseline.	Monitor patient's ongoing respiratory status, including respiratory rate, breath sounds, depth of respirations. Monitor ABGs for increasing carbon dioxide and decreasing PaO_2. Encourage patient to cough and deep breathe. Perform chest physiotherapy, e.g., percussion, vibration, suctioning, as needed. Administer oxygen as ordered according to clinical assessment. Administer sedatives and analgesics cautiously so as not to impair respiratory effort. Monitor fluid status and treat ascites; maintain accurate intake and output records, measure abdominal girth every 4 h, monitor daily weights, restrict fluids and sodium, administer diuretics as ordered. Assist with paracentesis as needed.
Altered thought processes related to impaired handling of ammonia, aggressive diuretic therapy, diet, medications that require liver metabolism, and decreased perfusion states.	Hepatic encephalopathy will be absent or resolved. BUN level will be stable.	Prevent increased ammonia production via protein restriction; prevent and treat infection, dehydration, electrolyte or acid-base disturbances; use sedatives, narcotic tranquilizers judiciously; cautiously administer diuretic therapy. Administer lactulose and neomycin and monitor results. Reduce risk of gastrointestinal bleeding through antacid and H_2 histamine blocker administration. Monitor patient response to therapy by checking ammonia levels and through ongoing neurological assessments. Reorient patient and provide for safety during periods of impaired mentation; prevent hazards related to immobility.

RESEARCH APPLICATION

Article References

Metheny, N., Reed, L., Wiersema, L., McSweeny, M., Wehrle, M. A., & Clark, J. (1993). Effectiveness of pH measurements in predicting tube feeding placement: An update. *Nursing Research, 42*(6), 324–331.

Metheny, N., Reed, L., Berglund, B., & Wehrle, M. A. (1994). Visual characteristics of aspirates from feeding tubes as a method for predicting tube location. *Nursing Research, 43*(5), 282–287.

In both of these articles, Metheny *et al.* reported on results from an ongoing study that began in 1989. The 1993 study was designed to evaluate the effectiveness of using pH readings (paper versus meter) to distinguish between gastric and intestinal feeding tube placement. Preliminary results indicated that the pH method was useful in differentiating gastric from intestinal placement. The 1994 study, which was a continuation of the previous study, evaluates the effectiveness of using the appearance of feeding tube aspirates to predict tube location. This research is important because nurses are primarily accountable for initial verification of correct feeding tube placement as well as ongoing monitoring of the tube. The current practice of abdominal auscultation to verify feeding tube placement is not always reliable; therefore, a more accurate method of verification is needed.

Study Overview

The purpose of the 1993 study by Metheny *et al.* was to find an effective way of verifying feeding tube placement so that the number of x-ray studies needed to ensure proper placement could be decreased. Two hypotheses were tested: (1) The pH of aspirates can be tested with a pH meter in order to differentiate between gastric and intestinal feeding placement, and (2) the pH aspirate can be used to differentiate between gastric and respiratory placement of newly inserted feeding tubes.

Subjects ranged in age from 16 to 94 years; 58% were older than 60 years. A little more than half of the patients received acid inhibitors, usually H_2 histamine blockers. To control extraneous variables, the researchers used readings rather than subjects as units of analysis. The sample consisted of a total of 794 pH meter readings: 389 from nasointestinal tubes and 405 from small-bore nasogastric tubes.

Data collection consisted of two phases. Phase I aspirates were taken within 5 minutes of x-ray study verification for initial tube placement, and phase II aspirates were taken after 1 or 2 days of tube feedings.

The data supported the first hypothesis. Gastric aspirates were differentiated from intestinal aspirates in the presence and in the absence of acid inhibiting agents. The researchers found that 80.2% of gastric aspirates were correctly classified, and 90.5% of the intestinal aspirates were correctly classified. The pH ranged from zero to 4.0 in 63.5% of nasogastric readings. The nasointestinal pH was greater than 6.0 in 87.1% of the readings. The low number (*n* = 4) of feeding tubes initially placed in the respiratory tract made it impossible to adequately test the second hypothesis. The researchers used random samples of pleural fluid obtained by thoracentesis and compared pH meter readings with analysis of the two random gastric samples. The pH of fluid from the respiratory tract ranged from 6.24 to 8.79; the mean was 7.92 for pleural fluid and 7.81 for tracheobronchial fluid. Gastric sample pH ranged from 1 to 8; the mean was 3.88.

The researchers discussed the importance of using pH meter readings in conjunction with the appearance of aspirates and x-ray studies to help determine feeding tube placement. Gastric aspirates are usually cloudy, off-white, green, brown, or colorless. Intestinal aspirates are usually clear yellow or gold. Readings from the pH meter tended to be more subjective and may be altered by formulas and added food coloring.

Critique

Verifying feeding tube placement is an important nursing responsibility in any setting. The risk for misplacement, particularly in the respiratory tract, is more probable when small-bore soft tubes are used. It is important therefore to study effective ways for nurses to correctly verify tube placement at the patient's bedside. Metheny et al. (1993) provided a well-designed quantitative study. They used a large sample size with subject age range of 18 to 24 years. Although no age-related differences were found, it is important to consider the changes in gastric mucosa and acid secretion that accompany aging. The researchers also considered the effects of acid-inhibiting agents on pH and incorporated this variable into the study.

Although the study was initially designed to compare readings using pH meters and three types of pH papers, the results presented were based only on meter readings. Inconsistencies between meter and paper readings, and accuracy of meter readings, support the decision to use pH meter readings in this study. It would be appropriate for future studies to compare the reliability and the accuracy of different types of pH papers.

The researchers compensated for the lack of adequate respiratory fluids for testing the second hypothesis by comparing random gastric samples with pleural fluid samples. Although results showed statistically significant differences in pH readings, caution must be taken in drawing conclusions from the small ($n = 23$) sample size tested. Perhaps one of the most obvious weaknesses of this study is the absence of an explanation of how pH values (zero to 4.0 for gastric; greater than 6.0 for intestinal) which were used to determine categories for comparison, were chosen. The thorough literature review cited numerous studies that reported a variety of pH values for gastric, intestinal, and tracheobronchial aspirate. Previous research offered some support for using a pH range of zero to 6.0 for gastric aspirate and a pH of greater than 6.0 for respiratory tract aspirate in the testing for initial tube placement. The use of a pH value of 4.0 as a cutoff in differentiating between gastric and intestinal fluid in subjects not receiving acid-inhibiting agents was not strongly supported by the presented literature.

The purpose of the 1994 follow-up study by Metheny et al. was to evaluate whether feeding tube placement could be accurately determined by assessment of the visual characteristics of aspirate. The authors were also interested in using visual characteristics for detecting correct tube placement in the gastrointestinal tract versus accidental placement in the respiratory tract. The results suggested that the appearance of feeding tube aspirate is not helpful in differentiating gastrointestinal placement from respiratory tract placement. However, some evidence indicates that visual characteristics can be used to help differentiate between gastric and intestinal feeding tube placement.

Results from both the 1993 and the 1994 studies are being used to develop future studies that question the use of pH, visual characteristics, and bilirubin and enzyme content to predict feeding tube placement.

Implications for Nursing Practice

Correct feeding tube placement is essential for patients who are at high risk for pulmonary aspiration. The current practice of abdominal auscultation to verify tube placement is not always reliable. More trustworthy methods must be identified for nurses to use in verifying feeding tube placement. Results support the use of the pH method to help determine correct feeding tube placement. The authors of these research studies do not recommend that pH testing replace radiographic verification of initial tube placement but rather help confirm placement until radiographic confirmation is obtained. The pH method would also be useful in verifying feeding tube placement before intermittent feedings and at regular intervals during continuous feedings. It is advisable to continue to use aspirate appearance in conjunction with the pH method in order to establish correct tube placement after feedings are started. Because continuous feedings alter the pH of the gastric or intestinal environment, further research is being conducted regarding the time period needed to interrupt continuous feedings in order to obtain accurate pH values. Continued research would also be helpful for determining more specific pH values for gastric, intestinal, and tracheobronchial aspirate; this information would help guide nursing interventions.

a. What are your priority nursing and medical interventions?

b. What is the suspected medical diagnosis?

2. A patient is admitted with acute abdominal signs that suggest the presence of acute peritonitis.
   a. What is the correct ordering of a thorough abdominal assessment?
   b. What are the cardinal signs of acute peritonitis?

3. A 50-year-old anxious patient is admitted with hematemesis and reports having dark stools for the past 12 hours. Which of the following admission data is the best indicator of the amount of blood lost: blood pressure, 95/60 mm Hg (supine); heart rate, 125 beats/min; respiratory rate, 28 breaths/min; Hct value, 27%; Hgb value, 14 g/dl; white blood cell count, 12,000; potassium level, 3.4 mEq/L; BUN level 40 mg/dl; creatinine level, 1.9 mg/dl; and glucose level, 220 mg/dl.

4. A patient you are caring for was admitted 24 hours ago and has not had anything to eat since leaving home. Which of the following parameters would be used to most accurately assess this patient's nutritional status?
   a. Weight
   b. Glucose level
   c. Nitrogen balance
   d. Albumin level
   e. Caloric needs

5. A 45-year-old business executive is admitted to your unit. He tells you that he travels a lot for business and has recently returned from a trip to Mexico. During your initial assessment, he tells you that he is not married and he relates stories about some of the women he has met and dated on his many trips. His history includes persistent abdominal pain, nausea with occasional vomiting, fatigue, and decreased appetite. Initial vital signs and laboratory results include heart rate, 70 beats/min; urine, clear and dark yellow; liver function test results increased (aspartate transaminase level, 20 IU/L; alanine transaminase level, 70 IU/L); albumin level, 3.2 mg/dl; and total bilirubin level, 1.5 mg/dl. What is the most likely diagnosis and what precautions should you take while caring for this patient?

REFERENCES

Aach, R., Hirschman, S. Z., & Holland, P. V. (1992). The ABC's of viral hepatitis. *Patient Care, 26*(13), 34–50.

Adams, L., & Soulen, M. C. (1993). TIPS: A new alternative for variceal bleeding. *American Journal of Critical Care, 2*(3), 196–200.

Agarwal, N., & Pitchumoni, C. S. (1991). Assessment of severity in acute pancreatitis. *American Journal of Gastroenterology, 86*(10), 1385–1391.

Alexander, J. W. (1993). Immunonutrition: An emerging strategy in the ICU. *Journal of Critical Care Nutrition, 1*(1), 21–32.

Brown, A. (1991). Acute pancreatitis. *Focus on Critical Care, 18*(2), 121–130.

Carey, W. D., & Patel, G. (1992). Viral hepatitis in the 1990's: Part I. Current principles of management. *Cleveland Clinic Journal of Medicine, 59*(3), 317–325.

Dudek, S. G. (1993). *Nutrition handbook for nursing practice.* Philadelphia: J. B. Lippincott Co.

Goff, J. S. (1993). Gastroesophageal varices: Pathogenesis and therapy of acute bleeding. *Gastroenterology Clinics of North America, 22*(4), 779–796.

Guyton, A. C. (1991). *Textbook of medical physiology* (8th ed.). Philadelphia: W. B. Saunders Co.

Henderson, J. M., Carey, W. D., Vogt, D. P., et al. (1993). Management of variceal bleeding in the 1990's. *Cleveland Clinic Journal of Medicine, 60*(6), 431–438.

Keithley, J. K., & Eisenberg, P. (1993). The significance of enteral nutrition in the intensive care unit patient. *Critical Care Nursing Clinics of North America, 5*(1), 23–29.

Lieberman, D. (1993). Gastrointestinal bleeding: Initial management. *Gastroenterology Clinics of North America, 22*(8), 723–735.

McFadden, D. W. (1991). Organ failure and multiple organ system failure in pancreatitis. *Pancreas, 6*(1), S37–S43.

Metheny, N. (1993). Minimizing respiratory complications of nasoenteric tube feedings: State of the science. *Heart and Lung, 22*(3), 213–223.

NIH Consensus Development Panel on *Helicobacter pylori* in Peptic Ulcer Disease. (1994). *Helicobacter pylori* in peptic ulcer disease. *Journal of the American Medical Association, 272*(1), 65–69.

Panteghini, M. & Pagani, G. (1991). Clinical evaluation of an algorithm for the interpretation of hyperamylasemia. *Archives of Pathologic Laboratory Medicine, 115*, 355–357.

Ranson, J. C. (1985). Risk factors in acute pancreatitis. *Hospital Practice, 20*(4), 69–73.

Reishtein, J. (1993). Liver failure: Case study of a complex problem. *Critical Care Nurse, 13*(5), 36–44.

Soll, A. H. (1990). Pathogenesis of peptic ulcer and complications for therapy. *New England Journal of Medicine, 322*(13), 909–916.

Young, L. M. (1993). Managing the patient with liver failure. *Medical-Surgical Nursing, 2*(4), 275–281.

RECOMMENDED READINGS

Caraceni, P., & Van Thiel, D. H. (1995). Acute liver failure. *Lancet, 345*, 163–169.

Douglas, D., & Rakela, J. (1992). Fulminant hepatitis. In N. Kaplowitz (Ed.), *Liver and biliary diseases.* Baltimore: Williams & Wilkins.

Gusten, P. K., & Fleischer, D. E. (1993). Nonvariceal upper gastrointestinal bleeding. *Medical Clinics of North America, 77*(5), 973–992.

Isaacs, K. L. (1994). Severe gastrointestinal bleeding. *Clinics in Geriatric Medicine, 10*(1), 1–16.

Jarvis, C. (1992). *Physical examination and health assessment.* Philadelphia: W. B. Saunders Co.

Krumberger, J. M. (1993). Acute pancreatitis. *Critical Care Nursing Clinics of North America, 5*(1), 185–202.

Waite, L. G., & Krumberger, J. M. (1993). *Noncardiac critical care nursing.* New York: Delmar Publishers.

15

Endocrine Alterations

Joanne M. Krumberger, M.S.N., R.N., CCRN
Linda G. Waite, M.N., R.N.

OBJECTIVES

- Identify disorders resulting from hormones secreted by the pancreas and the adrenal, thyroid, and posterior pituitary glands.
- Describe the feedback mechanisms for regulation of cortisol, antidiuretic hormone, thyroid hormone, and insulin.
- Compare pathophysiology, assessment, nursing diagnoses, outcomes, and interventions for hyperglycemic crisis,

hypoglycemic crisis, adrenal crisis, thyroid storm, myxedema coma, diabetes insipidus, and syndrome of inappropriate antidiuretic hormone.
- Compare and contrast diabetic ketoacidosis and hyperosmolar hyperglycemic nonketotic coma.
- Formulate plans of care for patients with endocrine alterations.

Introduction

The endocrine glands form a communication network that links all body systems. Hormones from these glands control and regulate metabolic processes governing such activities as energy production, fluid and electrolyte balance, and stress reactions. This system is closely linked to and integrated by the nervous system. In particular, the hypothalamus and pituitary gland play a major role in hormonal regulation. The hypothalamus manufactures and secretes several releasing or inhibiting hormones that are conveyed to the pituitary and stimulate or inhibit the release of specific hormones. This system is governed by feedback control mechanisms that regulate the level of hormones within the body. Positive feedback systems stimulate release of a controlling hormone when serum hormone levels are low. Negative feedback systems

inhibit the release of controlling hormones when hormone levels are high. Figures 15–1 and 15–2 provide examples of how these feedback systems work to control circulating levels of cortisol and thyroid hormones. These same feedback systems also control the secretion and inhibition of hormones outside of hypothalamic-pituitary control, such as insulin (Fig. 15–3).

Diseases involving the hypothalamus, the pituitary gland, or the primary endocrine organs (i.e., pancreas, adrenal gland, and thyroid gland) can interfere with normal feedback mechanisms and the secretion of hormones. Crisis states can occur when these diseases are untreated or undertreated, when the patient is stressed, or as the result of a multitude of other factors. This chapter deals with crises that occur as a result of dysfunction of hormones from the pancreas, adrenal gland, thyroid gland, and posterior pituitary gland.

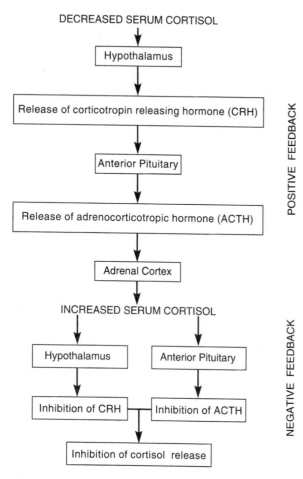

Figure 15–1. Feedback systems for cortisol regulation.

Pancreatic Endocrine Emergencies

REVIEW OF PHYSIOLOGY

The three major endocrine disorders associated with the pancreas are diabetic ketoacidosis (DKA), hyperosmolar hyperglycemic nonketotic coma (HHNC), and hypoglycemia, which are acute complications of diabetes mellitus (DM). An understanding of the normal physiology of insulin as well as of the pathophysiology, critical assessments, and collaborative treatment regimens of the above-mentioned disorders is essential to the management and nursing care of these patients.

Insulin is normally released from the pancreas by beta cells of the islets of Langerhans in response to increases in blood glucose. Other stimulants of insulin secretion include gastrin, secretin, cholecystokinin, and arginine. Insulin is essential to normal carbohydrate, protein, and fat metabolism. Table 15–1 summarizes

the physiological activity of insulin. Insulin is necessary for cellular uptake of glucose by most cells in the body, including muscle, fibroblasts, mammary glands, anterior pituitary, lens of the eye, and aorta. These cells constitute the largest percentage of body mass and expend the most energy. Insulin is not required for glucose to enter liver cells, kidney tubules, nerve tissue, erythrocytes, and intestinal mucosa.

Without insulin, glucose fails to enter cells, accumulates in the blood (hyperglycemia), and triggers a variety of physiological processes as the cells without glucose begin to starve. Insulin is also anabolic, in that it works with other hormones (thyroid, sex, and growth hormones) to promote growth. Levels of circulating insulin that exceed the body's requirement result in decreased serum glucose and changes in the level of

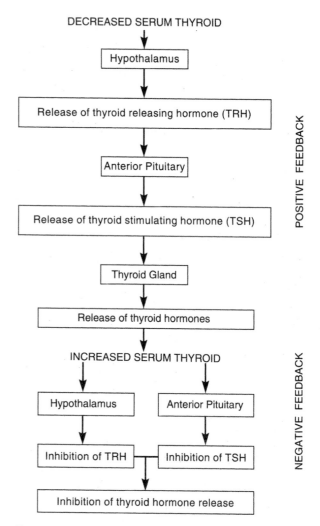

Figure 15–2. Feedback systems for thyroid hormone regulation.

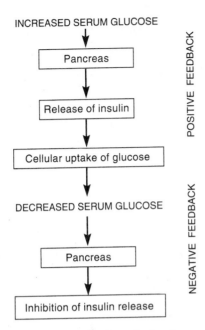

Figure 15–3. Feedback systems for insulin regulation.

consciousness, because glucose is the preferred fuel of the central nervous system.

DM is a metabolic disease that is caused by ineffective uptake of glucose by cells. There are several types of diabetes, the two most common being insulin-dependent DM (Type I, IDDM) and non–insulin-dependent DM (Type II, NIDDM). Type I DM usually has a juvenile or early adult onset and is characterized by little or no endogenous insulin production. Type II DM usually occurs in older adults and is associated with below-normal, normal, or above-normal insulin production.

HYPERGLYCEMIC CRISES

Pathophysiology of Diabetic Ketoacidosis

DKA is an endocrine emergency resulting from a sustained relative or absolute insulin deficiency (Fig. 15–4). It is also frequently associated with increased levels of insulin-antagonistic hormones (glucagon, cortisol, catecholamines, and growth hormone). The physiological consequences of insulin deficiency include increased fatty acid release, decreased glucose uptake by cells, and increased amino acid release from cells. Hyperglycemia also causes an osmotic diuresis. High extracellular glucose levels produce an osmotic gradient between the intracellular and extracellular spaces, causing fluid to move out of the cells. When the serum glucose exceeds the renal threshold, glucose is lost through the kidneys (glycosuria). This causes an osmotic diuresis, with urinary losses of water, sodium, potassium, magnesium, calcium, and phosphorus. With decreased insulin levels, metabolism of ketones formed by the liver as a result of fatty acid oxidation is impaired. These ketoacids accumulate in the blood and body fluids—a condition called ketosis. Metabolic acidosis results from an accumulation of ketoacids.

Protein stores are broken down by the liver into amino acids and then into glucose and nitrogen to provide energy. Without insulin, the liberated glucose cannot be used, and this further increases serum blood glucose, increases urine glucose (glycosuria), and

Table 15–1. PHYSIOLOGICAL ACTIVITY OF INSULIN

Carbohydrate metabolism
  Increases glucose transport across cell membrane in muscle, fat, and hepatic tissue
  Within liver and muscle, promotes formation of glycogen, the storage form of glucose
  Inhibits gluconeogenesis in liver, thus sparing amino acids and glycerol for protein and fatty acid synthesis

Fat metabolism
  Increases triglyceride synthesis
  Increases fatty acid transport into adipose tissue
  Inhibits lipolysis of triglycerides stored in adipose tissue
  Stimulates fatty acid synthesis from glucose and other substrates

Protein metabolism
  Increases amino acid transport across cell membrane of muscle and liver
  Augments protein synthesis
  Inhibits proteolysis

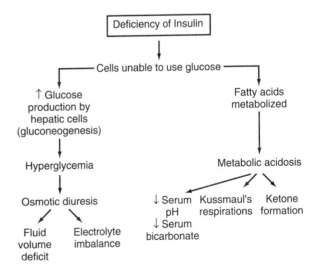

Figure 15–4. Pathophysiology of diabetic ketoacidosis.

worsens osmotic diuresis. As nitrogen accumulates in the periphery, blood urea nitrogen (BUN) rises. Breakdown of protein stores also stimulates the loss of intracellular potassium, increasing potassium in the serum. Potassium may accumulate in the serum (hyperkalemia) due to potassium shifts from the cell to the serum with acidosis, or it may be lost due to osmotic diuresis (hypokalemia). It is important to note that no matter what the serum level of potassium, total body potassium deficits are common and must be considered in the overall management of DKA.

Osmotic diuresis causes an increase in serum osmolality, further fluid shifts from the intracellular to the extracellular space, and worsening dehydration. It is also thought that this hyperosmolarity further impairs insulin secretion and promotes insulin resistance. The glomerular filtration rate in the kidney decreases in response to these severe fluid volume deficits. Decreased glucose excretion (which increases serum glucose) and hyperosmolality result. The altered neurological status frequently seen in these patients is partly due to cellular dehydration and the hyperosmolar state.

The absence or lack of insulin causes an enhanced decomposition of fat (lipolysis), increased free fatty acid mobilization from peripheral adipose tissue stores, and the development of ketosis from impaired metabolism of ketones. As ketone and hydrogen (H^+) ions accumulate and acidosis worsens, the body attempts to buffer this. Normally, this would be done by bicarbonate, but a patient with DKA often has diminished bicarbonate levels because of osmotic diuresis. Carbonic acid then accumulates. Acidosis in DKA characteristically develops very quickly. The respiratory system attempts to compensate for excess carbonic acid by blowing off carbon dioxide, which is also an acid. This explains the rapid, deep breathing seen in these patients, which is called *Kussmaul's respiration.* In addition to carbonic acid, patients with DKA may have an accumulation of lactic acids (lactic acidosis) from the loss of volume from the osmotic diuresis. Dehydration may cause decreased perfusion to core organs, causing hypoxemia and worsening of the lactic acidosis.

Excess lactic acid results in what is called an increased anion gap (increased body acids). Sodium, potassium, chloride, and bicarbonate are responsible for maintaining a normal anion gap, which is normally less than 18 mEq/L. Ketone accumulation causes an increase in the anion gap above 18 (Table 15–2).

Many enzymatic reactions within the body function only within a limited range of pH. As the patient becomes more acidotic and enzymes become more ineffective, body metabolism slows. This causes a further decrease in ketone metabolism, and acidosis becomes worse. The stress response also contributes to

Table 15–2. CALCULATION FOR ANION GAP

$$(Na^+ + K^+) - (Cl^- + HCO_3^-)$$

Normal value 8–18 mEq/L; elevated value indicates accumulation of acids associated with diabetic ketoacidosis.

the metabolic alterations as the liver is stimulated by hormones (glucagon, catecholamines, cortisol, and growth hormones) to break down protein stores, increasing serum glucose and nitrogen. Some of these hormones also decrease cells' ability to use glucose for energy, compounding the problem. The central nervous system alterations seen in DKA are thought to be influenced by the acidosis.

In summary, cells without glucose starve and begin to use existing stores of fat and protein to provide energy for body processes (gluconeogenesis). Fats are broken down faster than they can be metabolized, which results in an accumulation of ketone acids, a by-product of fat metabolism in the liver. Ketone acids accumulate in the bloodstream, where H^+ ions dissociate from the ketones, causing a metabolic acidosis. The more acidotic the patient becomes, the less able he or she is to metabolize these ketones. Acetone is also formed during this process and is responsible for the "fruity breath" found in these patients.

Etiology of DKA. A number of factors can trigger DKA (Table 15–3), the most common being infections and severe stress states. Many patients present with DKA as the initial indication of previously undiagnosed DM Type I. The condition may also occur in patients with known DM who fail to administer enough insulin or have increased insulin requirements. Patients using insulin pumps may develop DKA because of a malfunctioning pump system or infection of the catheter. Lack of knowledge regarding the disease process or insulin administration or lack of compliance with the therapeutic regimen must also be considered as possible etiologies. DKA characteristically develops over a short period, and patients seek medical help early because of the pathophysiological effects.

Pathophysiology of HHNC

HHNC, also known as hyperglycemic nonacidotic diabetic coma, is a pancreatic endocrine emergency characterized by profound hyperglycemia, hyperosmolality, and severe dehydration, which is associated with minimal ketosis resulting from insulin deficiency (Fig. 15–5).

Hyperglycemia results from decreased utilization and increased production of glucose. The hyperglycemic state causes an osmotic movement of water from

Table 15–3. PRECIPITATING FACTORS FOR DIABETIC KETOACIDOSIS

Infections
  Pneumonia
  Urinary tract
  Upper respiratory
  Meningitis
  Pancreatitis
  Cholecystitis

Vascular disorders
  Myocardial infarction
  Cerebrovascular accident

Drugs
  Thiazide diuretics
  Phenytoin
  Steroids
  Epinephrine
  Psychotropics
  Analgesics
  Beta-blockers

Insulin
  Omission (new-onset diabetes mellitus, noncompliance in a known diabetic, inadequate dosage of insulin)
  Increased demand (e.g., increased growth in children)
  Malfunction of insulin pump
  Infection at catheter site (infusion pump)

Stress (unmet increased requirements for insulin due to physical or emotional stress; also associated with increased secretion of insulin-antagonistic hormones)
  Infection
  Trauma
  Surgery
  Growth spurts
  Acute illness

Development of insulin resistance
  During menstruation
  During pregnancy

Endocrine disorders
  Hyperthyroidism
  Cushing's disease
  Pheochromocytoma

of HHNC is higher than that of DKA. Additionally, these patients are older and commonly have other medical problems that affect morbidity and mortality.

Ketoacidosis is usually not seen in patients with HHNC. It is believed that insulin levels in these patients may remain high enough to prevent lipolysis and ketone formation. Glucose counterregulatory hormones that promote lipolysis are lower in patients with HHNC than in those with DKA.

Etiology of HHNC. HHNC is usually precipitated by inadequate insulin secretion or action and is more commonly seen in newly diagnosed Type II non–insulin-dependent diabetics. Some patients may have no history of DM. The majority of patients are elderly, with decreased compensatory mechanisms to maintain homeostasis in hyperosmolar states. A major illness mediated through glucose overproduction due to the stress response may contribute to the development of HHNC. High-calorie parenteral and enteral feedings that exceed the patient's ability to metabolize glucose have been known to induce HHNC. Several drugs have also been associated with the development of the disorder. The major etiologic factors of HHNC are reviewed in Table 15–4.

Assessment

Clinical Presentation. The presenting symptoms of DKA and HHNC are similar (Table 15–5). Signs of DKA and HHNC are related to the degree of dehydra-

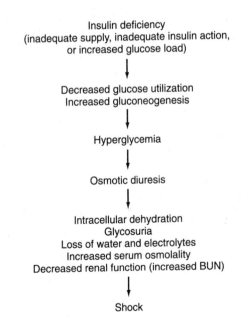

Figure 15–5. Pathophysiology of hyperosmolar hyperglycemic nonketotic coma. BUN = blood urea nitrogen.

a higher concentration of solutes (intracellular space) to a lesser concentration of solutes (extracellular space). This results in expansion of the extracellular fluid volume and intracellular dehydration. The osmotic diuresis and resultant intracellular and extracellular dehydration in HHNC are generally more severe than that found in DKA because HHNC generally develops insidiously over a period of weeks to months. By the time these patients seek medical attention, they are profoundly dehydrated and hyperosmolar. Alterations in neurological status are common and are due to cellular dehydration. As a result, the mortality rate

Table 15–4. CAUSES OF HYPEROSMOLAR HYPERGLYCEMIC NONKETOTIC COMA

Newly diagnosed non–insulin-dependent diabetes
Elderly
Major illnesses
  Sepsis
  Pancreatitis
  Uremia
  Stroke
  Burns
  Acute myocardial infarction
  Gastrointestinal hemorrhage
Stress
High-calorie parenteral or enteral feedings
Medications
  Thiazide diuretics
  Glucocorticoids
  Sympathomimetics
  Phenytoin
  Chlorpromazine
  Cimetidine
  Calcium channel blockers
  Immunosuppressive agents
  Beta-blockers
  Diazoxide

tion present and the electrolyte imbalances. The osmotic diuresis that occurs from hyperglycemia results in signs of increased thirst (polydipsia) and increased urine output (polyuria). Increased hunger (polyphagia) may also be an early sign. It is important to point out that the elderly have a decreased sense of thirst, so this may not be seen in patients who typically develop HHNC. Signs of intravascular dehydration are also common as these disease processes continue and may include:

- Hypotension (orthostatic)
- Tachycardia
- Warm, dry skin
- Dry mucous membranes
- Loss of skin turgor
- Sunken eyeballs

As intracellular and intravascular volumes are depleted, vomiting can occur, which worsens total body dehydration. As a result, urine output falls. Patients also report symptoms of weakness and anorexia. The lungs are clear to auscultation, even in the presence of pneumonia. Abdominal pain and tenderness are also common presenting symptoms, particularly in DKA, and are associated with dehydration and underlying pathophysiology, such as pyelonephritis, duodenal ulcer, appendicitis, and metabolic acidosis. Pain associated with DKA most commonly disappears with treatment of dehydration. Weight loss may also occur because of fluid losses and an inability to metabolize glucose.

Typically, dehydration is more profound in patients with HHNC because of the length of illness and the patient's age. The hypotonic osmotic diuresis also tends to be more severe, causing profound losses of water and electrolytes and resulting in intracellular and extracellular fluid volume deficits.

Altered states of consciousness range from restlessness, confusion, and agitation to somnolence and coma. Generally, altered states of consciousness are more pronounced in patients with HHNC. The level of consciousness is related to the severity of hyperglycemia and serum hyperosmolarity. Deep tendon reflexes may be decreased. Seizures and focal neurological signs may also be present and often cause misdiagnosis in patients with HHNC. Aphasia, paresis, and a positive Babinski's reflex may also be present with HHNC.

In DKA, because of the absence of sufficient insulin, glucose utilization is profoundly impaired and inhibits the peripheral uptake of glucose as well as protein synthesis and lipogenesis. Glucose can still be used in non–insulin-dependent tissues, and free fatty acids are mobilized and transported to the liver for metabolism. The liver becomes overwhelmed and is unable to oxidize the excessive amount of ketones. The excessive production and decreased metabolism of ketone bodies result in ketonuria and loss of bicarbonate, resulting in metabolic acidosis. Nausea is an early sign of DKA and is thought to be a result of retained ketones. Increases in the rate and depth of breathing (Kussmaul's respiration) are common as the patient attempts to compensate for the metabolic acidosis. Later in the disease process, the respiratory status of the patient may be influenced by the neurological status, precipitating impaired breathing patterns of gas exchange. Acetone breath from fat metabolism may also be noted. A decreased level of consciousness is also associated with the severe acidotic state (pH less than 7.15). The flushed face associated with DKA is common in carbonic acid accumulation and is due to superficial vasodilatation.

Laboratory Evaluation. A number of diagnostic studies are ordered by the physician to evaluate for DKA and HHNC, to rule out other diseases, and to detect complications.

In DKA, the serum glucose is generally greater than 300 mg/dl. A well-hydrated patient in ketoacidosis may present with a serum glucose less than 300 mg/dl. Glycosuria is present with a serum glucose greater than 170 to 200 mg/dl. Serum osmolality is increased from the high concentration of glucose. Increased serum and urine ketones are also present from

Table 15–5. MANIFESTATIONS OF DIABETIC KETOACIDOSIS (DKA) AND HYPEROSMOLAR HYPERGLYCEMIC NONKETOTIC COMA (HHNC)

	DKA	HHNC
Pathophysiology	Insulin deficiency resulting in cellular dehydration and volume depletion, acidosis, and protein catabolism	Insulin deficiency resulting in dehydration, hyperosmolality, and impaired renal function
Health history	History of Type I diabetes mellitus (DM) (use of insulin) Signs and symptoms of hyperglycemia prior to admission Can also occur in Type II DM in severe stress	History of Type II DM (non–insulin-dependent) Signs and symptoms of hyperglycemia prior to admission Occurs most frequently in elderly, with preexisting renal and cardiovascular disease
Onset	Develops quickly	Develops insidiously
Clinical presentation	Flushed, dry skin Dry mucous membranes Decreased skin turgor Tachycardia Hypotension Kussmaul's respirations Acetone breath Altered level of consciousness Polydipsia Polyuria Nausea and vomiting Anorexia	Flushed, dry skin Dry mucous membranes Decreased skin turgor (may not be present in elderly) Tachycardia Hypotension Shallow respirations Altered level of consciousness (generally more profound and may include absent deep tendon reflexes, paresis, and positive Babinski's sign)
Diagnostics	Elevated plasma (average: 675 mg/dl) and urine glucose levels Arterial pH <7.30 Decreased bicarbonate Positive serum and urine ketoacids Azotemia Electrolytes vary with state of hydration; often hyperkalemic Plasma hyperosmolality increased due to hemoconcentration	Elevated plasma glucose (usually >1000 mg/dl) Arterial pH >7.30 Bicarbonate >15 mEq/L Absence of significant ketosis Azotemia Electrolytes vary with state of hydration; often hypernatremic Plasma hyperosmolality (>330 mOsm/kg)

fat metabolism. Dehydration from osmotic diuresis is reflected by hemoconcentration (increased blood values due to decreased plasma volume). Therefore, the hematocrit, hemoglobin, and creatinine levels are often elevated. The BUN is also increased due to hemoconcentration and the breakdown of protein stores. The white blood cell count may be elevated from an infection or from the stress response.

Potassium (K^+) may be normal, elevated, or subnormal, depending on the hydration status of the patient. Most often, the patient presents with hyperkalemia, although total body stores of K^+ are quite depleted. Additionally, in an acidotic state—which is a hallmark of DKA—K^+ is forced out of the cell into the serum. It may accumulate there, causing hyperkalemia, or it may be lost via osmotic diuresis or from vomiting. Hyperkalemia can be life-threatening (greater than 6.5 mEq/dl), with the development of

heart blocks, bradydysrhythmias, sinus arrest, ventricular fibrillation, or asystole. During treatment of acidosis or with the administration of insulin, K^+ may be forced back into the cell and may cause a decrease in serum K^+, or hypokalemia. This is associated with ventricular dysrhythmias. Regardless of serum potassium levels, total body stores of potassium are generally low because of osmotic diuresis. Phosphate levels may also fall with treatment. Sodium (Na^+) may be elevated from hormonal effects during stress, low from the hyperglycemic state, or normal.

Arterial blood gas analysis commonly reflects a metabolic acidosis (low pH and low bicarbonate). The $PaCO_2$ may also be low, reflecting the respiratory system's attempt to compensate for the acidosis. As the patient's level of consciousness deteriorates, he or she may develop severe breathing disturbances that cause a precipitous increase in the $PaCO_2$ and a concurrent fall in pH. Severe acidosis is associated with cardiovascular collapse, which can result in death.

In HHNC, the laboratory results are similar to those in DKA, but with three major differences: (1) the serum glucose in HHNC is generally more elevated, (2) plasma osmolality is also higher than in DKA and is associated with the degree of dehydration, and (3) ketosis is usually absent or very mild in comparison to DKA. Serum electrolyte concentrations, as described above, may be low, normal, or elevated and generally are not reliable indicators of total body stores. Generally, profound total body electrolyte losses are expected. Table 15–6 summarizes the laboratory findings in DKA and HHNC.

Nursing Diagnoses

The nursing diagnoses that apply to a patient with DKA or HHNC based on assessment data include:

- Fluid volume deficit related to hyperglycemia and osmotic diuresis, effects of vomiting
- Ineffective breathing pattern or impaired gas exchange related to Kussmaul's respirations to compensate for acidosis (DKA only); effects of level of consciousness on respiratory status
- Sensory/perceptual alterations related to metabolic and electrolyte abnormalities
- Altered electrolyte balance related to hyperglycemia, osmotic diuresis, vomiting, acidosis, treatment regimen
- Altered acid-base balance: acidosis (DKA only) related to ketone and hydrogen ion accumulation, hypoperfusion from dehydration, decreased bicarbonate reserve
- Knowledge deficit related to disease process, monitoring, and treatment regimen

Nursing and Medical Interventions

The primary objectives in the treatment of DKA and HHNC include respiratory support, fluid and electrolyte replacement, administration of insulin to correct hyperglycemia, correction of acidosis in DKA, prevention of complications, and patient teaching and support.

Respiratory Support. Assessment of the airway, breathing, and circulation is the first priority in managing these life-threatening disorders. Airway and breathing may be supported through the use of oral airways and oxygen therapy. In more severe cases, the patient may be intubated. Prevention of aspiration is accomplished by elevating the head of the bed. Nasogastric tube suction may be considered in a patient with impaired mentation who is actively vomiting.

Table 15–6. DIAGNOSTIC FINDINGS IN DIABETIC KETOACIDOSIS (DKA) AND HYPEROSMOLAR HYPERGLYCEMIC NONKETOTIC COMA (HHNC)

Serum

Glucose	Elevated (generally higher in HHNC)
Potassium	Initially may be normal, elevated, or decreased, depending on hydration status
	Most commonly elevated in DKA, although body stores are depleted
	Decreased with initiation of therapy
Hydrogen ions	Elevated only in DKA, causing metabolic acidosis
Sodium	Normal, elevated, or decreased, depending on hydration status
	Most commonly elevated in HHNC
Phosphorus	Total body levels depleted
	Initial serum value may be normal, elevated, or decreased
	Serum level falls with treatment
Magnesium	Total body levels depleted
	Initial serum value may be normal, elevated, or decreased
	Serum level falls with treatment
Osmolality	Elevated due to dehydration (generally higher in HHNC)
Creatinine	Elevated due to hemoconcentration
BUN	Elevated due to protein breakdown and hemoconcentration
Chloride	Decreased with initiation of therapy
Amylase	Elevated due to hemoconcentration
Bicarbonate	Decreased (DKA only)
pH	Decreased due to accumulation of acids and dehydration (DKA only)
White blood cell count	Elevated due to infection or stress response
Anion gap	Elevated (DKA only)

Urine

Glucose	Elevated
Ketones	Elevated (DKA only)

Fluid Replacement. Dehydration may have progressed to shock by the time of admission. Immediate intravenous (IV) access and rehydration need to be accomplished. In DKA, the total water deficit approximates 3 to 4 L but may be as high as 10 L. In HHNC, fluid requirements are usually greater.

Monitoring for signs and symptoms of hypovolemic shock is a priority. Vital signs must be recorded at least every hour initially, along with the urine output. Unstable patients require constant monitoring and recording of hemodynamic parameters at least every 15 minutes. Central venous pressure or pulmonary artery pressure monitoring may also be instituted to evaluate fluid requirements and monitor the patient's response to treatment. This is particularly true of patients with HHNC, who tend to be elderly and have concurrent cardiovascular and renal disease. Accurate intake, hourly recording of urine output, and daily weights are also essential. Changes in mentation may also indicate a change in fluid status. Ongoing assessment of the level of consciousness, including response to pain, motor response, reflexes, and neurological signs, can alert the nurse to a change in mentation.

Normal saline (0.9% NS) is usually the fluid of choice for initial fluid replacement as long as the patient is hypotensive and in shock, because it best replaces extracellular fluid volume deficits. IV fluids are usually infused at rapid rates initially (1000 to 2000 cc in the first hour) (Sauve and Kessler, 1992). Once the patient has a normal blood pressure, hypotonic saline (0.45% NS) is used to replace intracellular fluid deficits. The goal is generally to replace half of the estimated fluid deficit over the first 8 hours. The second half of the fluid deficit should be replaced during the next 16 hours of therapy. Generally, IV fluid rates of 150 to 250 ml/h are tolerated hemodynamically (Lipsky, 1994). As the plasma glucose approaches 250 to 300 mg/dl, 5% glucose should be added to the replacement fluid. This prevents hypoglycemia and allows for the continued use of insulin. Glucose also prevents the development of cerebral edema, a complication of therapy.

Fluid overload from overaggressive fluid replacement can be prevented by monitoring breath sounds and performing cardiovascular assessments. Signs and symptoms of fluid overload are reviewed in Table 15–7. Rapid fluid administration may also contribute to cerebral edema, which is a complication associated with DKA. The rapid fall in plasma glucose, along with rapid fluid administration and concurrent insulin therapy (see next section), may result in movement of water into brain cells, causing brain swelling.

Insulin Therapy. Replacement of insulin is de-

finitive therapy for DKA and HHNC. The goal is to restore normal glucose uptake by cells while preventing complications of excess insulin administration—hypoglycemia, hypokalemia, and hypophosphatemia. Regular insulin IV is preferred. Low-dose insulin at a rate of 0.1 to 0.2 U/kg/h via constant infusion is recommended to achieve a steady decrease in serum glucose. The goal is to decrease the serum glucose 50 to 100 mg/dl/h (Sauve and Kessler, 1992).

Serum glucose levels need to be monitored every 1 to 2 hours while the patient is receiving continuous insulin drip therapy. Serum blood glucose, reagent pads, or glucometers can be used, as long as one consistent method is used. As soon as the serum glucose reaches 300 mg/dl, the insulin drip is usually decreased and the primary IV solution is changed to 5% glucose with hypotonic saline (D5/0.45 NS) to prevent hypoglycemia and cerebral edema and to replace intracellular fluid volume deficits. Once serum glucose levels stabilize, the patient is generally managed with IV insulin drips or with subcutaneous insulin based on a sliding scale. Serum glucose levels may then be monitored every 6 to 8 hours.

As discussed above, it is important that serum glucose not be lowered too rapidly, as cerebral edema may occur, resulting in seizures and coma. Any patient who exhibits an abrupt change in the level of consciousness after initiation of insulin therapy needs to have his or her blood glucose measured and protective steps instituted to prevent harm. Seizure precautions should also be started. Treatment of acute cerebral edema usually involves administration of an osmotic diuretic such as 20% mannitol solution and high-dose glucocorticoids.

Electrolyte Replacement. Potassium, phosphate, chloride, and magnesium replacement may be required, especially during insulin administration. Osmotic diuresis in DKA and HHNC results in total body potassium depletion ranging from 400 to 600 mEq. Potassium deficit may be greater in HHNC. In the absence of renal disease, potassium monitoring and replacement should begin with fluid therapy. Twenty to 40 mEq of potassium is usually added to each liter of fluid administered. This may be augmented by additional doses of potassium per minibag. Potassium therapy needs to be individualized for each patient (Lipsky, 1994).

Total body phosphorus levels are also depleted due to osmotic diuresis. This may result in impaired respiratory and cardiac functions. For this reason, potassium phosphate is often used in treating part of the potassium deficit. Phosphate replacements should not be used in patients with renal failure, because they are unable to excrete phosphate and typically suffer from hyperphosphatemia.

Table 15–7. SIGNS AND SYMPTOMS OF FLUID OVERLOAD

Tachypnea
Fine crackles
Neck vein distention
Tachycardia
Increased pulmonary capillary wedge and central venous pressures

Urinary losses of magnesium are also common. Replacements are usually given as 1 to 2 g magnesium sulfate 10% solution IV over 15 to 30 minutes.

Treatment of Acidosis. Acidosis is generally only a feature of DKA and is usually not treated with bicarbonate until the serum pH is 7.10 or less. Once fluid and electrolyte imbalances are corrected and insulin is administered, the kidneys will begin to conserve bicarbonate to restore acid-base homeostasis, and ketone formation will cease. When required, IV bicarbonate can be used to bring the pH up to 7.10, but not to correct pH. Usually, the bicarbonate is added to the hypotonic normal saline. Too rapid correction of acidosis may cause central nervous system acidosis and severe hypoxemia at the cellular level. Serum arterial blood gas (ABG) analysis should be done frequently to assess for changes in pH, bicarbonate, $PaCO_2$, and oxygenation status.

Patient and Family Education. Education of patients is key in the prevention of DKA in particular. Discharge goals for patients and family members include being able to:

- Describe the pathophysiology, diagnosis, and therapeutic regimen for diabetes
- Describe the early signs and symptoms of hyperglycemia and ketoacidosis
- Discuss signs and symptoms of infections that require medical attention
- Demonstrate prescribed therapies used to control diabetes (e.g., glucose monitoring, diet, exercise, insulin administration)
- Demonstrate documentation of serum glucose, insulin dosage and time, site of injection, diet, and exercise on therapy log
- List situations that may require an increase or decrease in insulin requirements

The teaching plan should be formulated with input from the patient and family. The importance of a regular eating schedule, exercise, rest and sleep, and relaxation needs to be emphasized. Teaching sessions may also be used to allow patients and family members to verbalize their feelings and discuss coping strategies related to the impact of diabetes on their lifestyle. The patient should also be encouraged to wear or carry a Medic-Alert bracelet or wallet card at all times.

Patient Outcomes

Outcomes for a patient with DKA or HHNC include:

- Fluid balance
- Electrolyte balance
- Hemodynamic stability
- Serum glucose less than 200 mg/dl
- Serum osmolality within normal limits
- Patient's mental status returned to baseline
- Patient's respiratory parameters returned to baseline
- Nutritional balance
- Verbalization of information needed to comply with discharge regimen
- ABGs within normal limits or returned to baseline (DKA)

See the Nursing Care Plan for the Patient with Hyperglycemic Complications of a Pancreatic Endocrine Disorder.

HYPOGLYCEMIA

Pathophysiology

A hypoglycemic episode is defined as a decrease in the plasma glucose level to 50 mg/dl or below. Glucose production falls behind glucose utilization, resulting in a change in the level of consciousness. Additionally, there is a rise in insulin-antagonistic hor-

NURSING CARE PLAN FOR THE PATIENT WITH HYPERGLYCEMIC COMPLICATIONS OF A PANCREATIC ENDOCRINE DISORDER		
Nursing Diagnosis	Patient Outcomes	Nursing Interventions
Fluid volume deficit related to osmotic diuresis and total body water loss, ketosis and increased lipolysis, vomiting.	Normal serum glucose. Hemodynamic stability: BP, HR, CVP, PCWP WNL. Normal sinus rhythm. Urine output >30 ml/h. Balanced I/O. Stable weight. Warm, dry extremities. Presence of normal skin turgor. Moist mucous membranes.	Assess fluid status: Vital signs every 1 h until stable. Intake/output measurements every 1–2 h. Skin turgor; signs of dehydration. Consider insensible fluid losses via skin and lungs. Daily weights. Initiate therapy for dehydration: IV fluid administration as ordered: monitor for signs and symptoms of fluid overload during administration; monitor effects. Monitor neurological status closely during fluid administration.

NURSING CARE PLAN FOR THE PATIENT WITH HYPERGLYCEMIC COMPLICATIONS OF A PANCREATIC ENDOCRINE DISORDER *Continued*

Nursing Diagnosis	Patient Outcomes	Nursing Interventions
Electrolyte imbalance related to lack of insulin, fluid shifts, acid/base imbalance, vomiting/NG suction.	Glucose 70–100 mg/dl. Serum electrolytes WNL: Sodium. Potassium. Calcium. Phosphorus. Osmolality.	Monitor blood glucose every 1 h via serum blood glucose or fingersticks, titrate insulin therapy; monitor for signs and symptoms of hypoglycemia. Serum electrolytes every 1–2 h until stable. Assess causes of electrolyte loss (e.g., diuresis, vomiting, NG suction). Replace electrolytes as needed, individualize according to serum values. Monitor for signs and symptoms of hypercalcemia (peaked *T* wave on ECG; ST-segment changes). Add glucose to maintenance IVs once blood sugar is at 300 mg/dl. Seizure precautions as necessary.
Ineffective breathing pattern or impaired gas exchange related to acidosis (DKA), decreased level of consciousness.	Normal respiratory rate and pattern: RR 10–25/min. Tidal volume >5 ml/kg. Normal $PaCO_2$ on ABG analysis (DKA).	Assess airway and breathing on admission. Provide support as appropriate (e.g., airway, intubation equipment). Assess respiratory status every 4 h; every 1–2 h in patients with impaired level of consciousness. Correlate ABG results with clinical examination. Prevent aspiration in patients with impaired level of consciousness; head of bed elevated; NG decompression.
Altered thought processes related to hyperglycemia, acidosis, electrolyte imbalance.	Patient is alert. Oriented to person, place, and time. Appropriate behavior.	Monitor neurological status every 1 h until stable, then every 2 h. Monitor for weakness, increasing confusion, lethargy, drowsiness, obtundation. Provide orientation cues. Seizure precautions as appropriate. Prevent complications related to immobility and alterations in consciousness: Provide mouth and skin care. Turn every 1–2 h. Perform passive ROM. Provide for elimination.
Knowledge deficit related to disease process, treatment regimen, complications of DKA.	Patient/family is able to: Describe pathophysiology and causes of DKA and HHNC. Discuss and follow diet, exercise regimen prescribed. List signs and symptoms of hypoglycemia, hyperglycemia. List signs and symptoms of infections that require medical follow-up. Demonstrate self–glucose monitoring. Demonstrate self-administration of insulin as appropriate.	Assess patient/family: ability to learn information; psychomotor and sensory skills if reagent strip monitoring or insulin self-administration is prescribed; use of insulin pump as appropriate. Design a teaching program that includes information on pathophysiology and causes of DKA or HHNC; diet and exercise restrictions; signs and symptoms of hyperglycemia and hypoglycemia, including interventions; signs and symptoms of infection. Demonstrate methods for blood glucose monitoring (i.e., fingersticks with glucometer or reagent strip, sugar and acetone of urine); have patient repeat demonstration until proficient. If patient is taking insulin, demonstrate method of insulin administration; discuss dosage, frequency, action, duration, sites, side effects; discuss situations that would require adjustment of insulin dose. Consult with dietitian if weight reduction program is appropriate. Encourage use of diabetic identification bracelet. Provide written materials for all content taught; provide means for the patient to get questions answered after discharge. Schedule follow-up teaching session after discharge.

mones, including glucagon, epinephrine, cortisol, and growth hormone.

Cognitive and perceptual changes are common, because glucose is the preferred energy source for the brain. Headache, impaired mentation, irritability, inability to concentrate, and dizziness are predominant findings. Prolonged hypoglycemia may lead to irreversible brain damage and coma.

Other systemic clinical manifestations of hypoglycemia are caused by activation of the sympathetic nervous system and the resultant release of epinephrine, which is triggered by a progressive decrease in the glucose supply to the brain. Systemic signs of epinephrine release include cool, clammy skin; pallor; tremors; palpitations; and tachydysrhythmias. The pathophysiological mechanisms associated with acute hypoglycemia are reviewed in Figure 15–6.

Etiology. Patients on insulin therapy need to be closely monitored for hypoglycemia or decreased serum glucose levels, especially when the insulin dose may be greater than the body's requirements or when injection sites are rotated from a hypertrophied area to one with unimpaired absorption. Other causes of hypoglycemia include insufficient caloric consumption due to a missed or delayed meal or snack; insufficient nutrition; and decreased intake due to nausea and vomiting, anorexia, or interrupted tube feedings or total parenteral nutrition. Weight loss and recovery from stress (infections, illness) decrease requirements for exogenous insulin. Strenuous exercise that is not compensated by an increased intake of food or a decrease in insulin dose can also precipitate hypoglycemia.

Careful assessment of a patient with renal and liver dysfunction and concurrent hypoglycemic medication administration is necessary. Decreased degradation or excretion of hypoglycemic medications prolongs or potentiates the effects of these medications. It is also important to keep in mind those drugs that potentiate the action of antidiabetic medications, such as propranolol and oxytetracycline.

In summary, hypoglycemia ensues when glucose uptake and utilization are too rapid (e.g., from exercise), when glucose release and availability are inadequate (e.g., from decreased intake), and when there is excessive insulin release (e.g., from taking too much insulin). The major etiological factors of hypoglycemia are reviewed in Table 15–8.

Assessment

Clinical Presentation. The most common signs and symptoms of hypoglycemia are summarized in Table 15–9. Symptoms of hypoglycemia can be categorized as (1) symptoms from autonomic nervous system stimulation, characteristic of a rapid decrease in serum glucose, and (2) symptoms reflective of an inadequate supply of glucose to neural tissues, associated with a slower, more prolonged decline in glucose. Subjective symptoms of impaired mentation predomi-

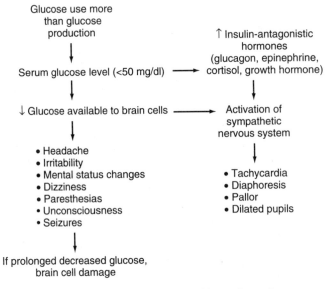

Figure 15–6. Pathophysiology of hypoglycemia.

Table 15–8. CAUSES OF HYPOGLYCEMIA

Excess Insulin/Oral Hypoglycemics

Dose of insulin or oral hypoglycemics too high
Islet cell tumors (insulinomas)
Liver disease (impaired metabolism of insulin)
Renal disease (impaired inactivation of insulin)
Autoimmune phenomenon
Drugs that potentiate action of antidiabetic
   medications (propranolol, oxytetracycline)
Elderly patients on sulfonylureas

Underproduction of Glucose

Heavy alcohol consumption
Poor nutrition
Drugs: aspirin, disopyramidine (Norpace), haloperidol
   (Haldol)
Decreased production by liver
Hormonal causes

Too Rapid Utilization of Glucose

GI surgery
Extrapancreatic tumor
Increased or strenuous exercise

nate because the brain requires constant glucose for energy.

With a rapid decrease in serum glucose levels, there is activation of the sympathetic nervous system, mediated by epinephrine release from the adrenal medulla. This compensatory "fight or flight" mechanism may result in symptoms such as tachycardia, diaphoresis, pallor, and dilated pupils. The patient may also report feelings of apprehension, nervousness, headache, tremulousness, and general weakness.

Slower and more prolonged declines in serum glucose result in symptoms related to an inadequate glucose supply to neural tissues (neuroglucopenia). These include restlessness and difficulty in thinking and speaking, and visual disturbances and paresthesias may be present. The patient may also have profound changes in the level of consciousness and/or convulsions. Personality changes and psychiatric manifestations have been reported.

Laboratory Evaluation. The confirming laboratory sign of hypoglycemia is a serum or capillary blood glucose level less than 50 mg/dl. The glucose level should be checked on all high-risk individuals with the above-mentioned clinical signs. In patients with a known history of DM, a thorough history of past experiences of hypoglycemia, including associated signs and symptoms, should be elicited during admission.

Nursing Diagnoses

The nursing diagnoses applicable to a patient with a hypoglycemic episode include:

- Electrolyte imbalance: hypoglycemia, related to excess circulating insulin as compared to glucose
- Altered thought processes related to decreased fuel (glucose) to brain cells
- Risk for injury (seizures) related to altered neuronal function associated with hypoglycemia
- Knowledge deficit related to prevention, recognition, and treatment of hypoglycemia

Nursing and Medical Interventions

After confirming plasma or capillary glucose levels, 10 to 20 g of carbohydrate needs to be administered. Common food substances that contain at least 15 g of carbohydrate are listed in Table 15–10. IV glucose is more commonly administered in the intensive care unit (50% dextrose injections). If venous

Table 15–9. SIGNS AND SYMPTOMS OF HYPOGLYCEMIA

Decrease in Blood Sugar	
Rapid	**Prolonged**
Activation of sympathetic nervous system	Inadequate glucose supply to neural tissues
Epinephrine release from adrenal medulla	Neuroglycopenia
Nervousness	Headache
Apprehension	Restlessness
Tachycardia	Difficulty speaking
Palpitations	Difficulty thinking
Pallor	Visual disturbances
Diaphoresis	Altered consciousness
Dilated pupils	Coma
Tremulousness	Convulsions
Fatigue	Change in personality
General weakness	Psychiatric reactions
Headache	Maniacal behavior
Hunger	Catatonia
	Acute paranoia

Table 15–10. FOOD SOURCES OF CARBOHYDRATES (15 g)

4 oz sweetened carbonated beverage
4 oz unsweetened fruit juice
1 cup skim milk
1 tablespoon honey
Glucose gels or tablets (follow manufacturer's instructions)

access is not available and the patient cannot take glucose by mouth, 1 mg glucagon can be administered intramuscularly (Mulcahy, 1992). Infusions of 10% dextrose may also be started to maintain serum glucose levels between 100 and 200 mg/100 dl. Glucose levels should be reassessed 15 to 30 minutes after treatment and repeated as necessary. Ongoing assessment of vital signs and electrocardiogram (ECG) during the acute phase is also a priority.

Neurological assessments should be done to detect any changes in cerebral function related to hypoglycemia. It is important to document baseline neurological status, including mental status, cranial nerve function, sensory and motor function, and deep tendon reflexes. There is a potential for seizures related to altered neuronal cellular metabolism during the hypoglycemic phase, so patients should be assessed for seizure activity. Description of the seizure event and associated symptoms are important to note. Seizure precautions should be instituted, including padded side rails, oral airway, oxygen and suction available at the bedside, and removal of potentially harmful objects from the environment. Hypoglycemia is also associated with dysrhythmias in susceptible patients.

Patient and family education about hypoglycemic episodes may also be appropriate in the critical care setting. The patient and family need to be instructed on the causes, symptoms, treatment, and prevention of hypoglycemia. Principles regarding diet, insulin or oral hypoglycemics, and exercise may need to be incorporated into the teaching plan, as appropriate. Instruction on the use of home blood glucose monitoring may also be needed.

Patient Outcomes

Outcomes for a patient with a hypoglycemic episode include:

- Plasma or capillary glucose within normal limits
- Absence of signs and symptoms of hypoglycemia
- Mental status returned to baseline
- Absence of seizure activity
- Patient and family are able to identify causes of hypoglycemia, state symptoms of hypoglycemia, state type and amount of foods that may be used to treat hypoglycemia, and perform home blood glucose monitoring

Acute Adrenal Crisis

REVIEW OF PHYSIOLOGY

Acute adrenal crisis represents a life-threatening endocrine emergency. Individuals who have suppres-

sion of or an absolute lack of secretion of corticosteroids are potential candidates for this disorder. The manifestations of acute adrenal crisis result from insufficient secretion by the adrenal cortex of glucocorticoids (primarily cortisol) and/or mineralocorticoids (primarily aldosterone). The deficiency of glucocorticoids is especially significant, because their influence on the defense mechanisms of the body and its response to stress make them essential for life. An insufficiency of adrenal androgens may also exist, but the manifestations are not clinically significant.

Cortisol is normally released in response to stimulation by adrenocorticotropic hormone (ACTH) from the anterior pituitary gland (Fig. 15–7). ACTH is stimulated by corticotropin-releasing hormone (CRH) from the hypothalamus, which is influenced by circulating cortisol levels, circadian rhythms, and stress. Circadian rhythms affect ACTH, and thus cortisol levels, diurnally, creating peak levels of cortisol in the morning and the lowest levels around midnight. This normal rhythm can be overridden by stress. During stress, plasma cortisol may increase as much as 10 times its normal level. Increased release of cortisol increases blood glucose concentration by promoting glycogen breakdown and gluconeogenesis in the liver, increases lipolysis and free fatty acid production, increases protein degradation, and inhibits the inflammatory and

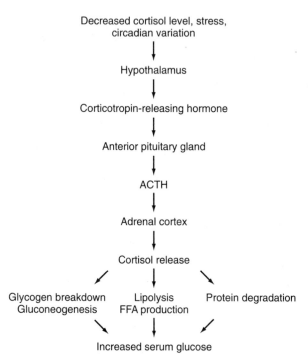

Figure 15–7. Physiology of cortisol release. ACTH = adrenocorticotropic hormone; FFA = free fatty acids.

Table 15–11. PHYSIOLOGICAL EFFECTS OF GLUCOCORTICOIDS (CORTISOL)

Protein metabolism: promotes gluconeogenesis; stimulates protein breakdown; and inhibits protein synthesis

Fat metabolism: increases lipolysis and free fatty acid production; promotes fat deposits in face and cervical area

Opposes action of insulin: decreases glucose transport and utilization in cells

Inhibits inflammatory response:
  Suppresses mediator release (kinins, histamine, prostaglandins, leukotrienes, serotonin)
  Stabilizes cell membrane and inhibits capillary dilatation
  Decreases formation of edema
  Inhibits leukocyte migration and phagocytic activity

Immunosuppression:
  Decreases proliferation of T lymphocytes and killer cell activity
  Decreases complement production and immunoglobulins

Increases circulating erythrocytes

GI effects: increases appetite; increases rate of acid and pepsin secretion in stomach

Increases uric acid excretion

Decreases serum calcium

Sensitizes arterioles to effects of catecholamines; maintains blood pressure

Increases renal glomerular filtration rate and excretion of water

immune responses. Additional effects are summarized in Table 15–11.

Aldosterone synthesis and secretion are regulated primarily by the renin-angiotensin system. Renin is an enzyme stored in the cells of the juxtaglomerular apparatus in the kidneys. Its release occurs in response to decreased plasma sodium, increased plasma potassium, decreased extracellular fluid volume, and decreased blood pressure. Once released, renin cleaves angiotensinogen in the plasma to form angiotensin I. Angiotensin I is then converted to angiotensin II, which stimulates the secretion of aldosterone by the adrenal cortex and is also a potent vasoconstrictor. Aldosterone acts in the kidneys on the ascending loop of Henle, the distal convoluted tubule, and the collecting ducts to increase sodium ion reabsorption and increase potassium and hydrogen ion excretion. Because reabsorption of sodium creates an osmotic gradient across the renal tubular membrane, antidiuretic hormone (ADH) is activated, causing water to be reabsorbed with sodium. The physiology of aldosterone release is summarized in Figure 15–8.

PATHOPHYSIOLOGY

Acute adrenal crisis is produced by an absolute or relative lack of cortisol (glucocorticoid) and aldoste-

rone (mineralocorticoid). A deficiency of cortisol results in decreased production of glucose, decreased metabolism of protein and fat, decreased appetite, decreased intestinal motility and digestion, decreased vascular tone, and diminished effect of catecholamines (Fig. 15–9). If a patient with deficient cortisol is stressed, this deficiency can produce profound shock because of significant decreases in vascular tone and the diminished effects of catecholamines.

Deficiency of aldosterone results in decreased sodium and water retention, decreased circulating volume, and increased potassium and hydrogen ion reabsorption. These effects are seen in patients with underlying primary adrenal insufficiency but not secondary adrenal insufficiency (decreased ACTH), because aldosterone secretion is not dependent on ACTH.

Etiology. Hypofunction of the adrenal gland results from either primary or secondary mechanisms that suppress corticosteroid secretion. Primary mechanisms, resulting in Addison's disease, are those that cause destruction of the adrenal gland itself. At least 90% of the adrenal cortex must be destroyed before clinical signs and symptoms appear. Primary disorders result in deficiencies of both glucocorticoids and mineralocorticoids. Some of the mechanisms that can cause primary adrenal deficiency include autoimmune destruction of the gland (idiopathic), infection, hemorrhagic destruction, and granulomatous infiltration.

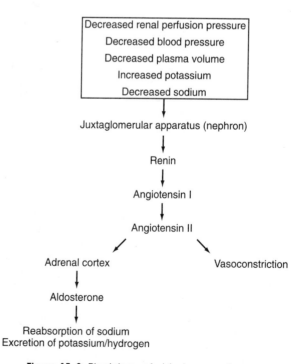

Decreased renal perfusion pressure
Decreased blood pressure
Decreased plasma volume
Increased potassium
Decreased sodium

↓

Juxtaglomerular apparatus (nephron)

↓

Renin

↓

Angiotensin I

↓

Angiotensin II

↙ ↘

Adrenal cortex   Vasoconstriction

↓

Aldosterone

↓

Reabsorption of sodium
Excretion of potassium/hydrogen

Figure 15–8. Physiology of aldosterone release.

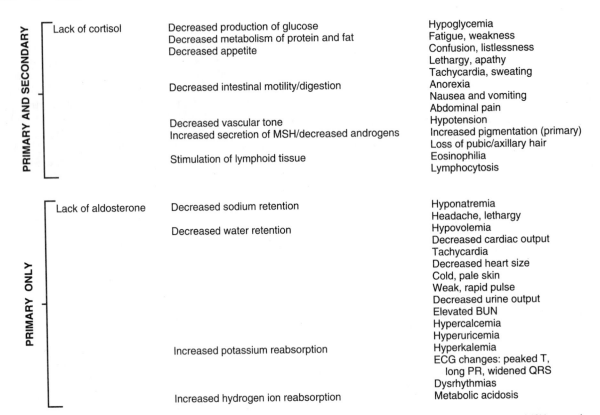

Figure 15–9. Pathophysiology of adrenal crisis. ECG = electrocardiogram; BUN = blood urea nitrogen; MSH = melanocyte-stimulating hormone.

Secondary mechanisms that can produce adrenal insufficiency are those that interfere with ACTH secretion or simply suppress normal secretion of corticosteroids. These generally result in deficiencies of only glucocorticoids, since stimulation of the mineralocorticoids is not dependent on ACTH secretion. Mechanisms that can produce secondary adrenal insufficiency include long-term steroid use and pituitary and hypothalamic disorders. A more detailed listing of possible causes of primary and secondary adrenal insufficiency is given in Table 15–12.

Patients experiencing acute adrenal crisis are most commonly those who are currently on or have recently been withdrawn from corticosteroid therapy. Corticosteroids are utilized in the treatment of various inflammatory, allergic, and immunoreactive disorders such as rheumatoid arthritis, asthma, lupus erythematosus, ulcerative colitis, and thrombocytopenic purpura. Other disorders in which corticosteroids are used are listed in Table 15–13. Chronic use of these steroids suppresses the normal CRH–ACTH–adrenal feedback systems (see Fig. 15–1). This can result in adrenal suppression, depending on the individual response, specific drug, dose, frequency, and duration of therapy.

Adrenal suppression can occur in patients receiving a dose of 20 mg hydrocortisone for more than 7 to 10 days (Lee and Gumowski, 1992). Longer-acting agents such as dexamethasone are more likely to produce suppression than are shorter-acting steroids such as hydrocortisone. It may take several months for normal secretion of corticosteroids to return in patients who have been tapered off corticosteroids in the previous 9 months. These individuals may be unable to respond adequately to stress. Thus, it is important to be familiar with disorders that may be treated with corticosteroids, because the resulting adrenal suppression may prevent a normal stress response in these individuals. This puts them at risk for the development of acute adrenal crisis.

Patients with human immunodeficiency virus (HIV) are a relatively new category of patients at risk for developing adrenal insufficiency. The adrenal glands may be the site of cytomegalovirus infection in as many as 50% of patients with HIV. Although adrenal involvement is common, it is rare for HIV patients to have over 90% destruction of the adrenal gland. However, some of the drugs utilized to treat HIV-positive patients, specifically trimethoprim and keto-

Table 15–12. CAUSES OF ADRENAL INSUFFICIENCY

Primary

Autoimmune disease (idiopathic and polyglandular)
Granulomatous disease (tuberculosis, sarcoidosis, histoplasmosis, blastomycosis)
Metastatic cancer
Hemorrhagic destruction (anticoagulation, trauma, sepsis)
Sepsis (meningococcal or staphylococcal)
Acquired immunodeficiency syndrome (AIDS)
Drugs: ketoconazole, aminoglutethimide, trimethoprim (suppress adrenals); phenytoin, barbiturates, rifampin (increase steroid degradation)
Developmental/genetic abnormality

Secondary

Long-term steroid use
Pituitary tumors, hemorrhage, radiation, metastatic cancer
Infiltrative disorders (sarcoidosis)
Postpartum hemorrhage (Sheehan's syndrome)
Trauma or surgery
Hypothalamic disorders

---

conazole, are also known to suppress adrenal function, placing them at risk (Epstein, 1992).

Addison's disease, or primary adrenal insufficiency, is a less common cause for adrenal insufficiency or adrenal crisis than either corticosteroid therapy or HIV infection. Damage to the adrenal gland in approximately 70% of individuals with Addison's disease is the result of idiopathic autoimmune destruction (Lee and Gumowski, 1992). Tuberculosis is now a rare cause of adrenal insufficiency in the United States. The autoimmune form of the disease is frequently associated with other autoimmune diseases such as Hashimoto's thyroiditis, pernicious anemia, idiopathic hypoparathyroidism, and Type I DM.

Hemorrhagic destruction of the adrenal gland has been reported with anticoagulation therapy, after surgical procedures, and during infection. Anticoagulation therapy with heparin can cause selective hypoaldosteronism and, more rarely, cases of hemorrhage resulting in both mineralocorticoid and glucocorticoid deficiencies. A common complication of meningococcal meningitis is massive adrenal hemorrhage, which can result in lethal adrenal insufficiency.

Acute adrenal crisis can be precipitated in any patient with chronic adrenal insufficiency by providing inadequate hormone replacement during times of acute stress such as infection, trauma, or surgery or after sudden withdrawal of steroids in a patient on long-term therapy. During periods of stress, the adrenal cortex is able to increase the production of cortisol up to 10 times the normal rate, if necessary. Individuals with inadequate adrenal cortex function are unable to increase production and thus go into an acute life-threatening crisis.

ASSESSMENT

Clinical Presentation. When collecting the patient database, look for patients who are at risk, have predisposing factors, or have physical findings associated with chronic adrenal insufficiency. Some of the historical data to look for includes:

- Drug history: steroids in past year, phenytoin, barbiturates, rifampin
- Illness history: infection, cancer, autoimmune disease, diseases treated with steroids, radiation to head or abdomen, HIV positive
- Family history: autoimmune disease, Addison's disease
- Nutrition: weight loss, decreased appetite
- Miscellaneous: fatigue, dizziness, weakness, darkening of skin, low blood glucose that does not respond to therapy, salt craving (dramatic craving such as drinking pickle juice or eating salt from the shaker)

Neurological System. Neurological signs and symptoms in acute adrenal crisis are related to de-

---

Table 15–13. THERAPEUTIC USES OF CORTICOSTEROIDS

Replacement therapy in patients with primary or secondary adrenal cortical insufficiency
Symptomatic treatment of inflammatory, allergic, or immunological disorders, including:
Rheumatic: rheumatoid arthritis, osteoarthritis, acute gouty arthritis, ankylosing spondylitis, systemic lupus erythematosus
Allergic: allergic rhinitis, bronchial asthma, dermatitis, serum sickness, drug hypersensitivity, anaphylactic shock
Ophthalmic: conjunctivitis, keratitis, iritis, uveitis, acute optic neuritis, chorioretinitis, allergic corneal marginal ulcers
Gastrointestinal: ulcerative colitis, regional enteritis, chronic active hepatitis
Hematological/neoplastic: thrombocytopenic purpura, hemolytic anemia, leukemia, Hodgkin's disease, multiple myeloma
Other: nephrotic syndrome, gout, hypercalcemia, multiple sclerosis, tuberculosis, meningitis
Supportive use in acute disorders, including:
Septic shock
Neurological emergencies (to treat cerebral edema): head trauma, cerebral hypoxia, tumors, hemorrhage, infection
Pulmonary disorders: asthma, chronic bronchitis, adult respiratory distress syndrome

creased glucose levels, decreased protein metabolism, decreased volume and perfusion, and decreased sodium. Patients may complain of headache, fatigue that worsens as the day progresses, and severe weakness. They may also suffer from mental confusion, listlessness, lethargy, apathy, psychoses, and emotional lability.

Cardiovascular System. Cardiovascular signs and symptoms in acute adrenal crisis are related to hypovolemia (decreased water reabsorption), decreased vascular tone (decreased effectiveness of catecholamines), and hyperkalemia. Assess the patient for hypotension (orthostatic or lying down); tachycardia; decreased cardiac output; weak, rapid pulse; dysrhythmias; and cold, pale skin. The chest x-ray study may show decreased heart size. Changes in the ECG may result if hyperkalemia is significant; these can include peaked T waves, widened QRS, prolonged PR interval, and/or decreased P wave amplitude. Hypovolemia and vascular dilatation may be severe enough in crisis to produce hemodynamic collapse and shock.

Gastrointestinal (GI) System. The GI signs and symptoms in acute adrenal crisis are related to decreased digestive enzymes and decreased intestinal motility and digestion. Anorexia, nausea, vomiting, and abdominal pain are present in the majority of patients (Epstein, 1992).

Genitourinary System. Decreased circulation to the kidneys from decreased circulating volume and hypotension causes a decrease in the glomerular filtration rate and decreased renal perfusion. Decreased urine output may occur as a result.

Integumentary System. Patients with chronic primary adrenal insufficiency may have hyperpigmentation, especially in the mucous membranes, in scars, and over joints. This is related to the increased secretion of melanocyte-stimulating hormone that occurs with increases in ACTH secretion. Women with chronic primary adrenal insufficiency may also suffer from loss of pubic and axillary hair related to decreased levels of adrenal androgens.

Laboratory Evaluation. Typical laboratory findings in a patient with acute adrenal crisis may include hypoglycemia, hyponatremia, hyperkalemia, increased BUN, and metabolic acidosis. Hypercalcemia or hyperuricemia are possible due to volume depletion. A summary of pathophysiological effects of adrenal insufficiency can be found in Figure 15–9.

Diagnosis of adrenal insufficiency is made by evaluating plasma cortisol levels. A decreased plasma cortisol level is indicative of adrenal insufficiency but does not differentiate between primary and secondary adrenal insufficiency. A plasma cortisol level of less than 10 μg/dl in a severely ill patient is consistent with the diagnosis of adrenal insufficiency (Claussen

---

Table 15–14. COSYNTROPIN STIMULATION TEST

Obtain baseline blood sample for cortisol level
Administer 0.25 mg cosyntropin (synthetic ACTH) IV
Obtain serum cortisol level 1 hr later
To cover adrenal insufficiency may give dexamethasone (Decadron) 8 mg IV (does not affect serum cortisol)
Normal response: Two- to threefold increase in cortisol over baseline, or cortisol level >20 μg/dl

Data from Knowlton, A. I. (1989). Adrenal insufficiency in the intensive care setting. *Journal of Intensive Care Medicine, 4*(1), 35–45; and Reasner, C. A. (1990). Adrenal disorders. *Critical Care Nurse Quarterly, 13*(3), 67–73.

---

et al., 1992). A "normal" plasma cortisol level in a stressed patient is considered abnormally low and may indicate adrenal insufficiency; it should be higher during stress. ACTH levels vary, depending on whether the adrenal insufficiency is primary (increased) or secondary (decreased), and can assist in diagnosis. In acute adrenal crisis, there is no time to wait for the laboratory results to confirm the diagnosis before beginning treatment. If possible, a cosyntropin (a synthetic ACTH; Cortrosyn) stimulation test is done to determine adrenal insufficiency. The technique for performing this test is outlined in Table 15–14. Notice that a corticosteroid, such as dexamethasone, is given to the patient during the test to provide the necessary glucocorticoid support while the test is being run.

Adrenal crisis features are nonspecific and may be attributed to other medical disorders. Signs and symptoms vary, depending on whether the patient is deficient in both glucocorticoids and mineralocorticoids (primary) or only glucocorticoids (secondary). Because of the emergent nature of this condition, the diagnosis should be considered in any patient acutely ill with fever, vomiting, hypotension, shock, decreased sodium, increased potassium, or hypoglycemia.

NURSING DIAGNOSES

The nursing diagnoses that may apply to a patient with acute adrenal crisis based on the assessment data include:

- Fluid volume deficit related to deficiency of aldosterone hormone (mineralocorticoid) and decreased sodium and water retention
- Altered tissue perfusion related to cortisol deficiency, resulting in decreased vascular tone and decreased effectiveness of catecholamines
- Altered thought processes related to decreased glucose levels, decreased protein metabolism, decreased perfusion, and decreased sodium

- Altered nutrition (less than body requirements) related to cortisol deficiency and resultant decreased metabolism of protein and fats, decreased appetite, and decreased intestinal motility and digestion
- Knowledge deficit related to long-term corticosteroid management
- Activity intolerance related to use of endogenous protein for energy needs and loss of skeletal muscle mass, as evidenced by early fatigue, weakness, and exertional dyspnea

NURSING AND MEDICAL INTERVENTIONS

Adrenal crisis requires immediate recognition and intervention if the patient is to survive. Primary objectives in the treatment of adrenal crisis include identifying and treating the precipitating cause, replacing fluid and electrolytes, replacing hormones, and educating the patient and family.

Fluid and Electrolyte Replacement. Fluid losses should be replaced with 5% dextrose and normal saline until signs and symptoms of hypovolemia stabilize. This not only reverses the volume deficit but also provides glucose to minimize the hypoglycemia. The patient may need as much as 5 L of fluid in the first 12 to 24 hours to maintain an adequate blood pressure and urine output and to replace the fluid deficit.

Hyperkalemia frequently responds to volume expansion and glucocorticoid replacement and may require no further treatment. In fact, the patient may become hypokalemic during therapy and require potassium replacement. The acidosis also usually corrects itself with volume expansion and glucocorticoid replacement. However, if the pH is less than 7.1 or HCO_3 is less than 10 mEq/L, the patient may require supplementary sodium bicarbonate.

Hormonal Replacement. If adrenal insufficiency has not been previously diagnosed and the patient is unstable, dexamethasone phosphate (Decadron) 4-mg IV bolus, then 4 mg every 8 hours, can be given until the cosyntropin test has been done. Dexamethasone does not interfere with serum cortisol levels.

Initially, glucocorticoid replacement is the most important hormonal replacement. Hydrocortisone sodium succinate (Solu-Cortef) is the drug of choice, because it has both glucocorticoid and mineralocorticoid activities in high doses. An initial IV bolus of 100 to 300 mg is given, followed by a continuous IV infusion to provide an additional 100 mg every 6 hours. Providing a continuous infusion is important, because the short half-life of the drug would leave the patient deficient if given only in bolus form. The infusion is usually continued for at least 24 hours or until the patient has stabilized. Cortisone acetate, 50

mg intramuscularly, may also be given every 12 hours until the patient is stable to provide coverage in case the IV route is faulty.

Once the patient improves, the dose of hydrocortisone is decreased 20 to 40% daily until a maintenance dose is achieved. The patient can be switched to oral replacement once oral intake is resumed. At these lower doses (less than 300 mg hydrocortisone/day), a patient with primary adrenal insufficiency may require mineralocorticoid replacement. Fludrocortisone 0.1 to 0.2 mg daily is then added. Table 15–15 describes in more detail the drugs utilized in the treatment of acute adrenal crisis.

Patient and Family Education. In a patient with known adrenal insufficiency and/or on corticosteroid therapy, adrenal crisis is preventable. Education of patients, family, and significant others is the key to prevention. In addition, patients should wear medical identification bracelets to facilitate treatment. Discharge goals include the patient and/or significant other being able to:

- Describe the pathophysiology and therapeutic regimen for chronic adrenal insufficiency
- Describe the rationale for and long-term effects of corticosteroid therapy
- Identify the signs and symptoms associated with acute adrenal insufficiency
- List minor stress situations that may require doubling of steroid administration
- List major stress situations that require notification of the physician
- Verbalize an understanding of the rationale for tapering doses of steroids rather than abruptly terminating administration
- Demonstrate administration of intramuscular doses of cortisol and describe situations in which this would be appropriate

Table 15–16 contains a summary of the treatment of adrenal crisis.

PATIENT OUTCOMES

Patient care outcomes for a patient with adrenal crisis include:

- Fluid and electrolyte balance
- Adequate central and peripheral perfusion
- Hemodynamic stability
- Mentation returned to baseline
- Normal protein and fat metabolism
- Adequate nutritional balance and stable weight
- Patient and family are able to state activities necessary to prevent adrenal crisis
- Increased physical activity

Table 15–15. DRUGS USED TO TREAT ADRENAL CRISIS

Drug	Action/Uses	Dosage/Route	Side Effects	Nursing Implications
Hydrocortisone sodium succinate (Solu-Cortef)	Same as cortisol (see Table 15–11) Anti-inflammatory and immunosuppressive effects Salt-retaining (mineralocorticoid) effects in high doses	Individualized: adrenal crisis—100–300 mg IV bolus; 100 mg every 6 hr in continuous infusion	Vertigo, headache, insomnia, menstrual abnormalities, fluid and electrolyte imbalance, hypertension, CHF, peptic ulcers, nausea and vomiting, immunosuppression, impaired wound healing, increased serum glucose, cushingoid state	Institute prophylactic measures against GI bleeding Be aware of multiple drug-drug interactions, especially with IV route: oral contraceptives, phenytoin, digoxin, phenobarbital, theophylline, insulin, anticoagulants, salicylates Avoid abrupt discontinuation Monitor serum glucose and electrolytes Watch for signs of fluid overload Watch for signs of infection (may mask) Maintain adequate nutrition to avoid catabolic effects Provide meticulous mouth care
Cortisone acetate (Cortone)	Same as hydrocortisone	Individualized: crisis—50 mg IM every 12 hr	Same as hydrocortisone	Same as hydrocortisone
Dexamethasone (Decadron)	Has only glucocorticoid effects	Give only during cosyntropin test; 4 mg IV bolus every 8 hr until test done	Same as hydrocortisone	Same as hydrocortisone
Fludrocortisone acetate (Florinef)	Increases sodium reabsorption in renal tubules and increases potassium, water, and hydrogen loss	0.1–0.2 mg/day po	Increased blood volume, edema, hypertension, CHF, headaches, weakness of extremities	Assess for signs of fluid overload, CHF Monitor serum sodium and potassium Use only in conjunction with glucocorticoids Restrict sodium intake if edema or fluid overload Not used to treat acute crisis, but added as glucocorticoid is decreased toward maintenance level

CHF = congestive heart failure.

Table 15–16. TREATMENT OF ADRENAL CRISIS

Identify and treat precipitating event

Replace fluid and electrolytes
    5% D/NS until hypotension improves
    Acidemia usually corrects with volume expansion; if pH <7.1, HCO_3 <10 mEq/L, give $NaHCO_3$
    Hyperkalemia responds to volume expansion and glucocorticoids (*Note:* Patient may become hypokalemic with volume expansion and may need replacement)

Hormonal replacement
    Hydrocortisone (Solu-Cortef) 100–300 mg IV immediately; add 100 mg to IV and give continuous infusion every 6 hr
    Cortisone acetate 50 mg IM every 12 hr (in case IV route faulty)
    Continue IV replacement at least 24 hr after recovery from acute phase
    After stabilized, decrease hydrocortisone dose 20–40%/day until maintenance dose reached (25.0–37.5 mg/day)
    When dose <100–150 mg/day, may need to add fludrocortisone acetate (oral mineralocorticoid)

Patient education
    ID bracelet
    Awareness of signs and symptoms of insufficiency
    Doubling dose with minor stress

See the Nursing Care Plan for the Patient in Acute Adrenal Crisis.

Thyroid Crises

REVIEW OF PHYSIOLOGY

Like adrenal insufficiency, thyroid disorders that have been previously diagnosed and adequately treated do not generally result in crisis states. However, if patients with thyroid disorders, especially undiagnosed thyroid disorders, are stressed either physiologically or psychologically, the results can be life-threatening.

Deficient or excessive thyroid hormones can produce dysfunction in all body systems. The thyroid hormones thyroxine (T_4) and triiodothyronine (T_3) are secreted by the thyroid gland under the influence of the anterior pituitary gland via secretion of thyroid-stimulating hormone (TSH) from the hypothalamus. Regulation of these hormones occurs via the positive and negative feedback mechanisms discussed earlier (see Fig. 15–2). T_4 accounts for 90% of circulating thyroid hormone, but half of all thyroid activity comes from T_3. T_3 is five times more potent, acts quicker, and enters cells more easily than T_4. T_3 is derived from conversion of T_4 in nonthyroid tissue. Certain

Table 15–17. CAUSES OF BLOCKAGE OF T_4 TO T_3 CONVERSION

Severe illness: chronic renal failure, cancer, chronic liver disease
Trauma
Malnutrition, fasting
Drugs: glucocorticoids, propranolol (Inderal), propylthiouracil, amiodarone
Radiopaque dyes

conditions and drugs can block the conversion of T_4 to T_3, creating potential thyroid imbalance. Possible causes for blocked conversion are listed in Table 15–17.

To understand the pathogenesis, clinical manifestations, and management of thyroid disease— particularly thyroid crises—it is necessary to understand the effects of thyroid hormones on the body. Table 15–18 lists some of the physiological effects of thyroid hormones.

THYROID STORM

Pathophysiology

The mechanisms that produce thyroid storm are not clearly understood. Thyroid hormones are highly bound to globulin, T_4-binding prealbumin, and albumin. Only the unbound (or free) fraction of circulating hormone is biologically active. In thyroid storm, the

Table 15–18. PHYSIOLOGICAL EFFECT OF THYROID HORMONES

Major Effects
Increases metabolic activities of all tissues
Increases rate of nutrient use for energy production
Increases rate of growth
Increases activities of other endocrine glands

Other Effects
Regulates protein synthesis and catabolism
Regulates body heat production and dissipation
Increases gluconeogenesis and utilization of glucose
Maintains appetite and secretion of GI substances
Maintains calcium metabolism
Stimulates cholesterol synthesis
Maintains cardiac rate, force, and output
Affects respiratory rate, oxygen utilization, and carbon dioxide formation
Affects red blood cell production
Affects central nervous system development and cerebration
Necessary for muscle tone and vigor and normal skin constituents

NURSING CARE PLAN FOR THE PATIENT IN ACUTE ADRENAL CRISIS

Nursing Diagnosis	Patient Outcomes	Nursing Interventions
Fluid volume deficit related to deficiency of aldosterone hormone (mineralocorticoid), decreased sodium, and water retention.	Fluid balance restored. Electrolyte balance restored: Na 135–145 mEq/L; K 3.5–5.0 mEq/L. Urine output >30 ml/h. BP WNL/returned to baseline. Warm, pink skin. HR 60–100 beats/min.	Administer IV fluids and electrolytes as ordered (5% D/normal saline) until signs and symptoms of hypovolemia stabilized; initial fluids will be administered rapidly; monitor for signs of overload. Monitor vital signs, orthostatic changes, hemodynamics (preload indicators with hemodynamic catheter in place; CVP/PCWP), central and peripheral perfusion (mean arterial pressure/cardiac output). Monitor fluid balance (intake and output)/daily weight. Monitor heart rate and rhythm at least every 1 h (every 15 min in unstable patients). Monitor glucose, potassium, and sodium every 2–4 h until stable. Monitor renal function: BUN, creatinine, urine output, specific gravity, urine sodium and potassium. Administer scheduled doses of IV glucocorticoids and assess response. Avoid abrupt changes in position (to upright) until fluid balance is restored. Explain diagnostic tests to patient/family. Prevent adrenal crisis by ensuring patients at risk receive exogenous cortisol in stress states.
Altered tissue perfusion (decreased) related to cortisol deficiency resulting in decreased vascular tone, decreased effectiveness of catecholamines.	Adequate central and peripheral perfusion and hemodynamic stability as evidenced by: Palpable peripheral pulses (2+) Warm/dry skin. Adequate urine output (30 ml/h). Usual mentation. Systolic BP >90 mm Hg; mean arterial pressure >60 mm Hg. CI >2.5 L/min/m². CVP 0–8 mm Hg. SVR 900–1400 dynes/sec/cm^{-5}. Absence of respiratory distress.	Monitor changes in mental status (anxiety, confusion, lethargy, coma), personality changes. Inspect skin for pallor, mottling, cyanosis; note color and temperature (especially in cannulated extremities). Provide skin care, change position every 1.5–2.0 h, keep skin clean, dry. Monitor respiratory rate. Monitor for changes in blood pressure. Assess GI function: decreased bowel sounds, nausea and vomiting, abdominal distention; anorexia; insert NG as needed. Monitor laboratory data: serum and urine electrolytes, BUN, creatinine. Note hourly changes in urine output; record specific gravity.
Altered thought processes related to decreased glucose levels, decreased protein metabolism, decreased perfusion, decreased sodium.	Mentation returned to baseline. Alert/oriented.	Assess level of consciousness, ability to speak, response to stimuli/commands. Observe behavioral responses: disorientation, confusion, irritability. Provide a quiet environment; speak in calm, quiet voice. Provide for consistent caregivers whenever possible. Encourage family/significant others to stay with patient. Provide frequent reality orientation. Provide for environmental safety, soft restraints; minimize stressful situations, promote rest. Monitor electrolytes, BUN, liver function tests. Administer and assess effects of drugs.

NURSING CARE PLAN FOR THE PATIENT IN ACUTE ADRENAL CRISIS *Continued*

Nursing Diagnosis	Patient Outcomes	Nursing Interventions
Altered nutrition (less than body requirements) related to deficiency of cortisol and resultant decreased metabolism of protein and fat, decreased appetite, decreased intestinal motility and digestion.	Normal protein and fat metabolism is restored. Adequate nutrition is reestablished as evidenced by positive nitrogen balance; weight WNL.	Note admission weight/height, daily weight. Document oral intake, food history, calorie counts. Promote optimal environment during attempts at oral intake; provide assistance with eating as necessary. Assess presence/character of bowel sounds; assess GI losses (i.e., vomiting, diarrhea). Assure parenteral/enteral nutrition solutions are delivered as prescribed; assess tolerance. Provide small frequent meals. Refer to nutritional team/registered dietitian. Provide antacids/histamine antagonists as ordered. Assess metabolic response to nutritional support; monitor lab studies.
Knowledge deficit related to long-term corticosteroid management.	Patient/family able to state activities necessary to prevent adrenal crisis: Pathophysiology and therapy for chronic adrenal insufficiency. Rationale for and long-term effects of corticosteroid therapy. Signs and symptoms of acute adrenal insufficiency. Doubling of corticosteroids during minor stress. Notification of physician during major stress situations Tapering of corticosteroids rather than withdrawing abruptly.	Provide medication instructions: action, name, dose, schedule, importance of adherence, lifelong need for drug. Instruct patient/family on administration of corticosteroids in stress states: Define stress: identification and reduction of; minor vs severe. Instruct patient to call physician for temporary increase in glucocorticoid dose; double dose for minor stress. If vomiting, instruct patient to call physician (for parenteral administration); instruct in parenteral hydrocortisone at home. Instruct patient to inform all health care providers of corticosteroid use; carry ID card. Instruct patient/family on importance of gradual corticosteroid tapering and to seek medical attention in event of stress state. (*Note:* Patients who have been on long-term corticosteroid therapy should receive glucocorticoids during periods of stress for at least 1 year after the drugs are discontinued.)
Activity intolerance related to use of endogenous protein for energy needs and loss of skeletal muscle mass as evidenced by early fatigue and weakness, exertional dyspnea.	Demonstrates increased physical activity as evidenced by: BP, HR, RR, WNL. Verbalizes decreased fatigue.	Provide passive/active ROM exercises to patient if bedridden. Assist with ambulation, ADLs. Monitor patient response to increased activity: monitor BP, heart rhythm, respirations; note tachycardia, dysrhythmias, dyspnea, diaphoresis, pallor. Check vital signs before and immediately after each activity. Assess for other causes of fatigue (i.e., treatments, medications). Restrict activity; space with rest periods. Provide for nutrition (see above). Encourage verbalization of feelings regarding limitations.

total levels of thyroid hormones may be no higher than those with uncomplicated hyperthyroidism, but recent studies indicate that free thyroid levels are higher in these patients (Tietgens and Leinung, 1995). It is believed that the rapidity with which hormone levels rise may be more important than absolute levels. Theories regarding the mechanisms that produce the sudden change in free thyroid hormone levels include (1) a sudden change in levels of binding proteins (noted postoperatively and in patients with nonthyroidal illness); (2) decreased binding affinity of thyroid hormones from the production of thyroid hormone–binding inhibitors (nonthyroidal systemic illness); or (3) saturation of hormone binding capacity, leading to rapid release of thyroid hormones into the bloodstream (radioactive iodine treatment, following thyroid surgery or thyroid hormone overdose) (Tietgens and Leinung, 1995). Another theory is that the tissues develop intolerance to thyroid hormones. Studies also indicate that part of the enhanced sympathetic activity that occurs may be due to an increased number of beta-adrenergic receptors (Tietgens and Leinung, 1995).

Certain enzymes may be the key to the dramatic increase in metabolic rate that occurs in thyroid storm. Thyroid hormones normally increase the synthesis of enzymes that stimulate cellular mitochondria and energy production. When excess thyroid hormones are present, as in thyroid storm, the increased activity of these enzymes produces excessive thermal energy and fever (Gavin, 1991).

Thyroid hormones play a major role in regulating body metabolism; as a result, they affect most body systems. Thus, hyperthyroidism can produce a hyperdynamic, hypermetabolic state that results in disruption of many major body functions. Understanding the pathophysiology of thyroid storm requires a knowledge of the disruptions that occur in hyperthyroidism. Thyroid crisis is really just a magnification of these disruptions. Common findings in patients with thyroid storm are listed in Table 15–19 and discussed below.

Etiology. Hyperthyroidism is a common and usually benign illness. The three most common types of hyperthyroidism are toxic diffuse goiter, toxic multinodular goiter, and toxic uninodular goiter. The vast majority of patients with hyperthyroid crises (thyroid storm) have either toxic diffuse goiter or an unusually large toxic multinodular goiter.

The most common form of hyperthyroidism is toxic diffuse goiter, also known as Graves' disease. It occurs most frequently in young (third or fourth decade), previously healthy women. A family history of hyperthyroidism is often present. Its cause is unknown, but it is believed to be an autoimmune disease, because all affected patients have abnormal immunoglobulins. These immunoglobulins attack thyroid tissue, producing thyroid inflammation, diffuse enlargement, and hyperplasia of the gland.

Toxic multinodular goiter is the second most common cause of hyperthyroidism. It also occurs more commonly in women, but they are generally older than those with toxic diffuse goiter (fourth to seventh decades). Crises in patients with toxic multinodular goiter are more commonly associated with heart failure or severe muscle weakness. These and other possible causes of hyperthyroidism are listed in Table 15–20.

Thyroid storm usually occurs in untreated or inadequately treated patients with hyperthyroidism. Few cases arise in patients who have had previously normal thyroids. Most of these individuals have had Graves' disease for at least several months. The crisis is often precipitated by stress related to an underlying illness, general anesthesia, or surgery. Nonsurgical causes are the most frequent precipitating events—DKA, trauma, burns, infection, or severe emotional stress. Mortality is more often the result of the underlying illness rather than the thyrotoxic state.

Assessment

Clinical Presentation. The signs and symptoms of thyroid storm are variable and nonspecific. Diagnosis may be delayed because it is difficult to see the relationship among the diverse signs and symptoms and attribute them to a hyperthyroid state. Thyroid storm has an abrupt onset and is best characterized as a state of unregulated hypermetabolism. The most prominent clinical features are severe fever, marked tachycardia, tremors, delirium, stupor, and coma. Untreated patients succumb in 1 to 2 days to extreme hyperpyrexia and cardiovascular collapse.

Neurological Disturbances. Thyroid hormones normally maintain central nervous system cerebration. The hypermetabolism and resulting increased cerebration produced by excess thyroid hormones cause hyperactivity of the nervous system both psychologically and physiologically. Patients may exhibit signs and symptoms such as increased irritability, decreased attention span, agitation, nervousness, wide mood swings, and fear or paranoia. Thyroid storm may be heralded by the onset of delirium, overt psychosis, convulsions, stupor, or coma. However, in an elderly patient, these signs and symptoms may be masked, and depression or apathy may be seen instead.

Muscle weakness is produced by increased protein catabolism. It can result in fine rhythmic tremors of the tongue, eyelids, or even eyeballs; peripheral tremors, especially with activity; thoracic muscle weakness, causing dyspnea; and proximal muscle weakness.

Temperature regulation is lost, resulting in increased cold tolerance, heat intolerance, fever, and

Table 15-19. CLINICAL MANIFESTATIONS OF THYROID STORM AND MYXEDEMA COMA

Thyroid Storm	Myxedema Coma
Increased metabolic rate	Decreased metabolic rate
Nervousness, delirium, emotional lability	Difficulty concentrating, lethargy, somnolence
Fine tremor	Perceptive hearing loss, vertigo
Exaggerated reflexes	Slow speech, coarse voice
Increased temperature, heat intolerance	Decreased temperature, cold intolerance
Increased perspiration	Decreased perspiration
Palpitations	Distant heart sounds
Tachycardia	Bradycardia
Widened pulse pressure	Pericardial effusion
Dysrhythmias	Mucinous edema
Dyspnea	Dyspnea on exertion
Increased respiratory rate	Decreased respiratory rate
Weight loss	Weight gain
Increased appetite	Decreased appetite
Increased bowel movements	Decreased bowel movements
Smooth, moist skin	Coarse, dry skin
Fine hair	Dry, brittle hair

excessive sweating. Cold tolerance is more common in young patients. Older patients may naturally lose their ability to shiver and may be less comfortable in the cold. The patient's body temperature may be elevated as high as 106°F (41.1°C).

Cardiovascular Disturbances. Thyroid hormones play a role in maintaining cardiac rate, force of contraction, and cardiac output. The increase in metabolism and the stimulation of catecholamines produced by thyroid hormones cause a hyperdynamic heart. Contractility, heart rate, and cardiac output increase. These effects are magnified by the body's increased demand for oxygen and nutrients. In thyroid storm, the increased demands on the heart may be so severe as to produce heart failure and cardiovascular collapse if the crisis is not recognized and treated.

The increase in heat production and metabolic end products also causes the blood vessels of the skin to dilate. This enhances oxygen and nutrient delivery to the peripheral tissues and accounts for the patient's warm, moist, pink skin.

Patients experience palpitations, tachycardia (out of proportion to the fever), and a widened pulse pressure. A prominent third heart sound may be heard as well as a systolic murmur over the pulmonic and/or aortic areas. Occasionally, a rub may be heard. The most common dysrhythmias are frequent premature atrial contractions, atrial fibrillation, and atrial flutter. In an elderly patient with underlying heart disease, thyroid storm may be heralded by worsening of angina or severe congestive heart failure. Hyperthyroidism should be suspected in a patient who has sinus tachycardia while asleep or in a patient with atrial fibrillation that does not slow in response to digoxin.

Pulmonary Disturbances. Thyroid hormones affect respiratory rate and depth, oxygen utilization, and CO_2 formation. Tissues need more oxygen as a result of hypermetabolism. This increased need for oxygen stimulates the respiratory drive, increasing respirations. However, increased protein catabolism reduces protein in respiratory muscles (diaphragm and intercostals), producing weakness and decreased lung vital capacity.

Table 15-20. CAUSES OF HYPERTHYROIDISM

Most common
Toxic diffuse goiter (Graves' disease)
Toxic multinodular goiter
Toxic uninodular goiter

Other causes
Factitious hyperthyroidism
T_3 toxicosis
Exogenous iodine in patient with preexisting thyroid disease: exposure to iodine load from radiographic contrast dyes, medications (amiodarone, organidine)
Thyroiditis (transient)

Rare causes
Metastatic thyroid cancer
Malignancies with circulating thyroid stimulators
TSH-producing pituitary tumors
Acromegaly

Associated with other disorders*
Pernicious anemia, idiopathic Addison's disease, myasthenia gravis, sarcoidosis, Albright's syndrome

*Presence of these disorders in a patient in crisis increases the likelihood that the patient has hyperthyroidism.
TSH = thyroid-stimulating hormone.

As a result, even with increased respirations, muscle weakness may prevent the patient from meeting the oxygen demand and cause hypoventilation, CO_2 retention, and respiratory failure.

GI Disturbances. Increased metabolism and accelerated protein and fat degradation increase appetite and cause weight loss. Thyroid hormones also increase GI motility, resulting in decreased absorption, especially of vitamins, and an increase in the frequency of stools. Diarrhea is not common but may occur; elderly patients may be constipated. Abdominal pain, nausea, jaundice, vomiting, and diarrhea may be prominent manifestations of a patient in thyroid storm.

Skeletal Muscle Disturbances. Muscle protein degradation in skeletal muscles exceeds protein synthesis, causing generalized muscle wasting, weight loss, fatigue, and weakness. The extreme energy expenditure of hypermetabolism also contributes to this process. The weakness tends to be most prominent in the proximal muscles of the limbs, making it difficult for patients to climb stairs or rise from chairs.

Integumentary Disturbances. Inadequate protein synthesis also affects the skin, hair, and nails. Patients with hyperthyroidism typically have thin, fine, silky, fragile hair; soft, friable nails; and thin skin. They can also develop petechiae caused by the rupture of fragile blood vessels. Some of these skin changes may vary with the age or sex of the patient. Young women generally have the more classic findings identified above. Young men may not notice texture changes in their skin but rather an increase in acne and sweating. An elderly patient with dry, atrophic skin may not have significant skin changes with hyperthyroidism.

Hematopoietic Disturbances. Thyroid hormones affect red cell production. Splenomegaly is present in up to half of patients with toxic diffuse goiter. Poor vitamin B_{12} absorption can produce pernicious anemia, resulting in weakness, fatigue, dyspnea, and pallor. The red blood cells being produced are abnormally large and may rupture as they pass through small capillaries and liberate free bilirubin, which causes the skin to turn pale yellow (jaundice). White blood cell and neutrophil counts vary. About 10% of patients have a decrease in neutrophils. Others have an increased white blood cell count, indicating underlying infection.

Ophthalmic Disturbances. Ophthalmic changes in hyperthyroidism most likely indicate thyroid disease but may be nonspecific. Exophthalmos is found almost exclusively in toxic diffuse goiter (Fig. 15–10), but the severity of eye findings is highly variable. Changes may be as mild as upper lid retraction and lid lag or as severe as extraocular muscle palsies and sight loss.

The patient's ability to survive thyroid storm is determined by the severity of the hyperthyroid state and the patient's general health. The severity of the hyperthyroid state is not necessarily indicated by the serum levels of thyroid hormones but rather by tissue and organ responsiveness to the hormones—i.e., the degree of impairment of key organ functions. General health factors that should be considered include age, nutritional status, chronic illness, underlying illness, stressful event, and concomitant drug therapy. In the elderly, some signs may be masked. A history of weight loss and the presence of such cardiac abnormalities as atrial fibrillation and congestive heart failure may be the only clues.

Laboratory Evaluation. There are no laboratory tests that separate thyroid storm from uncomplicated hyperthyroidism. Both T_3 and T_4 levels should be measured, as well as resin T_3 uptake. Resin T_3 uptake is an indirect measure of free T_4 levels (free T_4 is the portion that is biologically active) and is elevated in hyperthyroid states. Although an elevation of thyroid hormones is to be expected, these levels are generally no higher than those normally found in uncomplicated hyperthyroidism. In any event, the patient must be treated before these results are available.

Possible laboratory abnormalities that may result from thyroid storm are listed in Table 15–21.

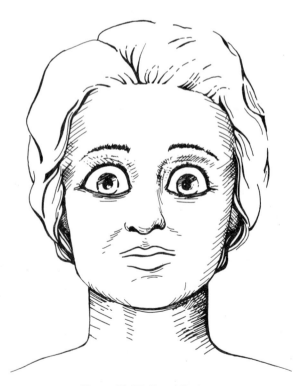

Figure 15–10. Exophthalmos.

Nursing Diagnoses

The nursing diagnoses that may apply to a patient with thyroid storm are based on assessment data and include:

- Decreased cardiac output related to increased metabolic demands on the heart, hyperthermia, extreme tachycardia, dysrhythmias, congestive heart failure
- Hyperthermia related to loss of temperature regulation, increased metabolism, increased heat production
- Ineffective breathing pattern related to muscle weakness and decreased vital capacity, resulting in hypoventilation, CO_2 retention, increased oxygen need
- Altered nutrition (less than body requirements) related to increased peristalsis, decreased absorption
- Risk for impaired skin integrity related to thin skin, fragile blood vessels
- Activity intolerance related to muscle weakness, muscle wasting, tremors, fatigue, extreme energy expenditure
- Altered thought processes related to hypermetabolism and increased cerebration, agitation, delirium, psychosis
- Knowledge deficit related to disease process, therapeutic regimen, prevention of complications

Nursing and Medical Interventions

Thyroid storm requires immediate intervention if the patient is to survive. The primary objectives in the treatment of thyroid storm are identifying and treating the precipitating cause, inhibiting thyroid hormone bio-

Table 15–21. LABORATORY MANIFESTATIONS OF THYROID STORM AND MYXEDEMA COMA

Thyroid Storm	Myxedema Coma
Increased T_3, T_4	Decreased T_3, T_4
Increased resin T_3 uptake	Decreased resin T_3 uptake
Anemia	Anemia
Hyperglycemia	Hypoglycemia
Leukocytosis	Leukocytosis absent
Increased/decreased sodium	Decreased sodium
	Respiratory acidosis
Decreased potassium	Decreased platelet count
Increased calcium	Increased cholesterol
Increased BUN	Increased triglycerides
Abnormal liver function tests	

synthesis, blocking thyroid hormone release, antagonizing peripheral effects of thyroid hormone, providing supportive care, and providing patient and family education.

Inhibition of Thyroid Hormone Biosynthesis. Two drugs may be used to inhibit thyroid hormone biosynthesis—propylthiouracil (PTU) and methimazole (Tapazole). Propylthiouracil is the drug of choice because in large doses it inhibits conversion of T_4 to T_3 in peripheral tissues, resulting in a more rapid reduction of circulating thyroid hormone levels. Neither of these drugs is available in IV form. A patient in thyroid crisis should receive propylthiouracil 600 to 1000 mg orally as a loading dose and then 200 to 250 mg orally every 4 hours until thyroid storm is controlled. Methimazole is administered in a 60- to 100-mg oral loading dose and then 20 mg orally every 4 hours. Both drugs can produce agranulocytosis and bleeding tendencies; other potential side effects include paresthesias, vertigo, drowsiness, nausea, and headaches.

The big drawback to both PTU and methimazole is that they lack immediate effect. They do not block the release of thyroid hormones already stored in the thyroid gland and may take weeks or even months to lower thyroid hormone levels to normal.

Blockage of Thyroid Hormone Release. Iodide agents have the ability to inhibit the release of thyroid hormones from the thyroid gland, and at high doses, they may also inhibit thyroid hormone production. Lugol's solution (30 drops a day in three to four doses) or saturated solution of potassium iodide (5 drops every 6 hours) is usually given. These drugs must be given 1 to 2 hours after antithyroid drugs (PTU or methimazole) to prevent the iodide from being used to synthesize more T_4. Possible side effects of iodide agents include metallic taste, inflammation of the salivary glands, rhinitis, headaches, diarrhea, and gastritis.

Ipodate (Oragrafin) and iopanoic acid (Telepaque) are radiographic contrast dyes that have also been used to block thyroid hormone release. Ipodate inhibits peripheral conversion of T_4 to T_3, blocks release due to its large iodide content, and may inhibit binding of thyroid hormones to cellular receptors. Ipodate is given at a dose of 0.5 to 3 g orally daily. Iopanoic acid 0.5 g twice a day may also be given.

Lithium carbonate also inhibits the release of thyroid hormones but is more toxic, so it is used only in patients with an iodide allergy. It can be given orally or by nasogastric tube at doses of 300 mg every 6 hours. Serum T_4 levels fall approximately 30 to 50% with any of these drugs, with stabilization in 3 to 6 days.

Antagonism of Peripheral Effects of Thyroid Hormones. Because it may take days or longer for the

Table 15–22. DRUGS USED TO TREAT THYROID STORM

Drug	Action/Use	Dosage/Route	Side Effects	Nursing Implications
Propylthiouracil (PTU)	Inhibits synthesis of thyroid hormones; inhibits peripheral conversion of T_4 to T_3	600–1000 mg PO loading dose; 200–250 mg PO every 4 hr	Granulocytopenia, thrombocytopenia, bleeding paresthesias, vertigo, drowsiness, depression, nausea and vomiting, epigastric distress, skin pigmentation, rash, loss of hair, edema	Monitor for bleeding tendencies, decreased platelet count Provide small, frequent meals if GI problems Monitor for neurological changes and provide safety measures Provide frequent skin care
Methimazole (Tapazole)	Inhibits thyroid hormone synthesis	60–100 mg PO loading dose; 20 mg every 4 hr	Same as above	Same as above
Lugol's solution, saturated solution of potassium iodide (SSKI)	Inhibit synthesis of thyroid hormones and their release into the circulation	Lugol's: 30 drops PO daily in 3–4 doses SSKI: 5 drops every 6 hr	Rash, metallic taste, burning mouth, sore teeth/gums, inflammation of salivary glands, headaches, gastritis, diarrhea, allergic reactions	Monitor for allergic reactions; acute toxicity (vomiting, abdominal pain, diarrhea, circulatory collapse) Provide frequent mouth care; dilute with fruit juice or water to improve taste Provide small, frequent meals if GI problems Give 1–2 hr after antithyroid drugs
Ipodate, iopanoic acid	Inhibit peripheral conversion of T_4 to T_3; blocks release into circulation; may inhibit binding of hormone to cell receptors	Ipodate: 0.5–3 g PO daily Iopanoic acid: 0.5 g bid	Flushing, warmth, tingling sensations, vertigo, nausea, metallic taste, allergic reaction, apprehension, restlessness, hypotension	Monitor for allergic reactions; acute toxicity (vomiting, abdominal pain, diarrhea, shock) Provide frequent mouth care Provide small, frequent meals if GI problems Give 1–2 hr after antithyroid drugs

Drug	Action	Dosage	Side Effects	Nursing Considerations
Propranolol (Inderal)	Blocks beta-adrenergic receptors in heart and juxtaglomerular apparatus; decreases sympathetic influence, causing decreased cardiac contractility, decreased heart rate, decreased renin release, and decreased blood pressure; also partially inhibits peripheral conversion of T_4 to T_3	IV: 1–2 mg bolus every 10–15 min up to 15–20 mg; PO: 160–480 mg daily in divided doses	Bradycardia, congestive heart failure, dysrhythmias, hypotension, dizziness, vertigo, tinnitus, bronchospasm, dyspnea, rhinitis; GI upset: pain, nausea, vomiting, anorexia	Contraindicated in patients with chronic lung disease, hypotension, pulmonary edema, or heart block; Caution in patients on insulin, oral hypoglycemic agents, and monoamine oxidase inhibitors and in pregnant women; Continuous cardiac monitoring and frequent blood pressure monitoring necessary when giving intravenously; Give with food if administering orally; Assess for side effects and consult with physician if they occur
Reserpine	Depletes catecholamine stores, reducing heart rate and blood pressure; also has sedative and tranquilizing effects	1–5 mg IM loading dose; then 1.0–2.5 mg every 4–6 hr	Cutaneous flushing, diarrhea, central nervous system depression, orthostatic hypotension	Monitor for central nervous system effects; Monitor blood pressure closely
Guanethidine (Ismelin)	Depletes catecholamine stores and blocks catecholamine release, reducing blood pressure	1–2 mg/kg PO daily	Dizziness, weakness, syncope, hypotension, diarrhea, fluid retention, edema	Same as reserpine

above treatments to have full effect, immediate action is necessary to minimize the dramatic effects of thyroid storm on the major organ systems. The mortality rate of thyroid storm has been significantly reduced with the introduction of beta-blockers to block the peripheral effects of thyroid hormones. The drug used most frequently is propranolol (Inderal); however, other beta-blockers such as esmolol hydrochloride (Brevibloc) or atenolol (Tenormin) may also be used. Beta-blockers markedly reduce the effects of thyroid hormones on the cardiovascular system, decreasing cardiac output, decreasing heart rate, and diminishing supraventricular dysrhythmias. They also have the ability to partially inhibit peripheral conversion of T_4 to T_3. Propranolol may be given in 1- to 2-mg IV boluses every 10 to 15 minutes, up to 15 to 20 mg. The IV route is indicated if the patient is comatose or is unable to take oral medications or if the heart rate is greater than 140 beats/min. Oral doses range from 160 to 480 mg daily in divided doses. The usual starting dose is 20 to 40 mg every 6 hours. The dose is individualized to the patient's response. Results should be seen within minutes using the IV route and within 1 hour using the oral route. IV effects should last 3 to 4 hours. Propranolol is contraindicated in patients with chronic lung disease (asthma, emphysema), hypotension, pulmonary edema, or heart block. Caution must also be used in patients who are on insulin or oral hypoglycemic agents, patients on monoamine inhibitors, and pregnant women.

If propranolol cannot be used, guanethidine and reserpine may be used instead. Reserpine decreases hyperthermia, tachycardia, and psychological aberrations within 4 to 6 hours. Problems with reserpine include its slow onset, nervous system depression, flushing, and diarrhea. Guanethidine takes several days to take effect and can produce orthostatic hypotension and deplete myocardial catecholamines.

Drugs used to treat thyroid storm are summarized in Table 15–22 (see pp. 500–501).

Supportive Care

1. Fluid and electrolyte deficits should be corrected with adequate hydration with glucose and multivitamins.
2. Fever should be treated with external cooling measures and acetaminophen. Aspirin should be avoided because it increases the level of free T_4. If shivering occurs, treat it with chlorpromazine, meperidine, or barbiturates.
3. Stress doses of glucocorticoids are given to cover possible adrenal insufficiency and minimize the effects of increased glucocorticoid turnover and degradation that occur in thyroid crisis. Hydrocortisone 200 to 300 mg IV initially, followed by 300 mg daily via

IV drip, is given. Dexamethasone 8 to 10 mg daily in three doses can also be used.
4. Digoxin is given to patients in congestive heart failure or with tachydysrhythmias. Calcium blockers such as verapamil and diltiazem may also be effective in controlling heart rate and rhythm.
5. If able to eat, patients should be given high-calorie, high-protein diets to support them during this state of hypermetabolism and protein catabolism. If patients are unable to eat, hyperalimentation or enteral feeding should be instituted.
6. Dialysis and plasmapheresis have been utilized with some success to remove large amounts of protein-bound thyroid hormones.

Patient and Family Education. Education of patients, families, and significant others is crucial in identifying and preventing episodes of thyroid storm. Teaching varies, depending on the long-term therapy chosen for each patient—e.g., drugs versus radioactive iodine or surgery. For a patient receiving drug therapy, discharge goals include the patient and/or significant other being able to:

• Describe the pathophysiology and therapeutic regimen for hyperthyroidism
• Identify the signs and symptoms associated with the development of hyperthyroid crisis
• Describe situations that require notification of the physician
• Describe the rationale for and appropriate administration of drugs used in treatment
• Identify signs and symptoms of side effects associated with the therapeutic regimen (agranulocytosis, hypothyroidism)

Table 15–23 contains a summary of the treatment of thyroid storm.

Patient Outcomes

Outcomes for a patient with thyroid storm include:

• Stable hemodynamic parameters and metabolic rate
• Temperature within normal range
• Effective breathing pattern
• Nutritional needs met and weight maintained
• Skin intact without petechiae
• Return to baseline activity level
• Return to baseline mentation and personality
• Patient/significant others will verbalize an understanding of the patient's illness, anticipated treatment, and potential complications

See the Nursing Care Plan for the Patient with Thyroid Storm.

Table 15–23. TREATMENT OF THYROID STORM

Identify and treat precipitating cause

Inhibit hormone biosynthesis
  Propylthiouracil (PTU) 600–1000 mg PO loading;
    200–250 mg every 4 hr until thyrotoxicosis controlled,
    or
  Methimazole (Tapazole) 60–100 mg PO loading dose;
    20 mg PO every 4 hr

Block thyroid hormone release

  Lugol's solution 30 drops daily PO in 3–4 doses
  SSKI 5 drops every 6 hr
  Ipodate 0.5–3 g PO daily
  Iopanoic acid 0.5 g PO twice daily
  Give 1–2 hr after PTU or methimazole loading dose

Antagonize peripheral effects of thyroid hormone

  Propranolol (Inderal) 1–2 mg IV boluses every 10–15
    min up to 15–20 mg IV; 160–480 mg daily PO;
    individualized to response; if beta-blocker
    contraindicated, give reserpine or guanethidine

Supportive therapy

  Correct fluid and electrolyte imbalance
  Treat hyperthermia (no aspirin)
  Hydrocortisone 200–300 mg IV loading, then 300 mg
    IV drip over 24 hr
  Digoxin for congestive heart failure or
    tachydysrhythmia; calcium blockers may be better
    at controlling heart rate and rhythm
  High-calorie, high-protein diet

Patient and family education

SSKI = saturated solution of potassium iodide.

MYXEDEMA COMA

Pathophysiology

Myxedema coma in the absence of an associated stress or illness is uncommon, with infection being the most frequent stressor. The addition of stress to an already hypothyroid patient accelerates the metabolism and clearance of whatever thyroid hormone is present in the body. Thus, he or she experiences increased hormone utilization but decreased hormone production, which precipitates a crisis state.

As in hyperthyroidism, low levels of thyroid hormones also disrupt the normal physiology of most body systems. Hypothyroidism produces a hypodynamic, hypometabolic state. Myxedema coma is a magnification of these disruptions initiated by some type of stressor, as indicated above. Myxedema coma takes many months to develop and should be suspected in patients with a known thyroid history, with a surgical scar on the lower neck, or in those who are unusually sensitive to medications or narcotics. Common findings in patients with myxedema coma are dis-

cussed below and contrasted with those of thyroid storm in Table 15–19.

Etiology. The underlying causes of myxedema coma are those that produce hypothyroidism. Most cases occur either in patients with long-standing autoimmune disease of the thyroid (Hashimoto's thyroiditis) or in patients who have received surgical or radioactive iodine treatment for Graves' disease and have received inadequate hormone replacement. It is rarely associated with hypothyroidism produced by pituitary or hypothalamic disorders. These and other less common causes of hypothyroidism are listed in Table 15–24.

Myxedema coma is the end stage of improperly treated, neglected, or undiagnosed hypothyroidism. It is a life-threatening emergency with a mortality rate as high as 50% despite appropriate therapy. Much of this mortality can be attributed to underlying illnesses. Most patients who develop myxedema coma are elderly females. It is rarely seen in young individuals. It occurs more frequently in winter as a result of the increased stress of exposure to cold in an individual unable to maintain body heat. It is also associated with other types of physiological or psychological stress or underlying illness. Known precipitating factors include exposure to cold, infection, trauma, critical illness, and administration of central nervous system depressants such as narcotics, barbiturates, or anesthesia. Common underlying illnesses include infection, anemia, heart failure, ascites, pleural and pericardial effusions, seizures, and aspiration.

Table 15–24. CAUSES OF HYPOTHYROIDISM

Primary Thyroid Disease

  Autoimmune (Hashimoto's thyroiditis)
  Radioactive iodine treatment of Graves' disease
  Thyroidectomy
  Congenital enzymatic defect in thyroid hormone
    biosynthesis
  Inhibition of thyroid hormone synthesis or release
    Antithyroid drugs
    Iodides
    Lithium carbonate
    Oral hypoglycemic agents
  Idiopathic thyroid atrophy

Secondary (Pituitary)/Tertiary (Hypothalamus) Disease

  Tumors
  Infiltrative disease (sarcoidosis)
  Hypophysectomy
  Pituitary irradiation
  Head injury
  Pituitary infarction

NURSING CARE PLAN FOR THE PATIENT WITH THYROID STORM

Nursing Diagnosis	Patient Outcomes	Nursing Interventions
Decreased cardiac output related to increased metabolic demands on heart, extreme tachycardia, dysrhythmias, congestive heart failure.	Stable hemodynamic parameters and metabolic rate as evidenced by: Cardiac output 4–8 L/min; cardiac index 2.8–4.2 L/min/m². Pulmonary artery pressures, wedge pressure, and CVP within normal range. Return to baseline BP for patient. Heart rate 60–100 beats/min. Control of dysrhythmias. Urine output >30 ml/h.	Control temperature (see nursing diagnosis of hyperthermia below). Assess/monitor for signs and symptoms of cardiac compromise: Blood pressure, pulse pressure. Apical pulse, resting heart rate. Pulmonary artery and wedge pressures, CVP. Cardiac output, cardiac index, SVR. Respiratory rate, breath sounds, secretions. Dysrhythmias. Heart sounds: S_1, S_2, gallop, murmur. Complaints of chest pain, palpitations, shortness of breath, signs of ischemia. Hourly urine output. Provide adequate hydration, monitor hemodynamic response to fluid therapy. Monitor electrolyte status: Monitor potassium and calcium levels. Watch for signs/symptoms of hypokalemia or hypercalcemia. Administer digoxin as ordered and monitor response. Minimize demand on heart by controlling activity. Assess for previous history of chronic lung disease, heart block, pulmonary edema (propranolol contraindicated). Administer and monitor effects of drugs utilized to combat thyroid hormone effects: Assess response to propranolol: BP, HR, CO, PAP, PCWP, CVP. Assess response to antithyroid drugs and monitor for toxic effects (see Table 15–22).
Hyperthermia related to loss of temperature regulation, increased metabolism, increased heat production.	Temperature return to normal range: 37°C (98.6°F).	Monitor patient's temperature every 1 h; continuously with probe if possible. Assess fluid status: hourly I/O, daily weights, diaphoresis, skin turgor, mucous membranes. Utilize cooling measures to decrease temperature: Administer acetaminophen (no aspirin). Ice packs (axillae and groin). Cooling mattress. Minimal covers. Control room temperature. Administer and monitor effects of drugs utilized to combat thyroid hormone effects. Administer antibiotics if infection a precipitator.

NURSING CARE PLAN FOR THE PATIENT WITH THYROID STORM *Continued*

Nursing Diagnosis	Patient Outcomes	Nursing Interventions
Ineffective breathing pattern related to muscle weakness and decreased vital capacity resulting in hypoventilation and CO_2 retention, increased oxygen need from hypermetabolism.	Effective breathing pattern as evidenced by: Normal respiratory rate, depth, and pattern. Normal $PaCO_2$ (35–45 mm Hg) and pH (7.35–7.45) and ABG analysis or return to patient baseline. PaO_2 >60 mm Hg. Normal vital capacity, tidal volume. Resolution of muscle weakness. Patient reports breathing easier.	Assess respiratory status every 4 h; every 1–2 h in patient with altered level of consciousness. Assess airway and breathing effort, use of accessory muscles. Assess rate and depth of respiration. Auscultate breath sounds. Obtain ABGs as ordered and PRN. Obtain pulmonary function parameters: tidal volume, vital capacity. Assess subjective complaints of shortness of breath, dyspnea on exertion. Provide supportive measures to facilitate respiratory effort: Airway, supplementary oxygen, suctioning, intubation equipment/ventilator. Position patient for ease of respiratory effort (i.e., head of bed elevated). Provide quiet, restful environment. Allow frequent rest periods. Minimize activity to decrease oxygen need. Send sputum for culture and sensitivity. Administer antibiotics if ordered. Administer and monitor effects of drugs utilized to combat thyroid hormone effects.
Altered nutrition (less than body requirements) related to increased peristalsis, decreased absorption, increased requirements.	Body weight will stabilize at patient's normal level. Nutritional needs met: Serum albumin 3.5–5.5 g/dl. Serum glucose 70–110 mg/dl.	Assess effects of thyroid hormone on GI system: Bowel sounds; abdominal pain. Nausea and vomiting. Increased number/frequency of bowel movements, diarrhea. Normal vs current weight (i.e., recent weight loss). Serum albumin level. Fatigue, weakness. Liver function tests, BUN. Provide adequate nutrition and calories: Provide high-calorie, high-protein diet. Avoid foods that increase peristalsis, such as tea, coffee, and fibrous and highly seasoned foods. Monitor adequacy of patient's intake; take measures to supplement if necessary (i.e., tube feedings, parenteral nutrition). Weigh patient daily on same scale at same time of day. Provide multivitamin and mineral supplements as needed. Provide frequent, small feedings. Monitor BUN, creatinine to assess positive nitrogen balance. Minimize activity to decrease energy requirement. Provide adequate glucose to support energy needs: Provide adequate dextrose in IV fluids. Administer hydrocortisone as ordered. Monitor for signs and symptoms of hyperglycemia (polyuria, polydipsia, weakness, fatigue, lethargy). Monitor serum glucose levels. Administer and monitor effects of drugs utilized to combat thyroid hormone effects.
Risk for impaired skin integrity related to thin skin, fragile blood vessels.	Skin intact without breakdown or petechiae.	Provide pressure relief measures (e.g., egg-crate, air mattress, heel pads). Turn and reposition every 2 h. Cleanse skin frequently to maintain minimal moisture. Check skin for signs of bleeding and pressure areas. Provide frequent mouth care.

Continued on following page

NURSING CARE PLAN FOR THE PATIENT WITH THYROID STORM *Continued*

Nursing Diagnosis	Patient Outcomes	Nursing Interventions

Activity intolerance related to muscle weakness, muscle wasting, tremors, fatigue, anemia, and extreme energy expenditure.	Patient will return to baseline activity level.	During acute crisis, minimize physical activity:
		  Provide all daily care for patient.
		  Maintain on bed rest.
		Allow for adequate rest/sleep periods:
		  Minimize group interruptions.
		  Assess patient's normal sleep patterns/habits and try to accommodate them.
		  Maintain quiet, calm environment.
		  Administer sedatives if ordered and assess effectiveness.
		  Assess for and provide patient with calming diversional activities.
		Provide adequate nutrition.
		Increase activity gradually after acute crisis abates; monitor physical response to activity.
		Administer oxygen during activity.
		Administer and monitor effects of drugs utilized to combat thyroid hormone effects.

Altered thought processes related to hypermetabolism and increased cerebration, agitation, delirium, psychosis.	Return to baseline mentation and behavior.
	Return to normal personality (per family/ significant others).
		Assess for degree of physiological/psychological dysfunction:
		  Orientation.
		  Irritability, nervousness, agitation.
		  Memory, attention span.
		  Mood swings, fear, paranoia.
		  Convulsions, stupor, coma.
		  Tremors: tongue, eyelids, peripheral.
		  Muscle weakness.
		Minimize effects of environment on mental status:
		  Reorient patient frequently.
		  Maintain quiet environment, minimizing extraneous stimuli.
		  Provide simple, brief explanations of activities, procedures, or equipment.
		  Provide meaningful, relaxing stimuli to patient.
		Minimize physiological effects of hypermetabolism:
		  Initiate protective measures for patient with convulsions/agitation/delusions: padded side rails, soft restraints, close supervision.
		  Provide all care if level of consciousness decreased.
		  Minimize physical exertion required by patient.
		  Assist patient with daily care as needed.
		Administer and monitor effects of drugs utilized to combat thyroid hormone effects.

Knowledge deficit related to disease process, therapeutic regimen, prevention of complications.	Patient/family member/ significant other will verbalize an understanding of the patient's illness, anticipated treatment, and potential complications.	Assess patient/family current level of knowledge and readiness to learn. Design teaching program that includes the following information as appropriate: Pathophysiology and hyperthyroidism. Signs of symptoms associated with hyperthyroid crisis. Situations that require notification of physician. Rationale for and appropriate administration of drugs. Signs and symptoms of side effects associated with therapeutic regimen (agranulocytosis, hypothyroidism). Provide written materials for all content taught; provide means for the patient to get questions answered after discharge. Schedule follow-up teaching session after discharge.

Assessment

Clinical Presentation. Many patients may have had vague signs and symptoms of hypothyroidism for several years. The earliest signs may be fatigue, weakness, muscle cramps, and intolerance to cold. Again, the clinical picture of myxedema coma varies with the rate of onset and severity. Diagnosis is based on the clinical signs and symptoms, a high index of suspicion, and a careful history and physical examination. Many of the manifestations are attributable to the development of mucinous edema. This interstitial edema is the result of water retention and decreased protein. It gives the face a puffy, pallid appearance, and the tongue may be enlarged. Fluid collection in joints and muscles may produce complaints of stiffness and muscle cramps. It can also produce pericardial effusion and contribute to weight gain.

Neurological Disturbances. The decreased metabolic rate and resulting decreased cerebration produce both psychological and physiological changes. Difficulty concentrating, slowed mentation, depression, lethargy, somnolence, and coma can all be seen. Grand mal seizures can occur. Speech may be slow and deliberate, and the patient may have a coarse, raspy, hoarse voice as a result of mucinous edema of the vocal cords. Mucinous edema can also produce hearing loss and vertigo. Personality changes such as paranoia and delusions may develop.

Patients with hypothyroidism are unable to maintain body heat due to the decreased metabolic rate and production of thermal energy. Because of this, patients may present in crisis after being stressed by exposure to cold. Hypothermia is present in 80% of patients in myxedema coma, with temperatures as low as 80°F (26.7°C) (Isley, 1993). Patients with temperatures less than 88.6°F (32°C) have a grave prognosis. If a patient with myxedema coma has a temperature greater than 98.6°F (37°C), underlying infection should be suspected.

Cardiovascular Disturbances. Cardiac function is depressed, resulting in decreased contractility, decreased stroke volume, decreased heart rate, and decreased cardiac output. The patient may develop a pericardial effusion, making heart tones distant. The ECG has decreased voltage as a result of the pericardial effusion. Because of the diminished adrenergic stimulation produced by low thyroid levels, hypotension may be present. However, these patients may also be hypertensive because of atherosclerotic disease.

Pulmonary Disturbances. Respirations are depressed, producing hypoventilation and CO_2 retention. Patients may experience dyspnea on exertion because they are unable to increase respiratory efforts with activity. As part of the picture of generalized mucinous edema and fluid retention, these patients may also develop pleural effusions or upper airway edema, further restricting their breathing.

GI Disturbances. Decreased thyroid levels decrease appetite, decrease peristalsis, and interfere with carbohydrate metabolism. Patients frequently experience anorexia, decreased bowel sounds, constipation, and paralytic ileus. Fluid retention and the decreased metabolic rate, however, result in weight gain and ascites.

Skeletal Muscle Disturbances. Slowed motor conduction produces decreased tendon reflexes and sluggish, awkward movements.

Integumentary Disturbances. Patients typically have dry, flaky, cool, coarse skin; dry, coarse hair; and brittle nails. They may also have a yellow tint to their skin that results from depressed hepatic conversion of carotene to vitamin A. Generalized mucinous edema develops, especially in the eyelids, periorbital tissue, and dorsa of the hands and feet. Ecchymoses may develop from increased capillary fragility and decreased platelets.

Laboratory Evaluation. Serum T_4 and T_3 levels and resin T_3 uptake are low in patients with myxedema coma. In primary hypothyroidism, TSH levels are high. If hypothyroidism is the result of disease of the pituitary gland or hypothalamus (secondary and tertiary hypothyroidism), TSH levels are inappropriately normal or low. However, as in patients with thyroid storm, if myxedema coma is suspected, treatment should not be delayed while awaiting these results to confirm the diagnosis.

Serum sodium levels may be low due to impaired water excretion and resultant water retention. Impaired water excretion is the result of the inappropriate ADH secretion and cortisol deficiency that frequently accompany hypothyroidism. The patient should be monitored for signs and symptoms related to hyponatremia such as weakness, muscle twitching, seizures, and coma.

Hypoglycemia is uncommon unless hypothyroidism is related to pituitary or hypophyseal disorders and/or coexists with adrenal insufficiency. Adrenal insufficiency may also result in serum cortisol levels that are inappropriately low for stress.

Complete blood count may show a normochromic normocytic anemia. Leukocytosis (elevated white count) is frequently absent, despite stress or underlying illness.

The slowed metabolism also causes elevated creatine phosphokinase, aspartate aminotransferase, lactate dehydrogenase, cholesterol, and triglycerides. Elevated cholesterol and triglycerides predispose individuals with hypothyroidism to the development of atherosclerosis.

Laboratory manifestations of myxedema coma are summarized in Table 15–21 (see p. 499).

Nursing Diagnoses

The nursing diagnoses that may apply to a patient in myxedema coma are based on assessment data and include:

- Fluid volume excess related to impaired water excretion
- Decreased cardiac output related to decreased contractility, decreased heart rate, decreased stroke volume, pericardial effusions, dysrhythmias
- Hypothermia related to the body's inability to retain heat
- Altered thought processes related to slowed metabolism, cerebration, hyponatremia
- Ineffective breathing pattern related to hypoventilation, muscle weakness, decreased respiratory rate, ascites, pleural effusions
- Risk for injury related to edema, decreased platelets
- Activity intolerance related to muscle weakness, anemia
- Altered nutrition (less than body requirements) related to decreased appetite, decreased carbohydrate metabolism, hypoglycemia
- Knowledge deficit related to disease process, therapeutic regimen, prevention of complications

Nursing and Medical Interventions

Myxedema coma requires immediate intervention if the patient is to survive. The primary objectives in the treatment of myxedema coma are identifying and treating the precipitating cause, providing thyroid replacement, restoring fluid and electrolyte balance, providing supportive care, and providing patient and family education.

Thyroid Replacement. The best method of thyroid replacement is controversial. Either liothyronine sodium (Cytomel; T_3) or levothyroxine sodium (Synthroid; T_4) can be used. T_3 is more potent than T_4, and most of T_3 comes from peripheral conversion of T_4 to T_3. Thus, liothyronine requires lower doses, and levothyroxine ultimately provides the patient with both T_4 and T_3 replacement.

Levothyroxine sodium is the more commonly used drug. It has a smoother effect and a longer activity, and a portion of it is converted to T_3 in peripheral tissues. A dose of 300 to 500 μg IV (2 μg/kg) is required to restore a patient in myxedema coma to a low-normal thyroid state. The preferred route is IV, because absorption of oral or intramuscular levothyroxine is variable. The initial dose may be decreased if the patient has underlying factors such as angina,

dysrhythmias, or other heart disease. These patients may receive only 300 μg initially. The initial bolus is followed by 50 μg IV or 100 to 200 μg orally daily.

Liothyronine sodium has heightened metabolic effects, a more rapid onset (6 hours), and a shorter half-life (1 day) than levothyroxine. The recommended dose is 25 μg IV every 8 hours for the first 24 to 48 hours, followed by 12.5 μg every 8 hours until the patient regains consciousness and can take oral medication. Because of liothyronine's potency, its administration may be complicated by angina, myocardial infarction, and cardiac irritability. Thus, it is generally avoided in older populations and is not used in myxedema coma.

The effects of levothyroxine are not as rapid as those of liothyronine, but its cardiac toxicity is lower. Serum levels of T_4 reach normal in 1 to 2 days. Levels of TSH begin to fall within 24 hours and return to normal in 7 to 10 days. Drugs used to treat myxedema coma are summarized in Table 15–25.

Fluid and Electrolyte Restoration. If the patient is hypotensive or in shock, thyroid replacement usually corrects this, but cautious volume expansion with saline also helps. Vasopressors should be used with extreme caution. Patients in myxedema coma are unable to respond to vasopressors until they have adequate levels of thyroid hormones available. Simultaneous administration of vasopressors and thyroid hormones is associated with myocardial irritability.

Hyponatremia usually responds to thyroid replacement and water restriction; the patient is able to get rid of free water once thyroid hormones are replaced. If hyponatremia is severe (less than 110 mEq/L) or patient is having seizures, hypertonic saline with or without furosemide (Lasix) may be administered, but only until symptoms disappear or the sodium level is 120 mEq/L.

Glucose should be added to IV fluids to provide support to a patient with hypoglycemia and/or concomitant adrenal insufficiency. Hydrocortisone 100 mg is given initially, followed by 50 to 100 mg every 6 hours in the first 24 hours. Subsequently, the dose is 50 to 100 mg every 8 hours for 7 to 10 days. The adrenal abnormality may last several weeks after thyroid replacement is begun, so this support should be continued during that time.

Supportive Care

1. Hypothermia is treated by passive methods, such as blankets. A more active method of rewarming such as a heating blanket can result in peripheral vasodilatation, circulatory collapse, and death. Thyroid replacement slowly returns the patient's temperature to normal.

2. Ventilatory support may range from oxygen

Table 15-25. DRUGS USED TO TREAT MYXEDEMA COMA

Drug	Action/Use	Dosage/Route	Side Effects	Nursing Implications
Levothyroxine sodium (Synthroid)	Same as thyroid hormone (see Table 15-18)	300–500 µg IV loading dose then 50 µg/day	Symptoms of hyperthyroidism, allergic skin reactions	Monitor for signs and symptoms of hyperthyroidism Monitor cardiac response closely
Liothyronine sodium (Cytomel)	Same as thyroid hormone (see Table 15-18)	25 µg IV every 8 hr for 24–48 hr; then 12.5 µg every 8 hr	Same as levothyroxine plus angina, myocardial infarction, cardiac irritability	Same as levothyroxine

supplementation to intubation and assisted ventilation. This depends on the severity of hypoventilation, hypoxia, and hypercapnia.

3. Avoid narcotics and sedative drugs. All drugs need to be administered cautiously due to the patient's hypometabolic state. As a result, he or she will have delayed drug turnover and degradation.

Patient and Family Education. The education of patients, family, and significant others is critical in identifying and preventing episodes of myxedema coma. Discharge goals include the patient and/or significant other being able to:

- Describe the pathophysiology and therapeutic regimen for hypothyroidism
- Identify the signs and symptoms associated with the development of hypothyroid crisis
- List stressors that can produce a hypothyroid crisis
- Describe situations that require notification of the physician
- Describe the rationale for and appropriate administration of drugs used in treatment
- Identify signs and symptoms of side effects and toxic effects associated with thyroid replacement drugs (hyperthyroidism, angina)

The treatment of myxedema coma is summarized in Table 15-26.

Patient Outcomes

Outcomes for a patient with myxedema coma include:

- Normal fluid volume
- Normal hemodynamics and metabolic rate
- Temperature within normal range
- Return to baseline mentation and personality
- Effective breathing pattern
- Intact skin without edema or bleeding

- Return to baseline activity level
- Adequate nutrition and stable body weight
- Patient and/or significant other able to verbalize understanding of disease, therapeutic regimen, and prevention of complications

See the Nursing Care Plan for the Patient in Myxedema Coma.

Antidiuretic Hormone Disorders

REVIEW OF PHYSIOLOGY

The primary function of ADH is regulation of water balance and serum osmolality. ADH (also known as arginine vasopressin) is produced in the supraoptic nuclei and paraventricular nuclei of the hypothalamus. These nuclei are positioned near the thirst center and osmoreceptors in the hypothalamus (Fig. 15–11). Once

Table 15-26. TREATMENT OF MYXEDEMA COMA

Identify and treat underlying disorder

Thyroid replacement: levothyroxine sodium 300–500 µg IV loading; 50 µg/day IV

Restore fluid and electrolyte balance
Administer vasopressors cautiously
Hyponatremia: <115 mEq/L, hypertonic saline; >120 mEq/L, fluid restriction
Hypoglycemia: IV glucose
Adrenal hormone replacement: hydrocortisone 100 mg IV bolus; 50–100 mg every 6 hr over first 24 hr up to 500 mg; then 50–100 mg IV every 8 hr for 7–10 days

Supportive care
Passive warming with blankets (do not actively warm)
Ventilatory assistance
Avoid narcotics and sedative drugs

Patient and family education

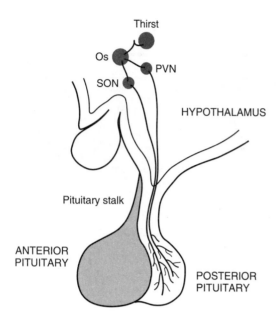

Thirst
Os
SON
PVN
HYPOTHALAMUS
Pituitary stalk
ANTERIOR PITUITARY
POSTERIOR PITUITARY

Figure 15–11. Hypothalamic-posterior pituitary system.

NURSING CARE PLAN FOR THE PATIENT IN MYXEDEMA COMA		
Nursing Diagnosis	Patient Outcomes	Nursing Interventions
Fluid volume excess related to impaired water excretion.	Normal fluid volume as indicated by: Urine output >30 ml/h. Blood pressure within 10 mm Hg of patient baseline. Weight close to patient baseline. No edema. No pericardial or pleural effusions.	Maintain fluid restriction. Monitor hourly I&O. Daily weight on same scale at same time of day. Monitor for signs and symptoms of hyponatremia. Monitor for signs and symptoms of cardiac failure (see nursing diagnosis for decreased cardiac output below). Institute protective measures to prevent injury related to edema (see nursing diagnosis for risk for injury below). Monitor blood pressure every 1 h. Administer and monitor effects of thyroid drugs.
Decreased cardiac output related to decreased contractility, decreased heart rate, decreased stroke volume, pericardial effusions, dysrhythmias.	Normal hemodynamics and metabolic rate as evidenced by: Cardiac output 4–8 L/ min; cardiac index 2.8–4.2 min/m². Pulmonary artery pressure, wedge pressure, and CVP within normal limits. Blood pressure within 10 mm Hg of patient baseline. Urine output >30 ml/h. Control of dysrhythmias. No pericardial effusion.	Assess and monitor patients for signs/symptoms of cardiovascular collapse: Cardiac output, cardiac index, SVR. Heart sounds: diminished, murmur, gallop. BP every 1 h. Urine output every 1 h. Chest pain, signs of ischemia. Heart rate and rhythm. Institute treatment to control dysrhythmias. Administer volume or vasopressors cautiously to maintain BP. Administer and monitor effects of thyroid replacement drugs.
Hypothermia related to inability of body to retain heat.	Temperature 37°C (98.6°F).	Warm patient passively with blankets (no active warming). Monitor temperature every 1–2 h or continuously with probe. Control room temperature; avoid exposure to cold. Administer and monitor effects of thyroid replacement drugs.

NURSING CARE PLAN FOR THE PATIENT IN MYXEDEMA COMA *Continued*

Nursing Diagnosis	Patient Outcomes	Nursing Interventions
Altered thought processes related to slowed metabolism and cerebration, hyponatremia.	Return to baseline mentation. Normal personality pattern (per family member/ significant other).	Protect patient if having seizures: padded side rails. Provide simple, clear explanations of all activities, procedures, and equipment. Reorient as needed. Minimize extraneous, meaningless stimuli. Monitor serum sodium and signs of hyponatremia. Administer and monitor effects of thyroid replacement drugs.
Ineffective breathing pattern related to hypoventilation, muscle weakness, decreased respiratory rate, ascites, pleural effusions.	Effective breathing pattern as evidenced by: Normal rate and depth of ventilation. $PaCO_2$ 35–45 mm Hg, pH 7.35–7.45. Patient reports no dyspnea with activity.	Assess effect of hypometabolism on breathing: Rate, depth, and rhythm of respiration. Breath sounds. ABGs. Pulmonary function tests: tidal volume, vital capacity. Minimize physical activity. Provide ventilatory support as needed: supplemental oxygen, airway, suctioning, intubation, mechanical ventilation. Monitor tidal volume and vital capacity. Draw ABGs as ordered and PRN. Minimize water retention (see fluid volume excess above). Monitor anemia. Administer and monitor effects of thyroid replacement drugs.
Risk for injury related to edema, decreased platelets.	Intact skin without edema or bleeding.	Provide frequent mouth care. Keep skin warm, dry. Turn patient every 2 h. Provide pressure relief measures: egg-crate mattress, air mattress, heel protectors. Inspect skin every 2 h for signs of reddening or breakdown. Assess extent of edema. Assess for signs of bleeding: Monitor/minimize puncture sites for signs of bleeding, guaiac stools. Assess gastric and pulmonary secretions and urine for signs of blood. Assess for easy bruising.
Activity intolerance related to muscle weakness.	Patient will return to baseline activity level.	During acute crisis, minimize physical activity: Provide all daily cares for patient. Maintain on bed rest. Allow for adequate rest/sleep periods: Minimize group interruptions. Assess patient's normal sleep patterns/habits and try to accommodate them. Maintain quiet, calm environment. Provide adequate nutrition. Increase activity gradually when patient able. Administer and monitor effects of thyroid replacement drugs.

Continued on following page

NURSING CARE PLAN FOR THE PATIENT IN MYXEDEMA COMA *Continued*

Nursing Diagnosis	Patient Outcomes	Nursing Interventions
Altered nutrition (less than body requirements) related to decreased appetite, decreased carbohydrate metabolism, hypoglycemia.	Body weight will stabilize at patient's normal level. Adequate nutrition as evidenced by: Serum albumin: 3.5–5.5 g/dl. Serum glucose: 70–110 mg/dl.	Assess effects of lack of thyroid hormone on GI system: Bowel sounds. Anorexia. Constipation. Normal vs current weight (i.e., recent weight gain). Serum albumin level. Ascites. Provide adequate nutrition and calories: Provide low-calorie diet with increased protein and moderate sodium. Monitor adequacy of patient's intake; take measures to supplement if necessary (i.e., tube feedings, TPN). Weigh patient daily on same scale at same time of day. Provide adequate glucose to support metabolism: Provide adequate dextrose in IV fluids. Administer hydrocortisone as ordered. Monitor for signs and symptoms of hypoglycemia. Monitor serum glucose levels. Administer and monitor effects of thyroid replacement drugs.
Knowledge deficit related to disease process, therapeutic regimen, prevention of complications.	Patient/family member/ significant other verbalizes understanding of disease, therapeutic regimen, and prevention of complications.	Assess patient/significant other's level of knowledge and readiness to learn. Design a teaching program that includes information on: Pathophysiology of hypothyroidism. Therapeutic regimen prescribed for patient. Signs and symptoms associated with development of hypothyroid crisis. Stressors that can precipitate hypothyroid crisis. Situations that require notification of the physician. Rationale for and appropriate administration of drugs. Signs and symptoms of side effects associated with thyroid replacement drugs and toxicity (angina, hyperthyroidism). Provide written materials for all content taught; provide means for patient/family member/significant other to get questions answered after discharge. Schedule follow-up session after discharge.

produced, ADH is stored in neurons in the posterior pituitary. If the supraoptic and paraventricular nuclei are stimulated (via mechanisms described below), their discharge stimulates the nerve endings in the posterior pituitary to release ADH. This stimulation occurs in response to both osmotic and nonsmotic forces: osmoreceptors in the hypothalamus respond to changes in extracellular osmolality; stretch receptors in the left atrium and baroreceptors in the carotid sinus and aortic arch respond to changes in circulating volume and blood pressure, respectively. Once released, ADH acts on the renal distal and collecting tubules to cause water reabsorption. In high concentrations, ADH also acts on smooth muscles of the arterioles to produce vasoconstriction. Normally, ADH is released in response to increased serum osmolality (primary stimulus), elevated serum sodium, decreased blood volume (10% drop), decreased blood pressure (5 to 10% drop), stress, trauma, hypoxia, pain, and anxiety. Certain drugs, such as narcotics, barbiturates, anesthetics, and chemotherapeutic agents, are also known to stimulate ADH release. The physiology of ADH release is summarized in Figure 15–12. Two common disturbances

of ADH are diabetes insipidus (DI) and the syndrome of inappropriate antidiuretic hormone (SIADH).

DIABETES INSIPIDUS

Pathophysiology

DI results from an ADH deficiency (neurogenic DI), ADH insensitivity (nephrogenic DI), or excessive water intake (secondary DI). Regardless of the cause, the result is impaired renal conservation of water and polyuria (greater than 3 L in 24 hours). As long as the thirst center remains intact and the person is able to respond to this thirst, fluid volume can be maintained. If the patient is unable to respond, severe dehydration can result if fluid losses are not replaced. This defect may be permanent or transient.

In neurogenic DI, absent or diminished release of circulating levels of ADH from the posterior pituitary produce free water loss, causing serum osmolality and serum sodium to rise. The posterior pituitary is unable to respond by increasing ADH levels, thus the kidneys are not stimulated to reabsorb water, resulting in exces-

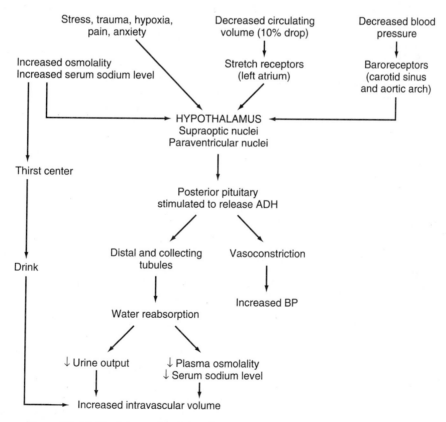

Figure 15–12. Physiology of antidiuretic hormone (ADH). BP = blood pressure.

sive water loss. Neurogenic DI occurs as the result of disruption of the neural pathways or structures involved in ADH production, synthesis, or release. A variety of disorders can produce neurogenic DI (Table 15–27), but the primary cause is traumatic injury to the posterior pituitary or hypothalamus as a result of head injury or surgery. Transient DI may occur after pituitary surgery or trauma due to manipulation of the pituitary stalk or cerebral edema. Permanent DI occurs when more than 80 to 85% of the supraoptic or paraventricular nuclei or the proximal end of the pituitary stalk is destroyed.

In nephrogenic DI, the kidney collecting ducts and distal tubules are unresponsive to ADH; thus, adequate levels of ADH may be synthesized and released, but the kidneys are unable to conserve water in response. Nephrogenic DI is usually acquired from chronic renal disease, drugs, or other conditions that produce permanent kidney damage.

Secondary DI is a syndrome characterized by excessive fluid intake. It results in a decrease in plasma osmolality and a decrease in ADH secretion and urine concentration. Water excretion rises to balance intake, and plasma osmolality stabilizes. In some patients, the excessive water intake seems to be due to an abnormal-ity in the regulation of thirst. In others, thirst is denied, and excessive drinking seems to be due to a more generalized cognitive dysfunction such as a mental illness. Secondary DI is often observed in psychotic patients motivated by factors other than thirst. Chronic polyuria in these patients leads to a reduction in urinary concentrating ability and water loss.

Assessment

Clinical Presentation. ADH suppression produces polyuria, as much as 5 to 40 L in 24 hours. The urine is pale and dilute. If the patient is unable to replace the water lost by responding to thirst, signs of hypovolemia will develop: hypotension, decreased skin turgor, dry mucous membranes, tachycardia, weight loss, and low central venous and pulmonary artery occlusion pressures. Neurological signs and symptoms may be produced by hypovolemia (decreased cerebral perfusion and cerebral dehydration) and hypernatremia: confusion, restlessness, irritability, lethargy, seizures, coma. A detailed listing of signs and symptoms of DI are found in Table 15–28.

Laboratory Evaluation. One of the classic signs of DI is the finding of an inappropriately low urine osmolality in the face of a high serum osmolality. Corresponding with the low urine osmolality is a decreased urine specific gravity. Serum osmolality is greater than 295 mOsm/kg and serum sodium is greater than 145 mEq/L. The presence of hypokalemia or hypercalcemia suggests nephrogenic DI. Other values such as BUN and creatinine may be elevated due to hemoconcentration. Plasma ADH may be measured to evaluate the cause of the DI. The level would be decreased in neurogenic DI, increased in nephrogenic DI, and normal in secondary DI.

If the cause of polyuria is unclear, additional diagnostic testing may be needed. A water deprivation test is typically done to determine whether the patient responds to hyperosmolality with the release of ADH. Water intake is restricted, and urine volume and serum osmolality are measured for 6 to 8 hours. If the urine remains dilute (urine osmolality less than 100 mOsm/kg, specific gravity less than 1.005) and polyuria continues in spite of increasing serum osmolality (greater than 300 mOsm/kg), the patient has DI. To differentiate neurogenic DI from nephrogenic DI, vasopressin 10 mU/kg^2 or 1 μg desmopressin is given. Urine is collected at 30-, 60-, 90-, and 120-minute intervals, and osmolality is measured. If urine volume decreases and the urine osmolality rises more than 50%, the patient has neurogenic DI. A patient with nephrogenic DI will not respond. Careful monitoring of the patient is mandatory during this testing to avoid dehydration and hypotension.

Table 15–27. CAUSES OF DIABETES INSIPIDUS (DI)

ADH Deficiency (Neurogenic DI)

Idiopathic; familial/congenital
Intracranial surgery, especially in region of pituitary
Tumors: craniopharyngioma, pituitary tumors,
  metastases to hypothalamus
Infections: meningitis, encephalitis
Granulomatous disease: tuberculosis, sarcoidosis,
  histiocytosis
Severe head trauma or any disorder that causes
  increased intracranial pressure

ADH Insensitivity (Nephrogenic DI)

Hereditary; idiopathic
Renal disease: pyelonephritis, polycystic kidney
  disease, obstructive uropathy, transplant
Multisystem disorders affecting kidneys: multiple
  myeloma, sickle cell disease, cystic fibrosis
Metabolic disturbances: chronic hypokalemia or
  hypercalcemia
Drugs: ethanol, phenytoin, lithium carbonate,
  demeclocycline, amphotericin, methoxyflurane

Secondary DI

Idiopathic
Psychogenic polydipsia
Hypothalamic disease: sarcoidosis
Excessive IV fluid administration
Drug induced: anticholinergic, tricyclic
  antidepressant

ADH = antidiuretic hormone.

Table 15–28. COMPARISON OF SIGNS AND SYMPTOMS OF ABNORMAL ANTIDIURETIC HORMONE SECRETION

System	Diabetes Insipidus	SIADH
Cardiovascular	Weight loss Hypotension Tachycardia Decreased skin turgor Dry mucous membranes CVP <2 mm Hg PCWP <8 mm Hg	Weight gain Hypertension CVP >10 mm Hg PCWP >12 mm Hg
Neurological	Confusion Restlessness Lethargy Irritability Seizures Coma	Confusion Restlessness Lethargy Weakness Difficulty concentrating Headache Seizures Coma
Renal	Pale, dilute urine Polyuria	Concentrated urine Decreased output
Gastrointestinal	Constipation	Nausea and vomiting Anorexia Muscle cramps Decreased bowel sounds
Pulmonary	Thick, tenacious secretions	Tachypnea Dyspnea Adventitious sounds Frothy, pink sputum
Laboratory values	Serum sodium >145 mEq/L Serum osmolality >295 mOsm/kg Urine osmolality decreased	Serum sodium <135 mEq/L Serum osmolality <275 mOsm/kg Urine osmolality increased

CVP = central venous pressure; PCWP = pulmonary capillary wedge pressure.

Nursing Diagnoses

The nursing diagnoses that may apply to a patient with DI include:

- Fluid volume deficit related to deficient ADH, renal cells insensitive to ADH, polyuria, and inability to respond to thirst
- Altered thought processes related to decreased cerebral perfusion, cerebral dehydration, and hypernatremia

Nursing and Medical Interventions

The primary goals of treatment are to identify and correct the underlying cause and restore normal fluid volume and osmolality. Identifying the underlying cause is a necessary part of determining appropriate treatment, particularly drug therapy.

Volume Replacement. As indicated earlier, if the patient is alert and able to respond to thirst, he or she will generally drink enough water to avoid symptomatic hypovolemia. However, patients in critical care units who develop DI are frequently unable to respond to or recognize thirst, so fluid replacement is essential.

If the patient already has symptoms of hypovolemia, the volume already lost must be replaced. In addition, fluid is replaced every hour to keep up with current urine losses. Correction of hypernatremia and replacement of free water are achieved using hypotonic dextrose in water solutions. However, if the patient has circulatory failure, isotonic saline may be administered until hemodynamic stability and vascular volume have been restored.

Monitoring for signs and symptoms of hypovolemia is a priority. Vital signs must be recorded at least every hour, along with urine output. Central venous pressure or pulmonary artery pressure monitoring may also be instituted to evaluate fluid requirements and monitor the patient's response to treatment. This is particularly important in elderly patients who are likely to have concurrent cardiovascular and renal disease. Accurate intake and output and daily weights are also essential. Measurement of urine specific gravity assists in evaluating the patient's response to treatment; once drug therapy has been instituted, the urine should become more concentrated and the specific gravity should increase.

Monitoring the patient's neurological status may indicate a change in fluid and/or electrolyte status (sodium). Ongoing assessment of level of consciousness, including response to pain, motor response, reflexes, and neurological signs, alerts the nurse to any change in mentation.

Fluid overload from overaggressive fluid replacement, particularly once drug therapy has been instituted, can be prevented by monitoring breath sounds and performing cardiovascular assessments. Signs and symptoms of fluid overload are reviewed in Table 15–7.

Hormone Replacement. Neurogenic DI is controlled primarily with exogenous ADH preparations. These drugs replace the absent or reduced ADH, enabling the kidneys to conserve water. They can be administered intravenously, intramuscularly, intranasally, or subcutaneously. Injectable forms are generally more potent than intranasal, and absorption is more reliable through the IV route.

The drug most commonly used for management is desmopressin (DDAVP), a synthetic analogue of vasopressin. Unlike aqueous vasopressin and lysine vasopressin, desmopressin is devoid of any vasoconstrictor effects and has a longer antidiuretic action (12 to 24 hours). It also has infrequent and mild side effects: headache, nausea, and mild abdominal cramps. See Table 15–29 for specific dosages of this and other drugs used to treat DI.

Aqueous vasopressin is used primarily for diagnostic purposes or in patients whose DI is expected to be temporary (such as those with head injuries). Its shorter duration of action (3 to 6 hours) enables detection of the return of ADH function (decreasing urine output and increased specific gravity without drug administration). Lysine vasopressin is generally used in patients who are refractory to desmopressin or demonstrate significant side effects.

Aqueous vasopressin and lysine vasopressin can cause vasoconstrictive side effects in high doses, but patients with preexisting vascular disease (particularly coronary artery disease) may experience these side effects even with small doses. Tachycardia, hypertension, dysrhythmias, angina, and myocardial infarction may occur in these patients. Careful hemodynamic and cardiac monitoring of these patients is required. When these drugs are used, a nitroglycerin drip may be started to counteract the potential cardiac effects.

Overmedication with an ADH preparation can also produce water overload. The patient should be monitored for signs of dyspnea, hypertension, weight gain, hyponatremia, headache, or drowsiness.

Table 15–29. DRUGS USED TO TREAT DIABETES INSIPIDUS

Drug	Dosage/Route	Side Effects	Nursing Implications
Aqueous vasopressin	IM/SC: 5–10 U every 8–12 hr IV: 102 mU/kg/hr Intranasal: individualized	Water intoxication, circumoral pallor, sweating, tremor, head pounding, abdominal cramps, gas, vertigo, nausea and vomiting Large doses or patients with cardiac history: hypertension, dysrhythmias, angina, myocardial infarction	Monitor for signs of water intoxication: lethargy, behavioral changes, disorientation, neuromuscular excitability Monitor I & O, daily weight, specific gravity Monitor BP, HR, ECG rhythm
Lysine vasopressin	Intranasal: 5–10 U several times a day	Same as above	Same as above
Desmopressin (DDAVP)	SC/IM/IV: 1–4 µg/day Intranasal: 10–25 µg bid	Infrequent and mild: headache, nausea, abdominal cramps	Monitor for signs of water intoxication Monitor I & O, daily weight
Chlorpropamide (Diabinese)	125–500 mg/day	Hypoglycemia, headache, weakness, dizziness, drowsiness	Monitor blood sugar Monitor I & O, daily weight Monitor for signs of water intoxication
Carbamazepine (Tegretol)	400–600 mg/day	Water intoxication, thrombocytopenia, leukocytosis, anemia, CHF, hypertension, syncope, edema	Monitor I & O, daily weight Monitor CBC and platelet count Monitor for signs of water intoxication
Clofibrate (Atromid-S)	2 g/day	Most common: nausea Less common: rash, myalgias, arthralgias, muscle weakness	Monitor renal/hepatic function (contraindicated in hepatic or renal disease) If GI symptoms, take drug with meals

IM = intramuscular, SC = subcutaneous; I & O = intake and output; BP = blood pressure; HR = heart rate; CHF = congestive heart failure; CBC = complete blood count; bid = twice a day; IV = intravenous; ECG = electrocardiogram; GI = gastrointestinal.

Additional Drugs. Thiazide diuretics combined with sodium restriction may also enhance water reabsorption. The effect is thought to be achieved by producing a negative salt balance, which diminishes delivery of fluid to the distal tubules of the kidneys, decreasing free water loss.

Other pharmacological agents have been used to treat neurogenic DI. Chlorpropamide (Diabinese) stimulates ADH release and potentiates its antidiuretic action. It may be particularly effective in patients who have partial DI (ADH is present but in inadequate amounts to prevent polyuria). However, due to chlorpropamide's antidiabetic properties, hypoglycemia is a significant risk, and chlorpropamide is generally used only in patients who cannot take ADH due to allergy or side effects. Drugs such as carbamazepine and clofibrate may decrease polyuria and polydipsia but are also rarely used.

Nephrogenic DI. Treatment of nephrogenic DI depends primarily on solute restriction and the administration of thiazide diuretics. Sodium depletion causes a fall in the glomerular filtration rate, enhanced reabsorption of fluid, and a reduced capacity to dilute the urine.

Secondary DI. Water restriction is usually all that is needed in secondary DI. Removal of the causative factor or treatment of the underlying cause is also necessary.

Patient and Family Education. Patients who have a permanent ADH deficit require education regarding:

- Pathogenesis of DI
- Dose, side effects, and rationale for prescribed medications
- Parameters for notifying the physician
- Importance of adherence to medication regimen
- Importance of wearing a Medic-Alert identification bracelet
- Importance of drinking according to thirst and avoiding excess drinking

Patient Outcomes

Outcomes for a patient with DI include:

- Normal circulating body fluid volume
- Serum osmolality 275 to 295 mOsm/kg
- Stable weight and balanced intake and output
- Return to baseline mentation
- Serum sodium 135 to 145 mEq/L

SYNDROME OF INAPPROPRIATE ANTIDIURETIC HORMONE
Pathophysiology

SIADH occurs when the body secretes excessive ADH unrelated to plasma osmolality; that is, there is a failure in the negative feedback mechanism that regulates the release and inhibition of ADH. The result is an inability to secrete a dilute urine, fluid retention, and dilutional hyponatremia. SIADH may result from a clinical disorder or may be pharmacologically induced. The primary categories of clinical disorders producing SIADH include malignancy, pulmonary disease, and central nervous system disorders.

The most common cause of SIADH is malignant disease, especially bronchogenic (oat cell) carcinoma. The malignant cells themselves actually synthesize, store, and release ADH, placing control of ADH outside the normal pituitary-hypothalamus feedback loops. Other types of malignancies known to produce SIADH include pancreatic, duodenal, and Hodgkin's lymphoma.

Nonmalignant pulmonary conditions such as tuberculosis, pneumonia, lung abscess, and chronic obstructive pulmonary disease can also produce SIADH. As with malignant cells, it is believed that benign pulmonary tissue is capable of synthesizing and releasing ADH in certain disease states.

Central nervous system disorders such as head injuries, infections, bleeds, surgery, and cerebrovascular accidents can produce SIADH, although DI is more frequently seen. SIADH is caused by stimulation of the hypothalamic and/or pituitary systems.

Many medications are associated with SIADH: antineoplastics, anesthetics, anticonvulsants, oral hypoglycemics, narcotics, and barbiturates. The mechanisms involved include increasing or potentiating the action of ADH (chlorpropamide, carbamazepine), acting on the renal distal tubule to decrease free water excretion (thiazide diuretics), or causing a central release of ADH (antineoplastics, oxytocin, nicotine). See Table 15–30 for a complete listing of etiological factors.

Assessment

Clinical Presentation. ADH stimulation produces a clinical picture of water intoxication. The clinical manifestations are primarily due to water retention, hyponatremia, and hypo-osmolality of the serum. The severity of the signs and symptoms is related to the rate of onset and the severity of the hyponatremia.

Central Nervous System. Manifestations such as weakness, lethargy, mental confusion, difficulty concentrating, restlessness, headache, seizures, and coma may occur in response to hyponatremia and hypo-osmolality. Hypo-osmolality disrupts the intracellular-extracellular osmotic gradient, causing a shift of water into brain cells, cerebral edema, and increased intracranial pressure. If the serum sodium falls below 120 mEq/L in 48 hours or less, there are usually serious

Table 15–30. CAUSES OF SIADH

Ectopic ADH Production

Bronchogenic cancer most common (oat cell)
Cancer of prostate, pancreas, or duodenum
Hodgkin's disease
Nonmalignant pulmonary disease: viral pneumonia,
    tuberculosis, chronic obstructive pulmonary disease,
    lung abscess

Central Nervous System Disorder

Head trauma
Infections: meningitis, encephalitis, brain abscess
Intracranial surgery, cerebral aneurysm, brain tumor,
    cerebral atrophy, cerebrovascular accident
Guillain-Barré syndrome, lupus erythematosus

Drugs

Chlorpropamide (Diabinese)
Antineoplastics: vincristine, cyclophosphamide,
    vinblastine, cisplatin
General anesthesia
Analgesics/narcotics: morphine, acetaminophen
Thiazide diuretics
Carbamazepine (Tegretol)
Isoproterenol
Pentamidine
Tricyclic antidepressants
Nicotine
Barbiturates

Positive Pressure Ventilation

---

neurological symptoms and a mortality rate as high as 50%. If hyponatremia develops more slowly, the body is able to protect against cerebral edema, and the patient may remain asymptomatic even with a very low sodium level.

GI System. Congestion of the GI tract and decreased motility due to electrolyte imbalance (hyponatremia) can produce nausea and vomiting, anorexia, muscle cramps, and decreased bowel sounds.

Cardiovascular System. In the cardiovascular system, water retention produces weight gain, increased blood pressure, and elevated central venous and pulmonary artery occlusion pressures.

Pulmonary System. Fluid overload in the pulmonary system can produce increased respirations, dyspnea, adventitious lung sounds, and frothy, pink sputum.

Laboratory Evaluation. The hallmark of SIADH is hyponatremia and hypo-osmolality in the presence of an inappropriately concentrated urine (a low serum osmolarity should trigger inhibition of ADH, resulting in the loss of water through the kidneys and a dilute urine). Hyponatremia (less than 135 mEq/L) and hypo-osmolality (less than 275 mOsm/kg) result from water retention.

High urinary sodium levels (greater than 20 mEq/L) help differentiate SIADH from other causes of hypo-osmolality, hyponatremia, and volume overload (such as congestive heart failure). In SIADH, renal perfusion (a major stimulus for sodium reabsorption) is usually adequate, so sodium is not conserved. In a disorder such as heart failure, renal perfusion is low due to decreased cardiac output, triggering reabsorption of sodium.

Hemodilution may also decrease other laboratory values such as BUN, creatinine, and albumin. SIADH should be suspected in a patient with evidence of hemodilution and urine that is hypertonic relative to plasma.

If the etiology of hyponatremia and hypo-osmolality is unclear, a water load test may be performed to establish the diagnosis of SIADH. In this test, an oral water load is administered over 15 to 20 minutes. Water volume and urine osmolality are then measured. Normally, 80% of the water load is excreted in 5 hours, and the urine becomes more dilute. If the patient has SIADH, less than 40% of the water is excreted in 5 hours, and the urine osmolality does not drop significantly. The serum sodium should be corrected to at least 125 mEq/L before performing this test.

Nursing Diagnoses

The nursing diagnoses that may apply to a patient with SIADH include:

- Fluid volume excess related to excess water retention from excess ADH
- Altered thought processes related to brain swelling, fluid shift into cerebral cells

Nursing and Medical Interventions

The primary goals of therapy are to treat the underlying cause, eliminate excess water, and increase serum osmolality. In many instances, treatment of the underlying disorder (e.g., discontinuation of a responsible drug) is all that is needed to return the patient to normal.

Fluid Balance. In mild to moderate cases (serum sodium 125 to 135 mEq/L), fluid intake is restricted to 800 to 1000 ml/d, with liberal dietary salt and protein intake. The patient's response is evaluated by monitoring serum sodium, serum osmolality, and weight loss.

In severe, symptomatic cases (coma, seizures, sodium less than 110 mEq/L), hypertonic 3 or 5% saline (200 to 300 ml) may be given over several hours, and fluid intake is restricted to 500 ml/day. Hypertonic saline may not be successful, however, because the additional sodium may be excreted rapidly. Hypertonic saline administration should be no faster than 1 to 2 ml/kg/h to raise the serum sodium no faster than 1 to 2 mEq/L/h. Sodium should be corrected to a serum level of 120 mEq/L (lower if the symptoms resolve) with hypertonic solutions. Administering hypertonic saline too rapidly and/or correcting serum sodium too rapidly can result in demyelination of nerves, cerebral edema, and seizures. The risk of heart failure is also significant. A diuretic such as furosemide may be given during hypertonic saline administration to promote diuresis and free water clearance. Loop diuretics decrease the effectiveness of ADH by impairing the kidney's ability to concentrate the urine.

Drug Therapy. For conditions that are not reversible (such as a malignancy), drugs may be prescribed. Demeclocycline is the treatment of choice and is more effective than lithium carbonate. Demeclocycline is an antibiotic that also decreases renal responsiveness to ADH. Doses of 900 to 1200 mg/d are given. Its onset is delayed for several days, however, and it may not be completely effective for 2 weeks. The major side effects are azotemia (nephrotoxicity) and risk of infection.

Urea, an osmotic diuretic, may be used in conjunction with a sodium supplement and water restriction to correct hyponatremia. It is administered orally, in doses of 30 g/d in 100 ml water and 15 g Maalox. The most common side effects are headache, nausea and vomiting, and gastric irritation. This treatment is contraindicated in patients with GI disturbances such as GI bleeding.

Lithium carbonate blocks the renal response to ADH but is less effective than demeclocycline and is limited by its toxic effects. If used, a dose of 600 to 1800 mg is provided daily. Its onset of action is also delayed.

The use of a loop diuretic in conjunction with increased salt and potassium intake is the safest method for treating chronic hyponatremia. The diuretic prevents urine concentration, and the increased salt and potassium intake increases water output by increasing delivery of solutes to the kidney.

Nursing. Prevention of SIADH may not be possible, but early detection and treatment may prevent more serious sequelae from occurring. Thus, being aware of the populations at risk and monitoring at-risk populations for clinical signs are key roles for the critical care nurse.

Close monitoring of fluid balance is required. Daily weight, intake and output, and urine specific gravity should be measured. Fluid overload may occur from hypervolemia or too rapid administration of hypertonic saline. Cardiovascular symptoms such as tachycardia, increased blood pressure, increased hemodynamic pressures, full bounding pulses, and distended neck veins are all indicators of fluid overload. Respiratory function should be monitored for signs of tachypnea, labored respirations, shortness of breath, or fine crackles.

Adherence to fluid restrictions is critical but very difficult for patients. The nurse should ensure that the patient and the family understand the importance of the restriction and that they are included in planning types and timing of fluids. Patients should be encouraged to choose fluids high in sodium content such as milk, tomato juice, and beef and chicken broth. Comfort measures that can relieve some of the discomfort caused by fluid restriction include frequent mouth care, oral rinses without swallowing, using chilled beverages, and sucking on hard candy.

Assessment of the patient's neurological status is also critical to monitor the effects of treatment and to watch for complications. The patient should be assessed for subtle changes that may indicate water intoxication, such as fatigue, weakness, headache, or changes in level of consciousness. Strict adherence to administration rates of hypertonic (3 to 5%) saline solutions and measurement of serial serum sodium levels are essential to prevent neurological sequelae. Seizure precautions should be instituted if the patient's sodium level falls below 120 mEq/L.

Patient and Family Education. In some patients, SIADH may require long-term treatment and/or ongoing monitoring. These patients and their families require instruction regarding:

- Early signs and symptoms to report to the physician: weight gain, lethargy, weakness, nausea, mental status changes
- The significance of adherence to fluid restriction
- Dose, side effects, and rationale for prescribed medications
- Importance of daily weights

Patient Outcomes

Outcomes for a patient with SIADH include:

- Normal fluid volume
- Serum osmolality 275 to 295 mOsm/kg
- Serum sodium 135 to 145 mEq/L
- Hemodynamic measurements within normal limits
- Vital signs returned to patient baseline
- Mental status returned to patient baseline
- Patient and family able to verbalize understanding of SIADH, therapeutic regimen, and prevention of complications

RESEARCH APPLICATION

Article Reference

Sylvain, H. F., Pokorny, M. E., English, S. M., et al. (1995). Accuracy of fingerstick glucose values in shock patients. *American Journal of Critical Care*, 4(1), 44–48.

Overview of Study

Fingerstick blood glucose measurement (FBGM) has become widespread in both hospital and prehospital settings. The objective of this study was to determine the accuracy of FBGM in patients with poor peripheral perfusion (shock). Results obtained from three methods of glucose analysis (FBGM, bedside, and laboratory) were examined prospectively for 38 patients from inpatient medical and surgical critical care units or the emergency department of a large tertiary care referral center. The means of the three glucose measurements were significantly different ($P = .005$). Univariate analysis of the mean laboratory glucose value versus the mean fingerstick glucose value was significantly different ($P = .1287$ and $.004$, respectively). The mean venous laboratory glucose value was not significantly different. These results suggest that fingerstick blood samples should not be used for bedside glucose analysis in patients who may have inadequate tissue perfusion.

Critique of Study

The use of bedside blood glucose monitoring in the critically ill has been introduced only recently. The literature clearly documents the cost effectiveness of bedside glucose measurement. This timely study addresses the clinically relevant topic of the accuracy of FBGM in patients in shock. Current manufacturer guidelines advise against the use of FBGM in patients with poor peripheral perfusion. This is a common problem in the critically ill patient population.

In this study, 38 patients with inadequate tissue perfusion were studied. The strengths of this study include an operational definition of shock, which helps when comparing the results to those of other studies, and the fact that each data collector was trained using a specific procedure for data collection. One limitation of the study was that 71% of the sample was receiving vasoactive agents; thus, the effect of the vasoactive drug, not the shock state itself, may have accounted for the observed differences. However, since the majority of shock patients receive vasoactive agents, excluding them from the sample would be clinically inappropriate. Another limitation was the small sample size, which limits the generalizability of the findings.

Implications for Nursing Practice

The results of this well-designed study are clinically significant, because the differences found in mean glucose measurements (177 fingerstick and 254 laboratory) would typically lead to different treatment. It is not unusual for insulin sliding scales to be written that begin administration of insulin only if the patient's blood sugar is greater than 200 mg/dl.

The results also support previous research showing that FBGM is inaccurate in patients with inadequate tissue perfusion. Therefore, fingerstick blood samples should not be used as the method for glucose analysis in patients with inadequate tissue perfusion.

CRITICAL THINKING QUESTIONS

1. Insulin therapy is a critical intervention in the treatment of DKA. What are the crucial parameters that need to be monitored to ensure optimal patient outcomes?
2. What is the critical assessment parameter to differentiate DKA from HHNC?
3. Which organ system is most affected by a slower, more prolonged fall in serum glucose, and what nursing interventions are most critical to prevent harm to the patient?
4. Adrenal crisis features are nonspecific and may be attributed to other medical disorders. What clinical indicators should make you consider this diagnosis? What would you look for in the patient's history?
5. The physician has ordered propylthiouracil 800 mg orally loading, then 250 mg orally every 4 hours,

and saturated solution of potassium iodide 5 drops every 6 hours for your patient in thyroid crisis. How should you time their administration, and why?

6. What are the major cardiac manifestations of myxedema coma, and what medical and nursing interventions are most important to prevent more serious sequelae?

REFERENCES

Baldwin, W. A., Allo, M. (1993). Occult hypoadrenalism in critically ill patients. *Archives of Surgery, 128*, 673–676.

Baylis, P. H. (1995). Vasopressin and its neurophysin. In L. J. DeGroot et al. (Eds.), *Endocrinology* (3rd ed.) (pp. 406–420). Philadelphia: W. B. Saunders Co.

Buonocore, C. M., & Robinson, A. G. (1993). The diagnosis and management of diabetes insipidus during medical emergencies. *Endocrinology Metabolism Clinics of North America, 22*(2), 411–423.

Claussen, M. S., Landercasper, J., & Cogbill, T. H. (1992). Acute adrenal insufficiency presenting as shock after trauma and surgery: Three cases and review of the literature. *Journal of Trauma, 32*(1), 94–100.

Coffland, F. I. (1993). Thyroid-induced cardiac disorders. *Critical Care Nurse, 13*(3), 25–30.

Epstein, C. D. (1992). Adrenocortical insufficiency in the critically ill patient. *AACN Clinical Issues in Critical Care Nursing, 3*(3), 705–713.

Gavin, L. A. (1991). Thyroid crisis. *Medical Clinics of North America, 75*(1), 179–192.

Holtzman, E. J., & Ausiello, D. A. (1994). Nephrogenic diabetes insipidus: Causes revealed. *Hospital Practice, 29*(3), 89–104.

Isley, W. L. (1993). Thyroid dysfunction in the severely ill and elderly. *Postgraduate Medicine, 94*(3), 111–128.

Knowlton, A. I. (1989). Adrenal insufficiency in the critical care setting. *Journal of Intensive Care Medicine, 4*(1), 35–45.

Ladenson, P. W. (1993). Thyrotoxicosis and the heart: Something old and something new. *Journal of Clinical Endocrinology and Metabolism, 77*(2), 332–333.

Lee, L. M., & Gumowski, J. (1992). Adrenocortical insufficiency: A medical emergency. *AACN Clinical Issues in Critical Care Nursing, 3*(2), 319–330.

Lipsky, M. S. (1994). Management of diabetic ketoacidosis. *American Family Physician, 49*(7), 1607–1612.

McMorrow, M. E. (1992). The elderly and thyrotoxicosis. *AACN Clinical Issues in Critical Care Nursing, 3*(1), 114–119.

Moore, J. M. (1994). Syndrome of inappropriate antidiuretic hormone secretion (SIADH). In J. Gross & B. L. Johnson (Eds.), *Handbook of oncology nursing* (2nd ed.) (pp. 701–713). Boston: Jones and Bartlett.

Mulcahy, K. (1992). Hypoglycemic emergencies. *AACN Clinical Issues in Critical Care Nursing, 3*(2), 361–369.

Mulloy, A. L., & Caruana, R. J. (1995). Hyponatremic emergencies. *Medical Clinics of North America, 79*(1), 155–168.

Reasner, C. A. (1990). Adrenal disorders. *Critical Care Nursing Quarterly, 13*(3), 67–73.

Reising, D. L. (1995). Acute hyperglycemia. *Nursing 95, 2,* 33–40.

Sauve, D. O., & Kessler, C. A. (1992). Hyperglycemic emergencies. *AACN Clinical Issues in Critical Care Nursing, 3*(2), 350–360.

Smallridge, R. C. (1992). Metabolic and anatomic thyroid emergencies: A review. *Critical Care Medicine, 20*(2), 276–291.

Snow, K., Jiang, N., Kao, P. C., & Scheithauer, B. W. (1992). Biochemical evaluation of adrenal dysfunction: The laboratory perspective. *Mayo Clinic Proceedings, 67,* 1055–1065.

Sorensen, J. B., Andersen, M. K., & Hansen, H. H. (1995). Syndrome of inappropriate secretion of antidiuretic hormone (SIADH) in malignant disease. *Journal of Internal Medicine, 238,* 97–110.

Tietgens, S. T., & Leinung, M. C. (1995). Thyroid storm. *Medical Clinics of North America, 79*(1), 169–184.

Woeber, K. A. (1992). Thyrotoxicosis and the heart. *New England Journal of Medicine, 327*(2), 94–98.

Yamamoto, T., Fukuyama, J., Hasegawa, K., & Sugiura, M. (1992). Isolated corticotropin deficiency in adults. *Archives of Internal Medicine, 152,* 1705–1712.

RECOMMENDED READINGS

Batcheller, J. (1994). Syndrome of inappropriate antidiuretic hormone secretion. *Critical Care Nursing Clinics of North America, 6*(4), 687–692.

Bell, T. N. (1994). Diabetes insipidus. *Critical Care Nursing Clinics of North America, 6*(4), 675–685.

Brody, G. M. (1992). Diabetic ketoacidosis and hyperosmolar hyperglycemic nonketotic coma. *Topics in Emergency Medicine, 14*(1), 12–22.

Coffland, F. I. (1994). Endocrine disorders affecting the cardiovascular system. *Critical Care Nursing Clinics of North America, 6*(4), 735–745.

Jordan, R. M. (1995). Myxedema coma: Pathophysiology, therapy, and factors affecting prognosis. *Medical Clinics of North America, 79*(1), 185–194.

Loriaux, D. L., & McDonald, W. J. (1995). Adrenal insufficiency. In L. J. DeGroot et al. (Eds.), *Endocrinology* (3rd ed.) (pp. 1731–1740). Philadelphia: W. B. Saunders Co.

Macheca, M. K. (1993). Diabetic hypoglycemia: How to keep the threat at bay. *American Journal of Nursing, 4,* 26–30.

Marshall, S. M. (1993). Hyperglycemic emergencies. *Care of the Critically Ill, 9*(5), 220–223.

Spittle, L. (1992). Diagnoses in opposition: Thyroid storm and myxedema coma. *AACN Clinical Issues in Critical Care Nursing, 3*(2), 300–308.

Toto, K. H. (1994). Endocrine physiology. *Critical Care Nursing Clinics of North America, 6*(4), 637–659.

16

Burns

Nancy C. Molter, M.N., R.N., CCRN
Elisabeth Greenfield, M.S., R.N., CCRN

OBJECTIVES

- Review the anatomy and physiology of the integumentary system.
- Discuss the pathophysiology of burns.
- Compare the types of burn injuries.
- Identify the assessment during resuscitation and the acute phases of burn management.

- Relate the nursing diagnoses, outcomes, and interventions for the burned patient.
- Formulate a plan of care for the patient with a burn injury.

Introduction

Historically, burn injuries have been one of the most lethal forms of trauma. Because of the major advances that have occurred in burn therapy, a patient who is admitted to the hospital with burn wounds covering less than 81% of the body has a high probability of survival (Saffle et al., 1995). However, morbidity remains significant in patients with burns on greater than 50% of their total body surface area, and older and younger patients with lower percentages of burned area remain at considerable risk for mortality. It is estimated that more than 500,000 emergency department visits and 70,000 inpatient admissions for burn injuries occur each year in the United States. Approximately 20,000 of the admissions are to hospitals with special capabilities for caring for extensive burn injuries (American Burn Association, 1990; Saffle et al., 1995).

The opinions or assertions contained herein are the private views of the authors and are not to be construed as official or as reflecting the views of the Department of the Army or Department of Defense.

The tissue damage that results from a major burn injury leads to two phases of dysfunction. In the first phase, a decreased response in organ function occurs, followed by a hypermetabolic and hyperfunctional response of all systems in the second phase. The responses are characteristic of those seen in any severe trauma and are proportional to the extent of the trauma. Thus, the burn patient can be viewed as the universal trauma model (Pruitt, 1984). Care of such patients requires a team that includes many disciplines in order to maximize favorable patient outcomes.

Traditionally, three treatment phases of burn care exist. The *resuscitative phase* is approximately 48 hours long and is the most crucial period for the patient. The primary goal is to prevent shock secondary to changes in capillary dynamics and fluid shifts.

With the onset of diuresis approximately 48 hours after the burn, the *acute phase* begins and lasts until wound closure occurs. This phase may continue for weeks or months. Nursing care focuses on the promotion of wound healing and the prevention of complications.

Although the critical care nurse is rarely involved in the *rehabilitative phase*, the care given in the first two phases is instrumental in achieving the final rehabilitative outcomes. The primary goal in this phase is to restore the patient's ability to function in society and to return to an established family role and vocation.

There is no greater challenge in critical care nursing than caring for a severely burned patient. Even with the expanded network of burn facilities that now exists, most patients are seen first in the community hospital. Therefore, it is crucial that emergency department and critical care nurses have the skills necessary to provide resuscitative care to burn-injured patients.

Review of Anatomy and Physiology of the Skin

The skin is composed of two layers, the epidermis and the dermis, with the outer, epidermal, layer being the thinner of the two. The dermis contains the sweat glands, the hair follicles, the sebaceous glands, and the sensory fibers for the detection of pain, pressure, touch, and temperature. The underlying subcutaneous tissue is a layer of connective tissue and fat deposits. The skin (or integumentary system) is the largest organ of the body, and it is crucial because of its many functions (Fig. 16–1).

Many physiological and psychological alterations place the patient in jeopardy when an extensive amount of skin is damaged because of injury. Such alterations in function include loss of body heat, fluids,

and thermoregulatory control; loss of protective barriers against infection and sensory contact with the environment; and loss of presentable cosmetic appearance.

Depth of Injury

The severity of burn injury depends on the duration of contact with the injuring agent, the temperature of the agent, the amount of tissue exposed, and the ability of the agent and tissue to dissipate the thermal energy. Although burn injuries have traditionally been classified as first-, second-, or third-degree burn injuries, they are currently described as partial-thickness or full-thickness burn injury.

Partial-thickness injury is subdivided into superficial and deep injury. Superficial partial-thickness injury may involve only the epidermis, such as occurs with a sunburn (often termed first degree injury), or it may involve a variable portion of the dermis (second-degree injury). A sunburn typically heals in 3 to 5 days. Burn injuries (first degree) that cause only erythema and do not involve the dermis are not included for calculation of fluid requirements. Superficial partial-thickness injury that involves the epidermis and a limited portion of the dermis usually heals within 21 days. Deeper, partial-thickness injury involves destruction of the epidermis and most of the dermis, and only the epidermal cells lining hair follicles and sweat glands remain intact. Although such wounds can heal

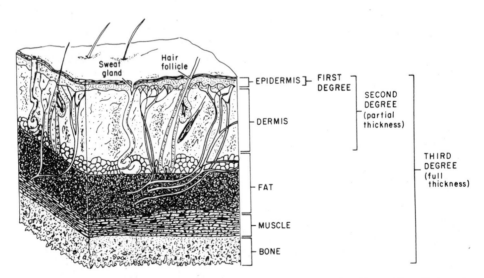

Figure 16–1. The depth of the injury determines whether a burn will heal or require skin grafting. First and second-degree burns heal because they are partial-thickness; thus, the elements necessary to generate new skin remain. Often, deep partial-thickness injuries are grafted for improved functional and cosmetic reasons. Full-thickness injury destroys all dermal appendages and requires skin grafting for achievement of coverage. (Adapted from Kravitz, M. (1988). Thermal injuries. In V. D. Cardona, et al. (Eds.), *Trauma nursing: From resuscitation through rehabilitation* (p. 709). Philadelphia: W. B. Saunders Co.)

Table 16–1. DEPTH OF BURN INJURY

Degree of Injury	Morphology	Healing Time	Characteristics of Wound
Superficial partial-thickness (first-degree)	Epidermal destruction only	Approximately 5 days	Red, dry, painful; blisters rarely present
Superficial partial-thickness (second-degree)	Destruction of epidermis and some dermis	Within 21 days	Moist pink or mottled red, painful, blisters
Deep partial-thickness (second-degree)	Destruction of epidermis and dermis; some skin appendages remain	Within 3–6 weeks	Pale, mottled, pearly white, mostly dry; often insensate; difficult to differentiate from full-thickness injury
Full-thickness (third-degree)	Destruction of epidermis, dermis, and underlying subcutaneous tissue	Requires skin grafting	Thick, leathery eschar; white, cherry-red or brown-black; insensate; thrombosed blood vessels; dry

spontaneously within 3 to 6 weeks, they are most often excised and grafted in order to achieve better functional and cosmetic results and to decrease the length of healing time and hospitalization. Destruction of all layers of the skin down to or past the subcutaneous fat, fascia, muscles, or bone is defined as full-thickness injury. The nerves are destroyed, resulting in a painless wound. These injuries always require skin grafting for permanent wound closure. Initially, differentiating partial-thickness from full-thickness injuries may be difficult, particularly in the elderly or in children. Table 16–1 describes the characteristics of partial-thickness and full-thickness burn injuries.

Three zones of thermal injury are used to describe the relationship of tissue effects to the severity of injury and the ultimate viability of the injured tissue (Fig. 16–2). The greatest area of tissue necrosis is the core of the wound. Peripheral to this area is a zone of stasis where vascular damage and potentially reversible tissue injury have occurred. Without adequate resuscitation, this area may progress to tissue death. The area of minimal injury is termed the *zone of hyperemia* and is similar to a superficial partial-thickness burn.

PATHOPHYSIOLOGY

Local Response

Significant hemodynamic, metabolic, and immunological effects occur locally and systemically as a result of cellular injury by heat. The release of cellular enzymes and vasoactive substances and the activation of complement result in altered vascular permeability.

A significant shift of protein molecules, fluid, and electrolytes occurs at the capillary level from the intravascular space to the extravascular space as a result of the increased membrane permeability of the vessels. Cellular swelling may also occur as a result of a decrease in cell transmembrane potential and a shift of extracellular sodium and water into the cell (Cope and Moore, 1947; Rue and Cioffi, 1991). In addition, the leaking of serum proteins eventually decreases or stops

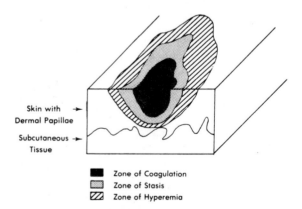

Figure 16–2. Zones of thermal injury. The zone of coagulation is the site of irreversible skin death. The zone of hyperemia is the site of minimal cell involvement and early spontaneous recovery. In the zone of stasis, infection or drying of the wound results in conversion of this potentially salvageable area to full-thickness skin destruction with irreversible cell death. (Redrawn from Army Burn Unit and adapted from Zawacki, B. (1974). *Reversal of capillary stasis and prevention of necrosis in burns. Annals of Surgery, 180,* 98.)

the lymph flow as a result of an obstruction in the lymphatic vessels (Pruitt and Goodwin, 1990).

In extensive burn injury (>25% total body surface area), the edema occurs in both burned and unburned areas as a result of the increase in capillary permeability and hypoproteinemia (Arturson and Jonsson, 1979) or as a result of the volume and oncotic pressure effects of the large fluid resuscitation volumes required (Mason, 1980). The magnitude of the response is proportionate to the extent of the injury. The maximum edema is seen 18 to 24 hours after the burn, and with adequate resuscitation, the transmembrane potential is restored within 24 to 36 hours after the burn (Rue and Cioffi, 1991).

Systemic Response

All organ systems are affected in burn injury; the response is manifested by two phases represented by hypofunction followed by hyperfunction. The degree of physiological change is proportionate to the extent of burn injury and reaches a maximum response in patients with burns of more than 50% total body surface area. When the wound heals or is closed, organ function returns to normal (Moylan et al., 1971; Pruitt and Goodwin, 1990; Pruitt et al., 1995). The specific organ system responses are summarized in the following sections (Fig. 16–3).

Cardiovascular Response. With a decreased cardiac output and an increased peripheral resistance, arterial blood pressure is maintained by the catecholamine-induced vasoconstrictive response producing the increased peripheral resistance. Redistribution of blood flow occurs early in the postburn period in order to perfuse essential viscera. With adequate fluid resuscitation, cardiac output is normalized toward the end of the first 24 hours after the burn and becomes supranormal thereafter until the burns are closed (Pruitt and Mason, 1971; Shea et al., 1973).

Host Defense Mechanisms. With the loss of skin, the primary barrier to microorganisms is gone. The mechanism for many of the immune defects that occur with extensive burn injury is unclear. It is postulated that complex interactions of several factors, including nutrition, hypermetabolism, and immunological alterations, may be caused by either an altered host environment, an injury-induced host-deficiency state, or both. The end result is overstimulation of suppressor T cells, activation of complement, and depression of other components, such as helper T cell and killer T cell activity and polymorphonuclear leukocyte activity. Patients who remain immunosuppressed without restoration of cell-mediated immune competence have higher sepsis-related morbidity and mortality (Ferrar et al., 1990; Kravitz, 1993).

Pulmonary Response. With any major burn, an initial transient pulmonary hypertension occurs that may be associated with a modest decrease in oxygen tension and lung compliance resulting from the release of vasoconstrictive agents (Pruitt et al., 1995). Lung injury secondary to the inhalation of smoke and products of incomplete combustion causes age-related and burn size–related increases in mortality greater than that caused by burn injury alone (Shirani et al., 1987; Carrougher, 1993). Inhalation injury is classified as (1) injury from carbon monoxide, (2) injury above the glottis, and (3) injury below the glottis (Nebraska Burn Institute, 1994). Table 16–2 summarizes characteristics of each type of injury. Inhalation injury may be the cause of admission to a burn unit, even when there are no surface burns.

Renal Response. The biphasic renal response manifests as an initial oliguria secondary to a decreased plasma flow and glomerular filtration rate, followed by a diuresis secondary to an increase in cardiac output. The diuresis may be modest because of the slow mobilization of edema fluid and the increase in evaporative water loss that occurs with the loss of skin (Pruitt et al., 1995).

Gastrointestinal Response. An ileus usually occurs secondary to hypovolemia and the neurological and endocrine responses to injury. Mucosal erosion and eventual ulceration may occur if the gastric mucosa is not protected with antacids and/or H_2 histamine receptor antagonists (Pruitt et al., 1995).

Table 16–2. TYPES OF SMOKE INHALATION INJURY

Type of Injury	Pathology
Carbon monoxide poisoning	Carbon monoxide binds to hemoglobin molecules more rapidly than oxygen molecules; tissue hypoxia results.
Inhalation injury above the glottis	Most often a thermal injury. Most heat absorption and damage occurs in the pharynx and larynx; may cause obstruction after resuscitation is initiated.
Inhalation injury below the glottis	Usually a chemical injury that produces impaired ciliary activity, erythema, hypersecretion, edema, ulceration of mucosa, increased blood flow, and spasm of bronchi and/or bronchioles.

Adapted from material from Nebraska Burn Institute. (1994). *Advanced burn life support course manual.* Lincoln, NB: Author.

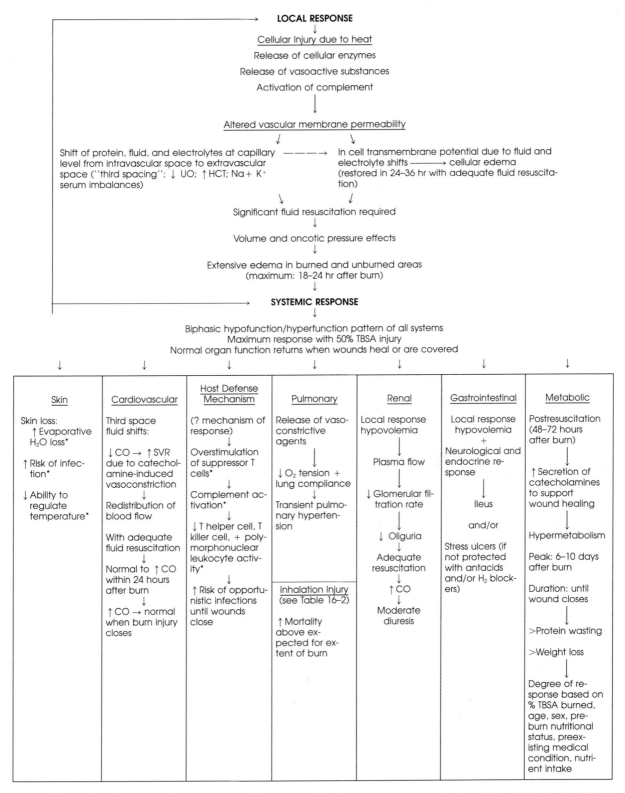

LOCAL RESPONSE
↓
Cellular Injury due to heat
Release of cellular enzymes
Release of vasoactive substances
Activation of complement
↓
Altered vascular membrane permeability
↓   ↓
Shift of protein, fluid, and electrolytes at capillary ———→ In cell transmembrane potential due to fluid and
level from intravascular space to extravascular   electrolyte shifts ———→ cellular edema
space (''third spacing''; ↓ UO; ↑HCT; Na+ K+   (restored in 24–36 hr with adequate fluid resuscita-
serum imbalances)   tion)
↓   ↓
Significant fluid resuscitation required
↓
Volume and oncotic pressure effects
↓
Extensive edema in burned and unburned areas
(maximum: 18–24 hr after burn)
↓
SYSTEMIC RESPONSE
↓
Biphasic hypofunction/hyperfunction pattern of all systems
Maximum response with 50% TBSA injury
Normal organ function returns when wounds heal or are covered

Skin	Cardiovascular	Host Defense Mechanism	Pulmonary	Renal	Gastrointestinal	Metabolic
Skin loss: ↑ Evaporative H_2O loss*	Third space fluid shifts: ↓	(? mechanism of response) ↓	Release of vaso-constrictive agents ↓	Local response hypovolemia ↓	Local response hypovolemia +	Postresuscitation (48–72 hours after burn) ↓
↑ Risk of infection*	↓ CO → ↑ SVR due to catecholamine-induced vasoconstriction ↓	Overstimulation of suppressor T cells* ↓	↓ O_2 tension + lung compliance ↓	Plasma flow ↓	Neurological and endocrine response ↓	↑ Secretion of catecholamines to support wound healing ↓
↓ Ability to regulate temperature*	Redistribution of blood flow	Complement activation* ↓	Transient pulmonary hypertension	↓ Glomerular filtration rate ↓	Ileus	Hypermetabolism
	With adequate fluid resuscitation ↓	↓T helper cell, T killer cell, + polymorphonuclear leukocyte activity* ↓		↓ Oliguria ↓	and/or	Peak: 6–10 days after burn
	Normal to ↑ CO within 24 hours after burn ↓	↑ Risk of opportunistic infections until wounds close	Inhalation Injury (see Table 16–2)	Adequate resuscitation ↓	Stress ulcers (if not protected with antacids and/or H_2 blockers)	Duration: until wound closes
	↑ CO → normal when burn injury closes		↑ Mortality above expected for extent of burn	↑ CO ↓		>Protein wasting
				Moderate diuresis		>Weight loss
						Degree of response based on % TBSA burned, age, sex, preburn nutritional status, preexisting medical condition, nutrient intake

Figure 16–3. Pathophysiology of extensive burn injury. Asterisk indicates injury to greater than 25% of total body surface area (TBSA). UO = urinary output; HCT = hematocrit; CO = cardiac output; SVR = systemic vascular resistance.

Metabolic Response. Hypermetabolism begins as resuscitation is completed and is one of the most significant alterations that occurs after burn injury. The rapid metabolic rate is probably mediated by the secretion of catecholamines and is required for wound healing. Peak hypermetabolic rates are reached between the sixth and tenth postburn days. The amount of protein wasting and weight loss that occurs is affected by several factors: percent of body surface burned, age, sex, preburn nutritional status, other health problems, and nutrient intake. When the wound is closed, oxygen consumption, protein mass, and weight begin to return to normal (Wilmore, 1987).

Types of Burn Injuries

Various injuries involving thermal trauma can result from exposure to heat, cold, electric current, or chemical agents. The focus of this chapter is on injuries resulting from heat, including electric and chemical burns. A limited discussion of the care of patients with toxic epidermal necrolysis is included because the extensive loss of skin that can occur with this condition may necessitate admission to a burn unit for specialized wound care.

THERMAL INJURIES

A heat source of less than 44°C (111.2°F) does not cause a burn, regardless of the length of exposure. The extent of damage increases with temperatures greater than this level in direct proportion to the duration of exposure. Full-thickness injury occurs when sufficient heat is applied to cause protein coagulation and cell death (Pruitt et al., 1995). Exposure to temperatures of 60°C (140°F) (which is the common setting for home water heaters) causes tissue destruction in as little as 3 to 5 seconds. Children and the elderly may be at greater risk for thermal injury from lower temperatures because of their thinner skin and their decreased agility in moving to avoid harm.

CHEMICAL INJURIES

Although chemical injuries account for only a small percentage of admissions to burn centers, they can be severe, causing both local and systemic effects. The severity of injury is related to the type of agent, the concentration of agent, the duration of contact, and the volume of agent. Chemical agents are part of our lifestyle; thus, the potential for injury from exposure is great. Unlike flame or scald injuries, with chemical burns, tissue damage continues until the chemical is completely removed or neutralized. Three categories of chemical agents exist: alkalies, acids, and organic compounds.

Commonly found in cleaning products used in the home and industry, alkalies produce liquefaction necrosis and loosening of tissue, thereby allowing the chemical to diffuse more deeply into the tissue. Therefore, this category of chemical agents can produce far more damage than acids.

Acids are also found in many household and industrial products, such as bathroom cleansers, rust removers, and acidifiers for home swimming pools. Acids cause coagulation necrosis of tissue and precipitation of protein.

Organic compounds, such as phenols and petroleum products, can produce chemical burns as well as systemic effects. Phenols cause severe coagulation necrosis. In addition, systemic effects, such as central nervous system depression, hypothermia, hypotension, pulmonary edema, and intravascular hemolysis, may be severe and can lead to shock and death. The solvent properties of hydrocarbons such as gasoline promote cell membrane injury and dissolution of lipids, with resulting skin necrosis. Chemical pneumonitis and bronchitis may occur as a result of hydrocarbon excretion from the lungs. Other complications observed with gasoline inhalation include hepatic and renal damage and sudden death (Nebraska Burn Institute, 1994; Mozingo et al., 1988).

ELECTRICAL INJURIES

Electrical injury is caused by contact with such varied sources as household current, car batteries, electrosurgical devices, high-tension electric lines, and lightning. Injuries are arbitrarily classified as high voltage (>1000 volts) or low voltage (<1000 volts) (Nebraska Burn Institute, 1994; Mozingo et al., 1994).

Tissue damage is the result of the electrical energy's conversion into heat. Many factors can affect the degree of injury, including the type of current, the pathway of current, the duration of contact, the environmental conditions, and the resistance offered by body tissues. The least resistance is in nerve tissue, and the greatest is in bone tissue. Current density, and thus the greatest heat, is at the point of entry or exit, which is often on the extremities. Injuries of the trunk are not as common. Although alternating and direct current are both dangerous, alternating current has a greater probability of producing cardiopulmonary arrest and has a tetanic effect that may "lock" the patient to the source of electricity. As high-voltage current ceases, the superficial tissues begin to cool more rapidly than the deeper tissues. Therefore, deep tissue necrosis commonly occurs beneath viable, more

Table 16–3. COMPLICATIONS OF ELECTRICAL INJURY

Complication	Cause
Early death	Cardiopulmonary arrest
Oliguria	Inadequate fluid resuscitation based on small surface injury
Acute renal failure	Hemochromogens in small volume of urine
Hyperkalemia	Muscle destruction
Deep tissue necrosis	Direct effect of electric current
Neurological deficits	Direct or delayed effect of current
Cataract formation	Immediate or delayed effect of current
Cholelithiasis	Unknown

Adapted from Pruitt, B. A., Jr., Goodwin, C. W., Jr. (1990). Burn injury. In E. F. Moore (Ed.), *Early care of the injured patient* (4th ed.) (pp. 286–306). Chicago: American College of Surgeons.

superficial, tissue. All patients with electric injury should be monitored closely for cardiac dysrhythmias. Many other severe complications related to electric injury are summarized in Table 16–3 (Pruitt et al., 1995; Mozingo et al., 1994).

The mechanism of lightning injury is a direct strike or a side flash that causes a flow of current between the person and a close object that is struck by lightning (Nebraska Burn Institute, 1994). Often, cutaneous injury is superficial because the current travels on the surface of the body rather than through it. Lightning injuries frequently result in cardiopulmonary arrest as well as transient but severe central nervous system deficits (Pruitt and Goodwin, 1990; Nebraska Burn Institute, 1994).

NONBURN INJURY

Toxic Epidermal Necrolysis. This condition is an exfoliative dermatitis that is usually associated with mucosal involvement of conjunctival, oral, or urogenital areas. The most common cause is a drug reaction, particularly to sulfa, phenobarbital, and phenytoin (Heimbach et al., 1987; DePew, 1991). In some cases, no apparent etiologic agent exists.

Staphylococcal Scalded Skin. This condition is caused by a reaction to staphylococcal toxin; it often presents with a clinical picture similar to that of toxic epidermal necrolysis. A low mortality (5%) exists with this condition, and skin slough occurs as a result of intraepidermal splitting. In contrast, toxic epidermal necrolysis is associated with a high mortality (25 to 50%), and the epidermal split occurs at the dermal-

epidermal junction. The differential or definitive diagnosis is made by microscopic examination of the denuded skin in order to determine the level of skin separation (DePew, 1991).

Although the massive fluid shifts seen in thermal injury do not occur in toxic epidermal necrolysis, immune suppression does occur and contributes to the life-threatening complications of sepsis and pneumonia. Patients present with fever and flulike symptoms, and erythema and blisters develop within 24 to 96 hours. As large bullae develop, the skin and mucous membranes slough, often resulting in significant and painful partial-thickness injury. Admission to a burn unit is advisable in order to ensure proper wound management (Heimbach et al., 1987).

ASSESSMENT

The critical care nurse must assess indices of essential organ function in order to prevent complications in patients with major thermal injury. Initially, monitoring occurs frequently in order to evaluate changes in the patient's condition that may occur rapidly during fluid resuscitation. Assessment in the resuscitative and acute care phases must focus on early detection or prevention of the following problems. It is often useful to use critical pathways or clinical guidelines as a guide to assessment and intervention during these phases (Greenfield, 1995). Figure 16–4 is an example of a critical pathway used for major burns during the resuscitative phase.

Resuscitative Phase

Respiratory. Upper and lower airway edema, pulmonary insufficiency, and decreased lung compliance may occur.

Cardiovascular. Decreased cardiac output occurs in the first 24 hours after injury. Low central venous pressure and pulmonary artery wedge pressure, significant alterations in vital signs (reflective of hypovolemia and the neuroendocrine response to injury), and absence of peripheral pulses in extremities (with circumferential burns) also occur.

Neurological. A decreased level of consciousness occurs that reflects the presence of hypoxemia, hypovolemia, or both.

Blood, Fluid, and Electrolytes. Loss of plasma volume, hyponatremia, hyperkalemia, hemoconcentration (typically, blood hematocrit values are in a range of 50 to 55%), hypoproteinemia, and hyperglycemia (except in children who do not have adequate glycogen stores and may become hypoglycemic) may occur.

Renal. Oliguria may occur in the absence of adequate resuscitation.

United States Army Institute of Surgical Research
Fort Sam, Houston, Texas 78234-5012

Critical Path
Major Burns: Resuscitation Phase

Attending M.D. _____   % 2nd Degree _____

Primary Nurse _____   % 3rd Degree _____

This path is a guideline only. Physicians' orders are required to implement specific treatment modalities.

	Day 1	Day 2	Day 3
Standard of care	Initiate: 1. Airway 2. Pain 3. Stress 4. Fluid volume 5. Skin integrity 6. Ineffective coping (record address and phone number of family and document initial assessment of family status) 7. Pediatric safety (if appropriate)	→ Ensure family has received ISR information booklet	Review all nursing orders related to standards of care and revise nursing care plan
Activities of daily living	Bedrest Bed bath Functional positioning devices initiated (slings, wedges, footboard, splints, etc.) Specialty bed initiated, if appropriate (obesity, fragile skin, other complications)		Review need for bedrest Review need for bed bath (is it possible to take the patient to the shower?)
Clinical monitoring parameters	Ensure *all* jewelry is removed NPO Vital signs every hour Urine output 30–50 ml/hour in thermal burns and 75–100 ml/hour with electrical injuries (adjust fluids as required) NG pH and guaiac every 2 hours Doppler pulse every hour in all extremities with circumferential burns Pain assessment Weights BID Maintain core body temperature at 99–101° Review special pediatric monitoring parameters with physician (i.e., serum sodium level, type of maintenance fluids, possible airway obstruction)	Assess possible need for feeding tube placement Assess need for continued Doppler pulse monitoring Assess need for P.M. weighings	

Figure 16–4 *See legend on opposite page*

	Day 1	Day 2	Day 3
Consults	Initiate social work service consultation Ophthalmology consultation	Record estimated discharge disposition.	Review results prior to the Multidisciplinary Rehabilitation and Discharge Planning Committee meeting during the first week of admission.
Wound care	Mafenide acetate (Sulfamylon) cream in A.M. Silver sulfadiazine (Silvadene) cream in P.M. (unless other wound care is ordered) Eye lubricants every hour Mafenide *only* on burned ears Silver sulfadiazine *only* on burned face (unless other wound care is ordered)		
Consents	5% silver sulfadiazine solution Blood transfusion HIV testing Donation of clinical excess specimens Photo (Admission photos are taken on the first duty day after admission. If the patient is expected to expire before the next duty day, the photographer is called in for admission photos.) Ask physician about other protocols		

Develop an individual path for each patient for the acute care phase.
Standard paths can be referenced for postoperative graft and donor site care as appropriate.

Figure 16–4 Critical pathway for major burns, resuscitative phase. This critical pathway was developed by the United States Army Institute of Surgical Research; it is used to guide nursing assessment and intervention for a patient with a major burn during the resuscitative phase. M.D. = physician; ISR = Institute of Surgical Research; NPO = nothing by mouth; NG = nasogastric; q = every; BID = twice a day; HIV = human immunodeficiency virus.

Gastrointestinal. Absent bowel sounds or ileus may occur.

Integumentary. Edema may occur in burned and nonburned tissue.

Psychosocial. Extreme patient or family anxiety, combative behavior, and severe pain (with partial-thickness injury) may occur.

Acute Phase

Respiratory. Tachypnea, dyspnea, abnormal breath sounds, and purulent secretions may occur.

Cardiovascular. Dysrhythmias, hypertension, or hypotension may occur.

Neurological. Restlessness, confusion, or lethargy may occur.

Blood, Fluid, and Electrolytes. Hyponatremia may occur, but this condition usually resolves within 1 week of onset. Hypernatremia may occur and is most commonly the result of inadequate replacement of evaporative water loss. Hypokalemia, hypoproteinemia, negative nitrogen balance, and metabolic acidosis may occur. Leukopenia may occur and is usually caused by silver sulfadiazine administration. Hyperchloremic metabolic acidosis may result from mafenide acetate. Hyperglycemia may occur as a result of infection or excessive carbohydrate loading. An increase in white blood cells may result from infection, as may prolonged coagulation times and decreased platelet count.

Renal. Excessive diuresis may occur (postburn diuresis should be moderate). Glycosuria may also occur and is a sign of early sepsis or preclinical diabetes.

Gastrointestinal. Stress ulcers may occur, as may an inability to maintain a gastric pH of greater than 5, the latter is a sign of impending sepsis.

Integumentary. The patient's temperature should be between 99° and 101°F—hyperthermia or hypothermia may indicate sepsis or extensive loss of heat from open wounds or from wounds in wet dressings. Wound biopsies may indicate bacterial or fungal invasion.

Psychosocial. Manipulation, regression, sleep deprivation, and pain and pruritus may occur. The patient may be unable to cope, and the family may be unable to cope and provide patient support.

NURSING DIAGNOSES

Resuscitative Phase

- Ineffective airway clearance related to tracheal edema secondary to inhalation injury.
- Impaired gas exchange related to interstitial edema manifested by hypoxemia and hypercapnia.
- Fluid volume deficit secondary to fluid shifts out of the vascular compartment into the interstitium.
- Altered tissue perfusion secondary to anaerobic metabolism leading to acid-base imbalance.
- Altered tissue perfusion related to impaired vascular perfusion in extremities with circumferential burns, manifested by decreased or absent peripheral pulses.
- Risk for infection related to loss of integument and invasive therapy (continues into acute care phase until wounds are closed).
- Altered tissue perfusion of bowel related to hypovolemia leading to ileus.
- Hypothermia related to injury-associated decrease in heat production and increased external heat loss (continues into acute care phase).
- Acute pain related to burn injury (continues into acute care phase).
- Risk for injury related to stress response manifested by gastrointestinal hemorrhage and hyperglycemia (must begin monitoring and prophylaxis treatment in resuscitative phase; continues in acute care phase).
- Ineffective individual/family coping related to acute stress of injury and potential life-threatening crisis (continues in acute care phase).

Acute Care Phase

- Fluid volume deficit related to diuresis and/or evaporative water loss.
- Impaired skin integrity related to burn wound.
- Altered nutritional (less than body requirements) related to increased metabolic demands secondary to physiological stress and wound healing.
- Impaired physical mobility and self-care deficit related to therapeutic splinting and/or contractures.
- Altered family processes related to acute illness and potential lifestyle or family role changes.
- Knowledge deficit related to discharge goals.

COLLABORATIVE INTERVENTIONS: RESUSCITATIVE AND ACUTE CARE PHASES

Prehospital Intervention

The first priority of care in the prehospital setting is stopping the burning process while preventing further injury to the patient and to staff (Nebraska Burn Institute, 1994; Pruitt and Goodwin, 1990). Flame burns may be extinguished by rolling the patient on the ground, smothering the flames with a blanket or other cover, or dousing the flames with water. The patient is kept in a supine position because flames may otherwise spread to the upper parts of the body, causing more extensive injury. Scald burns and tar or asphalt burns are treated by immediate cooling with water if available and/or immediate removal of the saturated clothing. Clothing that is burned into the skin is not removed, because increased tissue damage and bleeding may occur. No attempt is made to remove the tar at the scene. Chemical injuries differ from thermal injuries in that the burning process continues as long as the chemical is in contact with the skin. All clothing, including gloves and shoes, is immediately removed, and water lavage is instituted before and during transport. Powdered chemicals are first brushed from the clothing and skin before lavage is performed. Chemical burns of the eye are initially irrigated with water or physiological saline at the scene of injury, and lavage continues during transport to the emergency department. Cross-contamination of the opposite eye is avoided during lavage. When neutralizing agents come in contact with chemicals, the increased heat production that occurs could further increase the depth of injury. Therefore, no attempt is made to use such agents.

Immediate treatment for electrical injuries involves prompt removal of the patient from the electrical source while protecting the rescuer. Thermal injury can also occur if clothing is ignited.

As with any other type of trauma, the next priority at the scene of injury is to complete a primary survey of the patient's airway, breathing, and circulation (ABCs of patient management) and the cervical spine (Nebraska Burn Institute, 1994; Pruitt and Goodwin, 1990) (Fig. 16–5). After a burn injury, patients are normally alert. If they become confused or combative, hypoxia may be the cause. Hypoxia occurs with inhalation injuries or may occur after an electrical injury

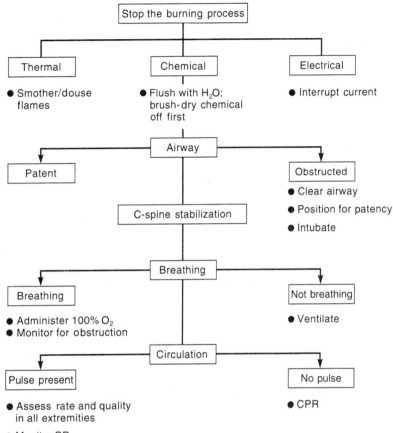

Figure 16–5. Major burn injury—primary survey. BP = blood pressure; CPR = cardiopulmonary resuscitation.

secondary to tetanic contractions of the respiratory muscles. Table 16–4 summarizes specific clinical findings that may be indicative of respiratory injury. All patients with suspected smoke inhalation are treated at the scene with 100% humidified oxygen delivered by face mask. If the patient exhibits respiratory stridor, which indicates airway obstruction, endotracheal intubation occurs at the scene.

Table 16–4. RESPIRATORY INJURY: CLINICAL INDICATORS IN BURN PATIENTS

- Facial burns
- Presence of soot around the mouth and nose and in sputum; singed nasal hairs
- Signs of hypoxemia (tachycardia, dysrythmias, anxiety, lethargy)
- Signs of respiratory difficulty (change in respiratory rate, use of accessory muscles for breathing, intercostal or sternal retractions, stridor, hoarseness)
- Abnormal breath sounds
- Abnormal blood gas values

Burn injury rarely results in hypovolemic shock in the early prehospital phase. If evidence of shock is present, then associated internal or external injury must be suspected. Cardiac arrest is a common complication of high-voltage electrical injury; it necessitates cardiopulmonary resuscitation. Peripheral pulses are assessed, especially in circumferential burns of the extremities, in order to confirm adequate circulation. All restrictive clothing and jewelry are removed and secured in order to prevent constriction and possible ischemia to distal extremities secondary to edema formation during resuscitation.

Potential spinal injury should be evaluated at the scene before the patient is moved. Patients with electrical injuries are at especially high risk for compression fractures resulting from tetanic contractions of the paravertebral muscles, or for fractures resulting from falls. Transport of the patient occurs only after the patient is placed on a back board with a cervical collar applied.

A rapid head-to-toe assessment to rule out any additional trauma is completed as part of the secondary survey (Fig. 16–6). An accurate history of the events that led to the burn injury is obtained, including the

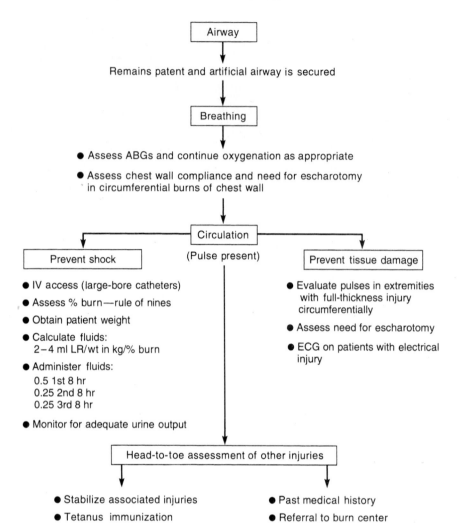

Figure 16–6. Major burn injury—secondary survey. ABG = arterial blood gas; IV = intravenous; LR = lactated Ringer's solution; ECG = electrocardiogram.

date and time of injury, the source of burns, and any events leading to the injury. Often, the patient is the most alert during this period after the injury; therefore, obtaining a brief medical history, including allergies, current medical problems and medications taken, past surgeries and/or trauma, time of last meal, history of tetanus immunization, and current weight, is beneficial (Nebraska Burn Institute, 1994).

In preparation for transport, the burned patient is covered with a clean, dry sheet and blankets in order to prevent further contamination of the wounds and hypothermia. Heat loss occurs rapidly in a major burn injury because the protective covering of skin is lost, thereby allowing heat to escape. Ice is never applied to the wounds, because further tissue damage may occur as a result of vasoconstriction and hypothermia. Intravenous therapy is not required unless the patient is greater than 45 minutes from the emergency department or unless other associated injuries resulting in

hemorrhage are present. Administration of narcotics is avoided during prehospital treatment because they may decrease the blood pressure, depress the respirations, and prevent the accurate assessment of level of consciousness. The patient should not receive anything by mouth before and during transport in order to prevent vomiting and aspiration. Vital signs are monitored en route to the nearest appropriate hospital (Pruitt and Goodwin, 1990).

Emergency Department Interventions: Resuscitative Phase

On arrival at the emergency department, the airway, breathing, and circulation are reassessed. If the patient is already intubated, accurate tube position is assessed. The nurse ensures that the endotracheal tube is securely tied in place with umbilical or tracheostomy cloth ties in order to prevent accidental extubation

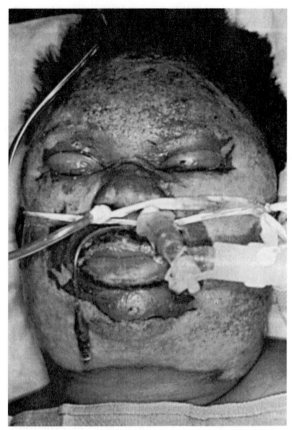

Figure 16–7. Facial edema. The massive edema that develops during fluid resuscitation in a major burn victim can lead to potential complications unless closely monitored by the critical care nurse. All facial tubes, such as endotracheal and nasogastric tubes, should be secured with the use of cloth ties to prevent dislodgment. Care must be taken to prevent ties from placing pressure on burned ear.

(Gordon, 1987) (Fig. 16–7). This measure is especially important with young children, who often require the use of uncuffed endotracheal tubes. If the patient has a circumferential full-thickness burn of the thorax, the nurse assesses for adequate ventilatory effort because edema may inhibit chest wall expansion. Young children, who have a more pliable thoracic wall, are more prone to this complication, and an immediate chest wall escharotomy may be indicated for the facilitation of breathing.

Special attention is given to circumferential full-thickness burns of the extremities. Pressure from the edema that develops as resuscitation proceeds may impair blood flow to underlying and distal tissue. Peripheral pulses are palpated or auscultated with an ultrasonic flow meter (Doppler) every hour, and upper extremities are elevated above the level of the heart.

Preparation is made for an escharotomy for relief of the pressure if pulses are absent or progressively decrease on serial examination. A fasciotomy may be indicated for deep electrical burns or severe muscle damage. If not yet removed, *all* jewelry and constrictive clothing must be removed and secured in order to prevent further injury as edema develops.

In determinations of fluid resuscitation requirements, the depth and extent of injury must be estimated. The quickest method to initially calculate the extent of injury is the rule of nines (Fig. 16–8), which recognizes that in the adult, the surface area of various anatomical parts represents 9% or a multiple thereof of the total body surface area. The rule of nines varies between adult and pediatric patients as a result of the significant difference in the proportion of surface area of the head in children compared with that in adults. In evaluations of the extent of injury in small, isolated burns, the rule of the palm may be used, whereby the size of the patient's palm equals 1% of the total body surface area. A surface area chart (Fig. 16–9) correlates body surface area with age, providing a more accurate determination of the extent of burn injury.

If the patient has a burn injury of greater than 20% of the body surface area, at least one, and preferably two, large-bore (#16- or #18-gauge) intravenous catheters are inserted peripherally in an unburned area of the extremities, if possible. They must be well secured. The nurse ensures that the catheters are not placed distal to circumferential burns. Central lines are not to be used unless other options are not available; if required, central lines are placed in a femoral vein. Lactated Ringer's solution is infused at 500 ml/h initially (Pruitt and Goodwin, 1990). All solution containers are numbered sequentially, and recording of intake and output is begun as soon as possible. An indwelling urethral catheter is inserted for hourly monitoring of urinary output. Several baseline laboratory studies are performed, including a complete blood count; determinations of serum electrolyte creatinine, glucose, and blood urea nitrogen levels; arterial blood gas values; carboxyhemoglobin level (if inhalation injury is suspected); and urinalysis.

Appropriate fluid resuscitation requirements for burned patients are estimated according to their body weight in kilograms, the percentage of total body surface area burned, and their age. The consensus fluid formula outlined in Table 16–5 specifies the fluid requirements for adults and children during the initial 24 hours after the burn (Nebraska Burn Institute, 1994). Half of the calculated amount is given over the first 8 hours after the injury, and the second half is given over the next 16 hours. The estimated fluid requirements serve only as a guide for the starting of resuscitation. Actual infusion rates are titrated in order to

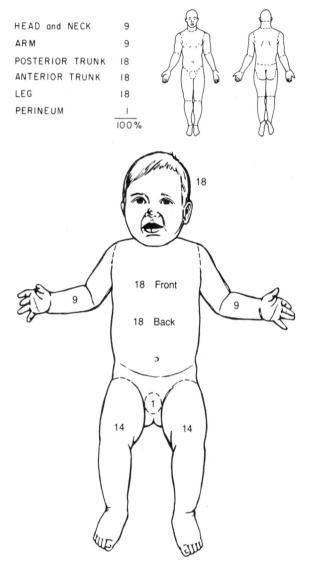

HEAD and NECK	9
ARM	9
POSTERIOR TRUNK	18
ANTERIOR TRUNK	18
LEG	18
PERINEUM	1
	100%

Figure 16–8. The rule of nines is a commonly used assessment tool that permits rapid estimation of the size and the extent of burn injury. Small children and infants have a proportionately larger head size related to lower extremities; therefore, an adjusted rule of nines is required.

ensure a urinary output of 30 to 50 ml/h in adults and 1 ml/kg of body weight per hour in children weighing less than 30 kg. Children require relatively more resuscitation fluid because they have a greater body surface area to mass ratio than that of adults. They may also require additional maintenance fluid, which is calculated by the physician (Nebraska Burn Institute, 1994; Pruitt et al., 1995).

Patients with high-voltage electrical burns or crush injuries may require larger volumes of resuscita-

tion fluids because of the hemochromogens released as a result of severe deep tissue damage (which often is not apparent). Urinary output for these patients is maintained at 75 to 100 ml/h (Nebraska Burn Institute, 1994; Mozingo et al., 1994; Pruitt and Goodwin, 1990). After the initial 24 hours after the burn, as capillary permeability returns to normal, the fluid requirements change, and colloids are commonly administered.

A chest film is obtained on admission to the emergency department, and other x-ray studies are ordered as indicated by the patient's condition. Spinal precautions are continued until all seven cervical vertebrae are clearly visualized on x-ray study with no evidence of injury. An electrocardiogram is obtained on admission, and serial evaluations are ordered for patients with electrical injuries (Nebraska Burn Institute, 1994).

Table 16–5. FLUID RESUSCITATION FOR BURN PATIENTS

First 24 Hours After Burn

Parameter	Instructions
Consensus formula	
Adults	2–4 ml LR/kg wt/% burn
Children	3 ml LR/kg wt/% burn
1st 8 h after burn	Administer 1/2 of total fluids
2nd 8 h after burn	Administer 1/4 of total fluids
3rd 8 h after burn	Administer 1/4 of total fluids

Use glucose-containing fluid if hypoglycemia develops in child. Titrate fluids to maintain urine output of 30–50 ml/h in adults and 1 ml/kg/h in children weighing < 30 kg.

EXAMPLE (using 2-ml value; 70-kg body weight; 50% burn): 2 ml × 50 × 70 = 7000 ml of LR in 24 h. Administer 3500 ml in first 8 h after burn

Second 24 Hours After Burn

Parameter	Instructions
Albumin diluted to physiological concentration in saline	0.3–0.5 ml/kg/% burn
Adults	Administer electrolyte-free water in order to meet metabolic needs and maintain urinary output
Children	Administer 5% glucose in half-normal saline in order to meet metabolic needs, maintain urinary output, and prevent hypoglycemia

' LR = lactated Ringer's solution.

BURN ESTIMATE AND DIAGRAM

AGE vs. AREA

AREA	Birth 1 yr	1 – 4 yr	5 – 9 yr	10 – 14 yr	15 yr	Adult	2°	3°	Total	Donor Areas
Head	19	17	13	11	9	7				
Neck	2	2	2	2	2	2				
Ant. Trunk	13	13	13	13	13	13				
Post. Trunk	13	13	13	13	13	13				
R. Buttock	2½	2½	2½	2½	2½	2½				
L. Buttock	2½	2½	2½	2½	2½	2½				
Genitalia	1	1	1	1	1	1				
R.U. Arm	4	4	4	4	4	4				
L.U. Arm	4	4	4	4	4	4				
R.L. Arm	3	3	3	3	3	3				
L.L. Arm	3	3	3	3	3	3				
R. Hand	2½	2½	2½	2½	2½	2½				
L. Hand	2½	2½	2½	2½	2½	2½				
R. Thigh	5½	6½	8	8½	9	9½				
L. Thigh	5½	6½	8	8½	9	9½				
R. Leg	5	5	5½	6	6½	7				
L. Leg	5	5	5½	6	6½	7				
R. Foot	3½	3½	3½	3½	3½	3½				
L. Foot	3½	3½	3½	3½	3½	3½				
						TOTAL				

BURN DIAGRAM

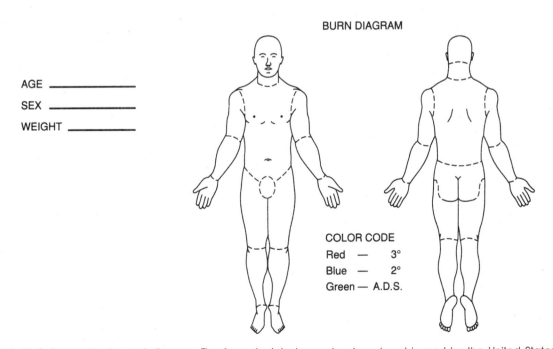

AGE _____

SEX _____

WEIGHT _____

COLOR CODE

Red — 3°

Blue — 2°

Green — A.D.S.

Figure 16–9. Burn estimate and diagram. The form depicted was developed and is used by the United States Army Institute of Surgical Research. Based on the Lund and Browder chart with Berkow's formula, it allows for more accurate assessment of the extent of burn injury based on age and depth of injury. Ant. = anterior; Post. = posterior; L. = left; R. = right; R.U. = right upper; R.L. = right lower; L.U. = left upper; L.L. = left lower; A.D.S. = available donor site.

Because patients with a major burn injury generally develop an ileus, a nasogastric tube is inserted and connected to low suction for the prevention of aspiration. The medical history and the history of the injury are conveyed to the medical team, and the patient receives tetanus immunization, if indicated. A short-acting narcotic, such as morphine sulfate, may be administered by an intravenous route only for pain relief. No intramuscular medications are given during the resuscitative phase because perfusion of edematous tissues is poor. As fluid is later mobilized, medication poorly absorbed from edematous tissue may re-enter the bloodstream and lead to an overdose (Pruitt and Goodwin, 1990).

Preparation for Transfer to a Burn Center

Caring for a patient who has sustained a major burn injury requires the availability and expertise of a specially trained multidisciplinary health care team. Factors such as the patient's age, health status, extent and depth of the burn, and body part burned significantly influence the severity of the injury. Small hospitals may not have the personnel or medical supplies needed to provide the specialized care that these patients require. The American Burn Association has developed guidelines for determining which burn-injured patients should be referred to a specialized burn center after initial stabilization has occurred (American Burn Association, 1990; Nebraska Burn Institute, 1994) (Table 16–6).

Once the patient is examined and transfer to a burn center is considered, the attending physician must make direct contact with a burn center physician. The burn center physician determines the mode of transportation and the treatment necessary for stabilizing the patient for transport (Treat et al., 1980). Accurate and timely communication between the staff at both facilities is essential and can be facilitated by the use of a patient transfer information sheet (Fig. 16–10).

Table 16–6. GUIDELINES FOR BURN CENTER REFERRAL

- > 5% total body surface area (TBSA) of full-thickness injury
- Partial-thickness and full-thickness burns involving
    10% TBSA: < 10 years of age or > 50 years of age
    20% TBSA: All other ages
- Burns involving the face, hands or feet, genitalia, perineum, or major joints
- Electrical and chemical burns
- Presence of inhalation injury
- Preexisting chronic disease
- Associated trauma

Safety is the prime concern during any type of transport. In either ground or aeromedical transport, environmental noise, vibration, poor lighting, limited space, and poor temperature control make emergency procedures, control of changes in the patient's condition, and management of supportive equipment difficult. In order to minimize risks, the following safeguards should be considered:

- Transfer should be expedited as soon as the patient is physiologically stable in order to reduce complications, which may surface later in postinjury management (Pruitt and Goodwin, 1990; Treat et al., 1980).
- Pulmonary and cardiac insufficiency, significant gastrointestinal bleeding, and hyperthermia exceeding 39.4°C are all contraindications to transport and should be controlled or corrected before the patient is moved (Pruitt and Goodwin, 1990).
- Trained personnel with essential equipment for safe transport should be available to adequately monitor and manage resuscitation en route (Pruitt and Goodwin, 1990; Treat et al., 1980).

To minimize complications during transport, the nurse has a vital role in assessing the patient. The nurse adheres to the following guidelines before transport:

- A secure, patent airway is present, with adequate gas exchange occurring. The endotracheal tube must be secured. If the tracheostomy tape is tied with a bow knot, it can be adjusted to accommodate facial edema. Chest x-ray studies are performed in order to rule out pulmonary disease and pneumothorax and to ensure proper tube placement (Pruitt and Goodwin, 1990). A Heimlich valve is attached to a chest tube and replaces the water seal drainage bottle. Arterial blood gas values are within acceptable limits during supplemental oxygen therapy. Suction and ventilation equipment are available at all times.
- Adequate circulatory support is established. Administration of resuscitation fluids and monitoring of response must continue during transport. Intravenous lines are secured by sutures, and connections are taped. Only plastic solution containers are used. The indwelling urethral catheter is anchored in order to prevent accidental displacement. Strong pulses must be present in all extremities with circumferential burns, with or without escharotomies.
- Mechanisms for the prevention of aspiration are initiated. The patient with a major burn is at significant risk for emesis and aspiration during

U. S. ARMY INSTITUTE OF SURGICAL RESEARCH

PATIENT TRANSFER INFORMATION SHEET

Date and time of call _____

Referring MD _____ Telephone _____

Hospital _____ City _____ State _____

PATIENT INFORMATION

Name _____ SSN _____ Status: Active Duty _____

Retired _____

Age _____ Sex _____ Pre-Burn Weight _____ Dependent _____

VAB _____

Date of burn _____ Cause _____ PHS _____

Civilian _____

Extent of burn _____ 3rd Degree _____

Areas burned _____

Inhalation Injury _____ Allergies _____

Association injury _____

Pre-existing diseases _____

TREATMENT CHECK-LIST

Resuscitation: Calculated need (2ml/Kg/% TBS) _____

Fluid in _____ Urine Output _____

Airway _____ Blood gases _____ E-T tube _____

Medication: Analgesics or sedatives _____ Tetanus _____

Antibiotics _____ Other Meds _____

Escharotomies: Arms _____ Legs _____ Chest _____

Wound Care: Wash and debride _____ Topical Agent _____

Lab tests: HCT _____ Electrolytes _____ BS _____ BUN _____

Request: Insert NG tube- Avoid general anesthesia or IM meds -Keep I&O

INFORMATION FOR FLIGHT PLAN

Burn Team _____ Family to accompany patient _____

Location of nearest airport with jet traffic _____

Transportation for team at destination _____

Figure 16–10. U.S. Army Institute of Surgical Research transfer information form. The use of transfer information form to summarize information concerning a burn patient's status promotes good communication between the referring and receiving facilities and ensures continuity of care. E-T = endotracheal; BUN = blood urea nitrogen; IM = intramuscular; I&O = intake and output; SSN = Social Security number; HCT = hematocrit; VAB = Veterans Affairs Beneficiary; BS = blood sugar; TBS = total body surface.

transport. Correct nasogastric tube placement is ensured, and the patient does not receive any oral intake.

- Thermoregulation is monitored. If the patient is transported within the first 12 hours after burn, the burn wounds are *not* cleansed and placed in a topical antimicrobial agent. Wounds are covered with a clean dry sheet or wrapped with a nonconstrictive gauze dressing. In order to minimize heat loss, the patient is wrapped in blankets, which are removed during transport if hyperthermia develops. Adequate absorbent padding is needed under the patient in order to accommodate large-volume plasma leakage from the burn wounds and to prevent pressure breakdown of skin.

- Comfort is maintained with adequate pain control. Morphine sulfate can cause nausea; therefore, careful evaluation is necessary during transport. If the patient is properly wrapped and kept warm, pain is minimized.

- All associated injuries are stabilized, and the patient is transported with appropriate splinting devices in place. Tetanus prophylaxis is given and documented.

- The patient and family are provided with support. Both the patient and the family must be kept informed on the details of the transfer. A brief assessment of family demographics can help the health care team determine special needs, especially for long-distance transfers.

• The nurse ensures that all records are complete and accurate and that an accurate summary of the events of the injury, the treatment given, and the patient monitoring and response accompanies the patient.

With careful anticipatory planning and appropriate preparation, the severely burned patient can be safely transported by ground or air to a burn center. Transport should occur early in the postburn period, based on guidelines provided by the receiving burn center.

Critical Care Burn Unit Interventions: Acute Care Phase

Once the patient has arrived in the burn critical care unit, the primary and secondary assessments are once again performed. Critical indices are monitored at least once an hour and include blood pressure, pulse, respiration, temperature, peripheral pulses, and urinary output. In addition, urine specific gravity, glucose and acetone levels, and gastric pH and heme test results are evaluated every 2 hours. All intravenous catheters are usually replaced, and the patient is weighed. Obtaining of weights continues once or twice daily until the patient's preburn weight is obtained after diuresis. Thereafter, weights are obtained daily, except during the immobilization period after skin grafting. All parameters must be documented, including hourly intake and output, for a careful analysis of trends.

Massive edema formation is an anticipated response to fluid resuscitation in an extensively burned patient. The upper extremities are elevated above the level of the heart in order to increase perfusion. Active or passive range-of-motion exercises may be performed for 5 minutes every hour in order to increase venous return and minimize edema. The patient's sensorium is evaluated hourly because increased agitation or confusion may be an indication of hypovolemia or hypoxemia. The head of the bed is elevated 30°, especially in children younger than 2 years of age, who are susceptible to cerebral edema from resuscitation fluid. Blood pressure measurements and, to some extent, heart rate are not reliable indicators of fluid resuscitation in burn patients. The burn patient often has a higher baseline heart rate of 100 to 120 beats per minute, and blood pressure readings (arterial or cuff measurements) may be altered by peripheral edema or vasoconstriction. Initially, urinary output is the only reliable indicator of adequate resuscitation. Titration of calculated fluid requirements according to hourly urine output is an essential function of the nurse during resuscitation. For patients with cardiopulmonary disease or for those who require excessive volumes of fluid, pulmonary artery pressure monitoring may be indicated, with frequent measurements of pulmonary capillary wedge pressures (Rue and Cioffi, 1991; Pruitt et al., 1995).

Serum electrolyte levels are determined at least two to four times a day during the resuscitative phase and as dictated by the patient's status during the acute care phase. Serum sodium levels typically approach the level of the resuscitation fluid being administered. Serum potassium levels may be increased as a result of release from injured tissue. Blood urea nitrogen level may also be increased when excessive protein catabolism occurs, and hyperglycemia may occur as a result of catecholamine release. Arterial blood gas values are evaluated frequently because metabolic acidosis may be indicative of inadequate tissue perfusion. A daily chest x-ray study is required during the first week for patients with extensive burns or inhalation injury.

Patients with suspected inhalation injuries who are not already intubated must be monitored frequently for hoarseness, stridor, or wheezing. These symptoms may not be apparent until after fluid resuscitation has been initiated. Carboxyhemoglobin levels should be determined when carbon monoxide poisoning is suspected. Injury above the glottis may be diagnosed by identification of edema of the oropharynx. Fiberoptic bronchoscopy or xenon-133 lung scanning may be indicated in order to provide a definitive diagnosis of injury below the glottis (Nebraska Burn Institute, 1994; Carrougher, 1993; Cioffi and Rue, 1991). All patients with inhalation injuries receive assistance with coughing, deep breathing, and repositioning at least every 2 hours. Humidifed oxygen is administered via a face tent or oxygen mask, while the patient is monitored for respiratory distress. If nasotracheal intubation is indicated, the patient is suctioned at least every 2 hours or as indicated. Oximetric monitoring of oxygen saturation and monitoring of end-tidal carbon dioxide levels occurs continuously as appropriate.

Patients with burns of greater than 20 to 25% of the body surface area have a nasogastric tube inserted. The acid content of the gastric secretions is buffered with prophylactic antacid, and/or histamine$_2$ receptor antagonists are administered in order to maintain a pH of greater than 5. Bowel sounds are assessed frequently for return of gastric motility so that enteral or oral feedings may be initiated.

Hypothermia is a potential problem for patients with major burns. Wound therapy, such as bathing and application of dressings, may potentiate heat loss. Patients are kept warm with external heat lamps or radiant heat shields. Temperatures are monitored closely until all burn wounds are closed.

Pain Control in Resuscitative and Acute Care Phases

The level of pain experienced in the resuscitative and acute care phases is related to the extent of partial-thickness injury and the amount of anxiety the patient experiences. Although full-thickness burns are insensate because cutaneous nerve endings have been destroyed, a patient usually has a mixture of full-thickness and partial-thickness burns. In addition, many painful procedures are necessary in order to facilitate the resuscitation process. The entire experience usually produces much anxiety, which can in turn increase the perception of pain intensity.

Pain control in the resuscitative phase is best achieved with the use of small doses of narcotics given intravenously at frequent intervals. Morphine (3 to 5 mg in adults) or meperidine (30 to 50 mg in adults) are the drugs of choice and are given at intervals established on the basis of the patient's physiological condition (Pruitt et al., 1995). A continuous infusion of morphine may be useful in maintaining a consistent level of analgesia. However, continuous infusions require close monitoring of the patient's response and are used most safely in patients who require mechanical ventilation. Subcutaneous or intramuscular injections are ineffective in this phase because of impaired circulation in soft tissue. If such injections are given, the potential for narcotic overdose is high because absorption increases with restored circulation during fluid resuscitation (Pruitt and Goodwin, 1990). Anxiety is generally lessened and pain relief from analgesics is enhanced by simple techniques, such as explaining all nursing care activities before performing them, talking in a quiet and calm voice, or using simple relaxation and guided imagery techniques (McCaffery and Beebe, 1989; Patterson, 1992). Anxiolytics may be required (Everett et al., 1994). If the patient is alert, patient-controlled analgesia may be helpful in maintaining a consistent level of analgesia and in providing the patient some control over pain relief, which could reduce anxiety (Choiniere et al., 1990; Cram and Kealey, 1990).

Many aspects of burn treatment in the acute phase produce pain: hydrotherapy, debridement, application of mafenide acetate, and physical therapy. Patient descriptions of perceived intensity of pain vary little, despite differences in the extent of burn, ethnicity, age, and socioeconomic status (Perry et al., 1981; Geisser,

1995). When the patient is hemodynamically stable and the ileus is resolved, analgesic medications can be given safely by intravenous, intramuscular, or oral routes. Although pain is reduced as the wounds heal or are covered with either temporary dressings or autograft skin, frequent surgeries and wound care procedures produce episodic periods of pain and anxiety until permanent wound closure or healing is completed. Despite the acute intermittent nature of the pain, the intensity of procedural pain and the mild-to-moderate pain that occurs with movement contribute to an overall perception of constant pain (Perry et al., 1981). Itching also becomes a major problem that contributes to the patient's overall discomfort. Several medications and soothing lotions can assist in controlling pruritus.

The elimination of most of the pain of burn injury has been shown to significantly increase the positive outcome for the patient. The first step is adequate assessment (Molter, 1991). In a recent study comparing pain assessment by burn patients and their nurses, the ratings of the two groups were highly correlated, but nurses accurately assessed the patient's pain only 53% of the time. Evidence indicated that providing descriptions of pain behavior was helpful in increasing the accuracy (Everett et al., 1994). Geisser (1995; see Research Box) found that nurses assessed patients' pain accurately only 37% of the time. The literature supports that there is much work to be done in improving assessment and intervention of severe burn pain (Molter, 1991; Agency for Health Care Policy and Research, 1992; Geisser, 1995). Greenfield and co-workers (1995) have been studying the types of pain assessment tools selected by burn patients. Despite the positive effects of appropriate pain control, a compromise must exist between the patient's pain perception, the pain state, and safe medical practice in managing severe burn pain (Loeser, 1987). The major paradox of burn pain management is that the nurses inflict pain and then must relieve it. It becomes a challenge for the critical care nurse to develop a pain management program that implements safe pharmacological therapy in combination with nonpharmacological pain control techniques. The goal should continue to be elimination of pain.

Infection Control

One of the most important nursing interventions in the care of burn patients is control of infection. As a result of improved formulas for fluid resuscitation, the use of topical antimicrobial agents, new antibiotics, improvements in nutrition, and more aggressive wound closure techniques, the survival of burn patients has significantly increased (Saffle et al., 1995). However, infection (primarily pulmonary) still remains the leading cause of morbidity and mortality in the burn population (Shirani et al., 1987; Weber and Tompkins, 1993; Rue et al., 1995). The immunosuppressive effects of burn injury, along with environmental and therapeutic factors, must be considered in the development of an infection control policy. Burn patients are at high risk not only for invasive burn wound infection but also for septic phlebitis secondary to intravenous therapy, urinary tract infections related to long-term catheterization, pneumonia, and septicemia (Waymack and Pruitt, 1990; Rue et al., 1995).

Burn eschar is normally colonized with various microorganisms. If these microorganisms invade underlying viable tissue, an invasive burn wound infection develops. Burn wound surface cultures should be performed on admission and several times a week in order to monitor changes in wound colonization, but a burn wound biopsy is the only definitive means of identifying an invasive burn wound infection (Waymack and Pruitt, 1990). Once invasion is diagnosed, appropriate local and/or systemic antibiotic therapy must be initiated.

Infection control policies differ between burn units, but all policies stress reverse isolation techniques, strict adherence to dress code policies, and hand washing as environmental priorities in the prevention of infection (McManus et al., 1987; Weber and Tompkins, 1993).

Wound Management

Before healing or excision and grafting of the burn wound, nursing care must focus on the prevention of burn wound infection. All wounds are cleansed at least once a day with a surgical detergent disinfectant and are rinsed with warm saline or sterile or tap water. This regimen is best accomplished in a shower or Hubbard tank, but bed baths may also be used for hemodynamically unstable patients. The patient is not immersed in water, because with immersion, there is a significant potential for cross-contamination of wounds in patients with significant body surface area injury, and hypothermia is more difficult to control. All necrotic tissue, exudates, and fibrous debris are removed from the wound bed in order to control bacterial proliferation and to promote healing. Loose eschar and wound debris are removed with gauze sponges or debrided with scissors and forceps during the bathing session. Hair is shaved 3 to 4 inches out from the

Table 16–7. TOPICAL ANTIMICROBIAL AGENTS FOR BURN WOUND MANAGEMENT

Agent	Indications	Nursing Considerations
Clotrimazole cream	Fungal colonization of wounds	Apply thin coat of agent to wound and wait 20 min before applying any dressings. Must use an antibacterial agent in addition to antifungal agent. Painless; may cause skin irritation and blistering.
Mafenide acetate (Sulfamylon)	Active against most gram-positive and gram-negative wound pathogens; drug of choice for electrical and ear burns.	Apply once or twice daily with sterile glove; do not use dressings that reduce effectiveness and cause maceration; monitor respiratory rate, electrolyte values, and arterial pH for evidence of metabolic acidosis; painful on application to partial-thickness burns for about 30 minutes.
Silver nitrate	Effective against wide spectrum of common wound pathogens and fungal infections; used in patients with sulfa allergy or toxic epidermal necrolysis. Poor penetration eschar.	Apply 0.5% solution wet dressings twice or three times a day; ensure that dressings remain moist by wetting them every 2 hours. Preserve solution in a light-resistant container. Protect walls, floors, and so on, with plastic in order to prevent black staining. Monitor for hyponatremia and hypochloremia.
Silver sulfadiazine (Silvadene)	Active against a wide spectrum of microbial pathogens. Use with caution in patients with impaired renal or hepatic function.	Apply once or twice a day with a sterile gloved hand. Leave wounds exposed or wrap lightly with gauze dressings. Painless.

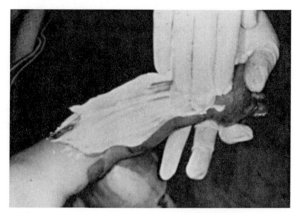

Figure 16–11. Application of topical agent to burn wound. A sterile gloved hand is used to apply a topical antimicrobial agent to the burn wound.

of the most common types and uses for biological and biosynthetic dressings. Research is currently being conducted related to the use of cultured epidermal sheets for permanent wound closure. The layered sheets of human epidermal cells (grown in a laboratory using tissue culture techniques to expand keratinocytes that are derived from a small, full-thickness skin biopsy specimen) provide hope for early wound coverage in extensively burned patients with limited donor sites (Rheinwald and Green, 1975; Phillips et al., 1990; Tompkins and Burk, 1992; Rue et al., 1993; Phillips, 1994).

Priority areas for autograft skin application include the face, the hands, the feet, and over the joints. Two approaches may be used for preparing a wound for grafting. Early eschar excision and application of

wound margin. Wet-to-wet or wet-to-dry dressings may also be used to aid in the debridement process in order to prepare the wound bed for grafting. All wounds are inspected closely, and their appearance is carefully documented so that changes across time can be readily noted.

After each hydrotherapy session, the unhealed or unexcised burn wound is covered with an antimicrobial topical agent or dressing (Fig. 16–11). Table 16–7 describes the most commonly used topical antimicrobial agents and nursing considerations. The topical agent not only assists in controlling infection but also prevents wound desiccation, which impedes the reepithelialization process (Kagan and Warden, 1994). Two common treatments of burn wounds are the open and the occlusive methods. With the open method, the burn wounds are left open to air after the antimicrobial agent is applied. With the occlusive method, the wound is covered with gauze dressings that have been saturated with a topical antimicrobial agent, or a thin layer of gauze is placed over an agent that is applied directly to the wounds. The dressings are then covered with a net bandage to hold the gauze in place. Each method has advantages and disadvantages, and specific protocols differ among burn units.

Any deep partial-thickness or full-thickness burn wound that requires more than 3 weeks for healing is a candidate for application of autograft skin. At present, autograft skin is the only permanent means of covering a burn wound. Biological or biosynthetic dressings are commonly used as temporary wound coverings for freshly excised burn wounds until autograft skin is available (Phillips, 1993; Cooper and Spielvogel, 1994). They may also be used as a dressing for partial-thickness burns, meshed autograft skin, or donor sites to promote healing. Table 16–8 provides descriptions

Table 16–8. BIOLOGICAL AND BIOSYNTHETIC DRESSINGS

Type of Dressing	Definition
Biological dressing	Temporary wound cover of human or animal species tissue
Allograft (homograft) skin	Temporary wound cover composed of a graft of skin transplanted from another human, living or dead.
Xenograft (heterograft) skin	Temporary wound cover to promote healing. A graft of skin, usually pigskin, is transplanted between animals of different species.
Biosynthetic dressing	A wound covering composed of both biological and synthetic materials
Biobrane	Bilaminate wound dressing composed of nylon mesh enclosed in a collagen derivative with a silicon rubber outer membrane. It is permeable to some antibiotic ointments.
Integra (``artificial skin'')	Wound dressing composed of 2 layers: a ``dermal'' layer made of animal collagen that interfaces with an open wound surface, and an ``epidermal'' layer made of Silastic that controls water loss from the dermis and acts as a bacterial barrier. The dermal layer biodegrades within several months and is resorbed. The epidermal layer may be removed and replaced with autograft skin when appropriate.

autograft skin constitute the more common treatment. Usually, excision and grafting are initiated within the first week after the burn, when the patient is hemodynamically stable. Advantages include earlier wound coverage, early return of function, decrease in scar formation, and decrease in length of hospitalization. The conservative approach involves wound treatment with antimicrobial agents, hydrotherapy, and debridement until partial-thickness burns are healed and full-thickness injury is ready for skin grafting. With the conservative approach, less blood loss and less potential risk of complications associated with blood replacement therapy exist (McManus et al., 1989).

Autograft skin is applied to the recipient bed,

dermal side down, and is secured with staples, surgical tape, fibrin glue, or sutures. Table 16–9 summarizes the types of skin graft used, along with nursing care requirements. Splinting of graft sites may be indicated in order to prevent movement and shearing of the grafts until healing is complete. Upper extremities are elevated in order to prevent pooling of blood, which can lead to increased pressure and thus graft loss (Waymack and Pruitt, 1990). A method of documenting wound treatment that facilitates day-to-day communication of care requirements should be used. Nursing interventions must also focus on the care of donor sites (Duncan and Driscoll, 1991). Once donor skin is harvested, the site must be covered with a dressing

---

Table 16–9. AUTOGRAFT SKIN: NURSING IMPLICATIONS

Type of Autograft	Definition	Nursing Implications
Split-thickness sheet skin graft	Sheet of skin composed of the epidermis and a variable portion of the dermis that is split at a predetermined thickness, allowing for transplantation to another area of the body.	Grafted area must be immobilized. Pockets of serous fluid must be evacuated by needle aspiration or rolling of the fluid with a cotton tip applicator toward the skin edges. If fluid is not evacuated, graft adherence is compromised.
Split-thickness meshed skin graft	Split-thickness sheet graft that is placed in a mesh dermatome, which expands the graft from 1.5 to 9 times its original size before being placed on a recipient bed of granulation tissue.	Grafted area is immobilized, often in splints. Skin graft is covered with fine mesh gauze, then coarse mesh gauze, and is then wrapped with absorbent gauze roll before being placed in a splint. Dressings must be kept moist with an antimicrobial solution, but not saturated, to prevent desiccation and promote epithelialization of the interstices of the meshed skin. The first dressing change is in 3–5 days.
Full-thickness skin graft	A skin graft that contains the full thickness of the skin down to the subcutaneous tissue.	Requires the same care as a sheet skin graft.
Cultured epidermal sheets	Layered sheets of human epidermal cells grown in the laboratory by use of tissue culture techniques to expand keratinocytes derived from a small full-thickness skin biopsy specimen. Allows for the potential of covering extensive wound areas more quickly without having to wait for healing of limited donor site skin surfaces.	In the first 7–10 days after surgery, daily dressing changes involve only the outer layer of fluffy gauze. The underlying coarse mesh gauze and petroleum jelly gauze, which are sutured over the graft, are not to be disturbed. Unlike care for meshed autograft skin, the outer dressing must remain dry. Many topical antimicrobial agents are toxic to the cultured epithelial autograft skin and should not come in contact with the graft dressings. Once the petroleum jelly gauze is loose (7–10 days), it can be removed, and wet saline dressings are used until approximately 21 days after grafting, when the skin graft is usually well adherent. Gentle passive range-of-motion exercises can begin once the petroleum jelly gauze is removed.

Table 16–10. TYPES OF DONOR SITE DRESSINGS

Dressing	Description
Fine mesh gauze	Cotton gauze is placed directly on a donor site. A crust or ''scab'' is formed as the gauze dries and epithelialization of the wound occurs under the dressing. The gauze peels away easily as the wound heals.
Fine mesh gauze	Cotton gauze is impregnated with a blend of lanolin, olive oil, petrolatum, and the red dye ''scarlet red.'' Healing occurs as with fine mesh gauze dressing.
Xeroform	Fine mesh gauze containing 3% bismuth tribromophenate in a petrolatum blend. Promotes healing as with other mesh gauze dressings.
Op-Site	A thin elastic film that is occlusive, waterproof, and permeable to moisture, vapor, and air. Fluid under dressing may need to be evacuated.
DuoDerm	A hydrocolloid dressing that interacts with moisture on skin, creating a bond that makes it adhere.
N-terface	A translucent, nonabsorbent, and nonreactive surface material used between the burn wound and the outer dressing.
Vigilon	A colloidal suspension on a polyethylene mesh support that provides a moist environment and is permeable to gases and water vapor.
Kaltostat	Hydrophylic, nonwoven fiber that converts to a firm gel when it is activated by wound exudate. Creates a warm, moist environment that is nonadherent to the wound.

until healing occurs. Many types of dressings can be used (Table 16–10), but any type should promote healing of the donor site within 8 to 14 days (Waymack and Pruitt, 1990).

Inherent in all wound care management is the necessity to improve and maintain function. Occupational and physical therapists are essential members of the burn team and are consulted from the day of admission. Often, the position of comfort for the patients is one that can lead to dysfunction or deformity. Specialized splints and exercises are required for the prevention of future complications (Hardin and Luster, 1991; Robson et al., 1992). Although the critical care nurse may not actually develop the plan for such

therapy, knowledge of and compliance with the plan are essential for positive patient outcomes.

Special Areas of Concern

Burns of the face, ears, eyes, hands, feet, genitalia, and perineum pose special concerns (Pruitt and Goodwin, 1990; Duncan and Driscoll, 1991).

BURNS OF THE FACE

Facial burns can lead to significant complications; thus, patients with such burns require hospitalization in a burn unit. The presence of facial burns may signal inhalation injury, and massive facial edema may lead to a compromised airway. Close monitoring of the patient's respiratory status is essential. The head of the bed is elevated in order to facilitate respiratory exchange and edema reabsorption. Special care must be taken in the cleansing of facial burns so that excessive bleeding and damage to new tissue growth are prevented. All hair is shaved from the wound each day. Once the wound is cleaned and debrided, a topical antimicrobial agent is applied per unit protocol. Because of the rich blood supply in the face, partial-thickness burns usually heal quickly as long as infection is prevented. Good oral hygiene is essential.

BURNS OF THE EARS

The ears are especially prone to inflammation and infection (chondritis) that could lead to complete loss of ear cartilage. Ear burns are treated with a topical antimicrobial agent, and application of any pressure to the ears must be prevented. Dressings are avoided, and cloth ties used for securing tubes to the face must not put pressure on the top of the ears. Pillows are not used, and a foam donut with a hole for the ear to rest in while the patient is in a lateral position is substituted.

BURNS OF THE EYES

Immediate examination of the eyes is necessary on arrival at the hospital because eyelid edema forms rapidly. Contact lenses are removed if present. The eyes are stained with fluorescein in order to rule out corneal injury, and the eyes are irrigated with copious amounts of physiological saline if injury is confirmed. A thorough examination by an ophthalmologist is mandatory for serious injuries. Once eyelid edema resolves, the cornea may become exposed as the eyelid retracts. Careful observation of eyelashes is also necessary because they may invert and scratch the cornea.

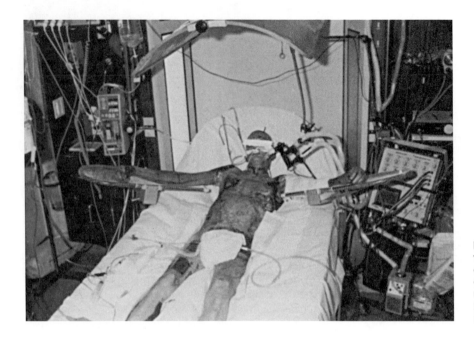

Figure 16–12. Slings used to elevate burned extremities. Slings can be devised to support and elevate burned extremities. The mesh on the slings pictured provides for air circulation that prevents wound maceration.

Nursing care involves the frequent application of ophthalmic ointment or artificial tears in order to protect the cornea and conjunctiva from drying.

BURNS OF THE HANDS OR FEET

Extensive burns of the hands and feet may cause permanent disability, necessitating a long convalescence. Nursing care is directed at preservation of function. Burned hands are elevated above the level of the heart on slings or wedges in order to reduce edema formation (Fig. 16–12). Although range-of-motion exercises may be painful, they must be initiated as soon as possible after the injury and must be performed frequently throughout each day. Active range-of-motion exercises prevent muscle atrophy, reduce or prevent the shortening of ligaments, and reduce edema. Passive range-of-motion exercises are indicated if patients are unable to move their extremities actively. Splinting may be required for the maintenance of function and the prevention of deformities of the affected part. An elastic bandage is applied over burn wounds of the feet and legs in order to prevent pooling of blood when the patient is ambulating or sitting, but the bandage is removed when the feet are elevated. In establishing a nursing plan of care, the nurse must remember that patients with bilateral burned hands are totally dependent on nursing personnel for all of their physical needs.

BURNS OF THE GENITALIA AND PERINEUM

Patients with perineal burns often require hospitalization for observation of urinary tract obstruction caused by edema formation, and they require meticulous wound management so that infection is prevented. Insertion of an indwelling urethral catheter may be indicated for the maintenance of urethral patency until the wounds are healed or grafted. Meticulous wound cleansing is essential because of the potential for fecal contamination with this type of burn. Perineal hair must be shaved as required. Scrotal edema is common, and the scrotum is elevated on towels. Antimicrobial topical agents are applied in order to prevent infection.

Nutritional Considerations

Adequate nutrition plays a critical role in the survival of extensively burned patients. For optimal wound healing to occur, the burn patient must be in a state of positive nitrogen balance. Because of the tendency toward catabolism that is mediated by the patient's hypermetabolic state, supplemental calories are essential in order to meet energy demands, and additional nitrogen is needed in order to replenish body protein stores. Inadequate nutrition may lead to significant body weight loss, delayed wound healing or skin graft loss, impaired immunologic responsiveness, sepsis, or even death (Carlson and Jordan, 1991; Reig, 1993).

Caloric needs are determined by use of metabolic studies for each burn patient with a major burn; these calculations take into consideration the percent of body surface area burned, the preburn nutritional status, and the presence of other complicating factors, such as inhalation injury (Curreri, 1990). Coordination of the nutritional plan is performed by a registered dietitian according to requirements delineated by the physician. The dietitian and the nursing staff provide vigorous nutritional support as soon as possible through the most appropriate method available. Enteral nutrition is the preferred route for any patient with a functioning gastrointestinal tract. Care must be taken to prevent aspiration if tube feedings are necessary. Parenteral nutrition is indicated only for patients whose clinical status precludes the use of enteric feedings.

Nursing assessment and intervention in assisting patients to meet nutritional requirements include accurate monitoring of daily weights; accurate measurement of intake and output, including bowel movements; and careful evaluation of nasogastric or enteric tubes to ensure proper placement and patency. Nurses can play an important role in ensuring that devices that facilitate self-feeding are available and that meal times are planned around other therapeutic requirements in order to provide a relaxed, pain-free environment (Fig. 16–13). Allowing family members to visit at meal times and to assist with feedings may also be beneficial to the patients and may be therapeutic for the family (Carlson and Jordan, 1991).

Psychosocial Considerations

Burn injury is one of the most psychologically devastating injuries to patients and their families. Not only is there a very real threat to survival, but the psychological and physical pain experienced, the fear of disfigurement, and the uncertainty of the long-term effects of the injury on future lifestyle and plans can precipitate a crisis for the patient and family. The patient may experience many stages of psychological adaptation before appropriate functioning returns (Table 16–11). Not all patients experience manifestations of all stages, but support and therapy are necessary for any patient and family experiencing a major burn injury. Some evidence indicates that psychosocial adaptation to burn injury lags behind improvement in physical performance. The critical care nurse needs to assess the patient and family in order to determine whether adequate support systems are available and whether appropriate coping mechanisms are being used. Interventions based on individual assessments are the most beneficial and may require assistance from consulting support personnel, such as chaplains, clinical nurse specialists, psychiatrists, and social workers. Interventions must include the family so that they can continue to support the patient (Summers, 1991). Recent research showed that several family needs continue to be perceived as important to the family up until the patient is discharged (Molter, 1993). As the patient moves out of the intensive care unit, support mechanisms need to continue in order to ensure continuity of care.

Discharge Planning

Discharge planning for critically ill burned patients must begin on the day of admission. Assess-

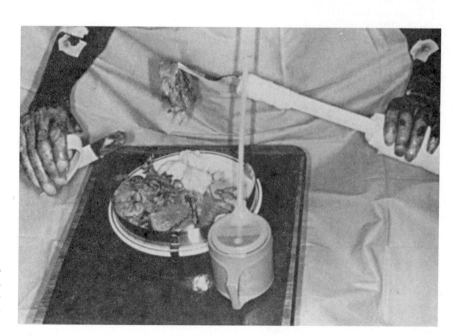

Figure 13. Adaptive devices for facilitation of self-feeding. Adaptive devices are provided in order to assist the patient to eat, thus promoting independence.

Table 16–11. STAGES OF POSTBURN PSYCHOLOGICAL ADAPTATION

Survival Anxiety

Often manifested by lack of concentration, easy startle response, tearfulness, social withdrawal, and inappropriate behavior. Instructions need to be repeated, and the patient has to be allowed time to verbalize concerns and fears. Increased reports of pain are frequently associated with high levels of anxiety.

Search for Meaning

During this phase, the patient repeatedly recounts the events leading to the injury, trying to determine a logical explanation that is emotionally acceptable. It is important to avoid judging the patient's reasoning and to listen actively and to participate in the discussions with the patient.

Investment in Recuperation

This is a period of increased cooperation with the treatment regimen. The patient is motivated to be independent and takes pride in small accomplishments. The nurse should educate the patient concerning discharge goals and involve the patient and family in planning for a program of increased self-care. The patient requires much praise and verbal encouragement in this phase.

Investment in Rehabilitation

As self-confidence increases, the patient is focused on achieving as much preburn function as possible. Depression may occur as new losses in function are realized. Staff support is limited in this phase, which usually occurs after the patient is discharged from the hospital and is undergoing outpatient rehabilitation. Praise, support, and continued information are beneficial.

Reintegration of Identity

The patient accepts losses and recognizes that changes have occurred. Adaptation is completed, and staff involvement is terminated.

Adapted from Watkins, P., Cook, E., May, S., & Ehleben, C. (1988). Psychological stages in adaptation following burn injury: A method for facilitating psychological recovery of burn victims. *Journal of Burn Care Rehabilitation, 9*(4), 376–384.

ments are made regarding patient survival, the potential or actual short-term or long-term functional disabilities secondary to the burn injury, the financial resources available, the family roles and expectations, and the psychological support systems. Patient and family education is essential for preparations for eventual discharge and for transfer from the intensive care unit. Patients and families who are returning home must understand how to care for their physical needs as well as their psychological and social needs. Nurses play an important role in multidisciplinary discharge planning by providing guidance for patient and family education and by evaluating the need for additional resources to plan for patient rehabilitative and home care requirements (Gordon, 1988).

PATIENT OUTCOMES

Expected patient outcomes for the burn-injured patient are summarized in the following sections.

Pulmonary

- Patient will have a patent airway with clear breath sounds on auscultation, after pulmonary hygiene.
- Arterial blood gas values and oxygen saturation will be normal.
- Dyspnea and work of breathing will be decreased with appropriate positioning.
- The patient will be able to cough effectively and produce clear secretions.

Fluid and Electrolytes

- Weight gain will be appropriate in first 48 hours, with diuresis occurring over next 8 to 10 days at a weight loss rate of no more than 10% of weight gain per day.
- Urine output in first 48 hours will be 30 to 50 ml/h (75 to 100 ml/h with electrical injuries) or 1 ml/kg/h for children weighing less than 30 kg.
- Urine specific gravity will normalize to 1.010 to 1.020 after diuresis. Urinary glucose and acetone levels will be normal.
- Electrolyte levels will be within normal limits after adequate replacement therapy.

Cardiovascular

- The patient's pulse will range from 80 to 120 beats/min.
- The patient's blood pressure will be adequate in relation to the patient's pulse and urinary output.
- The patient's cardiac output and pulmonary capillary wedge pressure will be low in the first 6 to 12 hours; then the cardiac output will be normal or supranormal and the capillary wedge pressure will be normal until wound closure.
- Patient will have strong, palpable pulses in all extremities and good capillary refill.

Pain

- Respirations will be adequate and hemodynamic stability will be achieved after narcotic analgesia is administered.
- Perceived pain level will be decreased based on a subjective scale or a change in physiological parameters.
- Patient will be able to identify factors that contribute to pain.

NURSING CARE PLAN: RESUSCITATIVE AND ACUTE CARE PHASES OF MAJOR BURN INJURY

Nursing Diagnosis	Patient Outcomes	Nursing Interventions
Ineffective airway clearance/impaired gas exchange related to tracheal edema or interstitial edema secondary to inhalation injury and manifested by hypoxemia and hypercapnia.	Partial pressure of arterial oxygen > 90 mm Hg, partial pressure of arterial carbon dioxide < 40 mm Hg, oxygen saturation > 95%. Respirations 16 to 20 breaths/min. Mentation will be clear. Patient will mobilize secretions. Clear to white secretions. Dyspnea will be absent, and work of breathing increased with appropriate positioning.	Assess respiratory rate and character q 1 h, breath sounds q 4 h, loss of consciousness q 1 h; evaluate need for chest escharotomy during fluid resuscitation. If patient is not intubated, assess for stridor, hoarseness q 1 h. Monitor oxygen saturation q 1 h, obtain and evaluate arterial blood gas values as needed (prn). Administer humidified oxygen as ordered. Assist patient in coughing, deep breathing q 1 h while he or she is awake. Suction q 1 to 2 h or prn, monitor sputum characteristics and amount. Elevate head of bed in order to facilitate lung expansion. Schedule activities to avoid fatigue, dyspnea. Turn patient q 2 h in order to mobilize secretions. Assist with obtaining chest x-ray study as ordered.
Fluid volume deficit secondary to fluid shifts to the interstitium and evaporative loss of fluids from the injured skin.	Weight gain based on volume of fluids administered in first 48 hours, followed by moderate diuresis over next 8 to 10 days with a weight loss rate of no more than 10 to 12% of weight gain per day. Hourly urine output 30 to 50 ml/h; 1 ml/kg/h in children < 30 kg of body weight; 75 to 100 ml/h in those with electrical injury. Specific gravity normal except during diuresis when it may be slightly decreased. Urine negative for glucose and acetone. Heart rate 80 to 120 beats/min, blood pressure adequate in relation to pulse and urine output. Sensorium clear. Laboratory values: sodium level will approach that of resuscitation fluid initially, then will return to normal with diuresis; potassium level initially high, Hct level 50 to 55% until adequate resuscitation is established; all other values within normal limits.	Titrate calculated fluid requirements in first 48 hours in order to maintain acceptable urinary output. Obtain and increase urine specific gravity and glucose and acetone levels q 2 h. Monitor vital signs q 1 h until patient is hemodynamically stable. Monitor mental status q 1 h for at least 48 h. Obtain and record weights daily or twice daily (bid). Record hourly intake and output measurements and evaluate trends. Monitor electrolyte, hematocrit (Hct), serum glucose, blood urea nitrogen, creatinine levels at least bid for first 48 hours and then as required by patient status.
Altered peripheral tissue perfusion related to impaired vascular perfusion in extremities with circumferential burns manifested by decreased or absent peripheral pulses.	No tissue injury in extremities secondary to inadequate perfusion related to vascular compression from edema.	Check peripheral pulses q 1 h × 72 h by palpation and/or ultrasonic flow meter; evaluate sensation of pain and capillary refill in extremities. Notify physician of changes in pulses, capillary refill, or pain sensation; be prepared to assist with escharotomy or fasciotomy. Elevate upper extremities.

Continued on following page

NURSING CARE PLAN: RESUSCITATIVE AND ACUTE CARE PHASES OF MAJOR BURN INJURY *Continued*

Nursing Diagnosis	Patient Outcomes	Nursing Interventions
Acute pain related to burn trauma.	Identifies factors that contribute to pain. Verbalizes improved comfort level. Physiological parameters return to normal. Respirations adequate, and hemodynamic stability achieved after administration of narcotic analgesia.	Medicate patient before bathing, dressing changes, major procedures, prn. Reduce anxiety: explain all activities before initiating them, talk to patient while performing activities; assess need for analgesic and/or anxiolytic medication using valid assessment tools, use nonpharmacological pain-reducing methods as appropriate. Monitor and document patient's response to analgesics or other interventions.
Risk for infection related to loss of skin, impaired immune response, and invasive therapies.	No inflamed burn wound margins. Sputum, blood, and urine cultures negative. There will be no wound biopsy evidence of burn wound invasion. Body temperature between 99° and 101°F. Glycosuria, vomiting, ileus, and/or change in mentation absent. White blood cell and platelet counts, coagulation times, and serum glucose level acceptable. Invasive catheter sites clean and dry with normal skin color and temperature. Autograft or allograft skin adheres to granulation tissue.	Assess burn wound and invasive catheter sites bid. Assess and document characteristics of urine and sputum q 8 h. Obtain wound, sputum, urine, and blood cultures as ordered. Assess and record temperature and vital signs q 1 to 4 h as appropriate. Provide protective isolation appropriate to method of wound care. Adhere to guidelines issued by Centers for Disease Control and Prevention for invasive catheter care. Provide wound care with antimicrobial topical agents as ordered.
Impaired skin integrity related to burn wound and/or the consequences of immobility.	No evidence of decubitus ulcers or other injury present in unburned skin. No evidence of progressive burn wound/donor site injury. Burn wound, donor site healing, and skin graft adherence occur within appropriate time frames.	Assess the following bid and document: skin over pressure areas, burn wounds, donor sites, pressure points under splints, dependent areas of unburned skin. Pad pressure areas: heels, elbows, sacrum, scapulae, and burned ears. Assess need for special beds, such as low-air-loss and air-fluidized beds; at a minimum, provide extra padding to mattress. Remove blood pressure cuff from areas of burned skin after each reading. Check circulation distal to restraints q 1 h; check circulation of digits in splinted extremities. Loosen securing devices for facial tube in order to accommodate changes occurring with edema; ensure that devices do not put pressure on ears. Promote drying of donor sites as appropriate: keep heat lamps at a safe distance in order to prevent injury. Immobilize skin graft sites for 5 to 7 days after grafting to promote graft adherence. Moisten meshed graft dressings as ordered or roll sheet grafts as ordered to promote skin graft adherence.

NURSING CARE PLAN: RESUSCITATIVE AND ACUTE CARE PHASES OF MAJOR BURN INJURY Continued

Nursing Diagnosis	Patient Outcomes	Nursing Interventions
Altered nutrition (less than body requirements) related to increased metabolic demands secondary to physiological stress and wound healing.	Daily requirement of nutrients, based on formulas for appropriate calorie calculation, consumed. Positive nitrogen balance. Progressive wound healing.	Monitor weights daily or biweekly. Assess abdomen, bowel sounds q 8 h. Record all oral intake. Activate enteral, parenteral feeding protocol as appropriate prn. Provide adaptive devices to facilitate self-feeding. Have family assist at mealtime.
Impaired physical mobility and self-care deficit related to therapeutic splinting and post skin graft immobilization requirements.	No evidence of permanent decreased joint function from preburn status unless it is directly related to trauma. Returns to vocation without functional limitations or will adjust to new vocation based on functional limitations.	Perform range-of-motion exercises to all extremities q 4 h. Progress patient's activity as tolerated. Promote the use of adaptive devices in order to decrease dependency. Provide pain relief measures before physical therapy.
Risk for hypothermia related to loss of skin and/or external cooling.	Rectal/core temperature 99° to 101°F.	Monitor and document rectal/core temperature q 1 to 2 h. For a temperature of less than 99°F: warm with heat lamps or shield; warm solutions used for dressing changes; cover patient with foil blanket or other substance in order to conserve heat.
Risk for ineffective individual/family coping related to acute stress of critical injury and potential life-threatening crisis; altered family processes related to critical injury.	Patient and family verbalize goals of treatment regimen. Patient and family demonstrate knowledge of support systems that are available. Patient and family able to express concerns and fears. Patient and family's coping functional and realistic for phase of hospitalization; family processes will be at precrisis level.	Support adaptive/functional coping mechanisms. Use interventions to reduce patient fatigue and pain. Promote use of group support sessions for patients and families. Orient patient and family to unit and support services and reinforce information frequently. Involve patient and family in treatment goals and plan of care.

Infection and Normothermia

- The body temperature will be between 99° and 101°F.
- Sputum, blood, and urine cultures will be negative.
- Wound biopsy will show no evidence of burn wound infection.
- White blood cell and platelet counts, coagulation times, and serum glucose level will be acceptable.
- Purulence, erythema, and pain around invasive catheter sites will be absent.
- Allograft or autograft skin will adhere to granulation tissue.

Tissue Integrity

- Skin will be intact in nonburned areas.

- Wound closure will be achieved within an appropriate time frame after burn injury or donor skin harvesting.

Gastrointestinal and Stress Response

- Aspiration will be absent.
- Gastric pH will be greater than 5.
- Stools and gastric contents will be heme negative.
- Patient will have formed stools.

Nutrition

- Patient will have a positive nitrogen balance.
- Patient will consume his or her daily requirement of nutrients, based on appropriate formulas for caloric calculations.

RESEARCH APPLICATION

References

Geisser, M. E., Bingham, H. G., & Robinson, M. E. (1995). Pain and anxiety during burn dressing changes: Concordance between patients' and nurses' ratings and relation to medication administration and patient variables. *Journal of Burn Care and Rehabilitation, 16,* 165–171.

Marvin, J. A., Carrougher, G., Bayley, E., Knighton, J., Rutan, R., & Weber, B. (1992). Burn nursing delphi study: Pain management. *Journal of Burn Care and Rehabilitation, 13,* 685–694.

Review of Study Methods and Findings

This study addressed three issues: (1) the agreement between patients' and nurses' ratings of pain and anxiety before and during burn dressing changes (107 measurements among 11 patients); (2) the correlation of burn injury variables, amount of analgesic and anxiolytic agents administered, and self-report of tension during the procedure on self-report of pain; and (3) the relationship between patient variables related to previous pain experiences, state and trait anxiety scores, and social desirability and self-report of pain and anxiety.

Pain and tension were measured by use of 10-cm visual analogue scales immediately after the dressing changes. If more than one nurse was involved, each provided a confidential measurement. An initial battery of tests assessing trait anxiety; trait anger; social desirability; and discriminability between, and attitude toward, imaginary painful situations was administered at the beginning of the study. A weekly evaluation of state anxiety, state anger, and depression was conducted.

As in several other studies, little agreement existed between the ratings of nurses and patients. Absolute differences ranged from 2.4 to 2.7. The percentage of agreement between ratings ranged from 25.2 to 37.4. Both sets of findings were based on nurse:patient ratings within 1 cm of one another. Within-subject variance of the interrater reliability coefficients was poorer than that reported in other studies (overall pain = 0.56 ($P < .01$); worst pain = 0.33 ($P = 0.07$); preprocedure tension = 0.42 ($P < .05$); during-procedure tension = 0.54 ($P < .01$)). The authors sug-

gested that the within-subject control of variance might have been partially responsible for the low correlations. Their conclusion was that either the instruments have little validity in this population or nurses do not accurately assess patients' pain and anxiety.

The amount of analgesic and anxiolytic agents given was positively related to patients' and nurses' ratings for overall pain and anxiety (patients: $r = 0.31$, $P < .01$ for analgesics and $r = 0.28$, $P < .01$ for anxiolytics; nurses: $r = 0.55$, $P < .001$ for analgesics and $r = 0.22$, $P < .05$ for anxiolytics). Similar findings were noted for worst pain and tension during the procedure. Correlations related to tension before the procedure were not significant. All patient ratings were significantly and inversely related to postburn day. Staff ratings were also negatively related, and all were statistically significant except the rating for tension before the procedure. No significant relationships existed between patient and nurse ratings and total body surface area burned (TBSA). Only initial admission TBSA percentage was used.

Multiple regression analysis was performed in two steps in order to predict self-report of pain. The first step, which used overall pain as the dependent variable, indicated that within-subject variance was not significant ($R^2 = 0.12$, $P = .17$). In the second step, significant variance ($R^2 = 0.40$, $P = < .0001$) was the result of tension during the procedure ($t = 4.2$, $P < .001$). It accounted for 12% of the variance in overall pain. Similar results were obtained when the dependent variable was worst pain. Tension during the procedure accounted for 8.4% of the variance ($t = 3.5$, $P < .001$) (within-subject variance: $R^2 = 0.15$, $P < .05$; step 2: $R^2 = 0.40$, $P = < .0001$).

The exploratory correlations gave some indication that the ability to discriminate between painful episodes, social desirability (or need of the patient to be liked by the staff), and trait and state mood may be important variables that contribute to the patient's self-report of pain and anxiety. The ability to discriminate between severe and mild pain using the scenarios on the instrument may have been difficult for a patient already experiencing severe burn pain. There were indications that if patients had a strong desire to be liked by the staff, the self-reports of pain were lower. Trait anxiety may be a factor in the level of anticipatory anxiety based on these preliminary findings.

RESEARCH APPLICATION *Continued*

Critique

The major strengths of this study were the evaluation of within-subject variance, the reliability and validity of the instruments, and the use of a non–care provider for unbiased data collection. The limitations included sample size and the ability of pain measurement tools to accurately measure the subjective phenomena of pain and anxiety. This is one of the more comprehensive studies in terms of the factors evaluated and the correlations explored.

Implications for Nursing Practice

Like most other studies correlating nurses' and patients' ratings of pain, the data reported that nurses do not very accurately estimate the level of pain that an individual patient experiences. The authors believed that the to ability to perform such an assessment is important because nurses make decisions about pain management based on their perception of the patient's pain. If health care providers truly embrace the definition of pain as being what the patient says it is, then only the patient's perception should be considered by the team in the development of pain management plans. The authors agree that the most important issue is assessment and modification of the patient's perception.

The interrater reliability coefficients of the assessment pain and anxiety scales used were lower than those reported on in other studies. Although within-subject variance may be an issue because of the subjectivity of the individual pain experience, continued research is needed related to the best types of assessment tools. This is a high priority of research identified by the burn nursing delphi study (Marvin et al., 1992).

This study also indicated that tension during the procedure was the strongest predictor of pain during the procedure. Additional findings suggested that trait anxiety levels may be a factor in anticipatory anxiety. It may be important to assess this trait as part of the routine admission assessment. The study of both pharmacological and nonpharmacological methods to reduce anxiety is greatly needed.

Finally, this study confirmed the results of several other studies that TBSA burned is not correlated with pain levels. Of interest is the observation made by the authors that it is usually initial TBSA measurements used. The pain of surgery, the impact of donor site pain, and the increase in healed areas were not taken into consideration in assessment of pain. Pain from these sources can have a significant effect on how a patient perceives any given dressing change. Therefore, assessing this impact is important in the planning of pain relief measures for each individual dressing change. What worked for previous changes may not be sufficient for the current procedure.

Pain and anxiety assessment is the first step in establishing an effective pain management program for the burn patient. Nurses should base their interventions on the patient's perception of pain and should use this perception as the ``gold standard'' for evaluating the effectiveness of therapy.

Physical Mobility

- Range of motion of all joints will be equal to the preburn level unless dysfunction is present that is secondary to associated trauma at the time of injury.

Patient and Family Coping

- Patient will be able to verbally describe goals of the treatment regimen.
- Patient will demonstrate knowledge of the support systems that are available.
- Patient will express concerns and fears.

Summary

The physiological response to a major burn injury is one of a biphasic pattern of multiorgan system hypofunction followed by hyperfunction. A major goal of resuscitative care is the prevention of burn shock. The critical care nurse's observations of the patient's responses are crucial for the prevention of complications related to the increased capillary permeability and massive fluid therapy required. In the acute phase, therapeutic goals include prevention of further tissue loss, maintenance of function, prevention of infection, and wound closure. As the patient progresses through various stages of wound care management, the nurse must not only provide the skilled care but also monitor the patient and family's response to the treatment experience. Psychosocial support is integral to the entire process.

Although providing care to the burned patient is a team effort, it is the critical care nurse who is with the patient 24 hours a day. The support and skill of the nurse make the critical difference in the patient outcome.

CRITICAL THINKING QUESTIONS

1. Mrs. J. is a 70-year-old woman who sustained a thermal burn injury in a house fire. An electric heater ignited her bedspread while she was asleep. She was trapped in the room approximately 15 minutes before being rescued by firefighters.
   a. Once Mrs. J. is removed from the fire, what priorities are essential in her initial management?
   b. She has singed nose hair and is coughing up sooty sputum. The emergency department is 15 minutes away. Based on this assessment, what should the paramedics do?
   c. What diagnostic tests and assessments do you anticipate once Mrs. J. reaches the emergency department?
2. Explain why patients with burns need extensive fluid resuscitation despite the fact that they are extremely edematous?
3. What interventions would you use to meet the high caloric needs of burn patients who can take foods by mouth?
4. What interventions can be used in the critical care unit to promote early rehabilitation of a burned individual?
5. Many burned patients must be treated at institutions far away from home. What interventions can be used to meet the psychosocial needs of these individuals and their families?

REFERENCES

Agency for Health Care Policy and Research (1992). *Clinical Practice Guideline: Acute Pain Management: Operative or Medical Procedures and Trauma.* (Publication No. 92-0032: 65–67). Rockville, MD: U.S. Department of Health and Human Services.
American Burn Association. (1990). Hospital and prehospital resources for optimal care of patients with burn injury: Guidelines for development and operation of burn centers. *Journal of Burn Care and Rehabilitation, 11,* 97–104.
Arturson, G., & Jonsson, C. E. (1979). Transcapillary transport after thermal injury. *Scandinavian Journal of Plastic and Reconstructive Surgery, 13,* 29–38.
Carlson, D. E., & Jordan, B. S. (1991). Implementing nutritional therapy in the thermally injured patient. *Nursing Clinics of North America, 3*(2):221–235.
Carrougher, G. (1993). Inhalation injury. *AACN Clinical Issues in Critical Care Nursing, 4*(2), 367–377.
Choiniere, M., Paquette, C., Grenier, R., & Paquin, M. J. (1990). A double blind study to determine the efficacy of patient controlled analgesia in burn patients. *Proceedings of the American Burn Association Meeting, 22,* Abstract No. 207.
Cioffi, W. G., & Rue, L. W. (1991). Diagnosis and treatment of inhalation injuries. *Critical Care Nursing Clinics of North America, 3*(2), 191–198.
Cooper, M. L., & Spielvogel, R. L. (1994). Artificial skin for wound healing. *Clinics in Dermatology, 12,* 183–193.
Cope, O., & Moore, F. D. (1947). The redistribution of body water in the fluid therapy of the burn patient. *Annals of Surgery, 126,* 1010–1018.
Cram, E., & Kealey, G. P. (1990). Patient controlled analgesia: A strategy for controlling acute burn pain. *Proceedings of the American Burn Association Meeting, 22,* Abstract No. 208.
Curreri, P. W. (1990). Assessing nutritional needs for the burned patient. *Journal of Trauma, 30*(Suppl), S20–S23.
DePew, C. L. (1991). Toxic epidermal necrolysis. *Critical Care Nursing Clinics of North America, 3*(2), 255–267.
Duncan, D. J., & Driscoll, D. M. (1991). Burn wound management. *Critical Care Nursing Clinics of North America, 3*(2), 199–220.
Everett, J. J., Patterson, D. R., Marvin, J. A., et al. (1994). Pain assessment from patients with burns and their nurses. *Journal of Burn Care and Rehabilitation, 15*:194–198.
Ferrar, J. J., Dyess, D. L., Luterman, A., Curreri, P. W. (1990). Transportation of immunosuppressive substances produced at the site of burn injury into the systemic circulation: The role of lymphatics. *Journal of Burn Care and Rehabilitation, 11,* 282–286.
Geisser, M. E., Bingham, H. G., & Robinson, M. E. (1995). Pain and anxiety during burn dressing changes: Concordance between patients' and nurses' ratings and relations to medication administration and patient variables. *Journal of Burn Care and Rehabilitation, 16,* 165–171.
Gordon, M. D. (Ed.) (1987). Burn care protocols: Anchoring endotubes on patients with facial burns. *Journal of Burn Care and Rehabilitation, 8*(3), 233–237.
Gordon, M. D. (Ed.) (1988). Burn care protocols: Discharge planning. *Journal of Burn Care and Rehabilitation, 9*(4), 414.
Greenfield, E. (1995). Critical pathways: What they are and what they are not. *Journal of Burn Care and Rehabilitation, 16*(2 Suppl.) 189–218.
Greenfield, E., Gordon, M., & Marvin, J. (1995). Pain assessment tool selection in patients with thermal injury. (Ongoing research funded in part by a grant from the International Firefighters Foundation.)
Hardin, N. G., & Luster, S. H. (1991). Rehabilitation considerations in the care of the acute burn patient. *Critical Care Nursing Clinics of North America, 3*(2), 245–253.
Heimbach, D. M., Engrav, L. H., Marvin, J. A., Harnar, T. J., & Grube, B. J. (1987). Toxic epidermal necrolysis: A step forward in treatment. *Journal of the American Medical Association, 257,* 2171–2175.
Kagan, R. J., & Warden, G. D. (1994). Management of the burn wound. *Clinics in Dermatology, 12*(1), 47–56.
Kravitz, M. (1993). Immune consequences of burn injury. *AACN Clinical Issues in Critical Care Nursing, 4*(2), 399–413.
Loeser, J. (1987). Conceptual framework for pain management. *Journal of Burn Care and Rehabilitation, 8*(4), 309–312.
Mason, A. D., Jr. (1980). The mathematics of resuscitation. *Journal of Trauma, 20,* 1015–1020.

McCaffery, M., & Beebe, A. (1989). *Pain: Clinical manual for nursing practice*. St. Louis: C. V. Mosby Co.

McManus, A. T., McManus, W. F., Mason, A. D., Jr., Aitcheson, A. R., & Pruitt, B. A., Jr. (1987). Microbial colonization in a new intensive care burn unit. *Archives of Surgery, 120*, 217–223.

McManus, W. F., Mason, A. D., Jr., & Pruitt, B. A., Jr. (1989). Excision of the burn wound in patients with large burns. *Archives of Surgery, 124*, 718–720.

Molter, N. C. (1991). Pain in the burn patient. In K. A. Puntillo (Ed.), *Pain in the critically ill: Assessment and management* (pp. 193–209). Rockville, MD: Aspen Publishers.

Molter, N. C. (1993). When is the burn injury healed?: Psychosocial implications of care. *AACN Clinical Issues in Critical Care, 4*(2), 424–432.

Moylan, J. A., Inge, W. W., & Pruitt, B. A., Jr. (1971). Circulatory changes following circumferential extremity burns evaluated by the ultrasonic flow meter: An analysis of 60 thermally injured limbs. *Journal of Trauma, 11*, 763–769.

Mozingo, J. W., Smith, A. A., McManus, W. F., Pruitt, B. A., Jr., & Mason, A. D., Jr. (1988). Chemical burns. *Journal of Trauma, 28*(5), 642–647.

Mozingo, D. W., Barillo, D. J., & Pruitt, B. A., Jr. (1994). Acute resuscitation and transfer management of burn and electrically injured patients. *Trauma Quarterly, 11*, 94–102.

Nebraska Burn Institute. (1994). *Advanced burn life support course manual*. Lincoln, NE: Author.

Patterson, D. R. (1992). Practical applications of psychological techniques in controlling burn pain. *Journal of Burn Care and Rehabilitation, 13*, 13–18.

Perry, S., Heidrich, G., & Ramos, E. (1981). Assessment of pain by burn patients. *Journal of Burn Care and Rehabilitation, 2*(6), 322–326.

Phillips, T. J., Bhawan, J., Leigh, I. M., et al. (1990). Cultured epidermal autografts and allografts: A study of differentiation and allograft survival. *Journal of the American Academy of Dermatology, 23*, 189–199.

Phillips, T. J. (1993). Biologic skin substitutes. *Journal of Dermatologic Surgery and Oncology, 19*, 794–802.

Phillips, T. J. (1994). Keratinocyte grafts for wound healing. *Clinics in Dermatology, 12*, 171–181.

Pruitt, B. A., Jr., & Mason, A. D. Jr. (1971). Hemodynamic studies of burned patients during resuscitation. In P. Matter, T. L. Barclay, & Z. Konickova (Eds.), *Research in burns*. Bern: Hans Huber Publishers.

Pruitt, B. A., Jr. (1984). The universal trauma model. *Bulletin of the American College of Surgeons, 70*(10), 2–13.

Pruitt, B. A., Jr., & Goodwin, C. W., Jr. (1990). Burn injury. In E. F. Moore (Ed.), *Early care of the injured patient* (4th ed.) (pp. 286–306). St. Louis: C. V. Mosby Co.

Pruitt, B. A., Jr., Goodwin, C. W., & Cioffi, W. G. (1995). Thermal injuries. In J. H. David, & G. G. Sheldon (Eds.), *Surgery: A problem solving approach* (pp. 642–720) St. Louis: C. V. Mosby Co.

Reig, L. S. (1993). Metabolic alterations and nutritional management. *AACN Clinical Issues in Critical Care Nursing, 4*(2), 388–398.

Rheinwald, J.G., & Green, H. (1975). Formation of a keratinizing epithelium in culture by a cloned cell line derived from a teratoma. *Cell, 6* (3):317–330.

Robson, M. C., Barnett, R. A., Leitch, I. O., et al. (1992). Prevention and treatment of postburn scars and contracture. *World Journal of Surgery, 16*, 87–97.

Rue, L. W. III, & Cioffi, W. G. (1991). Resuscitation of thermally injured patients. *Critical Care Nursing Clinics of North America, 3*(2), 181–189.

Rue, L. W., Cioffi, W. G., McManus, W. F., et al. (1993). Wound closure and outcome in extensively burned patients treated with cultured autologous keratinocytes. *Journal of Trauma, 35*, 662–672.

Rue, L. W. III, Cioffi, W. G., Mason, A. D., Jr, McManus, W. F., & Pruitt, B. A., Jr. (1995). The risk of pneumonia in thermally injured patients requiring ventilatory support. *Journal of Burn Care and Rehabilitation, 16*, 262–268.

Saffle, J. R., Davis, B., & Williams, P. (1995). Recent outcomes in the treatment of burn injury in the United States: A report from the American Burn Association Patient Registry. *Journal of Burn Care and Rehabilitation, 16*, 219–232.

Shea, S. M., Caulfield, J. B., & Burke, J. F. (1973). Microvascular ultrastructure in thermal injury: A reconsideration of the role of mediators. *Microvascular Research, 5*, 87–97.

Shirani, K. Z., Pruitt, B. A., Jr., & Mason, A. D., Jr. (1987). The influence of inhalation injury and pneumonia on burn mortality. *Annals of Surgery, 205*(1), 82–87.

Summers, T. M. (1991). Psychosocial support of the burn patient. *Critical Care Nursing Clinics of North America, 3*(2), 237–244.

Tompkins, R. F., & Burk, J. F. (1992). Burn wound closure using permanent skin replacement materials. *World Journal of Surgery, 16*, 47–56.

Treat, R. C., Sirinek, K. R., Levine, B. A., & Pruitt, B. A., Jr. (1980). Air evacuation of thermally injured patients: Principles of treatment and results. *Journal of Trauma, 20*, 275–279.

Waymack, J. P., & Pruitt, B. A., Jr. (1990). Burn wound care. *Advances in Surgery, 23*, 261–290.

Weber, J. M., & Tompkins, E. M. (1993). Improving survival: Infection control and burns. *AACN Clinical Issues in Critical Care Nursing, 4*(2), 414–423.

Wilmore, D. W. (1987). Metabolic changes after thermal injury. In J. A. Boswick, Jr. (Ed.), *The art and science of burn care* (pp. 137–144). Rockville, MD: Aspen Publishers.

SUGGESTED READINGS

Duncan, D. J. (Ed.) (1991). Burn management. *Critical Care Clinics of North America, 3*(2), 165–267.

Stotts, N. (1993). Wound healing. In M. Kinney, D. Packa, S. Dunbar (Eds.), *AACN's clinical reference for critical-care nursing* (3rd ed.) (pp. 1232–1242). St. Louis: C. V. Mosby Co.

Watkins, P., Cook, E., May, S., & Ehleben, C. (1988). Psychological stages in adaptation following burn injury: A method for facilitating psychological recovery of burn victims. *Journal of Burn Care and Rehabilitation, 9*(4), 376–390.

Waymack, J. P., & Rutan, R. L. (1994). Recent advances in burn care [Review]. *Annals of the New York Academy of Sciences, 720*; 230–238.

INDEX

Note: Page numbers in *italics* indicate illustrations; those followed by t indicate tables.

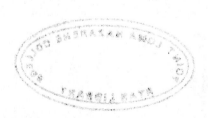